II. Post Procedure Protocol – Use clinical judgment regarding steps appropriate to skill you are performing

Follow these protocol steps at the end of a procedure. Use clinical judgment to individualize steps as necessary.

A. Remove any drape used to perform procedure.
B. Discard all soiled items in proper container. Note: Specific skills will note any special precautions to take related to that skill, e.g. if patient is on hazardous drugs.
C. Remove and discard gloves in proper container.
D. Assist patient in assuming a comfortable position.
E. Return bed to low and locked position.
F. Assist patient with gown, linens, call light, and other applicable items.
G. Discuss results of procedure with patient. Encourage questions.
H. Use Teach Back. Have patient/family caregiver explain back for you any education or instruction provided to evaluate their learning. Example: Nurse asks "Tell me what you understand about your new diet", and patient then responds.
I. Place nurse call system in an accessible location within patient's reach.
J. Perform Hand Hygiene and exit room
K. Return unused items to proper place (see agency policy).
L. Clean and return reusable items to proper place (see agency policy).

Potter & Perry's Pocket Guide to

Nursing Skills & Procedures

TENTH EDITION

Patricia A. Potter, RN, MSN, PhD, FAAN
Former Director of Research
Patient Care Services
Barnes-Jewish Hospital
St. Louis, Missouri

Anne Griffin Perry, RN, MSN, EdD, FAAN
Professor Emerita
School of Nursing
Southern Illinois University Edwardsville
Edwardsville, Illinois

ELSEVIER

Elsevier
3251 Riverport Lane
St. Louis, Missouri 63043

Potter & Perry's Pocket Guide to Nursing
Skills & Procedures, TENTH EDITION   ISBN: 978-0-323-87076-4

Notice

Practitioners and researchers must always rely on their own
experience and knowledge in evaluating and using any information,
methods, compounds or experiments described herein. Because of
rapid advances in the medical sciences, in particular, independent
verification of diagnoses and drug dosages should be made. To the
fullest extent of the law, no responsibility is assumed by Elsevier,
authors, editors or contributors for any injury and/or damage to
persons or property as a matter of products liability, negligence or
otherwise, or from any use or operation of any methods, products,
instructions, or ideas contained in the material herein.

Content Strategist: Brandi Graham
Content Development Specialist: Nicole Congleton
Publishing Services Manager: Deepthi Unni
Project Manager: Sindhuraj Thulasingam
Design Direction: Brian Salisbury

Printed in India

Last digit is the print number:
9   8   7   6   5   4   3   2   1

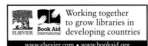

Working together
to grow libraries in
developing countries

www.elsevier.com • www.bookaid.org

Potter & Perry's Pocket Guide to Nursing Skills and Procedures, 10th edition, is a practical, portable reference for students and practitioners in the clinical setting. It is an ideal accompaniment to *Clinical Nursing Skills and Techniques*, 10th edition and the upcoming 11th edition. Grouped alphabetically, 83 commonly performed skills are presented in a clear, step-by-step format that includes:

- Purpose for performing each skill
- Safety Guidelines that emphasize principles for safe nursing practice
- Guidelines to help students in delegating tasks appropriately to assistive personnel
- Lists of equipment required for the skill
- Step-by-step format (including assessment, implementation, and evaluation) for each skill
- Rationales for each step to explain practical and scientific basis for why techniques are used
- Reporting and Recording guidelines found at the end of each skill
- Full-color photographs and drawings to provide visual reinforcement

In addition, Clinical Judgment alerts are included in the skills to highlight important steps within a skill where nurses should reflect on the safety of an approach and the clinical evidence for adapting or performing the step.

Current Standard Precautions guidelines from the Centers for Disease Control and Prevention are incorporated throughout. Preprocedure and postprocedure protocols are conveniently located on the inside back cover.

Features of This Edition

- Information is updated to incorporate new science into the skills.
- The addition of key assessment steps strengthens student's ability to make clinical decisions as part of skill performance.
- A step for "Evaluation of patient response" places greater emphasis on the importance of patient evaluation after skill performance.
- Unexpected Outcomes and Related Interventions present commonly occurring complications and the appropriate responses for patient care.
- Completely updated, full-color illustrations appear throughout.

This pocket guide is also available in formats compatible with handheld electronic devices. For a more complete discussion of information presented in this book, refer to Perry and Potter: *Clinical Nursing Skills and Techniques*, 10th edition and upcoming 11th edition.

TABLE OF CONTENTS

Acapella Device

The Acapella flutter valve is a handheld airway clearance device that uses positive expiratory pressure (PEP) to stabilize airways and improve aeration of the distal lung areas. During exhalation, pressure from the airways transmits to the Acapella device, causing PEP and airway vibration, which help mucus dislodge from the airway walls, making it easier for patients to expectorate mucus. Indications for use include (Respiratory Therapy Zone, 2021):

- Preventing or reducing atelectasis
- Removing secretions and clearing airways
- Reducing air trapping
- Maximizing delivery of aerosolized medications to patients receiving bronchial hygiene therapy

Safety Guidelines

- There are no contraindications to use of an Acapella device, but do confirm whether use is appropriate in patients with hemoptysis, intracranial pressure > 20 mmHg, acute dyspnea, and severe nausea.
- Verify that the correct device is selected to match patient's expiratory flow rate. There are two types of devices. The blue device is for patients who cannot maintain an expiratory flow greater than 15 L/min for longer than 3 seconds. The green device is for patients who can maintain expiratory flow greater than or equal to 15 L/min for at least 3 seconds.

Delegation

The skill of using an Acapella device can be delegated to assistive personnel (AP). The nurse is responsible for performing respiratory assessment, determining that the procedure is appropriate for patient situation, and evaluating a patient's response. Direct the AP to:

- Report immediately any changes in patient's breathing pattern or comfort level.
- Use specific patient precautions, such as positioning restrictions, related to disease or treatment.

Collaboration

- Respiratory therapy

Equipment

- Acapella device
- Stethoscope, pulse oximeter
- Water and glass, tissues, paper bag
- Chair
- Clear, graduated, screw-top container
- Suction equipment (if patient cannot cough and clear own secretions)
- Clean gloves
- Patient education materials

STEP	RATIONALE
1 Complete preprocedure protocol.	
Assessment	
• Review electronic health record for history of pulmonary conditions requiring Acapella device.	Indications for therapy allow you to anticipate patient response.
• Perform hand hygiene. Conduct respiratory assessment, including pulse oximetry and lung auscultation.	Reduces transmission of microorganisms. Determines baseline status and condition of lung segments requiring other therapies, e.g., vibration and percussion.
Implementation	
1 Prepare Acapella device (Fig. 1.1). Verify that the correct device selected matches the patient's expiratory flow rate.	
a Turn Acapella frequency adjustment dial counterclockwise to lowest resistance setting. As patient improves or is more proficient, adjust proper resistance level upward by turning dial clockwise.	This initial setting helps patient adjust to device and benefit from treatment.

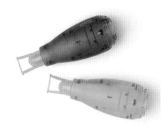

Fig. 1.1 Acapella device.
(Used with permission,
Smithmedical.com.)

STEP	RATIONALE
b If aerosol drug therapy is ordered, attach a nebulizer to the end of the Acapella valve.	
2 Instruct patient to:	
a Sit comfortably upright in bed or chair and take in a breath that is larger than normal but not to fill lungs completely.	Allows for maximal ventilation.
b Place mouthpiece into the mouth, maintaining tight seal.	
c Hold breath for 2 to 3 seconds.	Increases positive pressure to open airways.
d Try not to cough and exhale slowly for 3 to 4 seconds through the device while it vibrates.	Maximizes efficacy of therapy.
e Repeat cycle for 5 to 10 breaths as tolerated.	
f Remove mouthpiece and perform one or two "huff" coughs.	Removes any mucus in airways.
g Repeat Acapella therapy throughout day as ordered.	Frequency will be determined by patient condition.
3 Complete postprocedure protocol.	

Continued

STEP	RATIONALE
4 Evaluate patient response: a Auscultate lung fields; obtain vital signs and pulse oximetry.	Determines patient response to positive expiratory pressure.
b Inspect color, character, and amount of sputum. Help patient with oral hygiene.	Ongoing assessment determines thickness and consistency of mucus (hydration status) and whether infection has developed.

Recording and Reporting

- Record procedure, character and production of mucus, level of PEP resistance, and patient's tolerance.
- Record evaluation of patient learning.

UNEXPECTED OUTCOMES	RELATED INTERVENTIONS
• Patient develops severe dyspnea.	• Report to health care provider immediately. • Position patient in high Fowler position. • Monitor vital signs and continuous pulse oximetry. • Be prepared to administer oxygen as ordered.
• Patient develops changes in sputum.	• Increase patient hydration within any fluid restrictions. • If patient is receiving intravenous (IV) fluids consult with health care provider regarding increasing volume of infusion. • Consult with health care provider or respiratory therapist about possible use of nebulization or increased humidity with oxygen delivery.

Aquathermia and Heating Pads

Electric heating pads, water-flow pads such as aquathermia pads, and commercial heat packs are common forms of dry warm heat therapy. Dry warm heat reduces pain and increases healing by increasing blood flow in tissues and can be used at a low setting for a longer period than that used for moist heat with little chance of tissue injury (Petrofsky et al., 2016). Common indications for use include the following:

- Inflamed or edematous body part
- Infected wound
- Arthritis; degenerative joint disease; localized joint pain, muscle pain, muscle strains
- Low back pain
- Menstrual cramping
- Hemorrhoidal, perianal, and vaginal inflammation

Safety Guidelines

- Contraindications to dry heat include unstable cardiac conditions, active bleeding, nitroglycerin or other therapeutic medicinal patch, acute inflammatory reactions, recent (less than 72 h) musculoskeletal injury, persons with multiple sclerosis sensitivity to heat, and skin conditions with open lesions such as eczema.
- Older adults or patients who have diabetes mellitus, vascular disease, paralysis, peripheral neuropathy, or rheumatoid arthritis or who are taking certain cardiovascular medications are at greater risk for thermal injury (Ratliff, 2017).
- Because dry heat is applied to the skin, take extra precautions to prevent burns and/or skin and tissue injury. Cover area to be treated or the device itself with single layer of bath towel or pillowcase.
- Discourage patient use of conventional heating pad in the patient's home. However, if use is necessary, instruct on how to protect the skin. Never set such a device on a high setting.

Delegation

The skill of applying dry heat can be delegated to AP (see agency policy). The nurse must assess and evaluate the condition of the skin and tissues in the area that is treated. *If there are risks or expected complications, this skill cannot be delegated.* Direct the AP about:

- Proper temperature of the application.
- Specific positioning and time requirements to keep the application in place based on health care provider order or agency policy.
- Reporting any patient dizziness or light-headedness; change in heart rate or blood pressure; and burning, blistering, excessive redness, and pain of the skin during application.
- Reporting when treatment is complete so the patient's response can be evaluated.

Collaboration

- Physical therapists often use heat applications for treatment along with exercise.

Equipment

- Disposable aquathermia pad or commercial heat pack
- Heating unit for aquathermia pad
- Pillowcase
- Tape ties or gauze roll

STEP	RATIONALE
1 Complete preprocedure protocol.	
Assessment	
• Review patient's electronic health record (EHR) for medical indications for heat therapy and any documentation by other providers related to patient response to previous heat treatment.	Allows you to anticipate patient and ordered duration of response.
• Review EHR for contraindications or risks to heat therapy (see safety guidelines).	Will require precautions (e.g., more frequent assessments) during application or may contraindicate treatment.

STEP	RATIONALE
• Perform hand hygiene. Apply clean gloves, and assess condition of skin around area to be treated. Perform neurovascular assessments for sensitivity to temperature and pain by measuring light touch, pinprick, and temperature sensation.	Certain conditions alter conduction of sensory impulses that transmit temperature and pain, predisposing patients to injury from heat applications.
• When treating a wound, assess characteristics (e.g., redness, swelling edema).	Provides baseline to determine change in wound after heat application.
• Assess patient's level of consciousness and responsiveness (e.g., confusion, disorientation, dementia).	Patients with reduced level of consciousness are unable to sense or report reduced sensation or discomfort from therapy, thus requiring closer monitoring.
• Assess vital signs and ask patient to describe pain character and intensity on pain scale of 0 to 10	Provides baseline for response to therapy.
• Assess joint range of motion (ROM) if affected area involves joint. Perform hand hygiene.	Heat therapy will relieve muscle stiffness and potentially improve ROM. Reduces transmission of microorganisms.

Implementation

STEP	RATIONALE
1 Check electric plugs and heating unit cord for obvious fraying or cracking.	Prevents injury from accidental electric shock.
2 Determine patient and/or family member knowledge regarding risks of heat therapy related to procedure.	Determines extent of health teaching required.
3 Apply aquathermia pad a Cover or wrap area to be treated with single layer of pillowcase or bath towel.	Prevents heated surface from touching patient's skin directly and increasing risk for injury to patient's skin

Continued

STEP	RATIONALE
b Place pad over affected area (Fig. 2.1) and secure with tape, tie, or gauze as needed.	Pad should not slip onto different body part.
c Connect to heat source and turn on aquathermia unit. Check temperature setting. Tell patient when you will return to check on them (every 5 minutes, duration 20 minures).	Ensures temperature is safe to apply.

CLINICAL JUDGMENT *Do not pin the wrap to the pad, because this may cause a leak in the device.*

4 Apply commercial heat pad. a Break pouch inside larger pack (follow manufacturer's guidelines). Secure over area to be treated. (Commercial packs usually have outer covering that protects skin.)	Activates chemicals within pack to warm outer surface. Pad delivers dry warm heat to injured tissues. Pad should not slip onto different body part.
6 Complete postprocedure protocol.	
7 Evaluate patient response. a Return to patient room to monitor condition of skin every 5 minutes during application, and ask if patient feels a burning sensation.	Timely monitoring prevents burn, blistering, or other thermal injury to underlying skin.

Fig. 2.1 Aquathermia pad applied.

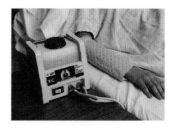

STEP	RATIONALE
b After no more than 20 minutes (or time ordered by health care provider), perform hand hygiene, apply clean gloves, remove pad, and store.	Safe time interval to reduce pain and spasm and increase blood flow and compliance of soft-tissue structures (Petrofsky et al., 2017a).

Recording and Reporting

- Record application type , skin condition before and after application, temperature and therapy duration.
- Document instruction given and patient and/orfamily caregiver's success in demonstrating procedure (when appropriate).
- Report procedure and patient response during shift change.
- Report incidence of thermal injury to health care provider and complete an agency occurrence report (thermal injury is reportable to risk management).

UNEXPECTED OUTCOMES	RELATED INTERVENTIONS
• Skin is reddened, sensitive to touch.	• Discontinue application immediately. • Verify proper temperature, or check device for proper functioning. • Notify health care provider and, if there is a burn, complete an occurrence report.
• Body part is painful to move.	• Discontinue application. • Observe for localized swelling. • Notify health care provider.
• Patient or family caregiver applies heat incorrectly or cannot explain precautions.	• Reinstruct patient and/or family caregiver as necessary. • Consider possible home health referral.

Aspiration Precautions

Dysphagia or difficulty swallowing is a sensation of food or liquid being delayed or hindered in its passage from the mouth to the stomach (Patel et al., 2017). Dysphagia occurs in patients with neurogenic (e.g., stroke), myogenic (e.g., myasthenia gravis), and obstructive conditions (e.g., head and neck cancer). Patients with dysphagia are at risk for aspiration. Conditions that suppress the cough reflex (such as sedation) also create risk for a patient (Metheny, 2021). Aspiration is the misdirection of oropharyngeal secretions or gastric contents into the larynx and lower respiratory tract (Metheny, 2021; O'Malley et al., 2018). Aspiration occurs when secretions in the oral pharynx enter the trachea, or may occur as a result of reflux of gastric content that enters the throat and then goes down the trachea. The risk of aspiration pneumonia is three times higher in patients with dysphagia (Lo Wen-Liang et al., 2019). Aspiration pneumonia can be a fatal complication of dysphagia, especially in older adults.

The primary approaches to managing dysphagia and preventing aspiration during oral intake include texture modification of food and liquids and positional swallowing maneuvers, such as chin-tuck or head rotation (Academy of Nutrition and Dietetics: Nutrition Care Manual, 2022). Appropriate food choices and consistency of liquids are individualized and based on which phase of swallowing is dysfunctional (International Dysphagia Diet Standardization Initiative [IDDSI], 2017). As of 2017 IDDSI completed standardization of the terminology for food textures and liquid consistencies for use around the world. The diet comprises eight levels (Table 3.1) (IDDSI, 2017).

Safety Guidelines

- The best way to prevent aspiration is to place a patient on NPO (nothing by mouth) until a dysphagia evaluation by a certified speech-language pathologist (SLP) can be performed and a safe diet resumed.
- Small-volume aspirations that produce no overt symptoms are common and are often not discovered until the condition progresses to aspiration pneumonia (Metheny, 2021).
- As patients with dysphagia age, their perception of the urge to cough decreases, which further increases the risk for silent aspiration.
- Assess a patient's level of consciousness and ability to swallow before attempting any oral feeding.
- Indicate in patient's health record that dysphagia/aspiration risk is present.

TABLE 3.1 International Dysphagia Diet Framework

Level and Description	Characteristics	Examples
0: Thin liquid	Flows like water, can be drunk easily from straw. *Rationale:* Functional ability to safely manage liquids of all types.	Coffee, tea, lemonade, juice, water
1: Slightly thick liquid	Thicker than water, requires more effort to drink, still flows through a straw or nipple. *Rationale:* Primarily used for the pediatric population to reduce flow speed.	Commercially available oral supplements similar in viscosity to an infant "anti-regurgitation" formula, nectars and thick juices
2: Mildly thick liquid	Flows off a spoon; effort is required to drink through a straw. *Rationale:* Suitable if tongue control is slightly reduced.	Milkshakes
3: Liquidized/ moderately thick	Can be drunk from a cup; some effort required to suck through a straw; cannot be eaten with a fork; will drip between prongs; no oral processing or chewing required. *Rationale:* Allows more time for oral control, needs some tongue propulsion effort.	Runny rice cereal; runny pureed fruit, sauces, and gravies; honey-thickened beverages
4: Pureed/ extremely thick	Cannot be drunk from cup; usually eaten with a spoon; cannot be sucked through a straw; does not require chewing; can be molded; contains no lumps; not sticky. *Rationale:* If tongue control is significantly reduced, requires less propulsion; no biting or chewing is required; appropriate if patient has missing teeth or poorly fitting dentures.	Pureed meat, vegetables, fruits, and thick cereals

Continued

TABLE 3.1 International Dysphagia Diet Framework—cont'd

Level and Description	Characteristics	Examples
5: Minced and moist	Can be eaten with a fork or spoon; soft and moist with no separate thick liquid; contains/consists of small lumps that are easy to squash with tongue. *Rationale:* Biting is not required; minimal chewing; tongue force alone can be used to break soft small particles; appropriate if patient has some missing teeth.	Finely minced or ground tender meats served in extremely thick, smooth, nonpouring sauce or gravy; mashed potatoes; mashed fruits; very thick cereals; pregelled soaked breads. Fluid or milk should NOT separate from items.
6: Soft and bite-sized	Can be eaten with a fork or spoon; can be mashed/broken down with pressure from utensils; knife is not required to cut; chewing is required before swallowing; soft, tender, and moist throughout. *Rationale:* Tongue force and control are required to move the food for chewing and to keep it within the mouth during chewing; tongue force is required to move the bolus for swallowing.	Soft cooked meat cut in small pieces, flaky fish, casseroles, stews, soft cooked vegetables in bite-sized pieces, mashed fruits
7: Regular	Normal, everyday foods of various textures. *Rationale:* Ability to bite hard or soft foods and chew all textures.	No restrictions

Data from the IDDSI framework and detailed level definitions. Available at https://iddsi.org/framework/.

Delegation

The skill of following aspiration precautions while feeding a patient can be delegated to assistive personnel (AP). However, the nurse is responsible for the ongoing assessment of a patient's risk for aspiration, determination of positioning, and the need for any special feeding techniques. Direct the AP to:

- Position patient upright (90 degrees or highest position allowed by patient's medical condition) during and after feeding.
- Use aspiration precautions while feeding patients who are experiencing dysphagia or who are at risk for aspiration. Explain feeding techniques that are successful for specific patients.
- Immediately report any onset of coughing, gagging, a wet voice, or food pocketing within the oral cavity.

Collaboration

- Refer to an SLP or a registered dietitian (RD).

Equipment

- Chair or bed that allows patient to sit upright in high Fowler position
- Thickening agents as designated by SLP (rice, cereal, yogurt, gelatin, commercial thickener)
- Tongue blade and penlight
- Oral hygiene supplies
- Suction equipment
- Clean gloves
- *Option:* Pulse oximeter

STEP	RATIONALE
1 Complete preprocedure protocol	
Assessment	
• Assess patient's current medications for use of sedatives, hypnotics or similar agents, calcium channel blockers, or diuretics) (Tan et al., 2018).	Medications may impair cough or swallowing reflex. Channel blockers and diuretics can dry oral secretions.

Continued

STEP	RATIONALE
• Assess patient for signs and symptoms of dysphagia. Use a screening tool if agency recommended. Refer to SLP or RD if findings are positive for dysphagia.	Patient symptoms help determine whether swallow evaluation is needed and appropriate approach to feeding.
• Assess patient's mental status: alertness, orientation, and ability to follow simple commands (e.g., open your mouth, stick out your tongue).	Disorientation and inability to follow commands present higher risk for dysphagia. Patients with progressive dementia develop dysphagia.
• Perform hand hygiene and apply gloves. Assess patient's oral cavity and level of dental hygiene; note missing teeth or poorly fitting dentures.	Poorly fitting dentures and absence of teeth can cause chewing and swallowing difficulties, increasing aspiration risk. Poor oral hygiene and periodontal disease can result in bacteria growth in oropharynx that, if aspirated, can lead to pneumonia (Thomas et al., 2019).
• *Option:* Obtain baseline assessment of oxygen saturation.	Research findings question whether oximetry can reliably detect aspiration (American Speech-Language-Hearing Association, 2020; Marian et al., 2017). A decline in SpO2). A decline in SpO2 $\geq$2% has been regarded as a possible marker of aspiration (Marian et al, 2017). (Marian et al., 2017).

Implementation

1 Prepare to observe patient during mealtime for signs of dysphagia (Box 3.1). Observe patient attempts to feed self; note type of food consistencies and liquids able to swallow. Note if patient tires.	Detects abnormal eating patterns such as frequent throat clearing or prolonged eating time. Chewing and sitting up for feeding bring on fatigue (Meiner and Yeager, 2019). Provides data for future planning of meal assistance.

BOX 3.1 Signs of Dysphagia

- Coughing during or right after eating or drinking.
- Wet or gurgling-sounding voice during or after eating or drinking.
- Extra effort or time needed to chew or swallow; food or liquid leaking from the mouth or getting stuck in the mouth after multiple attempts to swallow.
- Recurring chest congestion after eating.
- Weight loss or dehydration from not being able to eat enough.

Data from National Foundation of Swallowing Disorders, 2020. Available at https://swallowingdisorderfoundation.com/deciphering-dysphagia/.

STEP	RATIONALE
2 Provide patient 30 minutes of rest before feeding.	Fatigue increases aspiration risk.
3 Perform hand hygiene and have patient or family caregiver (if assisting with feeding) perform hand hygiene.	Prevents transmission of microorganisms.
4 Apply clean gloves. Provide thorough oral hygiene, including brushing tongue, before meal.	Risk for aspiration pneumonia has been associated with poor oral hygiene (Thomas et al., 2019).
5 Position patient upright (90 degrees or highest position allowed) in chair or bed. *Option:* Position side-lying if patient cannot have head elevated.	Position facilitates safe swallowing and enhances esophageal motility (Metheny, 2021; Thomas et al., 2019).
6 *Option:* Apply pulse oximeter to patient's finger; monitor during feeding.	
7 Use penlight and tongue blade to gently inspect mouth for pockets of food.	Pockets of food found inside cheeks may lead to aspiration (Zupec-Kania and O'Flaherty, 2017). Patient is usually unaware of pocketing.

Continued

STEP	RATIONALE
8 Provide appropriate thickness of liquids per SLP and type of liquids per RD (IDDSI, 2017) (Table 3.1). Encourage patient to feed self as much as possible.	Thin liquids are difficult to control in mouth and pharynx and are more easily aspirated.
9 Have patient assume chin-down position. Remind patient not to tilt head backward when eating or while drinking.	Position may help reduce aspiration (Metheny, 2021). One study suggests a head-turn-plus-chin-down maneuver may be more successful (Nagy et al., 2016).
10 Adjust the rate of feeding and size of bites to match patient's tolerance. If patient is unable to feed self, place ½ to 1 teaspoon of food on unaffected side of mouth, allowing utensil to touch mouth or tongue.	Small bites help patient swallow (Grodner et al., 2021; Metheny, 2021). Provides tactile cue to food being eaten; avoids food pocketing on weaker side.
11 Provide verbal coaching: remind patient to chew and think about swallowing. • Open your mouth. • Feel the food in your mouth. • Chew and taste the food. • Raise your tongue to the roof of your mouth. • Think about swallowing. • Close your mouth and swallow. • Swallow again. • Cough to clear your airway.	Verbal cueing keeps patient focused on normal swallowing (Metheny, 2021). Positive reinforcement enhances patient's confidence in ability to swallow.
12 Avoid mixing food of different textures in same mouthful. Alternate liquids and bites of food (Metheny, 2021).	Gradual increase in types and textures combined with constant monitoring helps patient to eat more safely.

STEP	RATIONALE
13 During the meal explain to patient and family caregiver the techniques being used to promote swallowing.	Enhances patient's and family caregiver's ability to use techniques in the home. Optimizes teaching time during patient contact.
14 Monitor swallowing and observe for any respiratory difficulty. Observe for throat clearing, coughing, choking, gagging, and food drooling; suction airway as needed.	Indications that suggest dysphagia and thus pose risk for aspiration.
15 Minimize distractions, do not talk (except for explanations being provided), and do not rush patient. Allow time for adequate chewing and swallowing. Provide rest periods as needed during meal.	Environmental distractions and conversations during mealtime and fatigue increase risk for aspiration.

CLINICAL JUDGMENT *If patient remains stable and continues eating without difficulty, this is good time to delegate continued feeding to AP so that you can attend to other patients and assigned priorities.*

16 Use sauces, condiments, and gravies (if part of dysphagia diet) to facilitate cohesive food bolus.	Helps to prevent pocketing or small food particles from entering the airway.
17 Ask patient to remain sitting upright for at least 30 to 60 minutes after a meal.	Reduces chance of aspiration by allowing food particles remaining in pharynx to clear (Metheny, 2021).
18 Provide thorough oral hygiene after meal.	Rigorous oral hygiene reduces plaque and secretions containing bacteria, with studies showing reduction in incidence of pneumonia (Thomas et al., 2019).

Continued

STEP	RATIONALE
19 Perform postprocedure protocol.	
20 Evaluate patient response:	
a Observe patient's ability to swallow food and fluids of various textures and thickness without choking.	Indicates if there is ease with swallowing and absence of signs related to aspiration.
b Monitor pulse oximetry readings (if ordered) for high-risk patients during eating.	Drop in oxygen saturation can indicate aspiration.
c Monitor patient's weight, intake and output, calorie count, and food intake.	Helps to detect malnutrition and dehydration resulting from dysphagia.
d Observe patient's oral cavity.	Determines presence of food pockets after any meal that included foods of various textures.

Recording and Reporting

- Record positioning for eating, assessment findings before and after feeding, patient's diet, tolerance of liquids and food textures, amount of assistance required, position during meal, absence or presence of any symptoms of dysphagia, fluid intake, and amount of food eaten.
- Document your evaluation of patient/family caregiver learning.
- Describe patient's tolerance to diet and degree of assistance required during hand off report.
- Report any coughing, gagging, choking, or other swallowing difficulties to SLP, RD, or health care provider.

UNEXPECTED OUTCOMES	RELATED INTERVENTION
• Patient coughs, gags, complains of food "stuck in mouth," and has wet quality to voice when eating.	• Stop feeding immediately and place patient on NPO. • Notify health care provider and suction orally as needed. • Anticipate consultation with SLP.
• Patient has weight loss over next several days/weeks.	• Discuss findings with health care provider and RD. Determine whether nutritional supplements are necessary.

Assisting with Use of Canes, Crutches, and Walkers

Regular physical activity and exercise contribute to individuals' physical and emotional well-being. Canes, crutches, and walkers are assistive devices that provide ambulation support for patients during walking when they have limited weight-bearing, muscular weakness, or balance problems. An assistive device is indicated to:

- Increase stability during ambulation
- Support weak extremities
- Reduce the load on such weight-bearing structures as hips, knees, or ankles.

Safety Guidelines

- When assisting patients with any form of ambulation, apply safe-patient handling techniques. Obtain extra personnel to help as needed.
- Obtain and become familiar with any type of assistive device designated for use by a patient. Know how to properly prepare and use the device so you can teach patients or family caregivers how to use it safely and correctly.
- Prepare patients for activity. Make sure that their vital signs are stable, they are rested and not overly tired, and their pain is under control.

Delegation

The skill of assisting patients with ambulation can be delegated to assistive personnel (AP). A nurse should conduct the initial assessment when patient is ambulating for the first time. Direct the AP to:

- Have a patient dangle the lower extremities over the side of the bed after lying in bed in preparation for ambulation.
- Immediately return a patient to the bed or chair if the patient develops a feeling of nausea, dizziness, or diaphoresis and report these signs and symptoms to the nurse immediately.
- Assist the patient to apply safe, nonskid footwear. Ensure that the environment is free of clutter and there is no moisture on the floor before ambulating patient.
- Report any incident of a fall immediately.

Collaboration

- A physical therapist (PT) determines appropriate assistive device and type of gait.

Equipment

- Ambulation device (crutch, walker, cane)
- Safety device (gait belt)
- Well-fitting, flat, nonskid footwear for patient
- *Option:* pedometer

STEP	RATIONALE
1 Perform preprocedure protocol	
Assessment	
• Review electronic health record (EHR) for patient's most recent activity experience: distance ambulated, use of assistive device, activity tolerance, balance, and gait. Note history of orthostatic hypotension or falling.	Baseline data helps determine patient's tolerance of walking with assistive device and precautions to use to prevent falling.
• Review patient's most recently recorded weight.	Patient's weight affects decisions regarding safe handling to prevent falls.
• Review health care provider's order for ambulation; note any mobility, range of motion, or weight-bearing restrictions.	Determines type of assistance patient will require. Collaborate with PT in gait selection.
• Assess baseline resting heart rate, BP, respirations, and oxygen saturation (when available).	Serves as baseline for assessing activity tolerance while walking.
• Ask whether patient feels excessively tired or is currently experiencing any pain.	Indicates activity tolerance and willingness or ability to ambulate.

Continued

STEP	RATIONALE
• Assess the patient's mobility: Administer the Banner Mobility Assessment Tool (Matz et al., 2019):	Assesses four functional tasks to identify the level of mobility a patient can achieve (Matz et al., 2019). The assessment helps determine a patient's level of mobility and recommends assistive devices needed to safely lift, transfer, and mobilize a patient.

a Sit and shake: From a semireclined position, ask patient to sit upright and rotate to a seated position at the side of the bed; patient may use the bed rail. Note patient's ability to maintain bedside position. Ask patient to reach out and grab your hand and shake, making sure patient reaches across his or her midline.

b If patient fails to sit and shake: Use total lift with sling and/or positioning sheet and/or straps, and/or use lateral transfer devices such as a roll board or friction-reducing (slide sheets/tube) or air-assisted device.

c Stretch and point: With patient in seated position at the side of the bed, have patient place both feet on the floor (or stool) with knees no higher than hips. Ask patient to extend one leg and straighten the knee, and then bend the ankle and point the toes. Repeat with the other leg.

d If patient fails to stretch and point: Use total lift for patient unable to bear weight on at least one leg; use sit-to-stand lift for patient who can bear weight on at least one leg.

STEP	RATIONALE
e Stand: Ask patient to elevate off the bed or chair (seated to standing) using an assistive device (walker, cane, bed rail). Patient should be able to raise buttocks off bed and hold for a count of five. May repeat once. Note patient's proprioception (awareness of position of body) and balance.	
f If patient fails to stand: Use nonpowered raising/stand aid (default to powered sit-to-stand lift if no stand aid available) or use total lift with ambulation accessories, or assistive device (cane, walker, crutches).	
g Walk (march in place and advance step). Ask patient to march in place at bedside, and then ask patient to step forward and back with each foot. Patient should display stability while performing tasks. Assess for stability and safety awareness.	
h If patient cannot walk: Use nonpowered raising/stand aid (default to powered sit-to-stand lift if no stand aid available) or use total lift with ambulation accessories or assistive device (cane, walker, crutches).	

Continued

STEP	RATIONALE
• Refer to patient's mobility status and safe-handling algorithm (available in most agencies) to determine whether patient needs to walk with assistance from a movable lift. Do not start procedure until all required caregivers are available.	Ensures safe ambulation assistance.
• Address a patient's fear of falling. Ask patients how they feel about walking, whether they have fallen recently, and how you intend to remove risks for falling.	Fear of falling may influence a patient's gait. Research has shown that the combination of fear of falling along with a history of falls is significantly associated with higher stride-to-stride variability (STSV) in community-dwelling older adults. This association depends on the level of walking speed; the increase in STSV at lower walking speed is mainly explained by a biomechanics effect, not fear of falling (Ayoubi et al., 2014).

Implementation

1 Explain and demonstrate specific gait technique.	Allows patient to partner in care.
2 Help patient from lying position to side of bed or up from chair. Explain safety precautions to prepare for ambulation.	Enhances learning and encourages cooperation.
3 Check for appropriate height and fit of assistive device (Table 4.1).	Ensures that patient is able to ambulate successfully without injury while using device.
4 Make sure device has rubber tips; check brakes on walker (if present).	Prevents device from slipping.

CLINICAL JUDGMENT *Remove obstacles from pathways, including throw rugs (in the home), fall pads, and electrical cords; wipe up any spills immediately. Avoid crowds.*

TABLE 4.1 Types of Assistive Devices

Device	Features	Measurement
Canes Lightweight, easily movable, extend approximately waist high, made of wood or metal. Three types: single straight-legged, tripod and quad.	• Straight canes provide support and balance. • Quad canes used for patients who have unilateral weakness from a neurologic event/disease (i.e., stroke) and require more support than a straight cane. • Tripods have smaller base than quad; better stability than straight cane. • Patient keeps the cane on the stronger side of the body (Fairchild et al., 2018). • Nurse stands on the patient's weak side for support.	• Have patient stand upright wearing normal shoes with arms relaxed and hanging lossely at sides. • Measure the distance from wrist to the floor (should be about the same as the distance from the floor to the point of greater trochanter). • Adjust cane so that the top of it is that same distance from the floor. • Have patient place hand on the cane handle. If the length is correct, there is a 20-degree to 30-degree bend in the elbow. • Cane handle should fit comfortably in palm of hand.
Crutches Wooden or metal staff. Two types: double adjustable Lofstrand or forearm crutch and the axillary wooden or metal crutch.	• Use of crutches is usually temporary (e.g., after ligament damage to the knee). • Patients with paralysis of the lower extremities need crutches permanently.	• Measurements include the patient's height, the angle of elbow flexion, and the distance between the crutch pad and the axilla.

Continued

TABLE 4.1 Types of Assistive Devices—cont'd

Device	Features	Measurement
	• Crutches remove weight from one leg; used by patients who must transfer more weight to their arms than is possible with canes.	• Measure standing: Position crutches with crutch tips at 15 cm (6 inches) laterally to side and 15 cm in front of patient's feet (tripod position). Crutch pads should be 3.75 to 5 cm (1 1/2 to 2 inches) or 2 to 3 finger widths) under axilla (see Fig. 4.1) with the elbows slightly flexed (American College of Foot and Ankle Surgeons, 2020). • Height of handgrips must be adjusted so patient's elbow is slightly flexed or grip sits at approximately height of wrist crease.

TABLE 4.1 Types of Assistive Devices—cont'd

Device	Features	Measurement
Walkers Extremely light, movable devices, positioned approximately waist high and made of metal tubing. They have four widely placed, sturdy legs. They can also have 2 to 4 wheels.	• Has a wide base of support, providing stability and security when walking.	• Have patient step inside walker. • See fitting for canes.

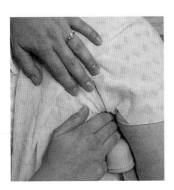

Fig. 4.1 Top of crutch.

STEP	RATIONALE
5 Apply gait belt around patient's waist. Belt should fit snugly, being sure two fingers fit between the belt and patient's body.	Belt controls patient's center of mass during mobility, assisting with balance.
6 Help patient stand at bedside fully erect with shoulders back and looking ahead (not at floor). Reassess height of assist device to make sure that it is correct size. Assess patient's ability to bear weight (e.g., does patient have discomfort, unsteady stance?) and balance.	Ensures that patient begins ambulation with correct posture and position.

Continued

STEP	RATIONALE
7 If patient is unsteady, place patient in chair or return patient to bed immediately.	Patient may require strengthening exercises or evaluation of balance by PT.
8 **Cane**	

CLINICAL JUDGMENT *Patients using a quad cane may walk slower. Gait will vary based on nature of patient's weakness or limited mobility.*

a Have patient hold cane on strong/unaffected side. Direct patient to place cane forward 10 to 15 cm (4 to 6 inches) and slightly to the side of the foot, keeping most of body weight on good foot. Allow approximately 15- to 30-degree elbow flexion.	Offers most support when on stronger side of body. Cane and weaker leg work together with each step.
b Have patient move cane and weak/affected leg forward together about 15 to 25 cm (6 to 10 inches). The cane and weak/affected leg swing and strike the ground at the same time.	Distributes body weight equally with weight supported by cane and strong leg.
c Next have patient advance strong/unaffected leg so that it is even with the cane. When first walking with the cane, this provides better balance.	Aligns patient's center of gravity. Returns patient body weight to equal distribution.
d Repeat sequences as patient tolerates. Once comfortable, have patient advance cane and weak/affected leg together and then the stronger/unaffected leg can advance 15 to 25 cm (6 to 10 inches) past the cane.	Mimics a more normal gait once patient has balance.

STEP	RATIONALE
9 Crutch walk using appropriate crutch gait. (Gait determined by PT.)	
a Four-point gait:	Most stable crutch gait. Provides at least three points of support at all times. Patient must be able to bear weight on both legs.
(1) Begin in tripod position (Fig. 4.2). Have patient lean slightly forward and place the crutch tips about 10 to 15 cm (4 to 6 inches) to the side and in front of each foot (American College of Foot and Ankle Surgeons, 2019) Have patient place weight on handgrips, not under arms.	Improves balance by providing wide base of support. Patient should have posture of erect head and neck, straight vertebrae, and extended hips and knees.

Continued

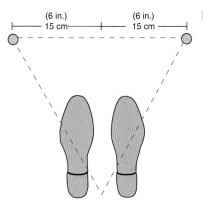

(6 in.) (6 in.)
├──── 15 cm ────┼──── 15 cm ────┤

Fig. 4.2 Tripod position.

STEP	RATIONALE
(2) Move right crutch tip forward 10 to 15 cm (4 to 6 inches) (Fig.4.3A).	Crutch and foot position is similar to arm and foot position during normal walking.
(3) Begin step as if patient were going to use the weaker foot or leg but, instead, shifts weight to the crutch. Move left foot forward to level of left crutch (Fig. 4.3B).	
(4) Move left crutch tip forward 10 to 15 cm (4 to 6 inches) (Fig. 4.3C).	
(5) Move right foot forward to level of right crutch (Fig. 4.3D).	
(6) Repeat above sequence.	
b Three-point gait:	Requires patient to bear all weight on the one strong foot. Weight is borne on strong/unaffected leg and then on both crutches. Weak/affected leg does not touch ground during three-point gait.
(1) Begin in tripod position, with patient standing on strong weight-bearing foot (Fig. 4.4A).	
(2) Advance both crutches 6 in (15 cm) and weak/affected leg, keeping foot of weak leg off floor (Fig. 4.4B).	
(3) Move weight-bearing strong leg forward, stepping on floor (Fig. 4.4C).	
(4) Repeat sequence.	
c Two-point gait:	Requires at least partial weight-bearing on each foot. Requires more balance because only two points support body at one time.

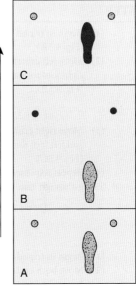

Fig. 4.4 Three-point gait with weight borne on unaffected right leg. Solid foot and crutch tips show weight-bearing in each phase.

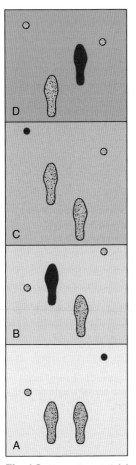

Fig. 4.3 Four-point gait. Solid feet and crutch tips show foot and crutch tip movement in each of the four phases. (A) Right tip moves forward. (B) Left foot moves toward left crutch. (C) Left crutch tip moves forward. (D) Right foot moves toward right crutch.

STEP	RATIONALE
(1) Begin in tripod position (Fig. 4.5A).	
(2) Move left crutch and right foot forward (Fig. 4.5B).	Crutch movements are similar to arm movement during normal walking: patient moves crutch at same time as opposing leg.
(3) Move right crutch and left foot forward (Fig. 4.5C).	
(4) Repeat sequence.	
d Swing-through gait:	Used by patients whose lower extremities are paralyzed or who wear weight-supporting braces on their legs.
(1) Begin in tripod position.	
(2) Move both crutches forward 6 in. (15 cm).	
(3) Lift and swing legs to crutches, letting crutches support body weight.	
(4) Repeat two previous steps.	
e Swing-to gait (Fig. 4.6):	Requires that patient can bear partial weight on both feet.
(1) Begin in tripod position with support on strongest leg.	
(2) Advance the left and right crutch, then the left and right legs are advanced.	Initial placement of crutches increases patient's base of support so when body swings forward, patient is moving center of gravity toward additional support provided by crutches.
(3) Lift and swing legs up to crutches.	
(4) Repeat previous steps.	

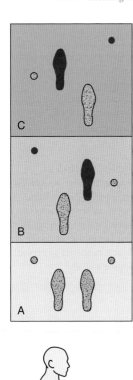

Fig. 4.5 Two-point gait. Solid areas indicate weight-bearing leg and crutch tips.

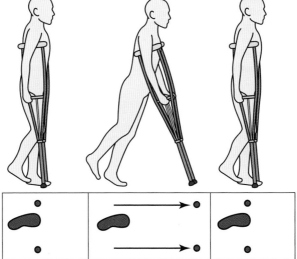

Fig. 4.6 Swing-through gait.

STEP	RATIONALE
10 Ambulate with walker:	Patients who are able to bear partial weight use walkers or rollators.
a Have patient stand straight in center of walker and grasp handgrips on upper bars. Do not allow patient to lean over walker.	Patient balances self before attempting to walk.
b Have patient move walker comfortable distance forward, about 15 to 20 cm (6 to 8 inches). Patient then takes step forward with weak/affected leg first and follows through with strong/unaffected leg into walker (Mayo Clinic, 2019). Instruct patient not to advance leg past the front bar of walker. If patient has equal strength in both legs, it makes no difference which leg advances first.	Provides broad base of support between walker and patient. Patient then moves center of gravity toward walker. Keeping all four feet of walker on the floor is necessary to prevent tipping walker.
c If patient is unable to bear weight on weak leg, have patient slowly hop to center of walker using strong leg, supporting weight on hands. *Caution:* Advise patient not to hop while using a rollator.	
d Instruct patient not to try to climb stairs with walker unless patient has specific walker for steps.	Patient should use handrails as alternative. Using walker could cause a fall.
11 Complete postprocedure protocol	
12 Evaluate patient response:	
a After ambulation, obtain patient's vital signs, observe skin color, and ask about their comfort and energy levels.	Evaluates tolerance to ambulation and whether there was progress.

STEP	RATIONALE
b Evaluate patient's subjective statements regarding experience.	Evaluates activity tolerance.
c Evaluate patient's gait pattern: observe body alignment in standing position and balance during gait.	Determines whether patient is using supportive aids for ambulation correctly.

Recording and Reporting

- Record assessment findings, type of assistive device and gait used, amount of help required, distance walked, and activity tolerance.
- Document your evaluation of patient and family caregiver learning.
- Immediately report to nurse in charge or health care provider any injury sustained during attempts to ambulate, alteration in vital signs, or inability to ambulate.

UNEXPECTED OUTCOMES	RELATED INTERVENTIONS
1 Patient is unable to ambulate because of fear of falling, physical discomfort, upper body muscles that are too weak to use ambulation device, or lower extremities that are too weak to support body.	• Consult with PT about possible exercise program to strengthen muscles or other alternative methods that patient can use for ambulation. • Provide analgesic for discomfort. • Discuss with patient fears or concerns about walking using assistive device.
2 Patient sustains an injury.	• Notify health care provider. • Return patient to bed if injury is stable. Otherwise have lift team transfer patient to bed. • Document per institution/agency policy.
3 When using cane or walker, patient bends over and does not stand straight.	• Reinforce correct posture. • Recheck to determine whether device measured correctly for patient.

Bladder Scan

A bladder scanner (Fig. 5.1) is a noninvasive portable 3D device that creates an ultrasound image of the bladder for measuring the volume of urine in the bladder. The device calculates urine volumes, especially lower volumes. The most common use for the bladder scan is to measure postvoid residual (PVR) urine (i.e., the volume of urine in the bladder after a normal voiding). To obtain the most reliable reading, measure PVR within 5 to 15 minutes of voiding (Huether et al., 2020). A volume less than 50 mL is considered normal. Two or more PVR measurements greater than 100 mL require further investigation. A bladder scan is indicated:

- When inadequate bladder emptying is suspected (e.g., postoperatively)
- After an indwelling urinary catheter is removed

Safety Guidelines

- Bladder distention can lead to a urinary tract infection if unrelieved. If a bladder scanner is not available, obtain a PVR by measuring urine emptied from the bladder after a straight catheterization.

Delegation

The skill of performing a bladder scan can be delegated to assistive personnel (AP). A nurse first determines the timing and frequency of the bladder scan measurement and interprets the measurements obtained. A nurse also assesses the patient's abdomen for distention if urinary retention is suspected. Direct the AP to:

- Follow manufacturer recommendations for the use of the device.
- Measure PVR volumes within 5 to 15 minutes after helping the patient to void.
- Report and record bladder scan volumes.

Collaboration

- Collaborate with wound ostomy care nurse before or after bladder measurement.

Equipment

- Bladder scanner (follow manufacturer instructions for use)
- Ultrasound gel; cleaning agent for scanner head such as an alcohol pad
- Urethral catheterization tray with single-use catheter for straight/intermittent catheterization
- Paper towel or washcloth

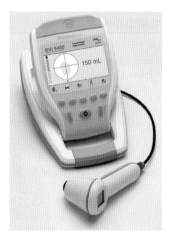

Fig. 5.1 Bladder scanner reading. (Courtesy Verathon, Inc., Bothell, WA.)

STEP	RATIONALE
1 Perform preprocedure protocol.	

Assessment

STEP	RATIONALE
• Review electronic health record to assess intake and output and most recent voiding.	Determines urine output trends and the timing for bladder scan measurement.
• Perform hand hygiene. Assess for abdominal pain and distention, a sensation of incomplete emptying, incontinence, constant dribbling of urine, and voiding in very small amounts. Perform hand hygiene.	Reduces transmission of microorganisms Signs and symptoms indicate inadequate bladder emptying.

Continued

STEP	RATIONALE

Implementation

2 Discuss procedure with patient. If measurement is for PVR, ask patient to void and measure voided urine volume. Measurement should be within 5 to 15 minutes of voiding. Follow infection control measures.

Ensures accurate measurement. Promotes understanding and cooperation.

3 Help patient to supine position with head slightly elevated. Have patient relax abdomen.

Provides access for scanner placement.

4 Measure PVR with the bladder scan:

  a Expose patient's lower abdomen.

  b Turn on scanner per manufacturer guidelines.

  c Set gender designation per manufacturer guidelines. Women who have had a hysterectomy should be designated as male.

Ensures accurate measurement.

  d Wipe scanner head with alcohol pad or other cleaner and allow to air-dry.

Reduces transmission of microorganisms.

  e Palpate patient's symphysis pubis (pubic bone). Apply generous amount of ultrasound gel (or a bladder scan gel pad, if available) to midline abdomen 2.5 to 4 cm (1 to 1.5 inches) above symphysis pubis.

Technique ensures accurate measurement.

STEP	RATIONALE
f Place scanner head on gel, ensuring that scanner head is oriented per manufacturer guidelines.	
g Apply light pressure, keep scanner head steady, and point it slightly downward toward bladder. Press and release the scan button (Fig. 5.2).	
h Verify accurate aim (refer to manufacturer guidelines). Complete scan and print image (if needed).	Image provides data for health care team members.
i Remove ultrasound gel from patient's abdomen with paper towel or moist cloth.	
5 Perform postprocedure protocol.	
6 Evaluate patient response:	
a Measure PVR after using straight/intermittent catheterization. Compare results with prevoiding scan; urine volume should be less. For patients with expected urinary retention, determine whether results reveal residual urine in bladder.	Determines need for urinary catheterization or continued monitoring.

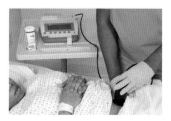

Fig. 5.2 Correct placement of bladder scanner head.

Recording and Reporting

- Record findings of scan, PVR, and patient tolerance of procedure.
- Report to health care provider outcome of bladder scan and need to catheterize for residual urine volume.

UNEXPECTED OUTCOME	RELATED INTERVENTION
1 Bladder scan shows little residual urine but patient continues to complain of bladder fullness.	• Use ultrasound as an alternative measure.

Blood Administration

Transfusion therapy or blood replacement is the intravenous (IV) administration of whole blood, its components (e.g., packed red blood cells(RBCs), cryoprecipitate, platelets), or a plasma-derived product for therapeutic purposes (Shaz et al., 2019). Transfusions restore intravascular volume with whole blood or albumin; restore oxygen-carrying capacity of blood with RBCs; provide clotting factors and/or platelets for patients with hematologic disorders, cancer, or injury, and treat diseases related to coagulation deficiencies (AABB, 2020). There are three primary blood-typing systems: ABO, Rh, and human leucocyte antigen (Table 6.1). These systems are used to crossmatch blood before transfusion to ensure the correct blood product is administered to a patient. Despite precautions taken to ensure the appropriate blood product is given, transfusion therapy carries risks. Compatibility of the patient and donor is essential. Blood transfusion can be a life-threatening procedure.

Safety Guidelines

- There are pretransfusion requirements to decrease transfusion-related errors (Teruya, 2020; Uhl, 2022):
  - Use proper labeling of the cross and match blood sample immediately on collection. Two separate specimens usually required.
  - The blood sample obtained for type and crossmatch should have a label identifying the patient's blood type and antibodies present in the plasma at the time of transfusion.
  - A blood sample for type and crossmatch must be sent to a laboratory within 72 h. If a patient has been pregnant in the last 3 months, the specimen must be less than 3 days old.
  - Compatibility testing is performed on plasma with blood drawn into a tube containing ethylenediaminetetraacetic acid (EDTA).
  - Pretransfusion testing routinely includes ABO and Rh(D) typing including antibody screening.
- Compatibility of blood unit with patient's blood is required. Human-related errors in transfusion include improper labeling, poor hand-off between nurses and the person transporting blood, and misuse of the method used to complete blood requisition.
- A health care provider's order is required for transfusion of any blood product.
- Follow blood delivery pathway:
  - Identify the patient with two unique identifiers.

TABLE 6.1 The ABO System

Patient Blood Type (Rh Factor)	Red Blood Cell Antigen	Transfuse With Type A	Transfuse With Type B	Transfuse With Type AB	Transfuse With Type O	Transfusion Options
A (+)	A	Yes	No	No	Yes	A+, A− O+, O−
A (−)	A	Yes	No	No	Yes	A−, O−
B (+)	B	No	Yes	No	Yes	B+, B− O+, O−
B (−)	B	No	Yes	No	Yes	B−, O−
AB (+)	AB	Yes	Yes	Yes	Yes	A+, A− B+, B− O+, O− Universal recipient
AB (−)	AB	Yes	Yes	Yes	Yes	A− B− O−
O (+)	None	No	No	No	Yes	O+, O−
O (−)	None	No	No	No	Yes	O− Universal donor

Data from Gorski L: Phillips's manual of I.V. therapeutics: evidence-based practice for infusion therapy, ed 7, Philadelphia, 2018. FA Davis.

- Connect the patient identifiers to all prepared lab samples, tests, and blood products by checking labels.
- Deliver the right blood product to the right patient at the right time, confirming patient identification again.

Delegation

The skill of initiating transfusion therapy cannot be delegated to assistive personnel (AP). The skill of initiating transfusion therapy by a licensed practical nurse (LPN) varies by state practice acts. After the transfusion has been started and the patient is stable, patient monitoring by AP does not relieve a registered nurse (RN) of the responsibility to continue to assess the patient during the transfusion. Instruct the AP about:

- Frequency of vital sign monitoring needed after RN determines stability.
- What to observe, such as complaints of shortness of breath, hives, and/or chills, and reporting this information to the nurse.
- Obtaining blood or blood components from the blood bank (check agency policy).

Collaboration

- Contact blood bank personnel for any guidelines regarding blood administration.

Equipment

- Y-tubing blood administration set (in-line filter) (*Note:* Depending on blood product, special tubing and filter are necessary.)
- Prescribed blood product
- 250-mL bag 0.9% NaCl (normal saline [NS]) IV solution
- 5- to 10-mL prefilled syringe with preservative-free 0.9% NS
- Antiseptic wipes (chlorhexidine based)
- Clean gloves
- Tape
- Vital sign equipment: thermometer, blood pressure cuff, and stethoscope
- Signed transfusion consent form
- *Optional:*
  - Rapid infusion pump
  - Electronic infusion device (Verify that pump can be used to deliver blood and blood products.)
  - Leukocyte-depleting filter (*Note:* Agency may irradiate blood products within the blood bank.)
  - Blood warmer
  - Pressure bag
  - Cardiac monitor for emergencies

STEP	RATIONALE
1 Perform preprocedure protocol.	

Assessment

STEP	RATIONALE
• Verify health care provider's order for specific blood product with appropriate date, time to begin transfusion, special instructions (e.g., irradiated, leukocyte depleted), duration, and any pretransfusion or posttransfusion medications to administer. If more than one blood product is ordered, the sequence of products should be specified.	Health care provider's order must be present before transfusion. Verification helps ensure that appropriate blood or blood component will be administered (Gorski, 2018). Pretransfusion medications may reduce transfusion sensitivity.
• Verify that any pretransfusion laboratory studies are completed and in patient's medical record. Review current laboratory values.	Baseline hemoglobin (Hgb), hematocrit (Hct), platelet count, and other laboratory studies are used to later evaluate patient's transfusion response.
• Obtain patient's transfusion history from electronic health record (EHR). Note any allergies or transfusion reactions. Be sure patient has allergy wrist band on arm. Verify type and crossmatch has been obtained within 72 h of transfusion.	Determines patient's prior response to transfusion of blood or blood component. If history of reaction identified, anticipate similar reaction and be prepared to intervene. Blood must be transfused within 72 h of testing.

Implementation

STEP	RATIONALE
1 Perform hand hygiene and apply clean gloves. Verify function of IV:	A patent IV ensures that transfusion will be initiated and infused within established time guidelines.

STEP	RATIONALE
a Assess the vascular access device (VAD) catheter–tubing junction site and surrounding area for catheter-related complications (e.g., infiltration, phlebitis): redness, tenderness, swelling, drainage.	Patent and functional IV ensures blood will be administered within established time guidelines.
b Assess the patency of the VAD by gently aspirating blood return or noting that existing IV fluids flow freely without signs of infiltration.	Ensures free-flow infusion as needed.
c If necessary place a new VAD for transfusion purposes. **(1)** Administer blood or blood components to an adult through a 14- to 24-gauge short-peripheral catheter with 18 to 20 gauge appropriate for the general population, and 14 to 18 gauge when rapid infusion is required (Gorski, 2018; Infusion Nurses Society [INS], 2021). **(2)** Transfuse a neonate, pediatric patient, or older adult using a 22- to 24-gauge device (Gorski, 2018; INS, 2021). **(3)** An appropriate gauge central vascular access device (CVAD) also may be used. **(4)** Remove and dispose of gloves. Perform hand hygiene.	Gauge of IV cannula should be appropriate for accommodating infusion of blood and/or blood components (INS, 2021). Large cannulas promote optimal flow of blood components. Use of smaller cannulas, such as 24 gauge, may require blood bank to divide unit so that each half can be infused within allotted time or may require pressure-assisted devices. The use of a CVAD for administration of blood depends on the catheter gauge and the manufacturer recommendations for use. (Gorski, 2018).

Continued

STEP	RATIONALE
2 Check that patient has properly completed and signed transfusion consent before retrieving blood.	Informed consent is required before transfusion. The consent form should include the risks, benefits, and treatment alternatives; the right to accept or refuse transfusion; and opportunity to ask questions (AABB, 2020; INS, 2021). Administration of albumin does not require an informed consent.
3 Determine patient's need for IV fluids or medications to be given during transfusion.	Need for additional therapies will require a second intravenous access. No other infusions/IV medications are to be given through same IV site as blood transfusion. Administer blood or blood components only with 0.9% NS (INS, 2021)
4 Obtain and record pretransfusion baseline vital signs (temperature, pulse, respirations, and blood pressure) within 30 minutes prior to transfusion. If patient is febrile (temperature greater than 37.8° C [100° F]), notify health care provider before initiating transfusion.	Change from baseline vital signs during infusion alerts you to potential transfusion reaction or adverse effect of therapy (Gorski, 2018; INS, 2021).
5 Preadministration:	
a Obtain blood/blood component from blood bank, following agency protocol (Fig. 6.1). Check patient and blood product identification.	Timely acquisition ensures product is safe to administer. Agency protocol has safeguards to ensure quality control throughout transfusion process.
b Observe and check blood bag for any signs of contamination (i.e., clumping/clots, gas bubbles, purplish color) and leaks.	Signs may indicate bacterial contamination or inadequate anticoagulation of stored blood/blood component. Presence of these attributes contraindicates infusion of that unit.

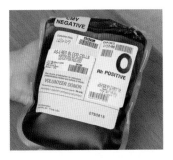

Fig. 6.1 Unit of blood with label.

STEP	RATIONALE
c At patient's bedside verbally compare and correctly verify patient, blood product, and type and transfusion order with another person considered qualified by your agency (e.g., RN or LPN). Check the following:	Strict adherence to verification procedures before administering blood or blood components reduces risk for administering wrong blood product to patient. Patient misidentification is one of the most important factors in transfusion errors (Gorski, 2018).
(1) Identify patient using two identifiers (e.g., name and birth date or name and medical record number) according to agency policy. Compare identifiers with information on patient's medication administration record or medical record.	Ensures correct patient. Complies with the Joint Commission requirements for patient safety (The Joint Commission, 2022).
(2) Confirm transfusion record number and patient's identification number match.	Prevents accidental administration of wrong component. Verifies correct patient.

Continued

STEP	RATIONALE
(3) Check that patient's name is correct on all documents. Check patient's identification number and date of birth on identification band and medical record.	
(4) Check unit number on blood bag with blood bank form to ensure that they are the same. Check expiration date and time.	Verifies correct blood product. Never administer expired blood because cell components deteriorate and may contain excess citrate. There is a higher rate of infection with expired blood (AABB, 2020).
(5) Confirm blood type matches on transfusion record and blood bag. Verify that blood type received from blood bank is the same component health care provider ordered.	Ensures that patient receives correct therapy. Misidentification and improper labeling result in transfusing the wrong ABO group.
(6) Check that patient's blood type and Rh type are compatible with donor blood type and Rh type.	Verifies accurate donor blood type and compatibility.
(7) Just before initiating transfusion check again the patient identification information with blood unit label. Do not administer blood to patient without identification bracelet or blood identification bracelet (see agency policy). (*Both nurses should confirm identification and record process*).	Serves as last check of patient and blood confirmation (Gorski, 2018). Documentation is legal medical record of procedure.

STEP	RATIONALE

CLINICAL JUDGMENT *If you notice a discrepancy during the verification procedure, do not administer the product. Notify blood bank and appropriate personnel as indicated by agency policy.*

d Ask patient to void. If patient has a catheter, don clean gloves and empty urine drainage collection device.	Ensures bladder is empty. If transfusion reaction occurs, urine specimen obtained at time of reaction will be obtained and sent to laboratory.
e Review purpose of transfusion and ask patient to report any changes they may feel during transfusion.	Signs and symptoms of transfusion reaction include chills, low back pain, shortness of breath, rash, hives, or itching (Gorski, 2018). Prompt notification aids in early detection.

CLINICAL JUDGMENT *Blood transfusion should be initiated within 30 minutes of time of release from blood bank. If this cannot be completed because of factors such as an elevated temperature, immediately return the blood to the blood bank and retrieve it when you can administer it (Gorski, 2018). It is important that the blood bag not be spiked until you ensure that no factors are present that would prevent immediate transfusion.*

6 Blood administration:

a Perform hand hygiene and don clean gloves. Reinspect blood product for leakage or signs of contamination.	Reduces risk for transmission of microorganisms. Continues blood product safety verification.
b Open Y-tubing blood administration set for a single unit. Use multiset Y tubing if multiple units are to be infused.	Y-tubing facilitates maintenance of IV access with NS in case patient will need more than one unit of blood.
c Set all clamps to "off" position.	Prevents accidental spilling and product waste.

Continued

STEP	RATIONALE
d Using aseptic technique, spike 0.9% NS IV bag with a Y-tubing spike. Hang the bag on an IV pole, and prime tubing. Open the upper clamp on NS side of tubing and squeeze the drip chamber until fluid covers the filter and one-third to one-half of the drip chamber (Fig. 6.2)	Primes tubing with fluid to eliminate air in Y-tubing. Closing the clamp prevents spilling and fluid waste.
e Maintain clamp on blood product side of Y-tubing in "off" position. Open common tubing clamp to finish priming the tubing to the distal end of tubing connector with NS. Close tubing clamp when tubing is filled with saline. All three tubing clamps should now be closed. Maintain protective sterile cap on tubing connector.	Priming the tubing with saline ensures that the IV line is ready to be connected to the patient's VAD.
f Prepare blood component for administration. Gently invert bag two or three times, turning back and forth. Remove protective covering from access port. Spike blood component unit with other Y connection.	Gentle agitation suspends the red blood cells in the anticoagulant. A protective barrier drape may be used to catch any potential blood spillage.

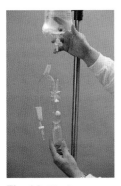

Fig. 6.2 Blood administration set is primed with normal saline.

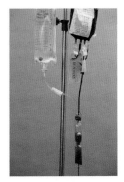

Fig. 6.3 Unit of blood connected to Y-tubing.

STEP	RATIONALE
g Close NS clamp above filter. Open clamp above filter to blood unit and prime tubing with blood (Fig. 6.3). Blood will flow into the drip chamber. Tap the filter chamber to ensure residual air is removed. Close clamp when tubing is filled. Apply sterile cap to end of tubing.	The tubing is primed with the blood unit and ready for transfusion into the patient.

CLINICAL JUDGMENT *NS is compatible with blood products, unlike solutions that contain dextrose, which causes coagulation of donor blood. Use only 0.9% NS to administer blood. No other solutions are to be administered as a secondary infusion along with blood products (AABB, 2020; INS, 2021).*

Continued

STEP	RATIONALE
h Insert infusion tubing into chamber of control mechanism of EID. Use EID indicated for blood administration. Roller clamp on IV tubing goes between EID and patient. Secure tubing through "air in line" alarm system. Close door and turn on power button. Select required administration rate.	Reduces transmission of microorganisms from catheter hub. Avoid using needleless connectors for rapid flow rates for RBC infusion; doing so can greatly reduce blood flow (INS, 2021).
i Maintaining asepsis, remove cap and attach primed tubing to patient's VAD by first cleansing the catheter hub with an antiseptic swab. Then connect primed tubing to VAD.	Initiates infusion of blood product into patient's vein.
j Open common tubing clamp and the clamp to blood bag, and regulate blood infusion to allow only 1 to 2 mL/min or 10 to 20 gtt/min (using macrodrip of 10 gtt/mL) to infuse in the initial 15 minutes. *Remain with patient during the first 15 minutes.*	Many transfusion reactions occur within first 15 minutes of transfusion (Gorski, 2018). Infusing a small amount of blood component initially minimizes the volume of blood to which the patient is exposed, thereby minimizing the severity of a reaction.

CLINICAL JUDGMENT *If signs of a transfusion reaction occur, stop the transfusion, start 0.9% NS with a new primed tubing attached directly to the VAD hub, and notify the health care provider immediately. Do not discard the blood product or tubing because they need to be returned to the blood bank. Do not infuse saline through existing tubing because it will cause blood in tubing to enter patient.*

STEP	RATIONALE
k Monitor patient's vital signs within 5 to 15 minutes of initiating the transfusion at the completion of the transfusion and for 1 h after transfusion completed (AABB, 2020; Gorski, 2018) or according to agency policy.	Frequently monitoring the patient helps to quickly alert you to transfusion reaction. The three most common causes of transfusion-related mortality are transfusion-related acute lung injury, acute hemolytic transfusion reaction, and transfusion associated circulatory overload (AABB, 2020).
l If there is no transfusion reaction, regulate rate of transfusion according to health care provider's orders. Check the drop factor for the blood administration tubing.	Maintaining the prescribed rate of flow decreases risk for fluid volume excess while restoring vascular volume. In most cases, drop factor for blood tubing is 10 gtt/mL.

CLINICAL JUDGMENT *Do not let a unit of blood hang for more than 4 h because of danger of bacterial growth. When a longer transfusion time is clinically indicated, the unit may be divided by the blood bank, and the portion not being transfused can be properly refrigerated (Gorski, 2018). Administration sets should be changed in conjunction with manufacturer's directions (INS, 2021). The AABB (2018) states that if the first unit requires 4 h for transfusion, the administration set is not reused.*

m After blood has infused turn off EID and the clamp to blood bag. Remove tubing from EID. Clear IV line with 0.9% NS by opening clamp to NS bag and infusing slowly. Once clear, regulate infusion by reinserting and regulating in EID. Discard blood bag according to agency policy.	Infusing IV NS allows remainder of blood in IV tubing to infuse and keeps IV line patent for supportive measures in case of transfusion reaction (Gorski, 2018). KVO must specify an infusion rate as required by the rights of medication administration.

Continued

STEP	RATIONALE
When consecutive blood units are ordered, maintain IV patency with 0.9% NS at keep-vein-open (KVO) rate as ordered by the health care provider and retrieve subsequent unit for administration.	
n Appropriately dispose of all supplies. Remove gloves, and perform hand hygiene.	Reduces transmission of microorganisms. Use appropriate disposal receptacle if patient is receiving hazardous drugs (Oncology Nursing Society, 2018)
7 Complete postprocedure protocol.	
8 Evaluate patient response: a Monitor IV site and infusion status each time vital signs are taken.	Detects presence of infiltration or phlebitis and verifies continuous and safe infusion of blood product.
b Observe for any changes in vital signs and signs of transfusion reaction (e.g., chills, flushing, itching, dyspnea, rash, or hypotension).	Compare presenting signs and symptoms with baseline patient assessment before transfusion. These are early signs of a transfusion reaction.
c Observe patient and monitor laboratory test results after transfusion.	Measures response to transfusion. Laboratory results may not reflect a transfusion reaction for several hours.

Recording and Reporting

- Before transfusion, record all pretransfusion medications, vital signs, location and condition of IV site, and patient education.
- Record the type and volume of blood component, blood unit/donor/recipient identification, compatibility, and expiration date according to agency policy, along with patient's response to therapy. Document on the transfusion record, nurses' notes in the EHR or

chart, medication administration record, flow sheet, and/or intake and output sheet, depending on agency policy.

- Record volume of NS and blood component infused.
- Record vital signs shortly after initiation and after transfusion.
- Document evaluation of patient learning.
- Report signs and symptoms of a transfusion reaction immediately to the health care provider.
- Report to health care provider any intratransfusion and posttransfusion deterioration in cardiac, pulmonary, and/or renal status.

UNEXPECTED OUTCOMES	RELATED INTERVENTIONS
1 Patient displays signs and symptoms of transfusion reaction e.g., chills, flushing, rash, hives, itching, fever, wheezing, tachycardia, hypotension.	• Stop transfusion immediately. • Disconnect blood tubing at VAD hub and cap distal end with sterile connector to maintain sterile system. • Connect NS-primed tubing at VAD hub to prevent any subsequent blood from infusing from tubing. • Keep vein open with slow infusion of NS at 1 to 2 mL/min to ensure venous patency and maintain venous access. Administer medications (e.g., antihistamines, antipyretics, epinephrine, corticosteroids) as ordered. • Notify health care provider and blood bank immediately. • Monitor vital signs and intake and output. • Provide oxygen support if ordered.

Continued

UNEXPECTED OUTCOMES	RELATED INTERVENTIONS
2 Patient develops infiltration or phlebitis at venipuncture site.	• Remove IV and insert new VAD at different site. Restart the blood product if remainder can be infused within 4 h of initiating transfusion. • Institute nursing measures to reduce discomfort at infiltrated or infected site.
3 Fluid overload occurs, and/or patient exhibits difficulty breathing or has crackles upon auscultation.	• Slow or stop transfusion, elevate head of bed, and inform health care provider of physical findings. • Administer diuretics, morphine, and/or oxygen as ordered by health care provider. • Continue frequent assessments, and closely monitor vital signs, intake, and output.

Blood Glucose Monitoring

Blood glucose monitoring is essential for diabetes self-management (American Diabetes Association [ADA], 2020). The ADA recommends a fasting blood sugar target of 80 to 130 mg/dL for most nonpregnant adults with diabetes (Campbell, 2020). However, desired ranges are individualized by health care providers based on patients' conditions. Blood glucose testing offers a current in-time measure of blood glucose. The test used to determine the amount of glucose available in the bloodstream over a 120-day life span of red blood cells is the glycosylated hemoglobin (HbA1c) test. The HbA1c provides an accurate long-term index of a patient's average blood glucose level drawn by venous puncture (Pagana et al., 2021). The ADA recommends an HbA1c level of 7% for an individual with diabetes (Campbell, 2020).

A variety of glucose meters are available on the market. Meters differ by the amount of blood needed for each test, testing speed, overall size, ability to store test results in memory, cost of the meter, and cost of test strips (United States Food & Drug Administration [USFDA], 2019).

Safety Guidelines

- Clean and disinfect a point-of-care blood glucose-testing meter after each patient use.
- Properly label all specimens with appropriate patient identifiers in front of patient. Also include date and time the specimen is obtained, name of the test, and source of the specimen/culture for each container when laboratory testing is ordered (The Joint Commission, 2022).
- Deliver specimens to the laboratory within the recommended time or ensure that they are stored properly for later transport.
- Follow precautions for collecting specimens from patients who are in protective isolation (see agency policy).

Delegation

Assessment of a patient's condition cannot be delegated to assistive personnel (AP). When the patient's condition is stable, the skill of blood glucose testing can be delegated to properly trained AP. Inform the AP by:

- Explaining appropriate sites to use for puncture and when to obtain glucose levels.

- Reviewing expected blood glucose levels and stating when to report unexpected glucose levels to the nurse so the nurse can retake blood glucose level as per agency policy.

Collaboration

- Diabetes nurse educator for diabetic counseling and education.

Equipment

- Antiseptic swab
- Cotton ball
- Lancet device, either self-activating or button activated
- Blood glucose meter (e.g., LifeScan, Accucheck III, OneTouch in example below)
- Blood glucose test strips appropriate for meter brand used
- Clean gloves
- Paper towel

STEP	RATIONALE
1 Perform preprocedure protocol.	
Assessment	
• Review patient's electronic health record (EHR) for health care provider's order for time or frequency of measurement.	Health care provider determines test schedule on basis of patient's physiological status and risk for glucose imbalance.
• Review EHR to determine whether there is risk to performing skin puncture (e.g., low platelet count, anticoagulant therapy, bleeding disorders).	Abnormal clotting mechanisms increase risk for local ecchymosis and bleeding.
• Determine whether specific conditions need to be met before or after sample collection (e.g., fasting, postprandial, after certain medications, before insulin doses).	Dietary intake of carbohydrates and ingestion of concentrated glucose preparations alter blood glucose levels.

STEP	RATIONALE
• Assess area of skin to be used as puncture site. Inspect fingers or forearms for edema, inflammation, cuts, or sores. Avoid areas of bruising and open lesions.	Sides of fingers are commonly selected because they have fewer nerve endings. Measurements from alternative sites are meter specific and may be different from those at traditional sites. Skin alterations can cause increased interstitial fluid and blood to mix and also increase risk for infection.
• For patient who performs test at home, assess knowledge and ability to handle skin-puncturing device and measure glucose. Patient may choose to self-test while in hospital.	Identifies level of patient knowledge and skill. Patient's physical health may change (e.g., vision disturbance, fatigue, pain, disease process), preventing them from performing test.
2 *Option:* Offer family caregiver opportunity to practice glucose-testing procedures.	Promotes understanding and assists caregiver in becoming a resource.

Implementation

1 Perform hand hygiene. Instruct patient to perform hand hygiene, including forearm (if applicable) with soap and water. Rinse and dry.	Promotes skin cleansing and vasodilation at selected puncture site. Reduces transmission of microorganisms.
2 Position patient comfortably in chair or in semi-Fowler position in bed.	Ensures easy accessibility to puncture site. Patient assumes position when self-testing.
3 Remove reagent strip from vial and tightly seal cap. Check code on test strip vial. Use only test strips recommended for glucose meter. Some newer meters do not require code and/or have disk or drum with 10 or more test strips.	Protects strips from accidental discoloration caused by exposure to air or light. Code on test strip vial must match code entered into glucose meter.

Continued

STEP	RATIONALE
4 Insert strip into meter (refer to manufacturer directions) (Fig. 7.1). Do not bend strip. Do not touch the sensor where the specimen of blood is to be obtained. Meter turns on automatically.	Some machines must be calibrated; others require zeroing of timer. Each meter is adjusted differently so follow manufacturer directions.
5 Remove unused reagent strip from meter and place on paper towel or clean, dry surface with test pad facing up (see manufacturer directions).	Moisture on strip can alter accuracy of final test results.

Fig. 7.1 Blood glucose monitor with loaded test strip. (Courtesy Lifescan, Milpitas, CA.)

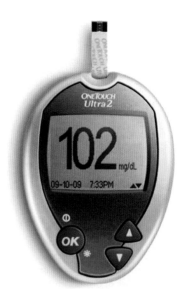

STEP	RATIONALE
6 Meter displays code on screen that must match code from test strip vial. Press proper button on meter to confirm matching codes. Meter is ready for use.	Codes must match for meter to operate. Meters have different messages that confirm that meter is ready for testing and blood can be applied.
7 Perform hand hygiene and apply clean gloves. Prepare single-use lancet or multiple-use lancet device. *Note:* Some meters recommend that this step be completed before preparing test strip. Remove cap from lancet device; insert new lancet. Some lancet devices have disk or cylinder that rotates to new lancet.	Reduces transmission of microorganisms. Never reuse a lancet because of infection risk.
a Twist off protective cover on lancet tip. Replace cap of lancet device.	
b Cock lancet device, adjusting for proper puncture depth.	Each patient varies as to depth of insertion needed for lancet to produce blood drop.
8 Obtain blood sample.	
a Wipe patient's finger or forearm lightly with antiseptic swab and allow to dry. Choose vascular area for puncture site. In stable adults select lateral side of finger. Avoid central tip of finger, which has denser nerve supply (Pagana et al., 2021).	Removes microorganisms from skin surface. Side of finger is less sensitive to pain.

Continued

STEP	RATIONALE
b Hold area to be punctured in dependent position. Do not milk or massage finger site.	Increases blood flow to area before puncture. Milking may hemolyze specimen and introduce excess tissue fluid (Pagana et al., 2021).
c Hold tip of lancet device against area of skin chosen for test site (Fig. 7.2). Press release button on device. Some devices allow you to see blood sample forming. Remove device.	Placement ensures that lancet enters skin properly.
d With some devices a blood sample begins to appear. Otherwise gently squeeze or massage fingertip until round drop of blood forms (Fig. 7.3).	Adequate-size blood sample is needed to test glucose.

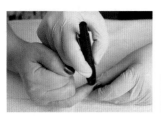

Fig. 7.2 Prick side of finger with lancet. (From Sorrentino SA, Remmert LN: Mosby's textbook for nursing assistants, ed 10, St. Louis, 2021, Elsevier.)

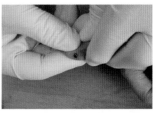

Fig. 7.3 Gently squeeze puncture site until drop of blood forms.

STEP	RATIONALE

9 Obtain test results.

   a Be sure that meter is still on. Bring test strip in meter to drop of blood. Blood will be wicked onto test strip (Fig. 7.4). Follow specific meter instructions to be sure that you obtain adequate sample.

Blood enters strip, and glucose device shows message on screen to signal that enough blood is obtained.

CLINICAL JUDGMENT *Do not scrape blood onto the test strips or apply it to wrong side of test strip. Doing so prevents accurate glucose measurement.*

---

   b Blood glucose test result will appear on screen (Fig. 7.5). Some devices "beep" when completed.

Continued

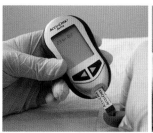

Fig. 7.4 Touch test strip to blood drop. Blood wicks into test strip. (From Sorrentino SA, Remmert LN: Mosby's textbook for nursing assistants, ed 10, St. Louis, 2021, Elsevier.)

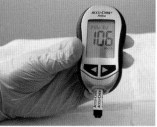

Fig. 7.5 Results appear on meter screen. (From Sorrentino SA, Remmert LN: Mosby's textbook for nursing assistants, ed 10, St. Louis, 2021, Elsevier.)

STEP	RATIONALE
10 Turn meter off. Some meters turn off automatically. Dispose of test strip, lancet, and gloves in proper receptacles.	Meter is battery powered. Proper disposal reduces risk for needlestick injury and spread of infection.
11 Discuss test results with patient. Encourage questions and eventual participation in care if this is a new diabetes mellitus diagnosis.	Promotes participation and adherence to therapy.
12 Perform postprocedure protocol	
13 Evaluate patient response:	
a Inspect puncture site for bleeding or tissue injury.	Site can be source of discomfort and infection.
b Compare glucose meter reading with recommended range for patient and with patient's baseline glucose readings.	Determines whether glucose level is appropriate for patient.

Recording and Reporting

- Record procedure and glucose level; any actions taken for abnormal range; patient response, including appearance of puncture site. (In some systems glucose value is automatically downloaded to EHR.)
- Document your evaluation of patient and family caregiver learning.
- Report abnormal blood glucose levels to patient's health care provider.

UNEXPECTED OUTCOMES	RELATED INTERVENTIONS
1 Blood glucose level is above or below target range.	• Continue to monitor patient. • Check whether there are medication orders for deviations in glucose level. • Notify health care provider. • **Administer insulin or carbohydrate source as ordered, depending on glucose level.**
2 Glucose meter malfunctions.	• Review instructions for troubleshooting glucose meter. Repeat test.

Blood Pressure by Auscultation: Upper Extremities, Lower Extremities, Palpation

The common indirect method of blood pressure (BP) measurement is by auscultation with a sphygmomanometer and stethoscope, or an automated oscillometric device without auscultation. Accuracy by auscultation depends on proper preparation of the patient, sphygmomanometer cuff placement, and listening for Korotkoff sounds. As a cuff is deflated, the five different sounds heard over an artery are called Korotkoff phases, and the sound in each phase has unique characteristics (Fig. 8.1). The BP is recorded with the systolic reading (first Korotkoff sound) before the diastolic (beginning of the fifth Korotkoff sound). The difference between systolic and diastolic pressure is the pulse pressure (e.g., if BP is 120/80 mm Hg, the pulse pressure is 40 mm Hg).

Select the proper sized cuff for a patient. Ideally the width of the cuff should be 40% of the circumference (or 20% wider than the diameter) of the midpoint of the limb on which the cuff is to be used. The bladder enclosed within the cuff should encircle at least 80% of the upper arm of an adult.

Safety Guidelines

- Several factors can contribute to errors in BP measurement (Table 8.1). If unsure of a reading, have a colleague reassess BP.

Delegation

The skill of BP measurement can be delegated to assistive personnel (AP) unless the patient is considered unstable (i.e., hypo/hypertension). Instruct the AP about:

- The appropriate limb to use for measurement, BP cuff size, and equipment (manual or electronic) to be used.
- The frequency of measurement and factors related to the patient's history such as risk for orthostatic hypotension.
- The patient's usual/baseline BP values and when to report changes/abnormalities.

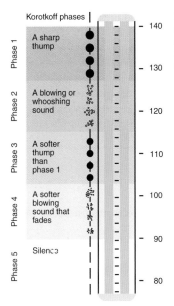

Fig. 8.1 The sounds auscultated during blood pressure measurement can be differentiated into five Korotkoff phases. In this example, the blood pressure is 140/90 mm Hg.

Korotkoff phases

Phase 1 — A sharp thump

Phase 2 — A blowing or whooshing sound

Phase 3 — A softer thump than phase 1

Phase 4 — A softer blowing sound that fades

Phase 5 — Silence

TABLE 8.1 Common Errors in Blood Pressure Assessment

Error	Effect
Bladder or cuff too wide	False-low reading
Bladder or cuff too narrow or too short	False-high reading
Cuff wrapped too loosely or unevenly	False-high reading
Deflating cuff too slowly	False-high diastolic reading
Deflating cuff too quickly	False-low systolic and false-high diastolic reading
Arm below heart level	False-high reading
Arm above heart level	False-low reading
Arm not supported	False-high reading
Stethoscope that fits poorly or impairment of examiner's hearing, causing sounds to be muffled	False-low systolic and false-high diastolic reading
Stethoscope applied too firmly against antecubital fossa	False-low diastolic reading

Continued

TABLE 8.1 Common Errors in Blood Pressure Assessment—cont'd

Error	Effect
Inflating too slowly	False-high diastolic reading
Repeating assessments too quickly	False-high systolic reading
Inadequate inflation level	False-low systolic reading
Multiple examiners using different sounds for diastolic readings	False-high systolic and false-low diastolic reading

Equipment

- Aneroid sphygmomanometer
- Cloth or disposable vinyl pressure cuff of appropriate size for patient's extremity
- Stethoscope
- Antiseptic swab
- Pen and vital sign flow sheet or electronic health record (EHR)

STEP	RATIONALE
1 Perform preprocedure protocol.	
Assessment	
• Review electronic health record (EHR) for factors that influence BP: age, gender, daily (diurnal) variation, position, exercise, weight, medications, smoking, race/ethnicity.	Acceptable values for BP vary throughout life. BP varies throughout the day.
• Assess EHR for history of following conditions: cardiovascular or renal disease, diabetes mellitus, increased intracranial pressure, recent rapid infusion of IV fluids, hypertensive disorders of pregnancy and/or preeclampsia.	Conditions listed place patients at risk for abnormal BP.

STEP	RATIONALE
• Assess patient for headache, facial flushing, fatigue, nosebleed, dizziness, mental confusion, or cool, mottled skin over extremities.	Signs and symptoms indicating possible hypo/hypertension.
• Determine best site for BP assessment. Avoid applying cuff to extremity where IV fluids are infusing, an arteriovenous shunt or fistula is present, a cast or bulky bandage is present, or on the side of body where breast or axillary surgery has been performed. Also, avoid applying cuff to traumatized or diseased extremity. Use lower extremities when brachial arteries are inaccessible. Select appropriate cuff size (Fig. 8.2).	Inappropriate site selection may result in poor sound amplification, causing inaccurate readings. Pressure from inflated bladder temporarily impairs blood flow and can further compromise circulation in extremity that already has impaired blood flow.

Continued

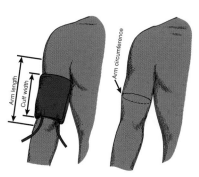

Fig. 8.2 Guidelines for proper blood pressure cuff size. Cuff width is 20% more than upper arm diameter, or 40% of circumference and two-thirds of upper arm length.

STEP	RATIONALE

Implementation

1 Perform hand hygiene. Clean stethoscope earpieces and diaphragm with antiseptic swab.

Reduces transmission of microorganisms.

2 Position patient:

a Upper extremity: Patient sitting or lying; place forearm at heart level with palm turned up. Support arm on table or under your arm. If sitting, have patient keep feet flat on floor without legs crossed. If lying down, do not cross legs.

b Lower extremity: With patient supine or prone, have patient flex knee slightly bent/flexed.

If arm unsupported, patient can inadvertently perform isometric exercise that increases diastolic pressure. Arm placement above level of heart causes false- low reading; below level of heart creates false-high reading (Gunes and Efteli, 2016; Kallioinen et al., 2017). Crossing the legs can increase BP (Kallioinen et al., 2017).

3 Expose extremity (arm or leg) fully by removing constricting clothing. Cuff may be placed over a sleeve as long as stethoscope rests on the skin (Kallioinen et al., 2017).

Ensures proper cuff application.

4 Palpate brachial artery (Fig. 8.3) or popliteal artery. With cuff fully deflated, apply cuff bladder above artery by centering arrows marked on cuff over artery. If cuff has no center arrows, estimate center of bladder and place this center over artery. Position cuff 2.5 cm (1 inch) above site of pulsation (antecubital or popliteal space) (Fig. 8.4). With cuff fully deflated, wrap it evenly and snugly around upper arm.

Placing bladder directly over artery ensures that you apply proper pressure during inflation. Loose-fitting cuff causes false-low readings. Popliteal artery is just below patient's thigh, behind knee.

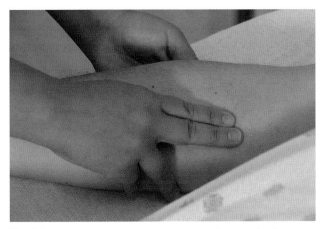

Fig. 8.3 Palpating brachial artery. (From *Clinical skills: essentials collection*, 2021, Elsevier.)

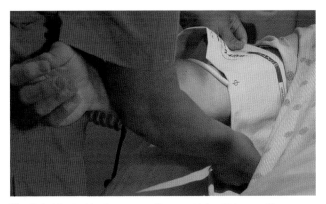

Fig. 8.4 Aligning blood pressure cuff arrow with brachial artery. (From *Clinical skills: essentials collection*, 2021, Elsevier.)

STEP	RATIONALE
5 Position manometer gauge vertically at eye level. You should be no farther than 1 meter (approximately 1 yard) away.	Looking up or down at scale can result in distorted readings.

6 Measure BP
  a Two-step method:
    (1) Relocate brachial or popliteal pulse. Palpate artery distal to cuff with fingertips of nondominant hand while inflating cuff rapidly to a pressure 30 mm Hg above point at which pulse disappears. Slowly deflate cuff and note point when pulse reappears. Deflate cuff fully and wait 30 seconds.
	Estimating prevents false-low readings. Determines maximal inflation point for accurate reading. If unable to palpate artery because of weakened pulse, use an ultrasonic stethoscope. Completely deflating cuff prevents venous congestion and false-high readings.

(2) Place stethoscope earpieces in ears and be sure that sounds are clear and not muffled.	Ensure that each earpiece follows angle of ear canal to facilitate hearing.
(3) Relocate artery, and place bell or diaphragm chest piece of stethoscope over it (Fig. 8.5). Do not allow chest piece to touch cuff or clothing.	Proper placement ensures best sound reception. Improper position causes muffled sounds that often result in false-low systolic and false-high diastolic. Diaphragm easier to secure with fingers and covers a larger area. Placing stethoscope under cuff increases systolic and decreases diastolic BP (Kallioinen et al., 2017).

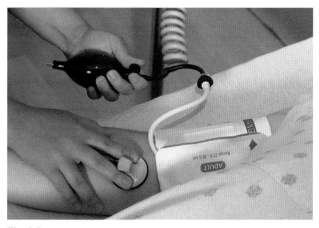

Fig. 8.5 Blood pressure cuff wrapped around upper arm with bell of stethoscope over brachial artery. (From *Clinical skills: essentials collection*, 2021, Elsevier.)

STEP	RATIONALE
(4) Close valve of pressure bulb clockwise until tight. Quickly inflate cuff to 30 mm Hg above patient's estimated systolic pressure.	Tightening valve prevents air leak during inflation. Rapid inflation ensures accurate measurement of systolic pressure.
(5) Slowly release pressure bulb valve and allow manometer needle to fall at rate of 2 to 3 mm Hg/s.	Too rapid a decline decreases systolic and increases diastolic BP (Kallioinen et al., 2017).
(6) Note point on manometer at which you hear first clear sound. The sound will slowly increase in intensity.	First Korotkoff sound reflects systolic BP.

Continued

STEP	RATIONALE
(7) Continue to deflate cuff gradually, noting point at which sound disappears in adults. Note pressure to nearest 2 mm Hg. Listen for 20 to 30 mm Hg after last sound and allow remaining air to escape quickly.	Beginning of the last or fifth sound indicates diastolic pressure in adults (Thomas and Pohl, 2020). In children, distinct muffling of sounds indicates diastolic pressure (Thomas and Pohl, 2020).
b One-step method:	
(1) Place stethoscope earpieces in ears and be sure that sounds are clear, not muffled.	Earpieces should follow angle of ear canal to facilitate hearing.
(2) Relocate brachial or popliteal artery and place bell or diaphragm chest piece of stethoscope over it. Do not allow chest piece to touch cuff or clothing.	Proper stethoscope placement ensures optimal sound reception and less chance of error.
(3) Close valve of pressure bulb clockwise until tight. Quickly inflate cuff to 30 mm Hg above patient's usual systolic pressure.	Tightening valve prevents air leak during inflation. Inflation above systolic level ensures accurate measurement of systolic pressure.

STEP	RATIONALE
(4) Slowly release pressure bulb valve and allow manometer needle to fall at rate of 2 to 3 mm Hg/s. Note point on manometer at which you hear first clear sound. Sound will slowly increase in intensity.	Too rapid a decline decreases systolic and increases diastolic BP (Kallioinen et al., 2017). First sound indicates systolic reading.
(5) Continue to deflate cuff gradually, noting point at which sound disappears in adults. Note pressure to nearest 2 mm Hg. Listen for 10 to 20 mm Hg after last sound and allow remaining air to escape quickly.	Beginning of the last or fifth sound indicates diastolic pressure in adults (Thomas and Pohl, 2020). In children, distinct muffling of sounds indicates diastolic pressure (Thomas and Pohl, 2020).
7 The American Heart Association recommends average of two sets of BP measurement, 2 minutes apart. Use second set of BP measurements as baseline. If readings are different by more than 5 mm Hg, additional readings are necessary.	Helps to prevent false-positive readings based on patient's sympathetic response (alert reaction). Averaging minimizes effect of anxiety, which often causes first reading to be higher than subsequent measures (Kallioinen et al., 2017).
8 Remove cuff from patient's arm or leg unless condition requires repeated measurement.	

Continued

STEP	RATIONALE
9 Assess systolic BP by palpation:	
a Follow Steps 1 through 5 of auscultation method.	Ensures proper patient position and cuff placement.
b Locate and then continually palpate brachial, radial, or popliteal artery with fingertips of one hand. Inflate cuff to a pressure 30 mm Hg above point at which you can no longer palpate pulse.	Ensures accurate detection of true systolic pressure once pressure valve is released.

CLINICAL JUDGMENT *If unable to palpate artery because of weakened pulse, use a Doppler ultrasonic stethoscope.*

c Slowly release valve and deflate cuff, allowing manometer needle to fall at rate of 2 mm Hg/s. Note point on manometer at which pulse is again palpable.	Too rapid a decline decreases systolic and increases diastolic BP (Kallioinen et al., 2017). Palpation helps identify systolic pressure only.
d Deflate cuff rapidly and completely. Remove cuff from patient's extremity unless you need to repeat measurement.	Continuous cuff inflation causes arterial occlusion, resulting in numbness and tingling of extremity.
e Help patient return to comfortable position and cover extremity if previously clothed.	Restores comfort and promotes sense of well-being.
10 If assessing BP for the first time, establish baseline BP if it is within acceptable range.	Used to compare future BP measurements.
11 Discuss results with patient.	Patient needs to be informed about BP for proper self-care management.

STEP	RATIONALE

12 Complete postprocedure protocol.

13 Evaluate patient response:

   a Compare BP reading with patient's previous baseline and usual BP for patient's age.

Allows you to assess for change in condition. Provides comparison with future BP measurements.

Recording and Reporting

- Record BP, site and method assessed, and any signs of BP alterations on vital sign flow sheet or EHR.
- Document BP after administration of specific therapies.
- Document evaluation of patient learning.
- Report elevated or low BP, difference of more than 20 mm Hg between extremities, or more than 20 mm Hg drop in systolic, or a 10 mm Hg drop in diastolic when rising from sitting position.

UNEXPECTED OUTCOMES	RELATED INTERVENTIONS
1 Patient's BP is above acceptable range.	• Repeat measurement in other extremity and compare findings. When difference is greater than 10 mm Hg, use arm with higher pressure (American Association of Critical Care Nurses, 2016). • Verify correct cuff size and placement. • Have another nurse repeat measurement in 1 to 2 minutes. • Observe for physical signs and symptoms of hypertension: headache, facial flushing, fatigue. • Report BP to health care provider.

Continued

UNEXPECTED OUTCOMES	RELATED INTERVENTIONS
2 Patient's BP is below acceptable level.	• Repeat measurement and compare with baseline. • Position patient supine: enhance circulation and restrict activity that decreases BP further. • Assess for signs and symptoms associated with hypotension: tachycardia; weak, thready pulse; weakness; dizziness; confusion; and cool, pale, skin. • Assess for factors that contribute to a low BP, including hemorrhage, vasodilation from hyperthermia, anesthesia, or medication side effects. • Report BP to health care provider. • Increase rate of IV infusion or administer vasoconstriction drugs if ordered.
3 Unable to obtain BP.	• Assess pulse and respiratory rate. • Use alternative site, Doppler ultrasound, or have another RN check BP.
4 Patient has orthostatic hypotension.	• Return patient to safe position in bed or chair. • Initiate fall prevention protocol.

Blood Pressure: Automatic

Many different styles of electronic blood pressure (BP) machines are available to determine BP automatically. Electronic BP machines rely on an electronic sensor placed over an artery to detect the vibrations caused by the rush of blood through the artery. Although electronic BP machines are faster, you must consider the advantages and limitations of the devices. They are used when frequent assessments are required, such as in critically ill or potentially unstable patients, during or after invasive procedures, during postoperative recovery, or when therapies require frequent monitoring.

Safety Guidelines

- Choose the correct cuff size for a patient's arm circumference, ensure the artery marker is aligned over the patient's brachial artery, and ensure the cuff is wrapped snugly.
- Ensure that the BP cuff is secure enough that it does not move on the patient's arm. Any movement of the BP cuff can cause fluctuations of the pressure measured; such movement can cause serious distortion to the signal it is detecting.
- Routinely check air hose, connector, and cuffs for leaks.

Delegation

The skill of obtaining an electronic BP measurement can be delegated to assistive personnel (AP) unless the patient is considered unstable. Instruct the AP by:

- Explaining the frequency and extremity to use for measurement.
- Reviewing how to select proper cuff for extremity and for the machine being used.
- Reviewing the patient's usual BP values and the importance of reporting changes/abnormalities to nurse.

Collaboration

- If you find an unexpected automatic BP reading, have a second nurse measure patient's BP.

Equipment

- Electronic BP device
- BP cuff of appropriate size (recommended by manufacturer)
- Pen and vital sign flow sheet or electronic health record (EHR)

STEP	RATIONALE
1 Perform preprocedure protocol.	

Assessment

• Perform assessment steps in Skill 8.	Reveals factors indicating status of patient's BP and determines site selection for measurement.
• Review patient's EHR for history of an irregular heart rate, peripheral vascular disease, seizures, tremors, or shivering.	These factors contraindicate use of automatic BP machine.

Implementation

1 Perform hand hygiene. Assist patient to comfortable position, lying or sitting. Plug in and place device near patient, ensuring that connector hose between cuff and machine will reach.	Comfortable position with device in correct position promotes accurate reading.
2 Turn machine on at switch to enable device to self-test its computer system (display will appear) (Fig. 9.1).	Activates electronic system.

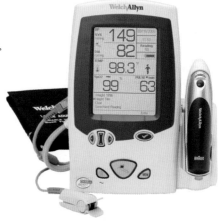

Fig. 9.1 Digital electronic blood pressure display. (Courtesy Welch Allyn, Skaneateles Falls, NY.)

STEP	RATIONALE
3 Select appropriate cuff size for patient and machine. Electronic BP cuff and machine must match. Not interchangeable.	Device will not function with inappropriate cuff.
4 Remove constricting clothing over extremity. Do not place BP cuff over clothing.	The cuff is the sensor and must be placed over skin.
5 Prepare BP cuff by manually squeezing out all the air and connecting cuff to connector hose.	Cuff must fit smoothly and firmly around extremity.
6 Wrap flattened cuff snugly around extremity. Make sure the "artery" arrow marked on outside of the cuff is placed over artery.	Ensures accurate reading.
7 Verify that connector hose between cuff and device is not kinked.	Kinking prevents proper inflation and deflation of cuff.
8 Following manufacturer's directions, set frequency control for automatic or manual and press the start button. The first BP measurement pumps cuff to a peak pressure of approximately 180 mm Hg. After this pressure is reached, the machine begins a deflation sequence that determines the BP. The first reading is peak pressure inflation.	When patient is to have frequent BP measurements, automatic mode is useful. Cuff can stay in place, but ensure cuff is fully deflated after each measurement.

CLINICAL JUDGMENT *When cuff is left in place, it must be removed every 2 h to assess condition of underlying skin. If possible alternate between measurement sites. Patients with bleeding tendencies may develop microvascular rupture from repeated inflation.*

Continued

STEP	RATIONALE
9 When deflation is complete, digital display shows most recent values of BP and time in minutes that have elapsed since last measurement.	
10 Set frequency of measurements and upper and lower alarm limits for systolic, diastolic, and mean BP. Intervals between measurements can be set from 1 to 90 minutes. Determine frequency and alarm limits based on patient condition, your clinical judgment, and health care provider order.	Unstable patients usually have a targeted range that health care providers want to achieve. Patients with no obvious cardiovascular problems will likely have normal limits set.
11 Obtain an additional reading at any time by pressing the start button. Pressing the cancel button immediately deflates the cuff.	
12 Discuss findings with patient.	
13 When patient no longer requires frequent monitoring, remove and clean cuff according to agency policy.	Reduces transmission of microorganisms.
14 Perform postprocedure protocol.	
15 Evaluate patient response:	
a Compare electronic readings with auscultatory readings (Skill 8).	Confirms accuracy of device.
b Compare electronic readings with patient's baseline or desired range.	Evaluates patient's clinical progress.

Recording and Reporting

- Record BP measurements and site used on vital sign flow sheet or EHR. Some devices automatically record results in patient's electronic data base.
- Record and report any signs of BP alterations.

UNEXPECTED OUTCOME	RELATED INTERVENTIONS
1 Unable to obtain BP with device.	• Check machine connections: plugged into electrical outlet, hose-cuff connection tight, machine on, correct cuff. • Repeat measurement and if still unable to obtain result, assess using auscultation method (Skill 8).

Cardiac Monitor Application

An electrocardiogram (ECG) is a graphic representation of the electrical activities, or conduction system, of the heart. An ECG is used for diagnostic and treatment purposes (e.g., determining type of cardiac arrhythmia and health care provider selection of appropriate medication). Accuracy depends on the correct placement and clean application of electrodes to a patient's skin. A cardiac monitor can be a bedside, hard-wired monitor or a wireless transmitter used with telemetry systems. A continuous ECG rhythm is obtained using three or five electrodes and leads. In the case of a bedside monitor, the electrodes deliver electrical impulses, allowing for detection of dysrhythmias. Most devices provide alarms when dysrhythmias appear or when heart rate limits are exceeded.

Safety Guidelines

- Know a patient's current medications. Beta blockers, calcium channel blockers, and other antiarrhythmics can cause dysrhythmias.

Delegation

The skill of applying a cardiac monitor can be delegated to assistive personnel (AP) who are specially trained. In some agencies the individual who applies a monitor is a specially trained telemetry technician. Direct the AP to:

- Immediately report alarms or patient complaints of pain, shortness of breath, or hypotension.
- Be sure the parameters for alarms and heart rate are set per health care provider's orders.

Collaboration

- Telemetry monitoring technicians observe ECG readings on multiple patients continuously. They notify RNs when dysrhythmias are identified.

Equipment

- Bedside cardiac monitor or telemetry transmitter
- Three or five ECG electrodes (disposable, self-adhesive)
- Three or five ECG leads with snap-on attachments
- Clean, dry towel, washcloth or gauze
- *Option:* Hair clippers if hair covers desired electrode site.

STEP	RATIONALE
1 Perform preprocedure protocol.	

Assessment

• Assess patient for dehydration, malnutrition, dermatologic conditions, or preexisting conditions that place patient at risk for skin injury, e.g., diabetes, infection, renal insufficiency, immune deficiency, and edema. Older adults also more at risk.	Risk factors for medical adhesive-related skin injury (MARSI) (Fumarola et al., 2020). The skin-contact surface of an electrode contains adhesive.
• Check skin at sites where electrodes are to be placed for excess oil or moisture. If present, wipe chest or limbs with clean, dry towel/gauze. If necessary, clean skin with soap and water, rinse, and dry thoroughly. *Option:* If hair covers chosen electrode site, clip hair.	Provides clean, dry contact surface for electrode; ensures more accurate recording.

Implementation

1 Perform hand hygiene	Reduces transmission of microorganisms.
2 Prepare patient by removing or repositioning gown to expose only patient's chest (or limbs). Keep abdomen and thighs covered.	Facilitates correct electrode placement and protects patient privacy.
3 Place patient in supine position.	Eases access to chest for electrode placement.

Continued

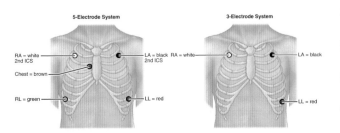

Fig. 10.1 Chest lead positioning in three-electrode and five-electrode systems. *ICS*, intercostal space; *LA*, left arm; *LL*, left leg; *RA*, Right arm; *RL*, Right leg.

STEP	RATIONALE

4 Apply electrodes in correct anatomic sites for either a three- or five-electrode system (Fig. 10.1).
 	
  a Three lead:
     RA: white lead placed along right midclavicular line just below clavicle
     LA: black lead placed along left midclavicular line just below clavicle
     LL: red lead placed over left lower sixth to seventh intercostal space along left midclavicular line.
  b Five lead: Same as three lead and also includes
     C: brown chest lead placed over fourth intercostal space right of sternum
     RL: green lead placed over right lower sixth to seventh intercostal space along right midclavicular line.
	Proper placement of leads is important for accurate dysrhythmia interpretation. Color of leads represent polarity: white is negative, black is positive, red is ground or neutral. Two additional leads of a five-lead system include green (positive or negative) and brown (positive).

STEP	RATIONALE
5 Check bedside monitor or telemetry station for any messages indicating electrode or lead issues. Troubleshoot placement and/or connections as needed.	Monitoring system may detect a bad electrode contact with skin or a loose lead connection.
6 Check that ECG rhythm can be seen on bedside monitor or central or remote viewing station.	Technicians watching monitor remotely communicate with nurse before they leave the room so any issues can be addressed quickly. Call to technician also notifies nurse that monitoring has started.
7 Change ECG electrodes daily or more often if electrode contact with skin is loose. Clean area of skin where electrode is removed.	Decreases number of false alarms. Routine skin care may reduce incidence of MARSI (Fumarola et al., 2020).
8 Customize alarm limits within 1 h of patient condition changing. Follow agency policy and health care provider orders.	Reduces false alarms and focuses on true alarms and/or reasons for monitoring.
9 Perform postprocedure protocol.	
10 Evaluate patient response:	
a Monitor patient for arrhythmias during care; electrodes stay in place regardless of patient activity (in bed, ambulating, in chair)	Detects possible cardiac changes or response.
b Review alarm trend/waveform at least once per shift or on the report of an alarm.	Ensures detection of arrythmia changes or new occurrences.

Recording and Reporting

- Record at least one rhythm strip per shift per agency policy, either on paper or saved in electronic format.
- Report any unexpected dysrhythmias to healthcare provider.

UNEXPECTED OUTCOMES	RELATED INTERVENTIONS
1 Monitor tracing cannot be interpreted. Absence of tracing on one or more leads. 2 Presence of artifact in ECG tracings.	• Inspect electrode for secure placement. Replace as needed with proper skin preparation. • Reposition any wires of the leads that move as result of patient breathing or movement. Do not reposition electrodes if in correct position. • If artifact looks like a thick lined waveform, unplug battery-operated equipment in room one item at a time to see whether interference disappears.

Central Vascular Access Device Care: Central and Peripherally Inserted

The need for safe and convenient intravenous (IV) therapy in seriously ill patients has led to the development of vascular access devices (VADs) designed for long-term access to the venous or arterial systems. A central vascular access device (CVAD) and a peripherally inserted central catheter (PICC) differ from short-peripheral or midline catheters in that the farthest tip of a central catheter ends in a large blood vessel. The tip of a CVAD should be placed in the upper body in the lower segment of the superior or inferior vena cava at or near the cavoatrial junction (Fig. 11.1). Those placed in the lower body should end in the inferior vena cava above the level of the diaphragm (Infusion Nurses Society [INS], 2021). A central catheter is typically inserted through the subclavian vein in adults (INS, 2021). In the case of a PICC, the insertion site is usually the antecubital space, using the median cubital, cephalic, basilic and brachial veins with sufficient size (INS, 2021). A venous site in adults where the catheter-to-vein ratio is equal to or less than 45% is recommended (INS, 2021).

A nurse's role is to anticipate a patient's need for a CVAD, assist the healthcare provider (HCP) in placing a CVAD, care for and maintain the device, administer solutions or medications correctly, and assess for signs and symptoms of IV-related complications. When accessing or manipulating a CVAD site use Aseptic Non-Touch Technique (ANTT), which is achieved by integrating standard precautions including hand hygiene, use of personal protective equipment (PPE) with appropriate aseptic field management, non-touch technique, and sterilized supplies (INS, 2021). There are similarities and differences between each CVAD (Table 11.1). Characteristics of the devices and the type of patient education affect care and maintenance of each CVAD.

CVADs have single or multiple lumens (Fig. 11.2). The choice of the number of lumens depends on a patient's condition and prescribed therapy. Patients requiring numerous infusions and blood samplings may have a device placed with more than one lumen, allowing simultaneous administration of solutions and medications. Multiple lumens also allow for administration of incompatible solutions or medications at the same time. A CVAD is accessed through the hub of the device located on the end of each external lumen.

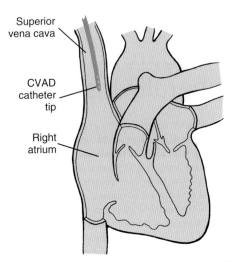

Superior
vena cava

CVAD
catheter
tip

Right
atrium

Fig. 11.1 Catheter tip from central vascular access device (CVAD) lies in superior vena cava.

TABLE 11.1 Central Vascular Access Devices

Short-Term Devices	Long-Term Devices
Nontunneled Percutaneous	**External Tunneled (Hickman, Broviac, Groshong)**
• Length of dwell: Days to several weeks • Insertion sites: Subclavian, external/internal jugular, and femoral veins • Can be placed at bedside; direct puncture into intended vein without passing through subcutaneous tissue • Held in place with sutures or securement device	• Length of dwell: Considered permanent until therapy no longer needed • Insertion sites: Chest region through subclavian or jugular vein • Insertion technique: Surgery required (Fig. 11.4) • Held in place by a Dacron cuff coated in antimicrobial solution; in 2 to 3 weeks, scar tissue forms around cuff, fixing catheter in place

TABLE 11.1 Central Vascular Access Devices—cont'd

Peripherally Inserted Central Catheters (Fig 11.2)	Implanted Venous Ports (Fig. 11.3)
• Length of dwell: As long as device functions properly with no evidence of IV-related complications • Insertion sites: Antecubital fossa or upper arm (basilic or cephalic vein) and advanced until catheter tip reaches superior vena cava • Can be inserted at bedside in any setting • Held in place with sutures or engineered securement device	• Length of dwell: Considered permanent until therapy no longer needed • Insertion sites: Chest, abdomen, or inner aspect of forearm • Insertion techniques: Surgery required. Catheter attached to reservoir located within a surgically created subcutaneous pocket (Fig. 11.3) • Sutured in place within surgically created pocket and accessed using a noncoring needle through the skin

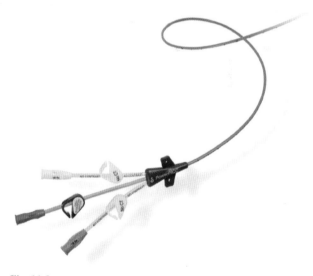

Fig. 11.2 Peripherally inserted central catheter. (Courtesy and copyright ©Bard Access Systems, Becton, Dickinson and Company, Franklin Lakes, NJ.)

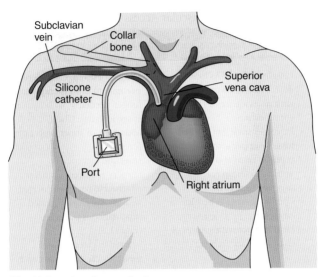

Fig. 11.3 Implanted port and catheter.

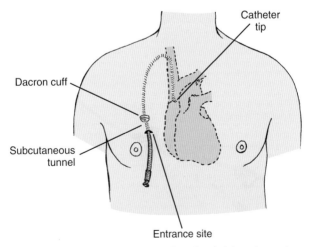

Fig. 11.4 Tunneled central catheter in place, threaded through superior vena cava.

TABLE 11.2 Common Central Vascular Access Device Complications

Complication	Assessment	Prevention	Intervention
Occlusion: thrombus, fibrin sheath, fibrin tail, precipitation, malposition	Assess insertion site and sutures. Assess for blood return. Assess for ability to infuse fluid. Assess for discomfort or pain in shoulder, neck, ear, or arm at insertion site. Assess for neck or shoulder edema.	Follow routine flushing protocol. Secure with catheter stabilization device to prevent tension on CVAD. Do not flush against resistance. Flush between medications. Flush vigorously after viscous solutions. Avoid kinking catheter.	Reposition patient and have cough and deep breathe. Raise patient's arm overhead. Obtain venogram if ordered. Administer thrombolytics if ordered. Remove catheter. Obtain x-ray film as ordered.
Infection and sepsis: catheter skin junction, tunnel, thrombus, port pocket, CLABSI	Assess catheter skin junction for redness, drainage, edema, or tenderness. Assess for signs of systemic infection. Monitor laboratory findings.	Prevent contamination of catheter hub. Adhere to dressing change technique. Apply TSM dressing over catheter skin junction.	Obtain blood cultures from peripheral and CVAD if ordered. Remove catheter. Replace catheter.
Dislodgement	Assess length of catheter daily. Identify edema at catheter skin junction or drainage. Palpate catheter skin junction and tunnel for coiling (catheter can feel cordlike underneath the skin). Assess for distended neck veins.	Loop and tape catheter securely. Use catheter stabilization device and TSM dressing. Avoid pulling on CVAD. Avoid manipulating catheter by hand.	Insert new catheter. Secure with catheter stabilization device. Teach patient not to manipulate catheter.

Continued

TABLE 11.2 Common Central Vascular Access Device Complications—cont'd

Complication	Assessment	Prevention	Intervention
Skin erosion (e.g., mechanical loss of skin tissue), hematomas (e.g., local collection of blood), cuff extrusion (e.g., tissue at edges of insertion site separate), scar tissue formation over port	Assess for loss of viable tissue over septum site. Assess for separation of exit site edges. Assess for drainage, redness, edema at catheter skin junction. Note if tunneled catheter is exposed (Dacron cuff is visible).	Maintain nutritional status. Avoid pressure or trauma. Rotate with each port access. Do not reinsert a noncoring needle in the same "hole" of a previous insertion. This creates a permanent hole in the septum. Do not use standard needle to access port.	Remove CVAD as ordered. Improve nutrition. Provide appropriate skin care.
Infiltration, extravasation	Assess for erythema, edema, spongy feeling, swelling around IV site and at termination of catheter tip. Assess for labored breathing. Assess for aspiration of fluid and/or blood. Assess for complaints of pain with infusion of solutions or medications (e.g., burning). Assess for non-free-flowing IV drip.	Immediately stop vesicant administration. Administer antidote or therapeutic medications to maintain tissue integrity according to protocol.	Apply cold/warm compresses according to specific vesicant protocol. Obtain x-ray film if ordered. Use antidotes per protocol. Discontinue IV solutions.
Pneumothorax, hemothorax, air emboli, hydrothorax	Assess for subcutaneous emphysema by inspecting and palpating skin around insertion site and along arm. Palpation reveals a crackling sensation such as popping plastic bubble wrap. Assess for chest pain, dyspnea, apnea, hypoxia, tachycardia, hypotension, nausea, confusion.	Use injection cap on distal end when not in use. Do not leave catheter hub open to air. If appropriate for device, be sure that clamps are engaged.	Administer oxygen as ordered. Elevate feet. Aspirate air, fluid. If air emboli suspected, place patient on left side with head down. Remove catheter as ordered. Help with insertion of chest tubes as ordered.

CLABSI, central line-associated bloodstream infection; *CVAD*, central vascular access device; *TSM*, transparent semipermeable membrane.

An implanted venous port has a reservoir placed in a pocket under the skin with the catheter inserted into a major vessel (e.g., subclavian) (Fig. 11.3). The port has no external lumen or hub. Instead, access to an implanted venous port is obtained by inserting a special 90-degree angle noncoring needle through the skin into the self-sealing injection port in the septum of the reservoir. It is common for a port not to be used for extended periods (i.e., weeks) between infusions, and it is not necessary that the port remain accessed during these periods. To maintain the patency of a port, it is necessary to flush monthly with heparin solution or 0.9% sodium chloride in accordance with agency policies and procedures and manufacturer directions for use (INS, 2021).

Safety Guidelines

- Complications of CVADs can include local or systemic infection. A local infection can develop around the catheter insertion site. A systemic infection may be caused by contamination of the catheter from the skin of the patient or poor infection-prevention practices during insertion, care, and maintenance (Gorski, 2018). Utilizing the Institute for Healthcare Improvement (IHI) Central Line Bundle prevents infection. Key components of the IHI Central Line Bundle are (Gupta et al., 2021):
  - Hand hygiene before catheter insertion or manipulation.
  - Maximal sterile barrier precautions with insertion. (Inserter wears a cap, mask, and sterile gloves and gown, and a large sterile drape is placed over patient during insertion.)
  - 0.5% Chlorhexidine gluconate (CHG) with Alcohol for skin antisepsis before insertion.
  - Disinfect catheter hubs, needleless connectors, and injection ports before accessing the catheter.
  - Necessity of daily review of the condition of the line and insertion site with prompt removal of unnecessary lines.

Delegation

Managing a CVAD cannot be delegated to assistive personnel (AP). Instruct the AP to:

- Report the following: bleeding or swelling around CVAD insertion site, shortness of breath, loosened or soiled dressing, elevated patient temperature, complaints of pain at the site, or catheter becomes dislodged.
- Report if the electronic infusion device alarm signals or if the fluid level in container is low or empty.
- Help with positioning patient during insertion and care.

Collaboration

- The health care provider (HCP), central supply and pharmacy services aid in the management of CVADs.

Equipment

Site Care and Dressing Change

- CVAD dressing change kit, which includes sterile gloves, mask, antiseptic swabs for skin disinfection (0.5% chlorhexidine with alcohol solution preferred), transparent semipermeable membrane dressing (TSM), 4 × 4-inch gauze pads, tape measure, sterile tape, and label for noting date/time/initials
- Engineered stabilization device (if not sutured) for PICC or nontunneled catheters
- Adhesive remover
- Clean gloves
- Needleless injection cap(s) for each lumen(s)
- Polymer-based skin protectant spray, wipe, or swab

Blood Sampling

- Clean gloves
- Antiseptic swabs (CHG solution preferred, or 70% isopropyl alcohol and povidone-iodine for chlorhexidine sensitivities)
- 5-mL Luer-Lok syringes
- 10-mL Luer-Lok syringes
- Vacuum system or blood transfer device (see agency policy)
- Blood tubes, including waste tubes; tube labels
- Needleless injection cap
- Syringe (5 mL or 10 mL; see agency policy) for discarded blood
- 10-mL syringe with 5 to 10 mL preservative-free 0.9% sodium chloride (normal saline [NS])
- 10-mL syringe with heparin flush solution
- Sterile cap to maintain sterility of distal end of IV tubing

Changing the Injection Cap

- Clean gloves
- Antiseptic swabs (CHG solution, or 70% isopropyl alcohol and povidone-iodine for chlorhexidine sensitivities)
- Needleless injection cap(s) and disinfection caps
- 10-mL syringe with 10 mL preservative-free 0.9% sodium chloride (NS)
- 10-mL syringe with heparin flush solution

Discontinuing a Nontunneled Central or Peripheral Catheter

- Personal protective equipment as indicated (goggles, gown, mask, and clean gloves)
- CVAD dressing change kit, which includes sterile gloves, mask, antiseptic swabs for skin disinfection, TSM dressing, 4 × 4-inch gauze pads, tape measure, sterile tape, label
- Petroleum-based ointment or petroleum-based gauze, sterile

- Suture removal kit (if sutures are in place)
- Stethoscope

STEP	RATIONALE
1 Perform preprocedure protocol.	

Assessment

• Review patient's electronic health record (EHR) for CVAD size and type, previous dressing changes, times for administration of IV solutions, medications, and blood sampling. Follow seven rights of medication administration.	Identifies patient's need for vascular access, evaluates response to therapy, and determines education needs.
• Review EHR to determine patient's age and history of dehydration, malnutrition, exposure to radiation therapy, underlying chronic conditions (e.g., diabetes mellitus, immunosuppression), and skin edema.	Common risk factors for medical adhesive—related skin injury (MARSI) (Fumarola et al., 2020)
• Confirm informed consent obtained properly.	Invasive procedure requires patient consent.
• Perform hand hygiene. Apply gloves. Assess patient's hydration status: skin turgor, mouth dryness, skin texture, and fluid intake and output.	Reduces transmission of microorganisms. Provides baseline to determine response to fluid therapy.
• Assess existing CVAD site for skin integrity (open lesions) and signs of infection (i.e., redness, pain, tenderness, swelling, bleeding, or drainage), phlebitis, and infiltration. Also assess skin temperature, color, moisture level, fragility, and overall integrity, including presence of irritation around potential IV site.	Compromised skin integrity contraindicates catheter insertion and can lead to secondary complications. Condition of skin creates risk for MARSI (Fumarola et al., 2020).

Continued

STEP	RATIONALE
• Ask patient to describe history of allergies: known type of allergies and normal allergic reaction. Compare information with health history. Focus on latex, iodine, lidocaine and chlorhexidine.	Allows prevention of exposure to allergic agent and anticipation of possible reactions.
• Review manufacturer directions concerning specific CVAD maintenance.	Care and management depend on type and size of catheter or port, number of lumens, and purpose of therapy.
• Assess for proper function of existing CVAD before therapy: catheter integrity, ability to flush or infuse solution, ability to aspirate blood. Remove and discard gloves. Perform hand hygiene.	Blood return should be obtained, and patency confirmed, before infusion of solutions or medications (INS, 2021).
• Assess whether any existing catheter lumens require flushing or CVAD site needs dressing change by referring to EHR, agency policies, and manufacturer-recommended guidelines for use.	Provides guidelines for maintaining catheter patency and preventing infection.

Implementation

1	Offer patient opportunity to void, and offer pain medication (if needed and ordered by provider).	Decreases anxiety, promotes cooperation, and prevents sudden movement during sterile procedures (may take several minutes).
2	Organize supplies and equipment on clean, clutter-free bedside stand or overbed table.	Reduces transmission of microorganisms and contamination of equipment (INS, 2021).

STEP	RATIONALE
3 Insertion site. care and dressing change	
a Position patient in comfortable position with head slightly elevated. Have arm extended for PICC in arm or midline device.	Provides access to patient.
b Prepare dressing materials.	TSM dressings have advantage of allowing visualization of IV site. Gauze dressings and TSM are associated with a lower rate of catheter tip infection (INS, 2021; Jacob, 2019).
(1) TSM dressing: change at least every 5–7 days.	
(2) Gauze dressing: change at least every 2 days.	
(3) Gauze under TSM: change at least every 2 days.	
c Perform hand hygiene and apply mask using ANTT. Have patient apply mask and turn head away from site during dressing change.	Reduces transfer of microorganisms; prevents spread of airborne microorganisms over CVAD insertion site.
d Apply clean gloves. Remove old TSM dressing following steps in Skill 18.	Prevents unintentional catheter removal.
e Remove catheter stabilization device if used and requires changing. Must use adhesive remover to remove adhesive stabilization devices.	Allows visualization of insertion site and allows for appropriate skin antisepsis (INS, 2021). Use of adhesive remover minimizes risk for MARSI (Fumarola et al., 2020).

CLINICAL JUDGMENT *If sutures are used for initial catheter stabilization and become loose or are no longer intact, use alternative stabilization measures. Using an engineered stabilization device is recommended because sutures are associated with increased risk of infection (INS, 2021).*

Continued

STEP	RATIONALE
f Inspect catheter, insertion site, and surrounding skin. Measure external CVAD length and compare with measurement from insertion if dislodgement is suspected. For PICC and midlines, measure upper-arm circumference 10 cm above antecubital fossa if clinically indicated and compare with baseline.	Insertion sites require regular inspection for early detection of signs and symptoms of IV-related complications and MARSI (INS, 2021; Fumarola et al., 2020). Measurement of external catheter length provides comparison to determine dislodgement; arm measurement with a 3-cm increase can indicate thrombosis (INS, 2021).
g Remove and discard clean gloves; perform hand hygiene. Open CVAD dressing kit using sterile technique and *apply sterile gloves* using sterile ANTT. Area to be cleaned should be same size as dressing.	Sterile technique is required to apply new dressing.
h Clean site:	Reduces incidence of catheter-related infections.
(1) Cleanse insertion site with CHG solution using friction in back-and-forth motion for 30 seconds and allow to dry completely.	Drying ensures complete antisepsis (INS, 2021).

STEP	RATIONALE
(2) Povidone-iodine and alcohol may be used if patient is sensitive to CHG (see agency policy). If using alcohol or povidone-iodine, clean in concentric circle, moving from insertion site outward with swab. Allow to dry completely.	
i Apply polymer-based skin protectant to insertion area. Allow to dry completely so that skin is not tacky. Skin protectant must be used if adhesive stabilization device will be used.	Protects irritated or fragile skin from dressing and stabilization device, if used, and minimizes risk for MARSI (Fumarola et al., 2020).
• *Option:* Use CHG-impregnated dressing for short-term CVADs.	Use with caution in premature neonates and patients with fragile skin and/or complicated skin pathologies (INS, 2021).
j Apply sterile TSM dressing over insertion site (see Skill 54).	Protects catheter insertion site and minimizes risk for infection (Gorski, 2023). Allows for clear visualization of catheter site between dressing changes (INS, 2021).

Continued

STEP	RATIONALE
k Apply new catheter stabilization device according to manufacturer directions for use if catheter is not sutured in place. Apply new injection caps to lumens of CVAD (see Step 6, below). Then apply disinfecting cap to end of injection caps of catheter.	Use of engineered stabilization devices that allow visual inspection of insertion site can reduce risk for VAD complications (INS, 2021). Injection caps provide non-Luer-Lok device for access to CVAD, Disinfecting caps reduces transmission of microorganisms.
l Apply label to dressing with date, time, and your initials.	Provides information about next dressing change.
m Have patient remove mask. Dispose of all contaminated supplies in appropriate receptacle, remove and dispose of gloves, and perform hand hygiene.	Reduces transmission of microorganisms. Use appropriate disposal receptacle if patient is on hazardous drugs (Oncology Nursing Society [ONS], 2018).
4 Blood sampling	
a Apply clean gloves and face mask.	Reduces transmission of microorganisms.
b Put the electronic infusion device on hold for at least 1 to 5 minutes before drawing blood. *Note:* If you cannot stop infusion, draw blood from peripheral vein.	Prevents dilution of sample. Use of peripheral vein prevents interruption of critical IV therapy.

STEP	RATIONALE
c Use the largest lumen for blood sampling from a multilumen CVAD (INS, 2021). When drawing through staggered multilumen catheters, draw from the lumen exiting at the point farthest away from the heart (or one recommended by manufacturer).	Distal lumen is typically largest-gauge lumen (Gorski, 2023).
d Clamp the CVAD lumen using the small slide clamp. *Exception:* valved catheter does not require clamping.	Prevents spillage. Valved catheters do not require clamping because clamp opens valve and allows reflux of blood into catheter.
e Syringe method	
(1) Remove disinfection cap from CVAD lumen. Scrub catheter injection cap hub with antiseptic swab for at least 15 seconds and allow to dry completely.	Reduces risk of infection. Drying ensures maximal antisepsis.
(2) Attach syringe containing 5 to 10mL of NS (see agency policy for volume) to end of hub. Unclamp CVAD (if necessary). Flush CVAD slowly with NS. Reclamp CVAD (if necessary).	Ensures patency of CVAD lumen. Clamping prevents spillage.

Continued

STEP	RATIONALE
(3) Clean catheter hub with antiseptic swab and allow to dry completely. Attach empty 5-mL syringe to hub and unclamp catheter (if necessary). To withdraw blood first aspirate gently, pulling back 1 to 2 mL. Pause and hold pressure to allow valve to open. Then continue pulling plunger slowly, staying just ahead of the blood flow until you obtain 2 to 25 mL of blood for discard sample depending on the internal volume of the CVAD (see agency policy) (Gorski, 2021).	Reduces transmission of microorganisms. A discard sample reduces risk of drug concentrations or diluted specimen (Gorski, 2018). Drawing specimens for international normalized ratio studies from heparinized lines is not recommended (INS, 2021).
(4) Reclamp catheter (if necessary); remove syringe with blood and discard in appropriate biohazard container.	Prevents spillage. Prevents transmission of microorganisms.
(5) Scrub catheter hub with another antiseptic swab for 15 seconds and allow to dry completely.	
(6) Attach syringe(s) to obtain required volume of blood needed for specimen(s) ordered.	Multiple syringes may be required, depending on specimens required and number of blood tubes needed.

STEP	RATIONALE

CLINICAL JUDGMENT *If multiple blood tests are ordered, anticipate timing so that accessing the CVAD is only necessary one time. Consult with laboratory about number of milliliters needed for any one sample (INS, 2021).*

- Unclamp catheter (if necessary) to withdraw blood. Obtain necessary blood volume for specimens.

  Minimum amount of blood is needed to perform any one blood test analysis.

- Once specimens are obtained, clamp catheter (if necessary) and remove syringe.

  Prevents spillage.

- Scrub catheter hub with antiseptic swab for 15 seconds and allow to dry completely.

- Attach prefilled syringe with 10 mL 0.9% sodium chloride (NS). Unclamp catheter (if necessary). Flush catheter using the appropriate flush/clamp/disconnect sequence based on the type of needleless connector (e.g., neutral, negative, or positive pressure displacement). Ensure that clamp is engaged (if available).

  Flush with minimum volume of twice the internal volume of catheter with 0.9% sodium chloride (NS) (INS, 2021). Refer to agency policy and procedure for flush volume requirements. Reduces risk for catheter clotting after procedure.

CLINICAL JUDGMENT *Always use a 10-mL syringe or syringe designed to generate lower injection pressure (i.e., 10-mL-diameter syringe barrel) on central lines in adults to minimize pressure during injection (INS, 2021).*

- Remove syringe and discard into appropriate biohazard container.

  Reduces transmission of microorganisms.

- Transfer blood from syringe into blood tubes using transfer vacuum device.

  Reduces risk of blood exposure.

Continued

STEP	RATIONALE
(13) *Option:* Flush catheter with heparin flush based on type of catheter and agency policy and procedure using appropriate flush/clamp/disconnect sequence. Ensure that clamp is engaged (if available).	Prevents clot formation. Heparin flush volume and concentration vary by agency and type of catheter. Valved catheters are flushed with 0.9% sodium chloride (NS) only and do not require heparin.
(14) Remove syringe. Scrub exposed hub with antiseptic swab for 15 seconds and allow to dry. Attach new injection cap (see Step 6, below) to accessed lumen. Apply disinfection cap to injection cap. Resume infusion as ordered.	Decreases risk of contamination.
(15) Dispose of all contaminated supplies in appropriate receptacle, remove and dispose of gloves and mask, and perform hand hygiene.	Reduces transmission of microorganisms. Use appropriate disposal receptacle if patient on hazardous drugs (ONS, 2018).

STEP	RATIONALE
5 Changing injection cap	Injection caps should be changed no more frequently than 96-h intervals.
	Primary administration set changed for continuous infusions if it is removed for any reason, if there is residual blood or debris in it, if it becomes contaminated, or according to agency policies and procedures (INS, 2021).
a Prepare new injection cap(s): determine type of device (e.g., positive, negative, or neutral displacement valves) (INS, 2021).	Ensures appropriate flush/clamp/disconnect sequence based on type of device (INS, 2021).
b Perform hand hygiene. Apply clean gloves and mask using ANTT. (*Option:* Have patient apply mask). Remove cap from package. Do not contaminate sterile injection port.	Reduces transfer of microorganisms. Maintains sterility.
c Keep protective cover on tip of injection cap.	Maintains sterility.
(1) Prime cap. Attach prefilled syringe to end of injection cap by pushing in and then turning clockwise. Prime injection cap by flushing with preservative-free 0.9% sodium chloride (NS) through cap until fluid escapes from tip of cap. Keep syringe attached to cap and keep connection sterile.	Removes air from system, preventing it from being introduced into vein.

Continued

STEP	RATIONALE
d Based on catheter type, clamp catheter lumen by using slide or squeeze clamp.	Prevents air from entering system when opened.
e Remove old injection cap by turning counterclockwise. Dispose of old injection cap using aseptic technique. Continue holding catheter lumen.	Reduces transmission of microorganisms.
f Scrub exposed catheter hub with antiseptic swab, twisting back and forth for 15 seconds, and allow to dry completely. Take the new injection cap and attached syringe, remove the protective cover from tip, and connect new injection cap(s) on catheter hub, turning clockwise just until you feel resistance. Remove and dispose of syringe. *Option:* Place disinfecting cap on end of injection cap.	Drying allows time for maximum antimicrobial activity of agents. Turning cap on too tightly makes it difficult to remove for subsequent cap change.
g Repeat procedure for additional CVAD lumens.	
h Dispose of all contaminated supplies in appropriate receptacle, remove and dispose of gloves and mask. Remove patient's mask (if worn) and perform hand hygiene.	Reduces transmission of microorganisms. Use appropriate disposal receptacle if patient is taking hazardous drugs (ONS, 2018).
i Perform postprocedure protocol.	

STEP	RATIONALE

6 Discontinuing nontunneled catheter

a Verify HCP's order to discontinue line. Check agency policy because most require HCPs to discontinue CVAD. In some settings advanced practice nurses or specially credentialed nurses can remove devices.

Verifies appropriateness of procedure. Only specially trained health care professional can remove CVAD.

b If IV solutions or medications are to continue, arrange placement of a short-peripheral or midline catheter before CVAD discontinuation. *Note:* Be aware of osmolarity of solution or medication for appropriateness of conversion to short-peripheral or midline catheter.

Prevents interruption of IV therapy.

c Position patient in supine flat or 10-degree Trendelenburg position unless contraindicated.

Position promotes venous filling and prevents air embolus during catheter removal.

d Perform hand hygiene using ANTT. Turn off IV solutions infusing through central line and convert to alternate VAD.

Prevents fluid loss during CVAD removal.

e Place moisture-proof pad under central line site. Apply gown, clean gloves, mask, and goggles.

Minimizes soil bed linen. Provides clean environment. Prevents transmission of microorganisms.

Continued

STEP	RATIONALE
f Gently remove CVAD dressing by stabilizing catheter with nondominant hand, pulling up one corner and gently pulling straight out and parallel to skin. Repeat on all sides until dressing has been removed.	Prevents skin tears. Allows inspection of CVAD insertion site before removal.
g If catheter securement device is present, carefully remove catheter from device and remove device with adhesive remover.	Aids in removal of securement device without causing skin tear (Fumarola et al., 2020).
h Remove gloves and perform hand hygiene; open CVAD dressing change kit and suture removal kit (if CVAD is sutured in place). Add items to sterile field. Apply sterile gloves.	Prevents transfer of organisms on soiled dressing to catheter insertion site.
i Cleanse insertion site with CHG solution using friction in back-and-forth motion for 30 seconds and allow to dry completely. *Option:* If CVAD is sutured in place, remove sutures.	Reduces risk of migration of microbes into catheter tract.

CLINICAL JUDGMENT *All CVADs require measurements of total length and external catheter on insertion. PICC lines also require measurement of upper-arm circumference.*

STEP	RATIONALE
j Using nondominant hand, apply sterile 4 × 4-inch gauze to site. Instruct patient to take a deep breath and bear down to perform Valsalva maneuver as catheter is withdrawn.	Valsalva maneuver reduces risk for air embolus by decreasing negative pressure in respiratory system.
k With dominant hand slowly remove catheter in smooth, continuous motion an inch at a time. Keeping fingers near insertion site, immediately apply digital pressure to site and continue until bleeding stops. Stop removal procedure if you meet any resistance while removing catheter (INS, 2016).	Gentle removal of catheter prevents stretching and breaking it. Damaged catheter may break off and leave piece in patient's arm. Direct pressure reduces risk for bleeding and hematoma formation.

CLINICAL JUDGMENT *It is often necessary to apply pressure longer if patient is receiving anticoagulation therapy or has prolonged clotting times.*

l When bleeding at site has stopped, apply sterile occlusive dressing, such as TSM dressing or sterile gauze to site. Change dressing every 24 h until healed.	Reduces chance of air embolism and seals skin-to-vein tract (Gorski, 2018). TSM dressing allows for inspection of site for bleeding and infection until it is healed.
m Label dressing with date, time, and your initials.	Identifies date of catheter removal and need for dressing change.

Continued

STEP	RATIONALE
n Inspect catheter integrity for intactness, especially along tip, and that length is appropriate for device. Discard in appropriate biohazard container. *Note:* Perform a catheter culture if patient suspected of having a catheter-related bloodstream infection. Catheter cultures should not be obtained routinely (INS, 2021).	If catheter tip is broken or compromised, place in container, label for possible follow-up, and notify HCP.
o Position patient in a supine position for 30 minutes after nontunneled CVAD removal (INS, 2021). Be sure that short-peripheral IV line or midline is infusing at correct rate.	Reduces chance of air embolism. Maintains prescribed IV solution therapy.
p Once stable, explain how patient can move or position and not pull on CVAD catheter or infusion line.	Prevents catheter dislodgement.
q Perform postprocedure protocol.	
7 Evaluate patient response:	
a Determine daily, in consultation with HCP, the continued need for the CVAD.	Daily review of need for line is a necessity. Prompt removal of unnecessary lines is practice recommended in the IHI central line–associated bloodstream infection prevention bundle (Gupta et al., 2021).

STEP	RATIONALE
b Evaluate for postinsertion complications (Table 11.2)	Complications after insertion can include pneumothorax, cardiac arrhythmias, and nerve injury (Gorski, 2018). Prompt identification can allow for treatment, repositioning of catheter, or removal if necessary.
(1) Pneumothorax: Auscultate breath sounds and evaluate for shortness of breath, chest pain, absent breath sounds.	Usually develops early during insertion if CVAD pierces intrathoracic space.
(2) Dysrhythmia: Monitor vital signs, including heart rate and rhythm.	Position of catheter tip may irritate myocardium.
(3) Nerve injury: Monitor patient for arm pain, numbness, tingling, or weakness.	Signs of nerve injury from catheter insertion.
c Evaluate laboratory values, input and output, patient weight, vital signs, and other postprocedural assessments.	IV solutions and additives maintain or restore fluid and electrolyte balance. Early recognition of complications leads to prompt treatment.
d Evaluate patient at established intervals for signs and symptoms of ongoing CVAD-related complications (see Table 11.2).	Prevents complications that compromise integrity of CVAD or that cause inaccurate IV solution flow rate, and allows for prompt intervention.
e Observe all connection points, ensuring that they are secure as directed by agency policy and procedure.	An intact system prevents accidental blood loss or entrance of air or microbes into the vasculature.

Recording and Reporting

- Record catheter type and site care, including catheter location; catheter size; number of lumens; condition of catheter insertion site and surrounding skin, external catheter length, mid-arm circumference for PICC; condition and type of securement device; date and time of dressing change; change of injection caps; catheter patency, including presence or absence of blood return or resistance; and patient's tolerance of the procedure.
- Record solution, volume, and concentration for catheter flushes.
- Record catheter removal: patient position, appearance of site, length of catheter removed, integrity of catheter after removal, integrity of skin around site, dressing applied, patient's tolerance of procedure, presence/absence of bleeding from site, and any problems with removal.
- Record blood draw: date, time, sample drawn, waste volume, and flushes used.
- Record unexpected outcomes and CVAD complications, interventions, and patient response to treatment.
- Record patient's and family caregiver's ability to explain instructions.
- Report to oncoming nursing staff signs or symptoms of observed or patient-reported IV-related complications, status of VAD and dressing, and patient condition.
- Report to HCP any CVAD-related complications, interventions, and response to treatment.

UNEXPECTED OUTCOMES	RELATED INTERVENTIONS
1 For catheter complications, see Table 11.2.	
2 Patient develops MARSI from securement device adhesive or tape.	Clean affected area, keep dry, but apply moisturizer. Use skin barrier if catheter remains in place and new securement device needed. Refer to wound care specialist for any tears or abrasions present.
3 Patient or family caregiver is unable to explain or perform CVAD care.	Indicates need for home care referral or additional instruction.

Chest Tube Insertion and Management

The purpose of a closed chest drainage system, with or without suction, is to promote air and/or fluid drainage from the pleural space. Lung reexpansion occurs after chest tube insertion as the fluid and/or air is removed, and the patient's oxygenation improves (Ritchie et al., 2017). When air enters the pleural space, a pneumothorax occurs. When blood enters the pleural space, a hemothorax occurs. Pleural effusions occur when fluid enters the pleural space in response to infection, inflammation, or cancer.

The location of the chest tube indicates the type of drainage expected (Fig. 12.1). Because air rises, chest tubes placed for removal of air are placed high, allowing air evacuation from the intrapleural space and lung reexpansion. Apical (second or third intercostal space) and anterior chest tube placement promotes air removal . The air is discharged into the atmosphere, and there is little or no drainage expected in the collection chamber.

Chest tubes for fluid removal are placed low (usually in the fifth or sixth intercostal space) and posterior or lateral. Fluid in the intrapleural space is affected by gravity and localizes in the lower part of the lung cavity. Tubes placed in these positions drain blood and fluid. A mediastinal chest tube is placed in the mediastinum, just below the sternum, and is connected to a drainage system. This tube drains blood or fluid, preventing its accumulation around the heart.

Safety Guidelines

- Infections occur rarely with chest tubes, but when they do, they can range from skin infections at the insertion site to empyema and even necrotizing infections (Pranit, 2020). Use sterile asepsis in management.
- Clogging of the chest tube can occur when small chest tubes are used and become blocked by blood clots and fibrin. Large-bore catheters (such as 28 Fr) safely remove any fluid or drainage (Waters, 2017).
- Milking or stripping chest tubes demonstrates no safety or efficacy benefits; it slightly increases intrathoracic pressure and risks tissue damage (Sasa, 2019).
- Constant bubbling in the water seal or a sudden, unexpected stoppage of water-seal activity is considered abnormal and requires immediate attention (Sasa, 2019; Waters, 2017).

115

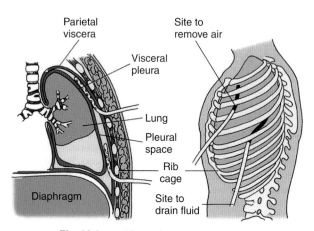

Fig. 12.1 Possible sites for chest tube placement.

- After 2 or 3 days, tidaling or bubbling on expiration is expected to stop, indicating that the lung has reexpanded and that the chest tube can be removed (Pickett, 2017; Sasa, 2019).
- Unexpected stoppage of chest tube activity may indicate a blockage. In these situations, immediate attention and correction are indicated.
- Notify a health care provider when there is a sudden increase of more than 100 mL of drainage over 1 h, or the drainage equals the volume indicated by health care provider order. This can indicate that fresh bleeding is occurring (Pickett, 2017; Sasa, 2019).

Delegation

The skill of chest tube management cannot be delegated to assistive personnel (AP). Instruct the AP about:

- Proper positioning of the patient with chest tubes to facilitate chest tube drainage and functioning of the system.
- Ambulating and transferring patient safely with a chest drainage system in place.
- Immediately reporting changes in vital signs, complaints of chest pain or sudden shortness of breath, or excessive bubbling in water-seal chamber.
- Danger of any disconnection of the drainage system, change in type and amount of drainage, sudden bleeding, or sudden cessation of bubbling.

Collaboration

- Advanced practice nurses and other health care providers are resources for chest tube management.

Equipment

- Prescribed chest drainage system: wet suction water seal or dry suction water seal. Disposable systems are available.
- Water-seal system or waterless (dry) suction system: sterile water or normal saline (NS) per manufacturer's directions
- Suction source and setup
- Sterile skin preparation solution (chlorhexidine solution preferred)
- Clean gloves
- Sterile gauze sponges
- Local anesthetic, if not an emergent procedure
- Chest tube tray (all items are sterile): knife handle (1), knife blade No. 10 or disposable safety scalpel No. 10, chest tube clamp, small sponge forceps, needle holder, size 3-0 silk sutures, tray liner (sterile field), curved 8-inch Kelly clamps (2), 4 × 4-inch sponges (10), suture scissors, hand towels (3), sterile gloves
- 1-inch adhesive tape for tubing.
- Dressings: petroleum or Xeroform gauze, split chest-tube dressings, several 4 × 4-inch gauze dressings, large gauze dressings (2), plastic tape for short-term wear (consider paper/cloth tape for long-time wear [Fumarola et al., 2020]) *Option:* Use skin barrier for area where dressing tape is to be applied to reduce risk of medical adhesive—related skin injury (MARSI) (Fumarola et al., 2020)
- Personal protective equipment: head cover, face mask/face shield, sterile gloves
- Two rubber-tipped hemostats for each chest tube
- 2.5-cm (1-inch) waterproof adhesive tape or plastic zip ties for securing connections
- Stethoscope, sphygmomanometer, and pulse oximeter

STEP	RATIONALE
1 Perform preprocedure protocol.	

Assessment

• Review patient's electronic health record (EHR) for significant medical history or injury, including chronic lung disease, spontaneous pneumothorax, pulmonary disease, therapeutic procedures, and mechanism of injury (Pickett, 2017).	Data may provide the reason for the occurrence of the pneumothorax, hemothorax, empyema, and/or pleural effusion.

Continued

STEP	RATIONALE
• Perform hand hygiene. Apply clean gloves.	Reduces transmission of microorganisms.
• Perform a complete respiratory assessment, baseline vital signs, and pulse oximetry (SpO$_2$). Note the following:	Baseline assessment and vital signs are essential for any invasive procedure. Chest tube insertion often causes respiratory distress.
a Decreased breath sounds over affected and unaffected lungs, marked cyanosis, asymmetrical chest movements, displaced trachea, shortness of breath, and confusion.	Signs and symptoms associated with respiratory distress from collapse of lung. Signs of hypoxia are related to inadequate oxygen to tissues.
b Sharp, stabbing chest pain or chest pain on inspiration, hypotension, and tachycardia. If possible, ask patient to rate level of pain on a scale of 0 to 10.	Sharp stabbing chest pain with or without decreased blood pressure and increased heart rate may indicate tension pneumothorax. Presence of pneumothorax or hemothorax is painful, frequently causing sharp inspiratory pain. When chest tube is present, discomfort is common. As a result, patients tend to not cough or change position in an effort to minimize this pain.
• Ask patient to describe history of allergies: known type of allergies and normal allergic reaction. Compare information with health history. Focus on latex, adhesive or any skin preparations.	Allows prevention of exposure to allergic agent and anticipation of possible reactions.

STEP	RATIONALE
• Review EHR to to determine patient's risk for developing MARSI using adhesive tape: age, dehydration, malnutrition, exposure to radiation therapy, underlying chronic conditions (e.g., diabetes, immunosuppression), and skin edema.	Common risk factors for MARSI (Fumarola et al, 2020)
• Review medication record for anticoagulant therapy, including aspirin, warfarin, heparin, or platelet aggregation inhibitors such as ticlopidine or dipyridamole.	Anticoagulation therapy can increase procedure-related blood loss.
• Review laboratory values for hemoglobin and hematocrit levels.	Parameters reflect whether blood loss is occurring, which may affect oxygenation.

Implementation

STEP	RATIONALE
1 Administer prescribed analgesics or sedatives as needed 30 minutes before insertion.	Reduces discomfort and anxiety experienced before insertion, facilitating patient cooperation and improving outcomes (Huggins et al., 2020).
2 Explain chest tube system and the patient's role. If applicable, teach patient how to move with chest tube in place.	Reduces anxiety and promotes cooperation. Self-care supports patient's sense of autonomy.
3 Check agency policy: Is informed consent needed? Complete time-out procedure (The Joint Commission, 2021b).	Invasive medical procedures typically require informed consent. Time-out is completed to determine right patient, procedure, and location of insertion or incision site (Pickett, 2017).
4 Review health care 'provider's order for chest tube placement.	Insertion of chest tube requires health care provider order.

Continued

STEP	RATIONALE
5 Perform hand hygiene. Apply clean gloves.	Reduces transmission of microorganisms.
6 Set up water-seal or dry system with suction; see manufacturer guidelines (Fig. 12.2).	The water-seal system contains two or three compartments or chambers. Fluid drains into the first chamber. The second chamber contains the water seal, which allows air to escape because of the force of expiration but not to reenter on inspiration. If suction is needed, a third chamber is used.

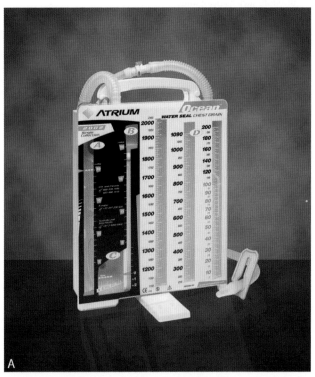

Fig. 12.2 (A) Disposable water-seal chest drainage system with suction.

(Continued)

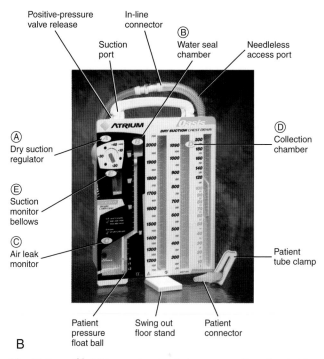

B

Fig. 12.2, cont'd (B) Dry suction chest drainage system. (Reproduced with permission from Atrium Medical Corp., Merrimack, NH.)

STEP	RATIONALE
a Remove wrappers.	Maintains sterility of system for use under sterile operating room conditions.
b While maintaining sterility of drainage tubing, stand system upright and add sterile water or NS to appropriate compartments.	Reduces possibility of contamination.

Continued

STEP	RATIONALE
(1) *Two-chamber water-seal system (without suction):* Add sterile solution to water-seal chamber (second chamber), bringing fluid to required level as indicated or ordered by health care provider.	Water-seal chamber acts as one-way valve so air cannot enter pleural space (Sasa, 2019).
(2) Three-chamber water-seal system (with suction): Add sterile solution to water-seal chamber (second chamber). Add amount of sterile solution prescribed by health care provider to suction-control chamber (third chamber), usually 20 cm H_2O pressure. Connect tubing from suction-control chamber to suction source.	Depth of fluid level dictates highest amount of negative pressure that can be present within system. For example, 20 cm of water is approximately 20 cm of water pressure. After chest tube is inserted, turn up the wall or portable suction source until water in suction-control bottle exhibits continuous, gentle bubbling.

Note: Suction-control chamber vent must not be occluded when suction is used.

CLINICAL JUDGMENT *When increasing suction, remember that increased bubbling does not result in more suction to the chest cavity, but serves only to evaporate the water more quickly.*

STEP	RATIONALE
(3) Dry suction system: Fill water-seal chamber with sterile solution. Adjust suction-control dial to prescribed level of suction; suction ranges from −10 to −40 cm of water pressure. Suction-control chamber vent is never occluded when suction is used. *Note:* On dry suction system, *DO NOT* obstruct positive pressure relief valve. This allows air to escape.	Automatic control valve on dry suction-control device adjusts to changes in patient air leaks and fluctuation in suction source and vacuum to deliver prescribed amount of suction.
7 Secure all tubing connections with adhesive tape in double-spiral fashion using 2.5-cm (1-inch) adhesive tape or zip ties (Parham-Martin bands) with a clamp (Pickett, 2017). Check system for patency by: a Clamping drainage tubing that will connect to patient's chest tube. b Connecting tubing from float ball chamber to suction source. c Turning on suction to prescribed level.	Prevents atmospheric air from leaking into system and patient's intrapleural space. Provides chance to ensure airtight system before connection to patient.

Continued

STEP	RATIONALE
8 Turn off suction source and unclamp drainage tubing before connecting patient to system. Suction source is turned on again after patient is connected.	Having patient connected to suction when it is initiated could damage pleural tissues from sudden increase in negative pressure. Tubing that is coiled or looped may become clotted and cause tension pneumothorax (Pickett, 2017).

CLINICAL JUDGMENT *During procedure, carefully monitor patient for changes in level of sedation.*

9 Provide psychological support to patient (Kirkwood, 2017). Reinforce preprocedure teaching, and coach and support patient throughout procedure.	Reduces patient anxiety and helps complete procedure efficiently.
10 Position patient for tube insertion so that side in which tube is to be inserted is accessible to health care provider.	For pneumothorax, place patient in lateral supine position. For hemothorax, place patient in semi-Fowler position.
11 Assist health care provider with chest tube insertion by providing needed equipment and local analgesic. Health care provider anesthetizes skin over insertion site, makes small skin incision, inserts clamped tube, sutures it in place, and applies occlusive dressing (using appropriate tape).	Ensures smooth insertion.

CLINICAL JUDGMENT *If patient is known to be sensitive to adhesive or at risk for sensitivity do not use adhesive tape to secure dressing.*

STEP	RATIONALE
12 Help health care provider attach drainage tube to chest tube; remove clamp. Turn on suction to prescribed level.	Connects drainage system and suction (if ordered) to chest tube.
13 Tape or zip-tie all connections between chest tube and drainage tube. (*Note:* Chest tube is usually taped by health care provider at time of tube placement; check agency policy.)	Secures chest tube to drainage system and reduces risk for air leakage that causes breaks in airtight system (Chotai, 2022).
14 Check systems for proper functioning. Health care provider will order chest x-ray film.	Verifies intrapleural placement of tube.
15 After tube placement, position patient: a Use semi-Fowler or high Fowler position to evacuate air (pneumothorax) (Chotai, 2022). b Use high Fowler position to drain fluid (hemothorax) (Chotai, 2022).	Permits optimum drainage of fluid and/or air.
16 Check patency of air vents in system. a Water-seal vent must have no occlusion.	Permits displaced air to pass into atmosphere.
b Suction-control chamber vent is not occluded when suction is used.	Provides safety factor of releasing excess negative pressure into atmosphere.
c Waterless systems have relief valves without caps.	Provides safety factor of releasing excess negative pressure.

Continued

STEP	RATIONALE
17 Position excess tubing horizontally on mattress next to patient. Secure with clamp provided so it does not obstruct tubing.	Prevents excess tubing from hanging over edge of mattress in dependent loop. Drainage collected in loop can occlude drainage system, which predisposes patient to tension pneumothorax (Pickett, 2017).
18 Adjust tubing to hang in straight line from chest tube to drainage chamber.	Promotes drainage and prevents fluid or blood from accumulating in pleural cavity.

CLINICAL JUDGMENT *Frequent gentle lifting of the chest tube drain allows gravity to help blood and other viscous material to move to the drainage bottle. Patients with recent chest surgery or trauma need to have the chest drain lifted based on assessment of the amount of drainage; some patients might need chest tube drains lifted every 5 to 10 minutes until drainage volume decreases. However, when coiled or dependent looping of tubing is unavoidable, lift the tubing every 15 minutes at a minimum to promote drainage (Pickett, 2017).*

19 Place two rubber-tipped hemostats (for each chest tube) in easily accessible position (e.g., taped to top of patient's headboard). These should remain with patient when ambulating.	Chest tubes are double-clamped under specific circumstances: (1) to assess for air leak (Table 12.1), (2) to empty or quickly change disposable systems, or (3) to assess whether patient is ready to have tube removed.

CLINICAL JUDGMENT *In the event of a chest tube disconnection and risk of contamination, submerge the tube 2 to 4 cm (1 to 2 inches) below the surface of a 250-mL bottle of sterile water or NS until a new chest tube unit can be set up (Harding et al., 2021).*

20 Dispose of all contaminated supplies in appropriate receptacle.	Reduces transmission of microorganisms
21 Perform postprocedure protocol.	

TABLE 12.1 Solving Problems Related to Chest Tubes

Assessment	Intervention
Air leak can occur at insertion site, at connection between tube and drainage device, or within drainage device itself. Determine when air leak occurs during respiratory cycle (e.g., inspiration or expiration). Continuous bubbling is noted in water-seal chamber that is attached to suction (Pickett, 2017).	Check all connections between chest tube and drainage system to make sure they are tight. When in doubt, remove tape without disconnecting the tube to inspect connections.
	Inspect the chest drainage unit for cracks or breaks that can allow air into the system.
	Leaks are corrected when constant bubbling stops.
	If present on a chest drainage system such as the Sahara S 1100a Pleur-Evac, observe the air-leak meter to determine the size of the leak.
Assess for location of leak by squeezing the chest drainage tubing between your hands. If the bubbling stops, air leak is inside patient's thorax or at chest insertion site.	Release the pressure on the drainage tube, reinforce chest dressing, and notify health care provider immediately. Leaving chest tube clamped can cause lung collapse, mediastinal shift, and eventual collapse of other lung from buildup of air pressure within the pleural cavity.
If bubbling continues, it indicates that leak is in the drainage system.	Change the drainage system.
Assess for tension pneumothorax: • Severe respiratory distress • Low oxygen saturation • Chest pain • Absence of breath sounds on affected side • Tracheal shift to unaffected side • Hypotension and signs of shock • Tachycardia	Make sure that chest tubes are patent: remove clamps, eliminate kinks, or eliminate occlusion.
	Notify health care provider immediately and prepare for another chest tube insertion.
	A one-way flutter (Heimlich) valve or large-gauge needle may be used for short-term emergency release of pressure in the intrapleural space.
	Have emergency equipment, oxygen, and code cart available because this condition is life-threatening.
Water-seal tube is no longer submerged in sterile fluid because of evaporation.	Add sterile water to water-seal chamber until distal tip is 2 cm under surface level. Most chest drainage units are marked at the 2-cm level to indicate the fill line.

STEP	RATIONALE
22 Care of patient after chest tube insertion:	
a Perform hand hygiene and apply clean gloves. Assess vital signs, oxygen saturation; pain; skin color; breath sounds; rate, depth, and ease of respirations; and insertion site every 15 minutes for first 2 h, and then at least every shift (see agency policy).	Provides immediate information about procedure-related complications such as respiratory distress and leakage. For severe pain, medicate with ordered analgesics and use complementary pain relief methods as needed (e.g., repositioning).
b Monitor color, consistency, and amount of chest tube drainage every 15 minutes for first 2 h. Indicate level of drainage fluid, date, and time on write-on surface of chamber.	Provides baseline for continuous assessment of type and quantity of drainage. Ensures early detection of complications.
(1) From mediastinal tube, expect less than 100 mL/h immediately after surgery and no more than 500 mL in first 24 h.	Sudden gush of drainage may result from coughing or changing patient's position (i.e., releasing pooled/collected blood rather than indicating active bleeding).
(2) From posterior chest tube, drainage is more blood-tinged during first several hours after surgery and changes to more serous consistency (Harding et al., 2021).	Acute bleeding indicates hemorrhage. Health care provider should be notified if there is more than 200 mL of bloody drainage in an hour (Harding et al., 2021; Pickett, 2017).

STEP	RATIONALE
(3) Expect little or no output from anterior chest tube that is inserted for a pneumothorax (Pickett, 2017).	
c Observe chest dressing for drainage. Inspect condition of skin around dressing.	Drainage around tube may indicate blockage. Inflammation or swelling of skin can indicate MARSI.
d Palpate around tube for swelling and crepitus (subcutaneous emphysema), as noted by crackling.	Indicates presence of air trapping in subcutaneous tissues. Most occurrences of crepitus are minor because small amounts are commonly absorbed. Large amounts are potentially dangerous, and the health care provider should be notified (Pickett, 2017; Sasa, 2019).

CLINICAL JUDGMENT *Some patients may develop subcutaneous emphysema (i.e., a collection of air under the skin after chest tube placement), which can occur if tubing is blocked or kinked. When this occurs, a crepitus (a crackling sensation) is felt on palpation of the skin where subcutaneous emphysema has occurred or spread.*

STEP	RATIONALE
e Check tubing to ensure that it is free of kinks and dependent loops.	Promotes drainage.
f Observe for fluctuation of drainage in tubing and water-seal chamber during inspiration and expiration. Observe for clots or debris in tubing.	If fluctuation or tidaling stops, it means that either the lung is fully expanded or system is obstructed (Pickett, 2017). In spontaneously breathing patient, fluid rises in water seal or diagnostic indicator (waterless system) with inspiration and falls with expiration. The opposite occurs in patient who is mechanically ventilated. This indicates that system is functioning properly.

Continued

STEP	RATIONALE
g Keep drainage system upright and below level of patient's chest.	Promotes gravity drainage and prevents backflow of fluid and air into pleural space.
h Check for air leaks by monitoring bubbling in water-seal chamber: Intermittent bubbling is normal during expiration when air is being evacuated from pleural cavity, but continuous bubbling during both inspiration and expiration indicates leak in system.	Absence of bubbling may indicate that lung is fully expanded in patient with pneumothorax. Check all connections and locate sources of air leak.
23 Instruct patient on how to regularly take deep breaths and to reposition as often as possible.	Maintains lung expansion.
24 Perform postprocedure protocol.	
25 Evaluate patient response:	
a Evaluate for decreased respiratory distress and chest pain. Auscultate patient's lungs and observe chest expansion.	Determines status of lung expansion.
b Monitor vital signs and SpO_2.	Determines whether level of oxygenation has improved.
c Reassess character of patient's pain and measure severity on scale of 0 to 10, comparing level with comfort before chest tube insertion.	Indicates need for analgesia. Patient with chest tube discomfort hesitates to take deep breaths and as a result is at risk for pneumonia and atelectasis.
d Evaluate patient's ability to use deep-breathing exercises while maintaining comfort.	Indicates patient's ability to promote lung expansion and prevent complications.

STEP	RATIONALE
e Monitor functioning of chest tube system (e.g., reduction in amount of drainage, resolution of air leak, and complete reexpansion of the lung).	Detects early signs of system complications or indicates possible need for chest tube removal.

Recording and Reporting

- Record respiratory assessment findings before and after insertion, type of chest tube system, amount of suction if used, amount of drainage in chamber, presence of bubbling, and presence or absence of an air leak.
- Record the integrity of the dressing and skin around tape for color, tenderness, presence of drainage.
- Record patient's tolerance of chest tube placement, comfort level, response to any analgesia and baseline vital signs, including oxygen saturation after tube insertion.
- Record patient teaching and validation of patient understanding.
- Report the quantity and quality of the chest tube drainage every shift.

UNEXPECTED OUTCOMES	RELATED INTERVENTIONS
1 Patient develops respiratory distress. Chest pain, decrease in breath sounds over affected and unaffected lungs, marked cyanosis, asymmetrical chest movements, presence of subcutaneous emphysema around tube insertion site or neck, hypotension, tachycardia, and/or mediastinal shift is critical and indicates severe change in patient status such as excessive blood loss or tension pneumothorax.	• Notify health care provider immediately. • Collect set of vital signs and SpO_2. • Prepare for chest x-ray examination. • Provide oxygen as ordered.

Continued

UNEXPECTED OUTCOMES	RELATED INTERVENTIONS
2 There is no chest tube drainage.	• Observe for kink in chest drainage system.
	• Observe for possible clot in chest drainage system.
	• Observe for mediastinal shift or respiratory distress (medical emergency).
	• Notify health care provider.
3 Chest tube is dislodged.	• Immediately apply pressure over chest tube insertion site.
	• Have assistant obtain sterile petroleum gauze dressing. Apply as patient exhales. Secure dressing with tight seal. Dressing with tape over three of four sides may allow air to escape if there is residual pneumothorax.
	• Notify health care provider.
4 Drainage system falls and becomes damaged.	• Immediately disconnect the tubing from the drainage system.
	• Insert the tubing below the surface of a bottle of sterile water and obtain a new system (Harding et al., 2021).
	• Notify the health care provider.

Cold Applications

Cold therapy is the superficial application of cold to the surface of the skin, with or without compression and with or without a mechanical recirculating device to maintain cold temperatures (Chou et al., 2016). It is designed to treat the localized inflammatory response of an injured body part that presents as edema, hemorrhage, muscle spasm, or pain. Cold therapy improves joint mobility by reducing pain, swelling, muscle spasm, enzymatic activity, tissue metabolism (Wang and Ni, 2021). and muscle tension and decreasing tissue metabolism, and reducing enzymatic activity (see Table 16.3) (Wang and Ni, 2021). Cold therapy is most commonly used immediately after soft tissue and musculoskeletal injuries such as sprains or strains; however, it has been used in the postoperative setting with patients who have undergone orthopedic surgeries, spinal fusion, and lumbar discectomy (Quinlan et al., 2017). Cold therapy should be used judiciously and only for the short term. Any cold therapy that reduces inflammation also delays healing since the process of inflammation is an essential aspect of recovery itself (Wang and Ni, 2021).

Safety Guidelines

- Assess a patient's risks for injury from a cold application.
- Older adults are more at risk for tissue damage because of altered responses to change in body temperature; therefore, they need frequent skin assessment during treatment (Touhy and Jett, 2020).
- Any patient with cognitive impairment should not be allowed to apply cold therapy independently.

Delegation

The skill of applying cold applications can be delegated to assistive personnel (AP) (see agency policy). The nurse assesses and evaluates the patient and explains the purpose of the treatment. If there are risks or possible complications, this skill is not delegated. Instruct the AP to:

- Keep the application in place for only the length of time specified in the health care provider's order.
- Immediately report any excessive redness of the skin, increase in pain, or decrease in sensation.
- Report when treatment is complete so that a nurse can evaluate the patient's response.

Collaboration

- Physical therapists often use cold therapy as a form of treatment.

Equipment

All Compresses, Bags, and Packs

- Clean gloves (if blood or body fluids are present)
- Cloth tape, ties, or elastic wrap bandage
- Soft cloth cover: towel, pillowcase, or stockinette
- Bath towel or blanket and waterproof absorbent pad

Cold Compress

- Absorbent gauze (clean or sterile) folded to desired size
- Basin
- Prescribed solution at desired temperature

Ice Bag or Gel Pack

- Ice bag
- Ice chips and water, or:
- Reusable commercial gel pack (cold pack)
- Disposable commercial chemical cold pack

Electronically Controlled Cooling Device

- Cool-water flow pad or cooling pad and electrical pump
- Gauze roll or elastic wrap

STEP	RATIONALE
1 Perform preprocedure protocol.	
Assessment	
• Refer to health care provider's order for type, location, and duration of application. Temperature of a cooling pad will be ordered or preset.	Order is required for all cold applications.
• Consider time elapsed since injury occurred. Follow these principles: Protect injured area, Rest (Reduce activity until cold can be applied), Ice injury in a timely manner, Compress (mild compression reduces edema), Elevate (Raise affected extremity to promote venous return)	Apply cold therapy as soon as possible after injury to reduce swelling, inflammation, tissue bleeding, and pain (Chatterjee, 2017; Quinlan et al., 2017).

STEP	RATIONALE
• Review medical history for peripheral vascular diseases (e.g., Raynaud disease, Buerger disease), diabetic neuropathy, rheumatoid arthritis, frostbite.	These conditions contraindicate use of cold therapy because they increase the risk for skin and tissue injury when exposed to cold.
• Perform hand hygiene and inspect condition of injured or affected part. Gently palpate area for edema (apply clean gloves if there is risk of exposure to body fluids).	Provides baseline for determining change in condition of injured tissues. Reduces transmission of microorganisms.
• Perform neurovascular check and inspect surrounding skin for integrity, circulation (presence of pulses), color, temperature, and sensitivity to touch. Remove and dispose of gloves. Perform hand hygiene.	Determines whether patient is insensitive to cold extremes, which increases risk for injury. Reduces transmission of microorganisms.

CLINICAL JUDGMENT *Keep injured part in alignment and immobilized. Movement can cause further injury to strains, sprains, or fractures.*

• Assess patient's level of consciousness and responsiveness.	Patients with reduced level of consciousness are unable to sense or report reduced sensation or discomfort.
• Ask patient to describe character of pain and rate severity on scale of 0 to 10 (or other pain scale when applicable). Assess range of motion (ROM) of affected extremity.	Provides baseline for determining pain relief and ROM with therapy.

Continued

STEP	RATIONALE

Implementation

1 Position patient in bed, keeping affected body part in proper alignment.

Limited mobility in uncomfortable position causes muscular stress.

2 Explain precautions regarding use of cold.

Improves likelihood of patient's adherence to using cold therapy correctly at home.

3 Perform hand hygiene and apply clean gloves.

Reduces transmission of microorganisms.

4 Place towel or absorbent pad under area to be treated.

Prevents soiling of bed linen.

5 Apply cold compress:

  a Place ice and water in basin and test temperature on inner aspect of your arm. Submerge gauze into basin filled with cold solution; wring out excess moisture.

Extreme temperature causes tissue damage. Dripping gauze is uncomfortable to patient.

  b Apply compress to affected area, molding it gently over site.

Ensures that cold is directed over site of injury.

  c Remove, remoisten, and reapply to maintain temperature as needed.

6 Apply ice pack or bag:

  a Fill bag with water, secure cap, and invert.

Ensures that there are no leaks.

  b Empty water and fill bag two-thirds full with small ice chips and water.

Bag is easier to mold over body part when it is not full.

  c Express excess air from bag, secure bag closure, and wipe bag dry.

Excess air interferes with cold conduction. Allows bag to conform to area and promotes maximum contact.

STEP	RATIONALE
d Squeeze or knead commercial ice pack according to manufacturer's directions.	Releases alcohol-based solution to create cold temperature.
e Wrap pack or bag with single layer of towel, pillowcase, or stockinette. Apply over injury. Secure with tape as needed. Always place a barrier (e.g., towel, pillowcase, ice pack covering) between cooling device and the patient's skin to avoid tissue injury.	Protects patient's tissue and absorbs condensation. Prevents direct exposure of cold against patient's skin.
7 Apply commercial gel pack:	
a Remove pack from freezer.	
b Wrap pack with towel, pillowcase, or stockinette. Apply pack directly over injury (Fig. 13.1).	Protects patient's tissue and absorbs condensation. Prevents direct exposure of cold against patient's skin.
c Secure with gauze, cloth tape, or ties as needed.	

CLINICAL JUDGMENT Do not reapply ice pack to red or bluish areas; continual use of ice pack makes ischemia worse.

Continued

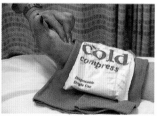

Fig. 13.1 Commercial ice pack.

STEP	RATIONALE
8 Apply electronically controlled cooling device:	
a Prepare device following manufacturer's directions. Some devices are gravity fed and require you to manually fill with ice water. Motorized units circulate chilled water.	
b Make sure that all connections are intact and temperature, if adjustable, is set (see agency policy).	Ensures safe temperature application.
c Wrap cool-water flow pad in single layer of towel or pillowcase.	Prevents adverse reactions from cold such as burn or frostbite.
d Wrap cool pad around body part.	Ensures even application of cold temperature.
e Turn device on and check correct temperature. (*Note:* Temperature is usually preset in health care settings [check agency policy].)	Ensures effective therapy. Preset temperature reduces risk of skin and tissue injury.
f Secure with elastic wrap bandage, gauze roll, or ties.	Ensures cold is distributed to correct body part.
9 Check condition of skin every 5 minutes for duration of application.	Reveals any adverse reactions to cold (e.g., mottling, redness, burning, blistering, numbness).
a If area is edematous, sensation may be reduced; use extra caution during cold therapy and assess site more often.	Prevents injury to skin and tissues.

STEP	RATIONALE
b Some numbness and tingling are common sensations with cold applications and indicate adverse reactions only when severe and coupled with other symptoms. Stop treatment when patient complains of burning sensation or increased sensation of numbness in the area of treatment.	When applying cold, skin will initially feel cold, followed by relief of pain. As cold continues, patient will feel burning sensation, then pain in skin, and finally numbness.
10 After 15 to 20 minutes (or as ordered by health care provider), remove compress or pad, and gently dry off any moisture.	Drying prevents skin maceration.

CLINICAL JUDGMENT *Areas with little body fat (e.g., knee, ankle, elbow) do not tolerate cold as well as fatty areas (e.g., thigh, buttocks) do. For bony areas, decrease time of cold application to lower range.*

---

11 Perform postprocedure protocol.	
12 Evaluate patient response:	
a Inspect affected area for integrity, color, temperature, and sensitivity to touch. Reevaluate 30 minutes after procedure,	Determines reaction to cold application.
b Palpate affected area gently and note any edema, bruising, and bleeding (apply gloves if needed).	Determines level of improvement.
c Ask patient to describe character of pain and rate pain level on scale of 0 to 10.	Determines whether pain has been relieved.
d Measure ROM of affected body part.	Determines whether edema or muscle spasm is relieved.

Recording and Reporting

- Record pain level, ROM of affected extremity, appearance and condition of skin and affected body part before and after treatment; type, location, and duration of application; and patient's response to therapy.
- Document your evaluation of patient and family caregiver learning.
- Report any sensations of burning, numbness, or unrelieved pain or skin color changes to health care provider.

UNEXPECTED OUTCOMES	RELATED INTERVENTIONS
1 Skin appears mottled, reddened, or bluish as a result of exposure to cold.	Stop treatment. Notify health care provider.
2 Patient complains of burning pain and numbness.	Stop therapy. Notify health care provider.
3 Patient or family caregiver is unable to describe or demonstrate therapy.	Provide further instruction and/or demonstration.

Condom and External Urinary Catheters

External urinary devices for men are designed to drain urine when patients are incontinent. A male urinary condom is a soft, pliable sheath that fits over the penis, providing a safe and noninvasive way to contain urine for men who have complete and spontaneous bladder emptying. Condom catheters are held in place by an adhesive coating on the internal lining of the sheath, a double-sided self-adhesive strip, brush-on adhesive applied to the penile shaft, or an external strap. **Never use tape to secure a condom catheter.** Disadvantages of condom catheters are urinary leakage, skin breakdown and, often, problems with sizing.

External urinary catheters (e.g., Men's Liberty brand) seal gently and securely to the tip of the penis with a 100% latex free hydrocolloid adhesive. The Men's LibertyAcute external male catheter has a seven-petal faceplate and faceplate strip that are easy to apply and form an occlusive seal around the urinary meatus for leakage protection. This device is helpful for patients with retracted anatomy, or a small penile tip, which can cause a traditional condom catheter to dislodge. Condoms and external catheters are made of soft silicone that reduces friction. They are clear to allow for easy visualization of the skin under the catheter. Both catheters attach to a small-volume (leg) urinary drainage bag or a large-volume (bedside) drainage bag, both of which need to be kept lower than the level of the bladder.

Safety Guidelines

- A patient who has a sensitivity to adhesive should not be given a condom catheter that uses adhesive.
- Condom catheters are still available in latex, so it is important to verify that a patient does not have a latex allergy before applying this type of catheter.

Delegation

Assessing the skin of a patient's penile shaft and patient allergies are done by a nurse before catheter application. The skill of applying a condom catheter can be delegated to assistive personnel (AP). Direct the AP to:

- Follow manufacturer directions for applying and securing the condom/catheter.

- Monitor urine intake and output and record if applicable.
- Immediately report any redness, swelling, or skin irritation or breakdown of glans penis or penile shaft.

Collaboration

- A wound ostomy care nurse is a resource for male patients who may need an alternative to a traditional condom catheter.

Equipment

- Male condom catheter kit: condom sheath of appropriate size, securing device (internal adhesive or strap), skin preparation solution (per manufacturer's recommendations)
- *Option:* External catheter with cleansing wipe
- Urinary collection bag with drainage tubing or leg bag and straps
- Basin with warm water and soap
- Towels, washcloth, bath blanket
- Clean gloves
- Scissors, hair guard, or paper towel

STEP	RATIONALE
1 Perform preprocedure protocol.	
Assessment	
• Review electronic health record and assess urinary pattern, ability to empty bladder effectively, and degree of urinary continence.	Urinary elimination pattern indicates whether patient is a candidate for a condom catheter.
• Ask patient to describe history of allergies: known allergies as well as typical allergic reaction or response. Ask if known sensitivity to adhesive. Check patient's allergy wristband.	Condoms are made of latex and can cause serious skin reaction. Adhesive in a catheter can result in medical adhesive--related skin injury (MARSI) (Fumarola et al., 2020)

CLINICAL JUDGMENT *Do not apply condom catheter with adhesive if patient has history of allergy to adhesive.*

• Perform hand hygiene and apply clean gloves. Assess skin of penis for rashes, erythema, and/or open areas. (This may be deferred until just before catheter application.)	Reduces transmission of microorganisms. Provides baseline to compare changes in condition of skin after applying condom catheter.

STEP	RATIONALE

CLINICAL JUDGMENT *Apply a condom catheter only when the skin on the penile surface is intact.*

STEP	RATIONALE
• Verify patient's size and type of male incontinence device, or use manufacturer measuring guide to measure length and diameter of penis in flaccid state. Remove and dispose of gloves and perform hand hygiene.	Identifies proper size of device needed. To measure the penile circumference, begin from the penile base where the diameter is the largest. To ensure accurate sizing of device, if it is between two sizes, choose the smallest size (Sinha et al., 2018). Reduces transmission of microorganisms.

Implementation

STEP	RATIONALE
1 Prepare urinary drainage collection bag and tubing (large-volume drainage bag or leg bag). Clamp off drainage bag port. Place nearby ready to attach to condom after applied.	Provides easy access to drainage equipment after applying catheter.
2 Help patient to supine or sitting position. Place bath blanket/sheet over upper torso. Fold sheets so that only penis is exposed.	Respects patient dignity and privacy; draping prevents unnecessary exposure of body parts.
3 Apply clean gloves. Provide thorough perineal care. Use a soap that does NOT contain a moisturizer. Dry thoroughly before applying condom or external catheter. In uncircumcised male: a Ensure that foreskin has been replaced to normal position before applying condom catheter b Be sure foreskin is pushed back for application of external catheter. Do not apply barrier cream.	Prevents skin breakdown from exposure to secretions. Removes any residual adhesives. Perineal care minimizes skin irritation and promotes adhesion of new external catheter. Barrier creams prevent sheath from adhering to penile shaft.

Continued

STEP	RATIONALE
4 Remove and dispose of gloves. Perform hand hygiene. Reapply clean gloves.	Reduces transmission of microorganisms.
5 Clip hair at base of penis as needed before applying condom sheath. Some manufacturers provide hair guard that is placed over penis before applying device. Remove hair guard after applying catheter. An alternative to hair guard is to tear a hole in a paper towel, place it over penis, and remove after applying the device.	Hair adheres to condom and is pulled during condom removal or may get caught in adhesive as external catheter is applied.

CLINICAL JUDGMENT *The pubic area should not be shaved because any microabrasions in skin increase risk for skin irritation and infection.*

6 Apply condom catheter. a With nondominant hand, grasp penis along shaft. With dominant hand, hold rolled condom sheath at tip of penis with head of penis in cone. Smoothly roll sheath onto penis. Allow 2.5 to 5 cm (1 to 2 inches) of space between tip of glans penis and end of condom catheter (Fig. 14.1).	Excessive wrinkles or creases in external catheter sheath after application may mean that patient needs smaller size.

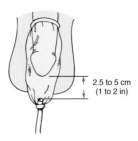

2.5 to 5 cm
(1 to 2 in)

Fig. 14.1 Distance between end of penis and tip of condom.

STEP	RATIONALE
b Apply appropriate securement device as indicated in manufacturer guidelines.	Condom must be secured firmly so that it is snug and stays on but not tight enough to constrict blood flow.
c Self-adhesive condom catheters: After application, apply gentle pressure on penile shaft for 10 to 15 seconds.	Ensures adherence of adhesive with penile skin. Secures catheter in place.
d Outer securing strip-type condom catheters: Use spiral wrap technique to wrap penile shaft with strip of supplied elastic adhesive. Strip should not overlap itself. Elastic strip should be snug, not tight (Fig. 14.2).	Using spiral wrap technique allows supplied elastic adhesive to expand so that blood flow to penis is not compromised.
7 Apply external catheter (Fig. 14.3).	Hydrocolloid material makes device less irritating to the skin and is suitable for patients with latex allergy (Bard Care, 2019). Allows the skin to breathe and the urine to be directed away from the body, making urination as natural as possible.

Continued

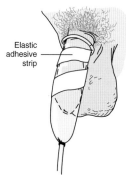

Elastic adhesive strip

Fig. 14.2 Tape applied in spiral fashion.

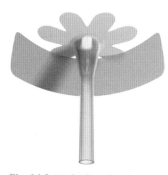

Fig. 14.3 Men's Liberty brand acute external urinary catheter for men. (Courtesy BioDerm, Inc., Largo, FL.)

STEP	RATIONALE
a Hold foreskin back. Wipe tip of penis with wipe supplied by manufacturer. (dry completely) (follow package directions).	Head of penis must be completely dry for device to adhere correctly.
b Position catheter with vent facing up. Then position so that flower portion of device faces the tip of penis. Line up catheter opening directly over urinary meatus.	Alignment is necessary for catheter to be applied correctly.
c Remove adhesive backing over petals, Then one by one, press petals down alternating sides, keeping catheter aligned over urinary meatus. Hold for 20 seconds.	Adheres catheter to penis and centers the device for drainage.
d Next allow winged adhesives to drop down. Pull off release papers as you wrap around head of penis one side at a time. Be sure that all of the petals are covered. Grasp head of penis and hold for 20 seconds.	Secure seal prevents urine leakage. Follow manufacturer's directions to ensure device covers and seals over tip of penis only.

CLINICAL JUDGMENT *Never use regular adhesive tape to secure a condom or external catheter. Constriction from tape can reduce blood flow to the penile tissues.*

STEP	RATIONALE
8 Remove hair guard if used. Connect condom/catheter to drainage tubing. Be sure that condom is not twisted. Place drainage bag either around leg, or attach drainage bag to bed below level of bladder. When using large drainage bag, secure drainage tubing to patient's leg (see manufacturer's directions).	Allows urine to be collected and measured. Keeps patient dry. Twisted condom obstructs urine flow, causing urine pooling, skin irritation, and weakening and deterioration of adhesive, causing catheter to come off. Drainage bag below level of bladder promotes drainage and reduces collection of urine around penis. Securing tubing prevents pulling.
9 Perform postprocedure protocol.	
10 Remove and reapply daily unless an extended-wear catheter is used (see manufacturer's directions). Reapply if becomes loose or soiled. Perform hand hygiene and apply clean gloves.	Prevents trauma and irritation to penile sheath. Reduces transmission of microorganisms. Gentle removal of device reduces irritation or abrasion to skin.
a To remove condom, wash penis with warm, soapy water and gently roll sheath and adhesive off penile shaft.	
b To remove catheter, gently roll adhesive bands away from skin. Then use adhesive remover recommended by manufacturer or warm, moist washcloth to loosen from tip of penis.	
c Perform postprocedure protocol.	

Continued

STEP	RATIONALE
11 Evaluate patient response:	
a Observe urinary drainage.	Twisted condom prevents urine from draining into collection bag.
b Inspect penis with device in place within 15 to 30 minutes after application. In the case of a condom device, assess for swelling and discoloration and ask patient if there is any discomfort.	Determines if condom is applied too tightly, impeding circulation to penis.
c Inspect skin on penile shaft for signs of breakdown or irritation at least daily, when performing hygiene, and before reapplying condom.	Signs of irritation may indicate MARSI (Fumarola et al., 2020). Changing external catheter decreases chance of infection.

Recording and Reporting

- Record condom/catheter application; condition of penis, skin, and scrotum; urinary output and voiding pattern; patient response to external catheter application; and patient learning.
- During hand-off reporting, communicate condition of skin and type of continence device in place.
- Report penile erythema, rashes, or skin breakdown to health care provider.

UNEXPECTED OUTCOMES	RELATED INTERVENTIONS
1 Skin around penis is inflamed, ulcerated, or denuded.	• Check again for latex allergy or allergy to adhesive. • Remove condom and notify health care provider. • Do not reapply until penis and surrounding tissue are free from irritation. • Ensure that condom is not twisted and urine flow is unobstructed after application.
2 Penile swelling or discoloration occurs.	• Remove external catheter. • Notify health care provider. • Reassess current condom size. See manufacturer size chart.
3 Incontinence device does not stay on.	• Ensure that catheter tubing is anchored and patient understands to not pull or tug on catheter. • Reassess catheter size. Refer to manufacturer guidelines for sizing. • Observe whether incontinence device outlet is kinked, and urine is pooling at tip of condom, bathing penis in urine; reapply as needed to avoid catheter obstruction. • Consult with wound ostomy care. • Assess need for another brand of incontinence device (i.e., one that is self-adhesive).

Continuous Subcutaneous Infusion

Continuous subcutaneous infusion (CSQI) is used for selected medications (e.g., opioids, insulin, and medicines used to stop preterm labor [e.g., terbutaline]) and to treat pulmonary hypertension (treprostinil sodium). The benefits of this route include providing a route for patients with poor venous access, providing pain relief to patients who are unable to tolerate oral pain medications, allowing patients greater mobility and better pain control (than intramuscular injections), and lowering the rate of infection (Harman et al., 2020). A drug given by CSQI usually has an onset of action about 20 minutes. One factor that determines the infusion rate of CSQI is the rate of medication absorption. Most patients can absorb 1 to 2 mL/h of medication or 62 mL/h of fluid, but the rate of absorption depends more on osmotic pressure than rate of administration (Caccialanza et al., 2018). Patients who most often use CSQI are those who have diabetes. A mini infusion pump is connected to a CSQI device for continuous insulin infusion.

The most common method for delivering CSQI is through the use of a commercially prepared Teflon cannula or a very fine 29-gauge needle (see infusion pump guidelines). In some cases winged IV needles can still be used. Teflon cannulas and fine-gauge needles are more comfortable for patients and have lower rates of complications than traditional winged IV needles. The cannulas are associated with fewer needlestick injuries. The choice of needle type should be based on pump parameters or patient preference. Use the needle with the shortest length and the smallest gauge necessary to establish and maintain the infusion.

Decision-making regarding site selection depends on a patient's activity level and the type of medication delivered. For example, pain medications given to ambulatory patients are best delivered in the upper chest so that a patient can move freely. In comparison, insulin is absorbed most consistently in the abdomen. When using this site, choose an injection point that is away from the waistline. Always avoid sites where the pump tubing could be disturbed. Rotate sites used for medication administration at least every 2 to 7 days, or whenever complications such as leaking occur (Infusion Nurses Society, 2021).

Safety Guidelines
- The CSQI route requires a computerized infusion pump with safety features, including lockout intervals and warning alarms.
- Avoid distractions while preparing a parenteral medication. No-interruption zones are recommended to reduce distractions during medication preparation and administration (Palese et al., 2019).

Delegation
The skill of administering CSQI medications cannot be delegated to assistive personnel (AP). Direct the AP to:
- Immediately report occurrence of medication side effects or reactions.
- Report complications (e.g., leaking, redness, discomfort) at the CSQI needle insertion site.
- Obtain any required vital signs and report unexpected findings.

Collaboration
- Agency pharmacist, diabetes educator, and pain specialist can assist with CSQI management.

Equipment
Initiating CSQI
- Clean gloves
- Antiseptic swab such as chlorhexidine
- CSQI-designed catheter/needle (e.g., Quick-set, Saf-T-Intima, or AutoSoft) with adhesive disk (Fig. 15.1) or small (25- to 27-gauge) winged IV catheter with attached tubing
- Infusion pump
- *Option:* Occlusive, transparent dressing
- Medication in appropriate syringe or transfer device for pump
- Medication administration record (MAR) or computer printout of same

Discontinuing CSQI
- Clean gloves
- Small, sterile gauze dressing
- Plastic tape
- Antiseptic swab
- Puncture-proof container

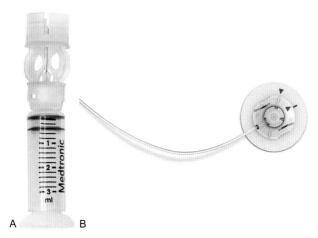

A   **B**

Fig. 15.1   MiniMed™ Quick-Set. **A,** Reservoir. **B,** tubing and inserter device. (Courtesy of Medtronic, Northridge, CA.)

STEP	RATIONALE
1 Perform preprocedure protocol	
Assessment	
• Review electronic health record (EHR) to assess patient's medical and medication history. Also note if patient has history of hemolytic disorders, reduced local tissue perfusion, extreme obesity.	Determines need for medication or possible contraindications for medication administration. Any existing coagulation disorder contraindicates heparin infusion. Reduced tissue perfusion interferes with medication absorption and distribution

STEP	RATIONALE
• Review EHR for these risk factors: neonate or and older adult; dry skin; dehydration; malnutrition; medications such as long-term use of corticosteroids, chemotherapeutic agents, and anti-inflammatory agents, dermatologic conditions, and underlying medical conditions that affect the skin (e.g., diabetes, immunosuppression).	Risk factors for developing medical adhesive-related skin injury (MARSI) from transparent dressing and/or adhesive patch (Fumarola et al., 2020). Presence of factors requires diligent monitoring of skin.
• Refer to drug reference for action, purpose, side effects, normal dose, time of peak onset, recommended infusion rate.	Allows safe medication administration, and monitoring of patient's response to therapy.
• Ask patient about allergy history and known reactions to allergens. Check patient's allergy wristband.	CSQI administration of medications may cause rapid allergic response.
• If an analgesic is being administered, assess character of patient's pain and rate severity using a scale from 0 to 10.	Provides an objective measure of pain severity.
• Perform hand hygiene. Assess adequacy of patient's adipose tissue to determine appropriate infusion site. If previous insertion site exists, assess for redness, maceration, or skin tear.	Physiologic changes of aging or patient illness influence amount of subcutaneous tissue, which affects choice of catheter insertion site. Signs of MARSI (Fumarola et al., 2020).

Implementation

1 Plan preparation to avoid interruptions or distractions.	Interruptions contribute to medication errors (Palese et al., 2019).

Continued

STEP	RATIONALE
2　Patients placed on CSQI infusion will require detailed instruction on how to prepare and administer an infusion. Include family caregiver as appropriate. Many agencies have diabetes educators available to assist with this teaching. Include patient in CSQI preparation and administration.	Patients who are placed on CSQI must be motivated and able to participate in medication management (determined by health care provider). Learning CSQI infusion procedure promotes self-care.
3　Review manufacturer directions for how to use pump and infusion set. *Note:* Insertion steps for infusion set will vary by type of device used.	Ensures proper use of equipment.
4　Perform hand hygiene. Check medication label carefully with MAR or computer printout when removing medication from storage and after preparation. *Note:* You will prepare the medication either by syringe (Fig. 15.2) or a reservoir transfer device (Fig. 15.1) (see Step 8, below) that comes with a commercial infusion set.	*These are the first two checks for accuracy,* ensuring that correct medication is administered.
5　At bedside, identify patient using at least two identifiers (e.g., name and birthdate or name and medical record number) according to agency policy. Compare identifiers with information on patient's MAR or medical record.	Ensures correct patient. Complies with The Joint Commission standards and improves patient safety (The Joint Commission, 2022). Some agencies use a barcode scanning system to help with patient identification.

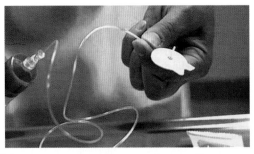

Fig. 15.2 Filling continuous subcutaneous infusion needle set using syringe. Image courtesy Nordic Infucare, Bromma, Sweden.

STEP	RATIONALE
6 At patient's bedside again compare MAR or computer printout with name of medication on medication label on syringe and patient name. Ask patient again if they allergies.	*This is the third check for accuracy* and ensures that patient receives correct medication. Confirms patient's allergy history.
7 Position patient comfortably, supine or sitting. Drape extremities.	Respects patient's dignity. Sitting facilitates patient instruction.
8 Perform hand hygiene. Program infusion pump. If not using a commercial infusion set device, prepare winged needle with tubing by priming with syringe filled with medication.	Ensures that medication dose administered is accurate. Reduces transmission of microorganisms. Prevents air from entering subcutaneous tissue.
9 Prepare commercial infusion set: a For a commercial device such as a Quick-set, use the transfer device and reservoir that comes with the set. Fill the reservoir with the prescribed medication per device directions.	Reservoir holds a dose of medication that will last usually 2 to 3 days (e.g., insulin).

Continued

STEP	RATIONALE
b When reservoir is full, remove the transfer device used to fill the reservoir. Discard in appropriate receptacle.	Reduces transmission of microorganisms.
c Connect the reservoir to the tubing of the infusion pump. Most pumps contain a compartment for the reservoir. Next turn on the pump and fill the tubing following manufacturer guidelines or directions shown on the pump screen. Most pumps will show a message when the pump is successfully filled.	Priming of tubing prevents air from entering subcutaneous tissue. Ensures proper pump function.
d Prepare the cannula/needle insertion device per manufacturer directions.	Insertion device ensures ease of cannula/needle insertion without contamination.
10 Initiate CSQI:	
a Perform hand hygiene and apply clean gloves. Select appropriate injection site free of irritation, away from bony prominences and waistline. Most common sites used are subclavicular and/or abdomen. Choose site easily accessible by patient. Note: condition of skin around proposed insertion site.	Ensures proper medication absorption. Provides baseline for condition of skin.

STEP	RATIONALE
b Clean injection site with antiseptic swab. Apply swab at center of site and rotate outward in circular direction for about 5 cm (2 inches). Allow to dry.	Reduces risk for infection at insertion site.
c Commercial device:	
(1) Remove guard to expose cannula/ needle in the insertion device. (*Note:* Some devices also require removal of adhesive backing from disk that will secure cannula/needle.)	Prepares needle for insertion. Ensures needle will enter subcutaneous tissue.
(2) Hold the insertion device against the prepared site on the patient's skin.	Delivers cannula/needle into subcutaneous tissue.
(3) Follow manufacturer's directions and push down on the device, inserting cannula/needle into the skin.	Secures cannula/needle.
(4) Once cannula/ needle is in place, pull inserter away from the body and press the adhesive disk surrounding the cannula/needle against the skin.	

Continued

STEP	RATIONALE
d Winged needle: 　　(1) If using a winged needle attached to prepared pump and tubing, pinch skin at insertion site. Then gently and firmly insert needle at 45- to 90-degree angle (Fig. 15.3). Refer to manufacturer's directions.	Decreases pain related to insertion of needle. Angle ensures subcutaneous tissue placement.
• Release skinfold and apply gentle pressure around adhesive disk. *Option:* Cover with transparent semipermeable membrane.	Secures needle.

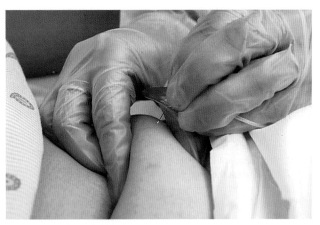

Fig. 15.3 Insert winged needle subcutaneously.

STEP	RATIONALE
11 Administer medication:	
a Commercial device: Be sure cannula/needle is secure. Turn pump on and check infusion rate.	Ensures correct dose administration.
b Winged needle: Attach tubing from needle to tubing from infusion pump and turn pump on. Check infusion rate.	
c Inspect site before leaving patient and instruct patient to report if site becomes red, swollen or begins to leak.	Initiate new site with new needle whenever erythema or leaking occurs. If site is free from complications, rotate needle every 2 to 7 days (Infusion Nurses Society, 2021). Adhesive may cause MARSI (Fumarola et al., 2020).
d Perform postprocedure protocol.	
e Discontinue CSQI:	
(1) Verify order and establish alternative method for medication administration if applicable.	If medication will be required after discontinuing CSQI, a different medication and/ or route is often necessary to continue to manage patient's illness or pain.
(2) Stop infusion pump.	Prevents medication from spilling.
(3) Perform hand hygiene and apply clean gloves.	Reduces transmission of microorganisms.

Continued

STEP	RATIONALE
(4) Remove disk: gently loosen a corner of the dressing. Lift off disk while removing needle from skin at same angle it was inserted.	Exposes needle. Minimizes risk of MARSI during removal.
(5) Remove transparent semipermeable membrane dressing: gently loosen corner and stretch it horizontally in the opposite direction of the insertion site. Walk fingers under the dressing to continue stretching it. One hand should continuously support the skin adhered to the dressing. The process can be repeated around the entire dressing (Fumarola et al., 2020). Lift off dressing and needle at same angle needle was inserted.	Minimizes risk of MARSI during removal.
	Prevents injury to patient and healthcare provider.
(6) Discard dressing and needle in puncture- and leak-proof receptacle	
(7) Apply gentle pressure at site until no fluid leaks out of skin.	Dressing adheres to site if skin remains dry.
h Apply small sterile gauze dressing or plastic bandage to site.	Prevents bacterial entry into puncture site. Plastic tape less likely to cause MARSI.
i Perform postprocedure protocol	

STEP	RATIONALE
12 Evaluate patient response: (1) Evaluate patient's response to medication.	Determines effect of therapy. Decreased or absent response to medication may indicate that patient is not receiving medication into subcutaneous tissue (e.g., pump malfunction, medication leaking at site).
(2) Assess site at least every 4 h for redness, pain, drainage, or swelling.	Indicates infection at insertion site. Inflammation and maceration can be result of MARSI (Fumarola et al., 2020).
(3) Evaluate patient's ability to fill pump, insert needle/cannula, and manage infusion pump.	Confirms learning and competency.

Recording and Reporting

- After initiating CSQI, immediately chart medication, dose, route, site, time, date, and type of medication pump in Medication administration record. If medication is an opioid, follow agency policy to document waste.
- Record patient's response to medication and appearance of site every 4 h or according to agency policy.
- Record patient teaching and validation of understanding.
- Report any adverse effects from medication or evidence of infection or MARSI at insertion site to patient's health care provider, and document according to agency policy. Patient's condition often indicates need for additional medical therapy.

UNEXPECTED OUTCOMES	RELATED INTERVENTIONS
1 Patient complains of localized pain or burning at insertion site; or site appears red or swollen or is leaking, indicating potential infection, MARSI, or needle dislodgement.	• Remove needle and place new needle in different site. • Continue to monitor original site for signs of infection and notify health care provider if you suspect infection. • Provide good skin care (Fumarola et al., 2020). • Avoid washing the skin too much and use a pH-balanced soap substitute to avoid drying the skin. • Hydrate the skin to ensure the patient drinks enough water to prevent dehydration. • Use emollient as a moisture barrier.
2 Patient displays signs of allergic reaction to medication.	• Stop delivering medication immediately and follow agency policy or guidelines for appropriate response to allergic reaction (e.g., administration of antihistamine such as diphenhydramine or epinephrine) and reporting adverse drug reactions. • Notify patient's health care provider of adverse effects immediately. • Add allergy information to medical record.

Dressings (Dry and Damp-to-Dry)

Dry gauze dressings are used to promote wound healing by primary intention with little drainage. Dry dressings protect a wound from injury, reduce discomfort, and speed healing. Dry gauze does not interact with wound tissues and causes little wound irritation. Gauze is used for wound cleansing and as a wick, a filter and a dressing. It can be moistened with various solutions. These dressings are commonly used for abrasions and nondraining postoperative incisions. Telfa gauze dressings contain a shiny, nonadherent surface on one side that does not stick to a wound. Drainage passes through the nonadherent surface to the outer gauze dressing.

Dry dressings are not appropriate for debriding wounds. When gauze adheres to drainage on a wound surface, the seal can pull off healthy tissue when the gauze is removed. If the old gauze dressing does adhere to a wound, moisten the dressing with sterile normal saline or sterile water before removing it to minimize wound trauma and pain.

Damp-to-dry dressings (also called moist or *moist-to-dry*) consist of gauze lightly moistened with an appropriate solution (i.e. normal saline). A damp-to-dry dressing has a moist contact layer that touches the wound surface. The moistened gauze increases the absorptive ability of the dressing to collect exudate and wound debris. When other forms of moisture-retentive dressings are not available, moist gauze is effective to mechanically debride a wound and promote wound healing (Bryant and Nix, 2024). Avoid applying excessively wet dressings on a wound surface, which causes moisture associated skin damage (MASD) (Jaszarowski and Murphree, 2022).

Safety Guidelines

- A wound is a break in skin integrity that increases a patient's risk for infection. Perform hand hygiene before and after a dressing change. Use appropriate gloves when changing a dressing.
- A favorable environment for wound healing is a moist wound bed; however, excessive moisture and/or exudate provides a medium for bacteria and MASD.
- Know the expected amount and type of exudate or drainage expected from the wound you are dressing.

Delegation

The skill of applying dry and damp-to-dry dressings can be delegated to assistive personnel (AP) if the wound is chronic (see agency policy). The nurse is responsible for wound assessments, care of acute new wounds, wound care requiring sterile technique, and evaluation of wound healing. Direct the AP about:

- Any unique modifications of the dressing change, such as the need for use of special tape or taping techniques to secure the dressing.
- Reporting pain, fever, bleeding, or wound drainage immediately.
- Reporting any potential contamination to existing dressing (e.g., patient incontinence or other body fluids, a dressing that becomes dislodged).

Collaboration

- Collaborate with a wound ostomy care nurse or wound care specialist when wounds do not heal or when a medical device–related pressure injury or other pressure injuries result.
- Collaborate with an infection control nurse when wounds are infected to determine what, if any, additional infection control measures are needed.

Equipment

- Clean and sterile gloves
- Sterile dressing set including sterile scissors and forceps (check agency policy)
- Sterile drape *(optional)*
- Necessary dressings: fine-mesh gauze, 4 × 4-inch gauze, abdominal (ABD) pads
- Sterile basin *(optional)*
- Antiseptic ointment (as prescribed)
- Wound cleanser (as prescribed)
- Sterile normal saline (or prescribed solution)
- Tape (nonallergenic tape, plastic tape recommended for short-term wear, and paper/cloth tape for long-time wear) (Fumarola et al., 2020)
- *Option:* Montgomery ties, or gauze roll bandages as needed
- Skin barrier (e.g., Stomahesive, liquid barrier, foam applicators, wipes or sprays)
- Measuring device: cotton-tipped applicator, measuring guide, camera
- Adhesive remover, scissors, or hair clipper *(optional)*
- Protective waterproof underpad
- Biohazard bag
- Personal protective equipment (i.e., gown, goggles, mask) if needed
- Additional lighting if needed (e.g., flashlight, treatment light)

STEP	RATIONALE
1 Perform preprocedure protocol.	

Assessment

• Review electronic health record (EHR), including health care provider's order and nurses' notes. Note previous dressing change, including equipment used and patient response.	Verifies dressing orders. Information can be applied to subsequent dressing changes.
• Review EHR; identify whether patient is at risk for wound-healing problems, including aging, premature infant, obesity, diabetes mellitus, circulation disorders, nutritional deficit, immunosuppression, radiation therapy, high levels of stress, and use of steroids.	Physiologic changes resulting from aging, chronic illness, poor nutrition, medications that affect wound healing, and cancer treatments have potential to affect wound healing (Doughty and Sparks, 2016). Presence of these factors raises your level of observation for healing problems.
• Identify whether patient is at risk for medical adhesive--related skin injury (MARSI) from adhesive tape: age, dehydration, malnutrition, exposure to radiation therapy, underlying chronic conditions (e.g., diabetes, immunosuppression) and edema of skin.	Common risk factors for MARSI (Fumarola et al., 2020). Factors raise your level of observation as long as patient has a dressing with adhesive closure.
• Ask patient to describe history of allergies: known type of allergies and normal allergic reaction. Check patient's allergy wristband. Focus on antiseptics, adhesive, or latex.	Reduces risk for exposing patient to allergens that can cause localized or systemic allergic reactions.

Continued

STEP	RATIONALE
• Ask patient to describe character of pain and rate severity on a scale of 0 to 10. *Administer prescribed analgesic as needed 30 minutes before dressing change.*	Superficial wounds with multiple exposed nerves may be intensely painful, whereas deeper wounds with destruction of dermis should be less painful (Bonham, 2022). A comfortable patient is less likely to move suddenly, causing wound or supply contamination. Serves as baseline to measure response to dressing therapy.
• Perform hand hygiene and apply clean gloves. Assess size, location, and presence of drainage on outer gauze. Remove and dispose of gloves. Perform hand hygiene.	Helps to plan for proper dressing type and securement of supplies needed and if help is needed during dressing procedure. Reduces transmission of microorganisms.

Implementation

1	Place biohazard bag within reach of work area. Fold top of bag to make a cuff.	Ensures easy disposal of soiled dressings. Do not reach across sterile field.
2	Position patient and drape to expose only wound site. Instruct patient not to touch wound or sterile supplies.	Draping provides access to wound while minimizing exposure. Dressing supplies become contaminated when touched by patient's hand.
3	Perform hand hygiene and apply clean gloves. Apply gown, goggles, and mask if risk for splashing exists.	Use of personal protective equipment reduces transmission of microorganisms.

STEP	RATIONALE
4 Remove tape strips by loosening edges and removing each side of tape toward the wound. Use fingers of opposite hand to push the skin down and away from the adhesive. When both sides are completely loosened, lift the strip up from the center of the wound. Use medical adhesive remover if needed to loosen the adhesive bond from skin (follow the manufacturer's instructions). If patient has hair growth in area of dressing, get patient's permission to clip area before applying new dressing (check agency policy).	Pulling tape toward dressing reduces stress on suture line or wound edges, irritation, discomfort, and risk of MARSI (Fumarola et al., 2020).

CLINICAL JUDGMENT *If surgical glue was used to close the wound, assess that the glue is intact. Do not remove the glue. Only replace the top dressing as needed.*

---

5 With gloved hand or forceps, remove dressing one layer at a time, observing appearance of drainage on dressing. Carefully remove outer secondary dressing first and then remove inner primary dressing in contact with wound bed. If drains are present (Fig. 16.1), slowly and carefully remove dressings and avoid tension on any drainage devices. Keep soiled undersurface from patient's sight.	Purpose of primary dressing is to remove necrotic tissue and exudate. Appearance of drainage may be upsetting to patient. Avoids accidental removal of drain.

Continued

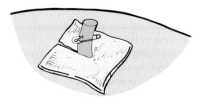

Fig. 16.1 Penrose drain with split gauze.

STEP	RATIONALE
a If bottom layer of damp-to-dry dressing adheres to wound, gently free dressing while alerting patient of possible discomfort.	Damp-to-dry dressing should debride wound (Bryant and Nix, 2024).
b If dry dressing adheres to wound that is not to be debrided, moisten with normal saline first, wait 1 to 2 minutes, then remove.	Prevents injury to wound surface and area around wound during dressing removal.
6 Inspect wound and area around wound for appearance, color, size (length, width, and depth), drainage, edema, presence and condition of drains, approximation (wound edges are together), granulation tissue, or odor. Use measuring guide or ruler to measure size of wound. Gently palpate wound edges for bogginess or patient report of increased pain.	Assesses condition of wound and area around the wound, indicating status of healing.

CLINICAL JUDGMENT *If drainage is observed or there is an odor from the wound, verify with health care provider regarding obtaining a wound culture.*

STEP	RATIONALE
7 Fold dressings with drainage contained inside and remove gloves inside out. With small dressings remove gloves inside out over dressing. Dispose of gloves and soiled dressing according to agency policy. Cover wound lightly with sterile gauze pad and perform hand hygiene.	Contains soiled dressings, prevents hand contact with drainage, and reduces cross contamination.
8 Describe appearance of wound and any indicators of wound healing to patient.	Wounds may be unsettling and frightening to patients. It helps patient to know that wound appearance is as expected and whether healing is taking place.
9 Create sterile field with sterile dressing tray or individually wrapped sterile supplies on overbed table. Pour any prescribed solution into sterile basin.	Sterile dressings remain sterile while on or within sterile surface. Preparing all supplies before dressing change prevents break in sterile technique.
10 Clean wound:	
a Apply clean gloves. Use gauze or cotton ball moistened in saline or antiseptic swab (per health care provider order) for each cleaning stroke or spray wound surface with wound cleaner.	Prevents transfer of microorganisms from previously cleaned area.
b Clean from least to most contaminated areas (Fig. 16.2).	Cleaning in this direction prevents introduction of microorganisms into wound.
c Clean around any drain (if present), using circular strokes starting near drain and moving outward and away from insertion site (Fig. 16.3).	Correct aseptic technique in cleaning prevents contamination.

Continued

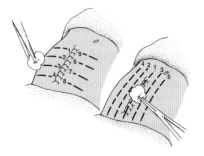

Fig. 16.2 Cleaning a wound from least to most contaminated area.

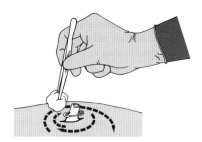

Fig. 16.3 Cleaning around a drain site.

STEP	RATIONALE
d Use sterile dry gauze to blot wound bed in same manner.	Drying reduces excess moisture, which could eventually harbor microorganisms.
11 Apply antiseptic ointment (if ordered) with sterile cotton-tipped applicator or gauze along wound edges. Remove and dispose of gloves. Perform hand hygiene.	Helps reduce growth of microorganisms.
12 Apply dressing (see agency policy): a Dry sterile dressing:	

CLINICAL JUDGMENT *Dry dressings are not appropriate for debriding wounds. In the presence of drainage, a dry dressing may adhere to the wound bed and surrounding tissue, causing pain and trauma on removal. Dry dressings have the disadvantage of moisture evaporating quickly, which can cause a dressing to dry out. As a result, frequent dressing changes are usually needed, and there are increased infection rates when compared with semiocclusive dressings (Thayer et al, 2022).*

STEP	RATIONALE
(1) Apply clean gloves (see agency policy).	Some agency policies or the condition of a wound may require sterile gloves.
(2) Apply loose woven gauze over simple closed wound as a contact layer (Fig. 16.4).	Promotes proper absorption of drainage.
(3) If drain is present, apply precut, split 4 × 4-inch gauze around drain.	Secures drain and promotes drainage absorption at site.
(4) Apply additional layers of gauze as needed for larger wound.	Ensures proper coverage and optimal absorption.
(5) Apply thicker woven pad (e.g., Surgipad, ABD pad) for the outermost dressing	This dressing is used on postoperative wounds when there is excessive drainage.
b Damp-to-dry dressing:	A damp-to-dry dressing has a moist primary contact dressing layer that touches the wound surface. The moistened gauze increases the absorptive ability of the dressing to collect exudate and wound debris.

Continued

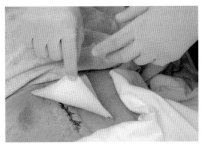

Fig. 16.4 Placing dry gauze dressing over simple wound.

STEP	RATIONALE

CLINICAL JUDGMENT *For patients at risk for MASD, use a moisture barrier, such as skin sealants, skin barrier ointments or paste and solid-wafer skin barrier to protect periwound skin (Earlam and Woods, 2022).*

(1)	Apply sterile gloves (see agency policy).	Reduces transmission of infection.
(2)	Place fine-mesh or loose 4 × 4-inch gauze in container of prescribed sterile solution. Wring out excess solution thoroughly.	Damp gauze absorbs drainage and, when allowed to dry, traps debris.

CLINICAL JUDGMENT *When using "packing strips," use sterile scissors to cut the amount of dressing that you will use to pack the wound. Do not let the packing strip touch the outside of the bottle. Place packing strip in container of prescribed sterile solution. Wring out excess solution.*

(3)	Apply damp fine-mesh or open-weave gauze as single layer directly onto wound surface. If wound is deep, gently pack gauze into wound with sterile gloved hand or forceps until all wound surfaces are in contact with damp gauze, including dead spaces from sinus tracts, tunnels, and undermining (Fig. 16.5). Be sure that gauze does not touch skin surrounding wound.	Inner gauze should be damp, not wet, to absorb drainage and adhere to debris. When packing a wound, gauze should conform to base and side of wound (Bryant and Nix, 2024). Wound is loosely packed to facilitate wicking of drainage into absorbent outer layer of dressing. Moisture that escapes dressing often macerates the area surrounding wound causing MASD.

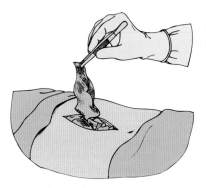

Fig. 16.5 Packing a wound with fine-mesh gauze.

STEP	RATIONALE

CLINICAL JUDGMENT *Count and record the number of pieces of gauze that are packed in the wound, especially deep wounds. This ensures that all gauze is removed from the wound with each dressing change.*

CLINICAL JUDGMENT *When packing the wound, do not forcibly overpack or underpack (Bryant and Nix, 2024). Packing should fill the wound but should not be above the level of the skin.*

STEP	RATIONALE
(4) Apply dry sterile 4 × 4-inch gauze over damp gauze.	Dry layer pulls moisture from wound.
(5) Cover with ABD pad, Surgipad, or gauze.	Protects wound from entrance of microorganisms.
13 Secure dressing.	
a Tape: Apply skin barrier 2.4 to 5 cm (1 to 2 inches) over surface of skin where tape is to be applied. Then apply tape over the gauze dressing, securing edges onto skin barrier. Use nonallergenic paper/cloth/plastic tape when necessary. Observe condition of skin where tape is placed.	Skin barriers form a protective interface between the skin and adhesive, reducing the risk of adhesive trauma (Fumarola et al., 2020). Supports wound and ensures placement and stability of dressing. Inspection allows for early detection of MARSI.

Continued

STEP	RATIONALE
b Montgomery ties (see Fig. 16.6).	Prevents skin irritation from repeated use of tape during dressing changes. However, most ties have adhesive backing. Observe for signs of MARSI.
(1) Be sure that skin is clean.	Moisture reduces adhesion.
(2) Apply a skin barrier (e.g., Stomahesive) over skin surface where tie is to be applied.	Skin barrier (Stomahesive) protects intact skin from stretch and tension of adhesive tape. Reduces incidence of MARSI (Fumarola et al., 2020).
(3) Expose the adhesive surface of Montgomery tape ends.	Prepares ties for application.
(4) Place ties on opposite sides of dressing over skin barrier.	
(5) Secure dressing by lacing ties across dressing snugly enough to hold it secure but without placing pressure on skin. Do not apply with tension or stretching (Fumarola et al., 2020).	

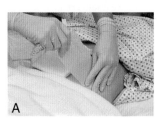 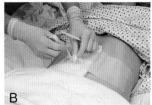

Fig. 16.6 Montgomery ties. (A) Each tie is placed at side of gauze dressing. (B) Securing ties encloses dressing.

STEP	RATIONALE
c For a protective window:	A protective window is an alternative to Montgomery ties for smaller wounds. There is less skin irritation by placing tape on window strips.
(1) Cut strip of Stomahesive or hydrocolloid pad into four strips, used to form a "window" around the wound.	Skin barriers form a protective interface between the skin and adhesive, thereby alleviating the risk of adhesive trauma (Fumarola et al., 2020).
(2) Use skin barrier to wipe areas of skin where strips will be applied.	
(3) Apply strips to frame a "window" around the wound, one on each side, one on the top, and one on the bottom of the wound (Fig. 16.7).	Window creates surface for placement of tape.
(4) Apply dressing inside window; secure tape ends to Stomahesive or hydrocolloid strips.	

Continued

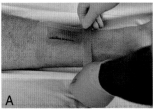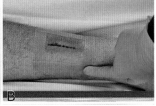

Fig. 16.7 Apply four adhesive strips to frame a "window" around wound.

STEP	RATIONALE
d For dressing on an extremity, secure with roller gauze or elastic net.	Roller gauze conforms to contour of foot or hand.
14 Label tape over dressing with your initials and the date dressing is changed.	Provides timeline for when next dressing change is to be scheduled.
15 Perform postprocedure protocol.	
16 Evaluate patient response: a Observe appearance of surrounding skin and wound for healing: measure size of wound; observe amount, color, and type of drainage and area surrounding wound for erythema, swelling, or patient-reported irritation.	Determines rate of healing and whether early signs of MARSI or MASD exist.
b Ask patient to describe character of pain and rate severity on a scale of 0 to 10.	Increased pain often indicates wound complications such as infection or results from dressing pulling tissue.
c Inspect condition of dressing at least every shift.	Determines status of wound drainage.

Recording and Reporting

- Record appearance and size of wound, characteristics of drainage, presence of necrotic tissue, condition of surrounding skin, type of dressing applied, patient's response to dressing change, and level of comfort.
- Record patient's and family caregiver's understanding of dressing change technique.
- Report any unexpected appearance of wound drainage, accidental removal of drain, bright red bleeding.
- Report any change in wound integrity (e.g., evidence of wound dehiscence or evisceration).

UNEXPECTED OUTCOMES	RELATED INTERVENTIONS
1 Wound appears inflamed and tender, drainage is evident, and/or odor is present.	• Monitor patient for additional signs of infection (e.g., fever, increased white blood cell count). • Notify health care provider. • Obtain wound cultures as ordered. • If there is yellow, tan, or brown necrotic tissue, notify health care provider to determine need for debridement.
2 Surrounding skin develops dermatitis, maceration, skin stripping or blistering, and folliculitis.	• Development of MARSI requires good skin care in daily routine (Fumarola et al., 2020): • Avoid washing the skin too much. • Use a pH-balanced soap substitute to avoid drying the skin. • Moisturize the skin daily and hydrate patient. • Avoid using alcohol-based products, perfumes, dyes, or harsh soaps. • Use emollients as a moisture barrier. • Handle skin with care: When drying the skin, lightly pat without rubbing.
3 Wound bleeds during dressing change.	• Observe color and amount of bloody drainage. If excessive, may need to apply direct dressing. • Inspect area along dressing and directly underneath patient to determine amount of bleeding. • Notify health care provider.

Continued

UNEXPECTED OUTCOMES	RELATED INTERVENTIONS
4 Patient reports sensation that "something has given way under the dressing." Drainage increases.	• Observe wound for dehiscence (partial or total separation of wound layers) or evisceration (total separation of wound layers and protrusion of viscera through wound opening). • If dehiscence or evisceration occurs, protect wound. Cover with sterile moist saline dressing. • Instruct patient to lie still. • Stay with patient to monitor vital signs. • Notify health care provider.

Dressings: Hydrocolloid, Hydrogel, Foam, and Alginate Dressing

A hydrocolloid dressing is a formulation of elastomeric adhesive and gelling agents. It promotes significantly better wound-healing outcomes compared with conventional gauze (Armstrong et al., 2022). These dressings absorb drainage and hydrate and debride wounds. When in contact with wound drainage, the hydrocolloid forms a gel that promotes a moist environment and facilitates autolytic and enzymatic debridement (Nazarko, 2018). These dressings cushion a wound surface to reduce pain and protect the wound and skin around the wound (periwound skin).

Hydrogel dressings are glycerin or water-based dressings that are moisture-retentive and designed to hydrate a wound, promoting moist wound healing and autolysis (Bryant and Nix, 2024). They have some absorptive properties. These dressings are similar to hydrocolloids and come in the form of sheets, amorphous gels, and impregnated gauze (Nazarko, 2018). A gel is nonadherent and less painful to remove.

Foam dressings absorb exudate in superficial or deep wounds, protect friable periwound skin, provide autolytic debridement, and cushion high trauma areas. Foam dressings manage chronic and infected wounds, pressure injuries and draining peristomal wounds. In addition, multilayered foam dressings aid in preventing heel and sacral pressure injuries (Haesler, 2017).

Alginate dressings are known for their absorptive properties, forming a gel over a wound surface to contain exudate. This dressing may come as a sheet or rope. An alginate dressing protects a wound and creates a moist environment, and promotes autolysis, granulation, and epithelialization of a wound bed (Nazarko, 2018). You can safely pack deep tracking wounds with calcium-sodium alginate preparation, which allows easy removal with little risk for retained dressing in a deep wound cavity (Bryant and Nix, 2024).

Safety Guidelines

- Hydrocolloid dressings are not intended for wounds with infection (Wound Care Society, 2016a).
- Hydrocolloid dressings can become dislodged in the case of heavy exudate (Wound Care Society, 2016a).

- Wound assessments can be made more difficult by opaque hydrocolloids (Wound Care Society, 2016a).
- Alginates should not be used on wounds with low drainage because they may dry them out completely, slowing down healing or even stopping it altogether (Wound Care Society, 2016b)
- A wound treated with foam or hydrogel dressings may dry out if there is little to no exudate to be absorbed, whereas maceration of the surrounding skin can occur if it becomes saturated with exudate.

Delegation

The skill of applying a hydrocolloid, hydrogel, foam, or alginate dressing cannot be delegated to assistive personnel (AP). Direct the AP to:

- Help position patient during dressing application.
- Immediately report any pain, fever, bleeding, wound drainage, or slippage of dressing.

Collaboration

- Collaborate with wound ostomy care nurse (WOCN) or wound specialist to determine the most effective dressing preparation for the patient's wound.

Equipment

- Clean gloves
- Sterile gloves *(optional)*
- Dressing set (items will vary): sterile scissors, sterile drape, face mask, sterile gloves, tape measure or other measuring guide, tape (nonallergenic tape), 4 × 4-inch gauze squares, dressing change label, antiseptic swabs
- Necessary primary dressings: gauze, hydrocolloid, hydrogel, foam, or alginate
- Secondary dressing of choice
- Tape (if not in kit): plastic tape recommended for short-term wear and paper/cloth tape for long-time wear (Fumarola et al., 2020)
- Montgomery ties
- Sterile saline or other cleaning solution (as ordered)
- Skin-barrier spray or wipe
- Biohazard bag
- Adhesive remover
- Debriding gel (as ordered)
- Irrigating solution if ordered
- Additional personal protective equipment (e.g., gown, goggles, and mask) as needed

STEP	RATIONALE
1 Perform preprocedure protocol.	

Assessment

- Review patient's electronic health record (EHR), including health care provider's order and nurses' notes for frequency and type of dressing change. *Do not use highly absorptive dressings, such as alginate or foam on nonexudative wounds.*

Indicates type of dressing or application to use.

- Review previous nurses' notes for type of dressing previously applied. Note whether a dressing requiring customization or a size to fit difficult body part has been used (e.g., sacrum, heels, elbows).

Information aids in selection of correct dressing materials. Customized shapes adhere more effectively.

- Review EHR; identify whether patient has risk for wound-healing problems, including aging, premature infant, obesity, diabetes mellitus, circulation disorders, nutritional deficit, immunosuppression, radiation therapy, high levels of stress, and steroid use.

Physiologic changes resulting from aging, chronic illness, poor nutrition, medications that affect wound healing, and cancer treatments have potential to affect wound healing (Doughty and Sparks, 2016). Presence of these factors increases the need for you to frequently observe wound for any healing problems

- Identify whether patient is at risk for medical adhesive—related skin injury (MARSI) from adhesive tape: age, dehydration, malnutrition, exposure to radiation therapy, underlying chronic conditions (e.g., diabetes, immunosuppression), and edema of skin.

Common risk factors for MARSI (Fumarola et al., 2020). Factors indicate the need for increased observation as long as patient has a dressing with adhesive closure.

Continued

STEP	RATIONALE
• Ask patient to describe history of allergies: known type of allergies and normal allergic reaction. Check patient's allergy wristband. Focus especially on allergies to antiseptics, adhesive, or latex.	Reduces risk for exposing patient to allergens that can cause localized or systemic allergic reactions.
• Ask patient to describe character of pain and rate severity on a scale of 0 to 10. *Administer prescribed analgesic as needed 30 minutes before dressing change.*	Patient may require pain medication before dressing change. Allows for peak effect of drug during procedure.
• Perform hand hygiene and inspect location, size, and condition of wound. Apply clean gloves if there is risk of contact with drainage. After assessment, remove and dispose of gloves and perform hand hygiene.	Reduces transmission of infection. Determines supplies and level of assistance needed.

Implementation

1	Place biohazard bag within reach of work area. Fold top of bag to make a cuff.	Ensures easy disposal of soiled dressings. Prevents reaching across sterile field.
2	Position and drape patient to expose only wound site. Instruct patient not to touch wound or sterile supplies.	Draping provides access to wound while minimizing exposure. Dressing supplies become contaminated when touched by patient.
3	Perform hand hygiene, apply clean gloves. Apply additional PPE as needed if there is a risk for splashing.	Reduced transmission of infectious organisms.

STEP	RATIONALE
4 Remove tape strips by loosening edges and removing each side of tape toward the wound. Use fingers of opposite hand to push the skin down and away from the adhesive. When both sides are completely loosened, lift the strip up from the center of the wound. Use medical adhesive remover if needed to loosen the adhesive bond from skin (follow the manufacturer's instructions). If patient has hair growth in area of dressing, obtain patient's permission to clip or shave area before applying new dressing (check agency policy).	Method for pulling tape toward dressing reduces stress on wound edges, irritation, discomfort, and risk of MARSI (Fumarola et al., 2020).
5 With gloved hand or forceps, remove old dressing one layer at a time. Note amount and character of drainage (Fig.17.1). Use caution to avoid tension on any drains.	Reduces irritation and possible injury to skin. Prevents accidental removal of drain.

CLINICAL JUDGMENT *Check removal directions for specific brand of dressing used. For some brands, soaking, irrigating, or moistening of the old dressing is needed to facilitate removal. If necessary, use adhesive remover to ease off dressing but avoid contact between the adhesive remover and the wound.*

Continued

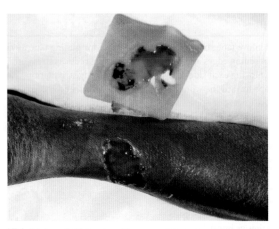

Fig. 17.1 Hydrocolloid dressing after removal from venous injury. Purulent-appearing exudate is present on dressing and wound. This is expected with autolysis under the dressing and is not evidence of infection. (From Bryant RA Nix DP: *Acute and chronic wounds: current management concepts*, ed 5, St Louis, 2016, Mosby.)

STEP	RATIONALE
6 Fold dressings inward so that drainage is contained inside and remove gloves inside out. With small dressings, remove gloves inside out to enclose dressing. Dispose of gloves and soiled dressing according to agency policy. Cover wound lightly with a sterile 4 × 4-inch gauze pad. Perform hand hygiene.	Contains soiled dressings; prevents contact of nurse's hands with drainage; reduces cross contamination.

CLINICAL JUDGMENT *Hydrocolloid dressings interact with wound fluids and form a soft whitish-yellowish gel, which is sometimes hard to remove and may have a faint odor. A residual gel substance occurs in wound beds with some absorption dressings. This is a normal occurrence; do not confuse these findings with pus or purulent exudate, wound infection, or wound deterioration (Bryant and Nix, 2024).*

STEP	RATIONALE
7 Prepare sterile field with sterile dressing kit or individually wrapped sterile supplies on overbed table. Pour prescribed cleansing solution into sterile bowl.	Creates sterile work area.
8 Remove gauze cover over wound.	
9 Clean wound: a Apply clean gloves. Sterile gloves are optional (see agency policy). Use 4 × 4-inch gauze cotton ball moistened in saline or an antiseptic swab (per health care provider order) for each cleaning stroke. *Option:* Spray wound surface with wound cleaner.	Reduces introduction of organisms into wound. Cleaning and irrigating effectively remove residual dressing gel without injuring newly formed delicate granulation tissue in healing wound bed.
b Clean in direction from least contaminated to most contaminated areas.	Cleaning in this direction prevents introduction of microorganisms into noncontaminated areas.
c Clean around any drain, using circular stroke starting near drain and moving outward away from insertion site.	
10 Use sterile dry gauze to completely blot dry the wound bed and skin around wound using same direction as Steps 9 b and c (Fumarola et al., 2020).	Dressing will not adhere to damp surface. Periwound maceration can enlarge wound and impede healing.

Continued

STEP	RATIONALE
11 Inspect appearance and condition of wound and periwound skin. Measure wound size and depth.	Appearance and measurement indicate state of wound healing and baseline for potential development of complications such as MARSI.

CLINICAL JUDGMENT *Thoroughly inspect the wound, periwound area and under adhesive material for signs of MARSI or MASD including contact dermatitis, maceration, blisters, excoriation, or skin tears (Hitchcock et al, 2021). Observe for subtle signs of infections: increased or altered exudate; friable, bright red granulation tissue; increased odor; increased pain; localized edema. Any combination of two or more is indicative of a local wound infection (Ramundo, 2022).*

STEP	RATIONALE
12 Remove and dispose of gloves and perform hand hygiene. Apply clean gloves. Sterile gloves are optional (see agency policy).	Reduces transmission of microorganisms.
13 Apply dressing (see manufacturer directions).	Ensures proper application of dressing. Different brands of dressings require different application techniques.
a Hydrocolloid dressings: (1) Select proper size wafer, allowing dressing to extend onto intact periwound skin at least 2.5 cm (1 inch) (Jaszarowski and Murphree, 2022) (Fig. 17.2). Apply skin barrier wipe to surrounding skin that will come in contact with any adhesive or gel.	Hydrocolloid design prevents shear and friction from loosening edges and circumvents need for tape along dressing borders (Bryant and Nix, 2024). Because of high water content of gels, care must be taken to protect periwound skin from MASD through use of skin barrier (Jaszarowski and Murphree, 2022).
(2) For deep wound, apply hydrocolloid granules, gauze soaked with gel, or paste before applying the wafer.	Functions as filler material to ensure contact with all wound surfaces.

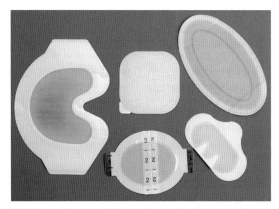

Fig. 17.2 Variety of sizes and shapes of hydrocolloid dressings. (Courtesy Bonnie Sue Rolstad.)

STEP	RATIONALE
(3) Remove paper backing from adhesive side and place over wound. *Do not stretch, and avoid wrinkles or tenting.* Hold dressing in place for 30 to 60 seconds after application.	Molds dressing at body temperature (Bryant and Nix, 2024).
(4) If cut from larger piece, tape edges with nonallergenic plastic/paper/ cloth tape to avoid rolling or adherence to clothing.	Selection of tape prevents MARSI

CLINICAL JUDGMENT *Edges may be notched to help mold around wound. Consider using custom shapes to better conform to certain parts of the body, such as heels, elbows, and sacrum.*

Continued

STEP	RATIONALE
b Hydrogel dressings:	
(1) Apply skin-barrier wipe or spray to surrounding skin that will come in contact with any adhesive or gel.	Protects periwound skin. Because of high water content of gels, care must be taken to protect periwound skin through use of skin barrier (Jaszarowski and Murphree, 2022). Prevents MARSI (Fumarola et al., 2020).
(2) Apply gel or gauze soaked in gel directly into wound, spreading evenly over wound bed (Fig. 17.3). Fill wound cavity with gel about one-third to one-half full or pack gauze loosely, including any undermined or tunneled areas. Cover with moisture-retentive dressing or hydrocolloid wafer.	Hydrogels hydrate and facilitate autolytic debridement of wounds. Filling wound cavity partially full allows for expansion with absorption of exudate (Jaszarowski and Murphree, 2022).
(3) Cut hydrogel sheet containing glycerin so that it extends 2.5 cm (1 inch) out onto intact periwound skin. Cover with secondary moisture-retentive dressing if needed.	Protects skin around wound from maceration.

CLINICAL JUDGMENT *Hydrogel sheets composed of water should be cut to size of wound only.*

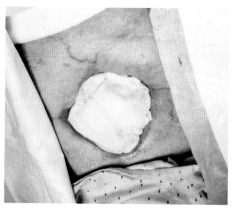

Fig. 17.3 Hydrogel-impregnated gauze used to maintain moist wound bed and fill dead space in this deep abdominal wound with undermining. (From Bryant RA, Nix DP: *Acute and chronic wounds: current management concepts*, ed 5, St Louis, 2016, Mosby.)

STEP	RATIONALE
(4) Secure dressing with nonallergenic plastic/paper/cloth tape if secondary dressing is not self-adhering.	The gel dressings are nonadherent and must be covered with a secondary dressing to hold them in place.
c Foam dressings:	
(1) Learn the removal and application characteristics of specific brands of foam (see manufacturer's directions). Foam is not for dry or wounds with eschar.	Foam dressings collect moderate to heavy wound exudate; however, some foam dressings contain an antimicrobial substance to reduce risk for bacterial colonization in wounds (Jaszarowski and Murphree, 2022)
(2) Apply skin-barrier wipe or spray to surrounding skin that will come in contact with thin foam dressing adhesive.	Protects periwound skin from maceration or irritation from adhesive. Prevents MARSI (Fumarola et al., 2020).

Continued

STEP	RATIONALE
(3) Cut foam sheet to extend 2.5 cm (1 inch) out onto intact periwound skin. (Verify which side of foam dressing should be placed toward wound bed and which side should be facing away from it; check product instructions.)	Ensures proper absorption and keeps wound exudate away from wound bed (Bryant and Nix, 2024).
(4) Cut foam to fit around drain or tube.	
(5) Cover with secondary dressing, such as loose gauze, as needed.	Some foam must be covered with secondary dressing (Bryant and Nix, 2024).

CLINICAL JUDGMENT *Foam dressings may macerate periwound skin and should be changed before they become overly saturated with exudate (Jaszarowski and Murphree, 2022).*

d Alginate dressings:	
(1) Cut sheet or rope to fit size of wound or loosely pack into wound space (Fig. 17.4), filling one-half to two-thirds full.	Highly absorptive product expands with absorption of serous fluid or exudate (Bryant and Nix, 2024).
(2) Apply secondary dressing, such as transparent film (Fig. 17.5), foam, or hydrocolloid	Secondary dressing prohibits drainage on bed linens and clothing.

CLINICAL JUDGMENT *Prior to applying new dressing material, fully irrigate the wound to remove all prior dressing residue (Jaszarowski and Murphree, 2022).*

14 Label dressing with your initials and date dressing changed.	Provides timeline for next dressing change.
15 Perform postprocedure protocol.	

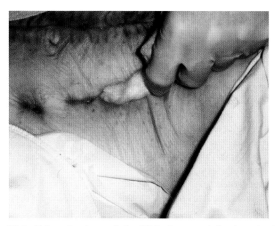

Fig. 17.4 Alginate dressing applied to fill dead space and absorb exudate in full-thickness abdominal wound. (From Bryant RA, Nix DP: *Acute and chronic wounds: current management concepts*, ed 5, St Louis, 2016, Mosby.)

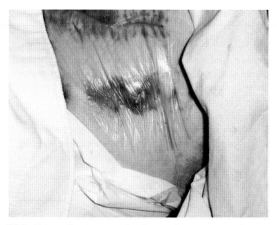

Fig. 17.5 Alginate dressing secured with secondary transparent dressing. (From Bryant RA, Nix DP: *Acute and chronic wounds: current management concepts*, ed 5, St Louis, 2016, Mosby.)

STEP	RATIONALE
16 Evaluate patient response:	
a Inspect appearance of wound: measure size of wound, observe amount and characteristics of drainage; observe presence of periwound edema, irritation, or erythema. Palpate around wound for tenderness.	Determines status of wound healing and whether MARSI is present.
b Evaluate patient's level of comfort, rating wound pain on scale of 0 to 10.	Documents patient's comfort level after procedure.
c Inspect condition of dressing at least every shift or as ordered.	Determines integrity of wound dressing.

Recording and Reporting

- Record size and appearance of wound, characteristics of drainage, presence of necrotic tissue, appearance of periwound skin, type of dressings applied, patient's response to dressing change, and comfort level.
- Document evaluation of patient learning.
- Report any unexpected appearance and character of wound and drainage/exudate (suggesting infection), bright-red bleeding, MARSI development, evidence of dehiscence or evisceration, or pain to health care provider.
- Report any change in wound management.

UNEXPECTED OUTCOMES	RELATED INTERVENTIONS
1 Wound develops more necrotic tissue and increases in size.	• In rare instances some wounds do not tolerate hypoxia induced by hydrocolloid dressings. In these patients discontinue use. Notify health care provider. • Evaluate appropriateness of wound care protocol. • Evaluate for other factors impairing wound healing. • Consult with wound care specialist.
2 Dressing does not stay in place.	• Evaluate size of dressing used to ensure it extends over wound for adequate margin (2.5 to 3.75 cm [1 to 1½ inches]) or dry skin more thoroughly before reapplication. • Consider custom shapes for difficult body parts. "Picture frame" edges of hydrocolloid dressing using tape. • Dressing may be secured with roll gauze, tape, transparent dressing, or dressing sheet.
3 Periwound skin is swollen, has tears, or is macerated, indicating MARSI.	• Assess moisture control property of dressing or application technique. May need new type of dressing. • Perform good skin care, keeping area dry and using skin emollients. Avoid harsh soaps or other applications.

Dressings: Transparent Dressing

A transparent film dressing is a clear, adherent, nonabsorptive, polyurethane sheet that is impermeable to fluids and bacteria (Bryant and Nix, 2024). Once the film is applied, a moist exudate forms over the wound surface that prevents tissue dehydration and allows for rapid, effective healing by speeding epithelial cell growth. The dressings are appropriate for prophylaxis when used on:

- High-risk intact skin (e.g., high-friction areas or patient's heels) (Haesler, 2017)
- Superficial wounds with minimal to no exudate
- Eschar-covered wounds when autolysis is indicated and safe

The synthetic permeable membrane acts as a temporary second skin, adheres to undamaged skin to contain exudate, minimizes wound contamination, and allows a wound to "breathe" (Armstrong et al., 2018; European Pressure Ulcer Advisory Panel et al., 2019b). A transparent dressing is commonly used to protect and secure an intravenous (IV) catheter insertion (see Skill 54).

Safety Guidelines

- A transparent membrane dressing has an adhesive border that secures the dressing to the skin around the wound (periwound skin). The adhesive increases the risk for medical adhesive--related skin injury (MARSI).

Delegation

The skill of applying a transparent dressing for select wounds can be delegated to assistive personnel (AP) (refer to agency policy). The assessment of the wound and care of sterile or new acute wounds cannot be delegated to AP. Direct the AP about:

- How to adapt the skill for a specific patient situation.
- Reporting any signs of bleeding, drainage, infection, or poor wound healing immediately.
- Reporting loosening of a dressing.

Collaboration

- Consult a wound ostomy care nurse or wound care specialist if a patient's skin shows signs of poor wound healing or early signs of pressure injury development.

Equipment

- Sterile gloves *(optional)*
- Clean gloves
- Dressing set *(optional)*
- Sterile saline or other cleansing agent (as ordered)
- Cotton swabs
- Biohazard bag for disposal
- Transparent dressing (size as needed)
- Sterile 4 × 4-inch gauze pads
- Skin barrier (e.g., liquid barrier film)
- Personal protective equipment (e.g., gown, goggles, mask) as needed

STEP	RATIONALE
1 Perform preprocedure protocol.	

Assessment

• Review patient's electronic health record (EHR), including health care provider's order for frequency and type of dressing change.	Health care provider orders indicate frequency of dressing changes and any special instructions.
• Review previous nurses' notes in EHR, noting wound location, recent assessments, size of wound, and patient response to transparent dressing changes.	Determines type of materials and size of transparent dressing needed for dressing change.
• Review EHR for patient's risk for impaired wound healing (e.g., aging, poor nutrition, immunosuppression, steroid use, or cancer).	Physiologic changes caused by aging, chronic illness, poor nutrition, medications, and cancer treatments can potentially affect wound healing (Doughty and Sparks, 2016).
• Ask patient to describe history of allergies: known types of allergies and typical allergic reactions. Check patient's allergy wristband. Be especially alert for allergies to antiseptics, adhesive, and latex.	Reduces risk for exposing patient to allergens that can cause localized or systemic allergic reactions.

Continued

STEP	RATIONALE
• Ask patient to rate level of wound pain using pain scale of 0 to 10 and assess characteristics of pain. Administer prescribed analgesic as needed 30 minutes before dressing change.	A patient who is comfortable is less likely to move suddenly, causing wound or supply contamination. Serves as baseline to measure response to dressing therapy.

Implementation

STEP	RATIONALE
1 Close door or cubicle curtains; gather and organize any equipment needed to perform procedure.	Protects patient's privacy and reduces anxiety. Ensures more efficiency when completing procedure.
2 Place biohazard bag within reach of work area.	Ensures easy disposal of soiled dressing.
3 Position patient and drape to expose only wound site. Instruct patient not to touch wound or sterile supplies.	Draping provides access to wound while minimizing additional exposure. Dressing supplies become contaminated when touched by patient.
4 Perform hand hygiene and apply clean gloves. Apply personal protective equipment as needed.	Reduces transmission of microorganisms.
5 Remove old dressing by loosening a corner of the dressing and stretching it horizontally in the opposite direction of the wound (stretch and relax technique). Walk fingers under the dressing to continue stretching it. One hand should continuously support the skin adhered to the dressing. The process can be repeated around the dressing	Stretching action gently breaks dressing seal (Bryant and Nix, 2024). Reduces excoriation, tearing, or irritation of skin during dressing removal (Fumarola et al., 2020).
6 Dispose of soiled dressing in waterproof bag. Remove gloves by pulling them inside out, then dispose in waterproof bag. Perform hand hygiene.	Reduces transmission of microorganisms.

STEP	RATIONALE
7 Pour saline or other prescribed solution over open package containing 4 × 4-inch sterile gauze pads.	Maintains sterility of dressing.
8 Apply clean gloves.	
9 Clean wound and periwound area gently with 4 × 4-inch sterile gauze pads moistened in sterile saline or wound cleaning spray. Clean wound and skin by moving from the least and then to the most contaminated area.	Reduces introduction of organisms into wound.
10 Pat skin around wound following same procedure as Step 9. Dry thoroughly with nonmoistened 4 × 4-inch sterile gauze pads.	Transparent dressing with adhesive backing does not adhere to damp surface (Bryant and Nix, 2024).
11 Inspect wound for tissue type, color, odor, and drainage; measure size if indicated. Inspect condition of surrounding skin.	Provides baseline for monitoring wound healing and early onset of MARSI.
12 Remove gloves and perform hand hygiene.	Reduces transmission of microorganisms.

CLINICAL JUDGMENT *If wound has a large amount of drainage, do not use a transparent dressing. Instead, choose another dressing that can absorb drainage. You may need to consult with a wound ostomy care nurse.*

---

13 Apply clean gloves. If patient's skin is fragile or if wound poses a risk for MARSI, apply a skin barrier (e.g., liquid barrier films available as foam applicators, wipes, and sprays) to skin surrounding wound.	Skin barriers form a protective interface between the skin and adhesive, thereby alleviating the risk of adhesive trauma (Fumarola et al., 2020)

Continued

STEP	RATIONALE
14 Apply transparent dressing according to manufacturer directions. *Do not stretch film during application and avoid wrinkles.*	Wrinkles provide tunnel for exudate drainage.
a Remove paper backing, taking care not to allow adhesive areas to touch one another.	
b Center film over wound and press down firmly without stretching. Use your fingers to smooth and adhere dressing . Remove paper edging. (Fig. 18.1).	Ensures coverage of wound. Prevents skin shearing from dressing that is too tight. Stretching can also break wound seal.
15 Label dressing with date, your initials, and time of dressing change on outer label of dressing	Provides record for determining when to next change dressing.
16 Perform postprocedure protocol.	
17 Evaluate patient response:	
a Inspect appearance of wound and characteristics and amount of drainage. Measure wound size.	Clear dressing allows you to observe wound and status of wound healing.
b Inspect condition of skin along periwound areas.	Identifies any injury to surrounding skin.

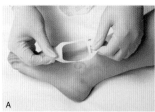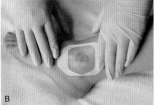

A   B

Fig. 18.1   (A) Transparent dressing placed over small wound on ankle. (B) Place film smoothly without stretching.

STEP	RATIONALE
c Ask patient to describe pain and rate severity on scale of 0 to 10.	Determines any change in pain during procedure.

Recording and Reporting

- Record appearance of wound, presence and characteristics of drainage, type of dressing applied, condition of skin surrounding wound, patient's response to dressing change, and level of comfort.
- Record patient's and family caregiver's understanding of how to apply dressing.
- Report any signs of infection, changes in skin integrity, or signs of MARSI to the health care provider.

UNEXPECTED OUTCOMES	RELATED INTERVENTIONS
1 Wound is inflamed, tender; accumulation of fluid with white, opaque appearance and erythema of surrounding tissue; increased drainage or change in the color of drainage; necrosis; and/or odor is present.	• Remove dressing and obtain wound culture according to agency policy. • A different type of dressing may be required. • Notify health care provider.
2 Dressing does not stay in place.	• Evaluate size of dressing selected to be sure it extends over wound margin (2.5 to 3.75 cm [1 to 1.5 inches]). • Assess for increased drainage from wound. • Dry patient's skin thoroughly before reapplication.
3 Skin surrounding wound becomes inflamed or blistered or outer layer of patient's skin tears on removal of dressing.	• Adhesive backing may be too strong for patient's skin. • Consider other transparent dressings that do not contain adhesive. • Provide thorough skin care, gently cleaning skin and using an emollient.

Ear Medications

Ear (otic) medications usually come in a liquid solution and are instilled by drops. Although structures of the outer ear are not sterile, sterile solutions should be used in case a patient's eardrum is ruptured. Do not occlude the ear canal with a medicine dropper because doing so can cause pressure within the canal during instillation and subsequent injury to the eardrum. When safety precautions are followed, eardrops instillation is a safe and effective therapy.

Safety Guidelines

- Because internal ear structures are sensitive to temperature extremes, administer eardrops at room temperature. Cold drops can cause vertigo (severe dizziness) or nausea and debilitate a patient for several minutes.
- Avoid forcing any solution into the ear.

Equipment

- Medication administration record (MAR) (electronic or printed)
- Medication bottle with dropper
- Cotton-tipped applicator, cotton balls
- Clean gloves if drainage is present

Delegation

The skill of administering ear medications cannot be delegated to assistive personnel (AP). Instruct the AP about:

- Potential side effects of medications and to report their occurrence.
- The potential for dizziness or irritation after administration of ear medications.

Collaboration

- Collaborate with healthcare provider to remove impacted cerumen before administering medication and/or if patient's ear condition worsens.

STEP	RATIONALE
1 Perform preprocedure protocol.	

Assessment

• Check accuracy and completeness of each MAR or computer printout with health care provider's written medication order. Check patient's name, medication name and dosage, route of administration, and time of administration.	Recopy or reprint any part of MAR that is difficult to read. The order sheet is the most reliable source and only legal record of medications to be received by patient. Ensures that patient receives correct medications (Palese et al., 2019). Transcription errors are a source of medication errors (Palese et al., 2019).
• Review electronic health record (EHR): assess patient's medical and medication history.	Determines need for medication or possible contraindications for medication administration.
• Review drug reference information for medication action, purpose, normal dose, side effects, time of peak onset, and nursing implications.	Allows you to administer medication safely and monitor patient's response to therapy.
• Ask patient to describe history of allergies: known type of allergies and normal allergic reaction. Check patient's allergy wristband.	Communication of patient allergies is essential part of safe medication administration.
• Determine whether patient has any symptoms of ear discomfort or hearing impairment.	Certain ear medications act to either lessen or increase these symptoms. External ear canal occlusion from swelling, drainage, or cerumen can impair hearing acuity and cause pain.
• Perform hand hygiene and assess condition of external ear structures. This may be done just before drug instillation (if drainage is present, apply clean gloves).	Provides baseline to determine whether local response to medications occurs. Also indicates need to clean ear before drug application.

Continued

STEP	RATIONALE
• Assess patient's level of consciousness and ability to follow directions.	There is a greater risk for accidental injury if patient becomes restless or combative during procedure.
• Assess patient's ability to manipulate and hold ear dropper.	Determines whether instruction is needed to prepare patient for self-administration of drug.

Implementation

1 Explain to patient purpose of each medication, action, indication, and possible adverse effects. Allow sufficient time for patient to ask any questions. Patients who self-instill medications may be allowed to give ear medications under nurse's supervision (check agency policy).

Makes patient a participant in care, which minimizes anxiety. Patient has the right to be informed, and patient understanding of each medication improves adherence with drug therapy. Prepares patient to self-administer drug, which increases feelings of independence.

2 Prepare medication without interruptions/distractions. Create a quiet environment. Keep all materials related to each patient's MAR separated and look at only one patient's electronic MAR at a time.

Interruptions contribute to medication errors (Palese et al., 2019).

3 Perform hand hygiene. Prepare medications for one patient at a time using aseptic technique. Complete two checks comparing label of medication carefully with MAR or computer printout when preparing medication.

Ensures that medication is sterile. *These are the first and second checks for accuracy* and ensure that correct medication is administered.

STEP	RATIONALE
4 Preparation usually involves taking eardrops out of refrigerator and allowing to warm to room temperature before administering to patient. Check expiration date on container.	Ear structures are sensitive to temperature extremes. Cold may cause vertigo and nausea. Administering eardrops at room temperature reduces risk for vertigo and nausea.
5 Take medication(s) to patient at correct time (see agency policy). Medications that require exact timing include stat, first-time or loading doses, and one-time doses. Give medications that are not scheduled time-critical within a range of 1 or 2 h of scheduled dose (Institute for Safe Medication Practices, 2011). During administration apply seven rights of medication administration.	Hospitals must adopt medication administration policy and procedure for timing of medication administration that considers nature of the prescribed medication, specific clinical application, and patient needs (United States Department of Health and Human Services Centers for Medicare and Medicaid, 2020; Institute for Safe Medication Practices, 2011).
6 Help patient to comfortable sitting position. Arrange supplies at bedside.	Ensures an organized procedure.
7 Identify patient using at least two identifiers (e.g., name and birthday or name and medical record number) according to agency policy. Compare identifiers with information on patient's MAR or medical record.	Ensures correct patient. Complies with The Joint Commission standards and improves patient safety (The Joint Commission, 2022).

Continued

STEP	RATIONALE
8 At patient's bedside, again compare MAR or computer printout with names of medications on medication labels and patient name. Reassess whether patient has allergies.	*This is the third check for accuracy* and ensures that patient receives correct medication. Confirms patient's allergy history.
9 Perform hand hygiene. *Option:* Apply clean gloves if ear drainage present. Position patient on side (if not contraindicated), with ear to be treated facing up. Alternatively, patient may sit in chair or at bedside. Stabilize patient's head with their own hand.	Facilitates distribution of medication into ear.
10 Straighten ear canal by pulling pinna up and back to 10 o'clock position (adult, or child older than age 3 years) (Fig. 19.1) or down and back to 6 to 9 o'clock position (child younger than age 3 years).	Straightening ear canal provides direct access to deeper ear structures. Anatomic differences in younger children and infants necessitate different methods of positioning ear canal (Hockenberry et al., 2019).

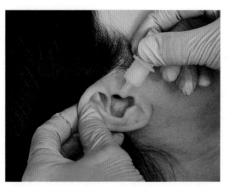

Fig. 19.1 Pull the pinna up and back for an adult, or a child older than 3 years.

STEP	RATIONALE
11 If cerumen or drainage occludes outermost part of ear canal, wipe out gently with cotton-tipped applicator. *Take care not to force cerumen into canal.*	Cerumen and drainage harbor microorganisms and can block distribution of medication into canal. Occlusion blocks sound transmission.
12 Instill prescribed drops holding dropper 1 cm (½ inch) above ear canal.	Avoiding contact with external ear canal prevents dropper contamination, which could further contaminate medication in container.
13 Ask patient to remain in side-lying position for a few minutes. Apply gentle massage or pressure to tragus with finger (Fig. 19.2).	Allows complete distribution of medication. Pressure and massage move medication inward.
14 If ordered, gently insert part of cotton ball into outermost part of canal. Do not press cotton into canal.	Prevents escape of medication when patient sits or stands.
15 Remove cotton after 15 minutes. Help patient to comfortable position after drops are absorbed.	Allows time for drug distribution and absorption.

Continued

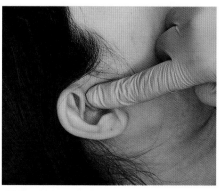

Fig 19.2 Apply gentle pressure to tragus after instilling drops.

STEP	RATIONALE
16 Perform postprocedure protocol.	
17 Evaluate patient response:	
a Observe response to medication by assessing hearing changes, asking if symptoms are relieved, and noting any side effects or discomfort felt.	Evaluates effects of medication.
b Ask patient to discuss purpose of drug, action, side effects, and administration technique.	Determines patient's level of understanding.

Recording and Reporting

- Record drug, concentration, dose or strength, number of drops, application site (left, right, or both ears), and time of administration on MAR immediately *after* administration, not before. Include initials or signature.
- Record patient teaching and validate understanding of how to administer medication.
- Record appearance of ear canal (e.g., drainage, tenderness, irritation), any subjective data (e.g., ear pain, ringing in ears, change in hearing acuity), and patient's response to medications.
- Report any adverse effects, patient response, and/or withheld drugs to charge nurse and/or health care provider.

UNEXPECTED OUTCOMES*	RELATED INTERVENTIONS
1 Ear canal remains inflamed, swollen, tender to palpation. Drainage is present.	• Hold next dose. • Notify health care provider for possible adjustment in medication type and dosage.
2 Patient's hearing acuity does not improve.	• Notify health care provider. • Cerumen may be impacted, requiring ear irrigation.

Ear Irrigation

Indications for irrigation of the external ear canal are the presence of foreign bodies, local inflammation, and buildup of cerumen (ear wax) in the canal. Irrigations are typically performed with solutions that have been warmed to body temperature to avoid vertigo or nausea in patients. It is important to adequately control the irrigating syringe and to prevent sudden moves by the patient to prevent damage to the external auditory meatus that occurs when the canal lining is scratched. Drying the ear properly is also essential to prevent acute otitis externa (infection of the outer ear).

Ear emergencies include the presence of foreign bodies, insect bites, or percussion injuries. A patient can have blood and drainage in the external ear from damage to the internal ear. Damage to the skull, brain, or spine may lead to cerebrospinal fluid leakage, resulting in bloody or clear drainage in the ear canal. If a head or neck injury is suspected, immobilize the patient. Cover the outside of the ear with a sterile dressing (if available), **do not irrigate** the ear, and get medical help immediately. In addition, **do not irrigate** the ear if the patient has any of the following conditions: anatomic abnormalities of the ear, a history of surgery involving the ear or ear canal (including myringotomy tubes), active dermatitis or infection of the ear canal and surrounding tissue, prior intolerance or adverse reaction to ear irrigation, or if the tympanic membrane is ruptured (Schwartz et al., 2017).

Safety Guidelines

- The greatest danger during ear irrigation is trauma to the tympanic membrane by forcing the irrigant into the ear canal under pressure

Delegation

The skill of performing ear irrigation cannot be delegated to assistive personnel (AP). Direct the AP to:

- Immediately report any potential side effects after an ear irrigation (e.g., pain, drainage, dizziness).
- Assist a patient when ambulating after the procedure because some light-headedness may be present, which increases a patient's risk for falling.

Collaboration

- Collaborate with the health care provider and audiology services as appropriate for a patient who requires ear irrigation.

Equipment

- Clean gloves
- Otoscope (optional)
- Irrigation or bulb syringe
- Basin for irrigating solution (Use sterile basin if sterile irrigating solution is used [i.e., when tympanic membrane is ruptured].)
- Emesis basin for drainage or irrigating solution exiting the ear
- Towel
- Cotton balls or 4 × 4-inch gauze
- Prescribed irrigating solution (e.g., normal saline) warmed to body temperature
- Cerumen softener: mineral oil or an over-the-counter softener
- Medication administration record (MAR) (print or electronic)

STEP	RATIONALE
1 Perform preprocedure protocol.	
Assessment	
• Review health care provider's order, including solution to be instilled and affected ear(s): right (AD), left (AS), or both (AU) to receive irrigation.	Ensures safe and correct administration of irrigant.
• Review electronic health record (EHR) for history of diabetes, eczema, or other skin problem in the ear canal, a weakened immune system, ruptured tympanic membrane, or placement of myringotomy tubes or other surgery of the auditory canal (American Academy of Otolaryngology–Head and Neck Surgery, 2021).	These conditions contraindicate irrigation.
• Perform hand hygiene and inspect pinna and external auditory meatus for redness, swelling, drainage, abrasions, and presence of cerumen or foreign objects. (Apply clean gloves if drainage present.)	Findings provide baseline to monitor effects of irrigation solution.

STEP	RATIONALE

CLINICAL JUDGMENT *Always try to remove foreign objects in ear by first simply straightening ear canal. This can cause object to fall out. If vegetable matter such as a dried bean or pea is occluded in the canal, do not perform irrigation. The material can swell on contact with water and cause further damage to the canal (Hockenberry et al., 2019).*

- Use otoscope to inspect deeper parts of auditory canal and tympanic membrane. *Caution:* If you visualize an object, do not push an object further into the ear canal.

  When auditory canal is unobstructed, this inspection verifies whether tympanic membrane is intact.

- Ask whether patient is having earache or fullness in the ear, partial hearing loss, tinnitus (ringing in the ear), itching or discharge from ear, or coughing (American Academy of Otolaryngology–Head and Neck Surgery, 2021).

  Common symptoms of cerumen impaction.

- Ask patient to describe any ear discomfort and rate severity on scale of 0 to 10.

  Provides baseline assessment. Pain is symptomatic of external ear infection or inflammation.

- Determine patient's hearing acuity by testing ability to hear your voice clearly.

  Occlusion of auditory canal by cerumen or foreign object can impair hearing.

Implementation

1 If irrigant contains medications other than normal saline, check accuracy and completeness of each MAR with health care provider's written procedure order. Check patient's name, drug name and dosage, route of administration, and time for administration. Compare MAR with label of ear irrigation solution.

   The order sheet is the most reliable source and only legal record of drugs or procedure that patient is to receive. Ensures that patient receives correct medication.

   First check for accuracy.

Continued

STEP	RATIONALE
2 If patient is found to have impacted cerumen, instill one or two drops of mineral oil or over-the-counter softener into ear twice a day for 2 to 3 days before irrigation (when possible).	Loosens cerumen and ensures easier removal during irrigation.
3 Inform patient that irrigation may cause sensation of dizziness, ear fullness, and warmth.	Promotes cooperation and prepares patient to anticipate effects of irrigation.
4 Assist patient into a sitting or lying position with head turned toward affected ear. Place towel under patient's head and ear. When possible have patient hold emesis basin.	Provides privacy. Positioning minimizes leakage of fluids around neck and facial area. Solution will flow from ear canal to basin.
5 Perform hand hygiene. Compare MAR with label of prescribed medicated irrigant (except when using normal saline). Pour irrigating solution into basin. Check label one more time. Check temperature of solution by pouring small drop on your inner forearm. *Note:* If sterile irrigating solution is used, sterile basin is required.	Reduces transfer of microorganisms; facilitates smooth performance of procedure. *Second and third check for medication accuracy.*
6 Apply clean gloves. Gently clean auricle and outer ear canal with gauze or cotton balls. Do *not* force drainage or cerumen into ear canal.	Prevents infected material from reentering ear canal. Forceful instillation of solution into occluded canal can cause injury to eardrum.
7 Fill irrigating syringe with solution (approximately 50 mL).	Enough fluid is needed to provide a steady irrigating stream.

STEP	RATIONALE
8 For adults and children over 3 years old, gently pull pinna up and back. In children 3 years or younger, pinna should be pulled down and back (Hockenberry et al., 2019). Adults can lie supine. Place tip of irrigating device just inside external meatus. Leave space around irrigating tip and canal.	Pulling pinna straightens external ear canal. This also prevents obstruction of canal with device, which can lead to increased pressure on tympanic membrane.
9 Slowly instill irrigating solution by holding tip of syringe 1 cm (½ inch) above opening to ear canal. Direct fluid toward superior aspect of ear canal. Allow fluid to drain out into basin during instillation. Continue until canal is cleaned or all solution is used (Fig. 20.1).	Slow instillation prevents pressure buildup in ear canal and ensures contact of solution with all canal surfaces.

Continued

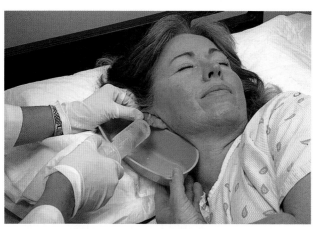

Fig. 20.1 Tip of syringe does not occlude ear canal during irrigation.

STEP	RATIONALE
10 Maintain irrigation flow in steady stream until pieces of cerumen or exudate flow from canal.	Constant flow of fluid loosens cerumen.
11 Periodically ask whether patient is experiencing pain, nausea, or vertigo.	Symptoms indicate that irrigating solution is too hot or too cold or instilled with too much pressure.
12 Drain excessive fluid from ear by having patient tilt head toward affected side.	Excess fluid may promote microorganism growth if not drained.
13 Dry outer ear canal gently with cotton ball. Leave cotton ball in place for 5 to 10 minutes.	Drying prevents moisture buildup that can lead to otitis externa.
14 Perform postprocedure protocol.	
15 Evaluate patient response:	
a Ask patient if discomfort is noted during instillation of solution.	Fluid instilled improperly under pressure causes discomfort.
b Ask patient about sensations of light-headedness or dizziness.	Instillation of fluid can cause these symptoms, which can put patient at risk for falling.
c Reinspect condition of meatus and canal.	Determines whether solution reduced inflammation and removed foreign materials.
d Assess patient's level of pain and hearing acuity, and assess for presence of preirrigation symptoms.	Determines whether cerumen is removed and hearing is improved.

Recording and Reporting

- Document indication for ear irrigation, symptoms of cerumen buildup or infection, condition of the tympanic membrane and ear canal before and after irrigation, characteristics of cerumen or other material removed, patient's hearing acuity before and after procedure, and patient's response to procedure.

- Record the type and amount of solution, time of administration, and the ear receiving the irrigation.
- Document evaluation of patient and family caregiver learning.
- Report indication for ear irrigation, which ear was irrigated, outcome of procedure, and any adverse effects, including change in hearing acuity.

UNEXPECTED OUTCOMES	RELATED INTERVENTIONS
1 Patient complains of increased ear pain during irrigation. Rupture of eardrum may have occurred.	• Stop irrigation immediately. • Notify health care provider immediately.
2 Ear canal remains occluded with cerumen.	• Repeat irrigation.
3 Foreign body remains in ear canal.	• Refer patient to otolaryngologist if foreign object remains after irrigation.

Obtaining a 12-Lead Electrocardiogram

Electrical impulses of the heart are conducted to the surface of the body and are detected by electrodes placed on the skin of the limbs and torso. The electrodes carry these impulses to either a continuous cardiac monitor or a 12-lead electrocardiograph machine. The appearance of the electrocardiogram (ECG) pattern or waveform helps to diagnose whether any abnormalities are affecting the electrical conduction through the heart. The 12-lead ECG provides a snapshot of the waveforms from 12 different angles or views of the heart. One electrode is placed on each of the four extremities, and six electrodes are placed at specific sites on the chest for a total of 10 electrodes on the patient's skin. They are bipolar limb leads I, II, and III; augmented limb leads a VR, aVL, aVF; and precordial chest leads V_1 to V_6. The leads view a specific part of the surface of the heart and can help determine which part of the heart has sustained or is sustaining damage and the origin and flow of the electrical impulse.

Safety Guidelines

- Patients with chest pain need to have their 12-lead ECG within 10 minutes of the assessment and onset of pain (Reeder and Kennedy, 2020). A 12-lead ECG will determine the next step in their treatment plan.
- Determine whether the patient took any nitroglycerin before admission because this may alter the ECG.

Delegation

The skill of obtaining a 12-lead ECG can be delegated to assistive personnel (AP) who are specifically trained in obtaining the measurement. Direct the AP to:

- Immediately report changes in the patient's cardiac status such as complaints of chest pain.
- Immediately deliver the completed 12-lead ECG recording to a health care provider for interpretation.
- Use specific patient precautions related to disease, mobility status, or position restrictions during care.

Collaboration

- Collaborate with the code team or cardiac catheterization laboratory personnel for possible emergency needs.

Equipment

- 12-lead electrocardiograph
- ECG leads with snap-on attachments or alligator clips
- ECG electrodes (disposable, self-adhesive)
- Clean, dry towel or sponge wipes
- Hair clippers (*optional*, depending on hair at electrode sites)

STEP	RATIONALE
1 Perform preprocedure protocol.	
Assessment	
• Review electronic health record (EHR) to determine indications for obtaining ECG. Assess patient's history and cardiopulmonary status (e.g., heart rate and rhythm, blood pressure, respirations).	If 12-lead ECG is ordered for chest pain or other ischemic signs and symptoms, obtain ECG within 10 minutes of patient's pain report.
• Assess for chest pain; rate acuity on scale of 0 to 10. Also note whether there are other sources of pain.	Determines level of chest discomfort, which may be warning for cardiac ischemia. Allows you to discriminate chest pain severity.
• Assess patient's ability to follow directions and remain still in a supine position.	Provides clear, accurate recording without artifact.
Implementation	
1 Perform hand hygiene and prepare patient for procedure.	Reduces transmission of microorganisms
2 Remove or reposition patient's clothing to expose only patient's chest and arms. Keep abdomen and thighs covered.	Facilitates correct placement of cardiac leads and maintains patient's modesty. Improper lead placement produces artifact, which necessitates repeating the test, or can cause interpretation errors.

Continued

STEP	RATIONALE
3 Place patient in supine position with head of bed no higher than 30 degrees.	Electrodes must be placed on anterior chest for standard 12-lead ECG (Prutkin, 2019a).
4 Instruct patient to lie still without talking and to keep legs uncrossed.	Body movement or talking produces artifact, which may necessitate repeating the test.
5 Turn on machine; enter required demographic information.	Turning machine on first helps to identify electrode and lead issues on application.
6 Clean and prepare skin for isolated electrode placement with soap and water. Wipe area with rough washcloth or gauze or use edge of electrode to gently scrape skin. Clip excessive hair from electrode area.	Proper skin preparation before ECG electrodes are placed decreases skin interference and signal noise, thereby producing a cleaner, more accurate recording. Do not use alcohol to clean area because it will dry out the skin. Electric clipping of hair in electrode area is preferred. Shaving leaves nicks that predispose to infection (Anderson and Sexton, 2020).

7 Apply electrodes in correct positions:
  a Chest (precordial) leads (Fig. 21.1):
    (1) V_1—Fourth intercostal space (ICS) at right sternal angle
    (2) V_2—Fourth ICS at left sternal border
    (3) V_3—Midway between V_2 and V_4
    (4) V_4—Fifth ICS at midclavicular line
    (5) V_5—Left anterior axillary line at level of V_4 horizontally
    (6) V_6—Left midaxillary line at level of V_4 horizontally
	Proper placement of leads is very important for accurate interpretation of 12-lead ECG. Ensure that the correct lead is in the correct location. If any leads are misplaced, ECG reading will be inaccurate (Prutkin, 2019a; Prutkin, 2019b).

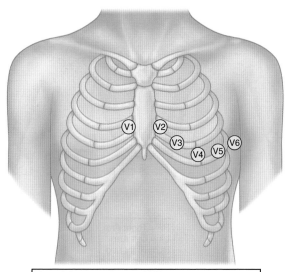

V1 – 4th intercostal space (ICS) at right sternal angle
V2 – 4th ICS at left sternal border
V3 – Midway between V2 and V4
V4 – Fifth ICS at midclavicular line
V5 – Left anterior axillary line at level of V4 horizontally
V6 – Left midaxillary line at level of V4 horizontally

Fig. 21.1 Chest electrode positioning for 12-lead ECG.

STEP	RATIONALE
b Extremities: One lead on each extremity (Fig. 21.2): right wrist, left wrist, right ankle, left ankle.	
8 Check 12-lead machine for messages indicating a need to correct electrode or lead issues. If no messages occur, press button to obtain 12-lead ECG. Allow to run for full 10 seconds.	Automatic machine calibration helps detect misconnections. Ten seconds is required for a standard rhythm strip.

Continued

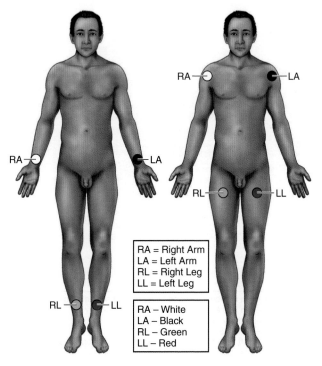

RA — LA

RA — LA

RL — LL

| RA = Right Arm |
| LA = Left Arm |
| RL = Right Leg |
| LL = Left Leg |

| RA – White |
| LA – Black |
| RL – Green |
| LL – Red |

RL — LL

Fig. 21.2 Limb electrode positioning for 12-lead ECG.

STEP	RATIONALE
9 Review tracing. If ECG tracing does not contain artifact, disconnect leads.	Ensures accurate reading. Promotes comfort and hygiene.
10 If ECG ordered stat, immediately deliver ECG tracing (if not computerized) to appropriate health care provider for interpretation.	If not a stat 12-lead ECG, place in patient's chart or designated area.

STEP	RATIONALE
11 Perform postprocedure protocol.	
12 Evaluate patient response:	
a Note and document if patient is experiencing any chest discomfort during procedure.	Helps correlate ECG changes to symptoms of chest pain.
b Discuss findings and results of 12-lead ECG with health care provider to determine next steps in patient's treatment plan.	If myocardial infarction is identified, immediate steps will need to be taken to get patient to cardiac catheterization laboratory or consider use of new medications (e.g., thrombolytics).

Recording and Reporting

- Record date and time ECG was obtained, reason for obtaining ECG, any symptoms patient experienced during procedure, and to whom ECG was given for interpretation.
- Document your evaluation of patient understanding of instructions/procedure.
- Report any chest pain or unexpected outcomes immediately.

UNEXPECTED OUTCOMES	RELATED INTERVENTIONS
1 ECG cannot be interpreted (absence of tracing on one or more leads, presence of artifact in ECG tracings).	• Inspect electrodes for secure placement. • Reposition any wires that move as a result of patient breathing, movement, or vibrations in environment. Do not reposition electrodes if in correct position. • If patient is moving, remind patient that lying still is necessary to obtain good tracing.

Continued

UNEXPECTED OUTCOMES	RELATED INTERVENTIONS
	• If artifact looks like 60-cycle interference (very thick-lined waveform), unplug battery-operated equipment in room one item at a time to see if interference disappears. *Note:* 60-cycle interference is rare.
	• Repeat tracing.
2 Patient has chest pain or anxiety.	• Continue to monitor patient.
	• Reassess factors contributing to anxiety or distress.
	• Follow specific orders related to findings.
	• Notify health care provider.

Enema Administration

An enema is the instillation of a solution into the rectum and sigmoid colon to promote defecation by stimulating peristalsis. Although the first choice of therapies includes dietary changes, bulk-forming laxatives, and non–bulk-forming laxatives to treat constipation, an enema may be prescribed for immediate relief. Other reasons to give an enema may be to prepare a patient for surgery or diagnostic procedures (Caffrey and Pensa, 2019). Enemas such as soap suds and saline act by stimulating peristalsis through the infusion of large volumes of solution. Oil-retention enemas act by lubricating the rectum and colon, allowing feces to absorb oil and become softer and easier to pass.

Medicated enemas contain pharmacologic therapeutic agents. Some are prescribed to reduce dangerously high serum potassium levels (e.g., sodium polystyrene sulfonate enema) or to reduce bacteria in the colon before bowel surgery (e.g., neomycin enema).

Safety Guidelines

- Do not repeat a tap water enema after first instillation because water toxicity or circulatory overload can develop.
- Remain near a patient's room after enema administration. Answer call light promptly to assist patient to bathroom. Slow response to call light is a common contributing factor to patient falls. Patients will try to independently get to bathroom when they have the urge to defecate.

Delegation

The skill of administering an enema can be delegated to assistive personnel (AP) (see agency policy). *Note:* If a medicated enema is ordered, it must be administered by a nurse. Instruct the AP about:

- How to properly position patients who have mobility restrictions or therapeutic equipment such as drains, intravenous (IV) catheters, or traction.
- Immediately reporting patient's new-onset abdominal pain (Exception: a patient reports cramping) or rectal bleeding.
- Immediately reporting the presence of blood in the stool or around the rectal area or any change in vital signs.

Equipment

- Clean gloves
- Water-soluble local anesthetic lubricant (Note: Some facilities require use of water-soluble lubricant without anesthetic when a nurse performs procedure.)

221

Fig. 22.1 Prepackaged enema container with rectal tip and cap.

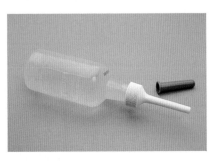

- Waterproof, absorbent pads
- Bedpan
- Bedpan cover (optional if available)
- Bath blanket
- Washbasin, washcloths, towels, and soap

Enema Bag Administration

- Enema container
- IV pole
- Tubing and clamp (if not already attached to container)
- Appropriate-size rectal tube (adult, 22 to 30 Fr; child, 12 to 18 Fr)
- Correct volume of warmed (tepid) solution (adult, 750 to 1000 mL; adolescent, 500 to 700 mL; school-age child, 300 to 500 mL; toddler, 250 to 350 mL; infant, 150 to 250 mL) (Hockenberry et al., 2019)

Prepackaged Enema

- Prepackaged enema container with lubricated rectal tip (Fig. 22.1)

STEP	RATIONALE
1 Perform preprocedure protocol.	

Assessment

STEP	RATIONALE
• Review health care provider's order for enema and clarify reason for administration.	Order by health care provider is usually required for hospitalized patient. Order states which type of enema patient will receive.
• Review electronic health record (EHR) or ask patient about last bowel movement, baseline/normal versus most recent bowel pattern, presence of hemorrhoids, and presence of abdominal pain or cramping.	Determines need for enema and type of enema used. Also establishes baseline for bowel function. Hemorrhoids may obscure rectal opening and cause discomfort or bleeding during evacuation.

STEP	RATIONALE
• Assess patient's mobility and ability to turn and position on side.	Determines whether you need assistance in positioning patient.
• Ask patient to describe history of allergies, with focus on allergies to active ingredients of Fleet enema. Have patient describe typical allergic reaction. List allergies on each page of medication administration record (MAR). Check patient's allergy wristband. Confer with health care provider about alternative enema.	Communication of patient allergies is an essential part of safe medication administration.
• Perform hand hygiene. Inspect and palpate abdomen for presence of distention and ask if patient feels discomfort.	Reduces transmission of microorganisms. Establishes assessment baseline before administering enema.

CLINICAL JUDGMENT *When "enemas until clear" is ordered, the water expelled may be tinted but should not contain solid fecal material. It is essential to observe contents of solution passed. A patient should typically receive only three consecutive enemas to prevent fluid and electrolyte imbalance (check agency policy).*

Implementation

1 Check accuracy and completeness of each MAR with health care provider's written order. (This applies to medicated enemas). Check patient's name, type of enema, and time for administration. Compare MAR with label of enema solution.	The health care provider's order is most reliable source and only legal record of drugs or procedure that patient is to receive. Ensures that patient receives correct enema.
2 Perform hand hygiene. Obtain medicated enema from medication storage system. Otherwise obtain enema from supply area.	

Continued

STEP	RATIONALE
3 Arrange supplies at bedside. Place bedpan or bedside commode in easily accessible position. If patient will be expelling contents in toilet, ensure that toilet is available and place patient's nonskid slippers and bathrobe in easily accessible position.	Bedpan is used if patient is unable to get out of bed. Toilet availability and nonskid slippers help prevent falls.
4 Perform hand hygiene.	Reduces transmission of microorganisms.
5 With side rail raised on patient's left side and bed raised to appropriate working height, help patient turn onto left side-lying (Sims) position with right knee flexed. Determine that patient is comfortable and encourage patient to remain in position until procedure is complete. *Note:* Place a child in the dorsal recumbent position.	Allows enema solution to flow downward by gravity along natural curve of sigmoid colon and rectum, thus improving retention of solution.

CLINICAL JUDGMENT *Patients with poor sphincter control require placement of a bedpan under the buttocks. Administering enema with patient sitting on toilet is unsafe because curved rectal tubing can cause abrasions to rectal wall.*

STEP	RATIONALE
6 Apply clean gloves and place waterproof pad, absorbent side up, under hips and buttocks. Cover patient with bath blanket, exposing only rectal area, clearly visualizing anus.	Pad prevents soiling of linen. Blanket provides warmth, reduces exposure of body parts, and allows patient to feel more relaxed and comfortable.

STEP	RATIONALE
7 Separate buttocks and examine perianal region for abnormalities, including hemorrhoids, anal fissure, and rectal prolapse.	Findings influence approach for inserting enema tip. Prolapse contraindicates enema.
8 Administer enema:	Verbalize to the patient when you will be touching their buttocks and inserting the enema tubing.
a Prepackaged disposable enema:	
(1) Remove plastic cap from tip of container. Tip may already be lubricated. Apply more water-soluble lubricant as needed	Lubrication provides for smooth insertion of rectal tube without causing rectal irritation or trauma. With presence of hemorrhoids, extra lubricant provides added comfort.
(2) Gently separate buttocks and locate anus. Instruct patient to relax by breathing out slowly through mouth. Inform patient when tip is to be inserted.	Breathing out promotes relaxation of external rectal sphincter.
(3) Hold container upright and expel any air from enema container.	Introducing air into colon causes further distention and discomfort.
(4) Insert lubricated tip of container gently into anal canal toward umbilicus (Fig. 22.2): *Adult:* 7.5–10 cm (3–4 inches)	Gentle insertion prevents trauma to rectal mucosa.

Continued

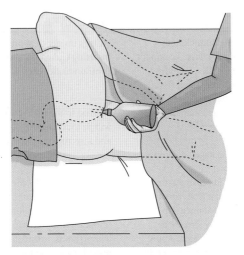

Fig. 22.2 With patient in left lateral Sims position, insert tip of commercial enema into rectum. (From Sorrentino SA: *Mosby's textbook for nursing assistants*, ed 7, St Louis, 2009, Mosby.)

STEP	RATIONALE
Adolescent: 7.5 cm–10 cm (3–4 inches) *Child:* 5–7.5 cm (2–3 inches) *Infant:* 2.5–3.75 cm (1–1½ inches)	

CLINICAL JUDGMENT *If pain occurs or you feel resistance at any time during procedure, stop and discuss with health care provider. Do not force insertion.*

STEP	RATIONALE
(5) Squeeze and roll plastic bottle from bottom to tip until all of solution has entered rectum and colon. Instruct patient to retain solution until urge to defecate occurs, usually in 2 to 5 minutes.	Prevents instillation of air into colon and ensures that all content enters rectum. Hypertonic solutions require only small volumes to stimulate defecation.
b Administer enema in standard enema bag:	
(1) Add warmed prescribed type of solution and amount to enema bag. Options: Warm tap water as it flows from faucet. Place saline container in basin of warm water before adding saline to enema bag. Check temperature of solution by pouring small amount of solution over inner wrist.	Hot water burns intestinal mucosa. Cold water causes abdominal cramping and is difficult to retain.
(2) If soapsuds enema (SSE) is ordered, add castile soap after water.	Reduces suds in enema bag.
(3) Raise container, release clamp, and allow solution to flow long enough to fill tubing.	Removes air from tubing.

Continued

STEP	RATIONALE
(4) Reclamp tubing.	Prevents further loss of solution.
(5) Lubricate 6–8 cm (2½–3 inches) of tip of rectal tube with lubricant.	Allows smooth insertion of rectal tube without risk for irritation or trauma to mucosa.
(6) Gently separate buttocks and locate anus. Verbalize when enema tip will be inserted. Instruct patient to relax by breathing out slowly through mouth. Touch patient's skin next to anus with tip of rectal tube.	Breathing out and touching skin with tube promotes relaxation of external anal sphincter.
(7) Insert tip of rectal tube slowly by pointing it in direction of patient's umbilicus. Length of insertion varies.	Careful insertion prevents trauma to rectal mucosa from accidental lodging of tube against rectal wall. Insertion beyond proper limit can cause bowel perforation.

CLINICAL JUDGMENT *If tube does not pass easily, do not force. Consider allowing a small amount of fluid to infuse, and then try to reinsert the tube slowly. The instillation of fluid relaxes the sphincter and provides additional lubrication. If fecal impaction is present, remove before administering the enema.*

STEP	RATIONALE
(8) Hold tubing in rectum constantly until end of fluid instillation.	Prevents expulsion of rectal tube during bowel contractions.
(9) Open regulating clamp and allow solution to enter slowly with container at patient's hip level.	Rapid infusion stimulates evacuation of tubing and can cause cramping.

STEP	RATIONALE
(10) Raise height of enema container slowly to appropriate level above anus: 30–45 cm (12–18 inches) for high enema; 30 cm (12 inches) for regular enema (Fig. 22.3); 7.5 cm (3 inches) for low enema. Instillation time varies with volume of solution administered (e.g., 1 L may take 10 minutes). You may use an IV pole to hold an enema bag once you establish a slow flow of fluid.	Allows for continuous, slow instillation of solution. Raising container too high causes rapid instillation and possible painful distention of colon. High pressure can result in bowel rupture.

CLINICAL JUDGMENT *Temporary cessation of infusion minimizes cramping and promotes ability to retain solution. Lower container or clamp tubing if patient complains of cramping or if fluid escapes around rectal tube.*

(11) Instill all solution and clamp tubing. Tell patient that procedure is completed and that you will remove tubing.	Prevents air entering rectum. Patient may misinterpret sensation of removing tube as loss of control.
9 Place layers of toilet tissue around tube at anus and gently withdraw rectal tube and tip.	Provides for patient's comfort and cleanliness.

Continued

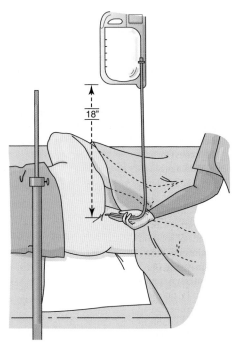

Fig. 22.3 Intravenous (IV) pole is positioned so
bottom of enema bag is 45 cm (18 inches) above anus.
(From Sorrentino SA: *Mosby's textbook for nursing
assistants*, ed 7, St Louis, 2009, Mosby.)

STEP	RATIONALE
10 Explain to patient that some distention and abdominal cramping are normal. Ask the patient to retain solution as long as possible until urge to defecate occurs. This usually takes a few minutes. **Stay at bedside**. Have patient lie quietly in bed if possible. (For infant or young child gently hold buttocks together for few minutes.) Keep call light within patient's reach.	Solution distends bowel. Length of retention varies with type of enema and patient's ability to contract rectal sphincter. Longer retention promotes stimulation of peristalsis and defecation.

STEP	RATIONALE
11 Help patient to bathroom or commode as needed. If using bedpan, apply clean gloves and help patient to as near a normal position for evacuation as possible.	Normal squatting position promotes defecation.
12 After patient has defecated, assist as needed to wash anal area with warm soap and water (use gloves for perineal care).	Fecal contents irritate skin. Hygiene promotes patient's comfort.
13 Perform postprocedure protocol	
14 Evaluate patient response: a Observe character of stool and solution (instruct patient not to flush toilet before inspection).	Determines whether enema was effective.
b Palpate for abdominal distention and ask if discomfort present.	Determines whether distention is relieved.

Recording and Reporting

- Record the time, type, and volume of enema administered; patient's signs and symptoms; response to enema; and results, including color, amount, and appearance of stool.
- Report failure of patient to defecate or any adverse reactions to health care provider.

UNEXPECTED OUTCOMES	RELATED INTERVENTIONS
1 Severe abdominal cramping, bleeding, or sudden abdominal pain develops and is unrelieved by temporarily stopping or slowing flow of solution.	• Stop enema. • Notify health care provider. • Obtain vital signs.
2 Patient is unable to hold enema solution.	• Slow rate of infusion.

Enteral Nutrition: Nasogastric, Nasointestinal, Gastrostomy, or Jejunostomy Tube

Enteral nutrition (EN), or tube feeding, is a method for providing nutrients to patients who are not able to meet their nutrition requirements orally. As a rule, candidates for EN must have a sufficiently functional gastrointestinal tract to digest and absorb nutrients. Examples of indications for enteral feeding include:

- Conditions in which normal eating is unsafe because of high risk for aspiration: altered mental status, swallowing disorders, impaired gag reflex, dependence on mechanical ventilation, unfavorable esophageal conditions, and delayed gastric emptying.
- Clinical conditions that interfere with normal ingestion or absorption of nutrients or create hypermetabolic states: surgical resection of oropharynx, proximal intestinal obstruction or fistula, pancreatitis, burns, and severe pressure injuries.
- Conditions in which disease or treatment-related symptoms reduce oral intake: anorexia, nausea, pain, fatigue, shortness of breath, or depression.

Gastric feedings are the most common type of EN, allowing tube-feeding formulas to enter the stomach and then pass gradually through the intestinal tract to ensure absorption. In contrast, small-bowel feeding occurs beyond the pyloric sphincter of the stomach, which theoretically reduces the risk for pulmonary aspiration, provided that feedings do not reflux into the stomach (Powers et al., 2021; VanBlarcom and McCoy, 2018). To avoid bloating, cramping, and diarrhea, using an enteral infusion pump controls the administration rate of small-bowel feedings and many continuous gastric feedings.

Nasally or orally placed feeding tubes are used for short-term feeding (less than 4 to 6 weeks) and are inserted with tips located in the stomach (nasogastric tube) or small bowel (nasointestinal tube). For long-term feeding (more than 4 to 6 weeks), feeding tubes may be inserted directly through a patient's abdominal wall into the stomach (gastrostomy, jejunostomy). Most patients will tolerate feeding into the stomach. Conversion to intestinal feeding should be done only when gastric feeding is poorly tolerated owing to ileus of the stomach, gastroparesis (delayed gastric emptying), high risk for aspiration, or mechanical issues (gastric resection) (McClave et al., 2016).

Feeding tubes that end in the stomach deliver feedings by gravity bolus or continuous infusion by infusion pumps. The small intestine does not have the storage capacity of the stomach, and therefore a tube feeding administered into the small intestine is delivered more slowly and continuously with an infusion pump.

Safety Guidelines

- Inserting air into a feeding tube while auscultating for abdominal sounds is **not recommended** to confirm tube placement.
  Sounds may be transmitted to the epigastrium whether the tube is positioned in the lung, esophagus, stomach, duodenum, or proximal jejunum (Fan et al., 2017).
- The most common complication of blindly inserted feeding tubes (tubes not confirmed by x-ray) is improper placement in the esophagus or pulmonary system (Irving et al., 2018; Metheny et al., 2019).
- Maintaining and monitoring enteral tube location during enteral feeding and keeping the head-of-bed (HOB) elevation at a minimum of 30 degrees (preferably 45 degrees) effectively reduces aspiration and subsequent pneumonia (Metheny et al., 2019; VanBlarcom and McCoy, 2018).
- Gastric residual volumes (GRVs) are measured routinely during tube feeding to identify risk for regurgitation and pulmonary aspiration of gastric contents.
- Nasal tubes are associated with sinusitis, otitis, vocal cord paralysis, and medical device–related pressure injury (MDRPI) to the nose. Use of adhesives to anchor tubes at nose may cause medical adhesive related skin injury (MARSI) (Fumarola et al., 2020).
- Use ENFit connectors for all EN sets, syringes, and feeding tubes to prevent instillation of feeding into a different device (e.g., IV line or drainage tube).

Delegation

The skill of administration of nasoenteric tube feeding can be delegated to assistive personnel (AP) in some settings (refer to agency policy). A registered nurse or licensed practical nurse must first verify tube placement and patency. Direct the AP to:

- Keep patient positioned with HOB elevated to 30 to 45 degrees or sit patient upright in bed or chair (unless contraindicated).
- Infuse feeding as ordered; do not adjust feeding rate.

- Report any difficulty infusing the feeding or any discomfort voiced by the patient.
- Report any gagging, paroxysms of coughing, or choking.
- Provide frequent oral hygiene.

Collaboration

- Registered dietitian (RD) and health care provider determine patient's caloric and protein requirements.

Equipment

- Disposable feeding bag, tubing, or ready-to-hang system
- 60-mL or larger ENFit syringe
- Stethoscope
- Enteral infusion pump for continuous feedings
- pH indicator strip (scale 1.0 to 11.0)
- Water for flushing tube; purified or sterile as indicated
- Prescribed enteral formula (standard polymetric, high protein or disease specific [Allen and Hoffman, 2019; McClave et al., 2016])
- Clean gloves
- ENFit connector

STEP	RATIONALE
1 Perform preprocedure protocol.	

Assessment

• Review electronic health record (EHR) for health care provider's order for type of formula, rate, route, and frequency.	Ensures that correct formula will be administered in appropriate volume. Enteral formulas are not interchangeable.
• Ask patient to describe history of allergies: known type of allergies and normal allergic reaction. Focus on foods and adhesives. Check patient's allergy wristband.	Do not administer tube-feeding formula if there is a known patient allergy. Communication of patient allergies is essential for safe patient care.
• Assess patient for factors that increase risk for aspiration: sedation, mechanical ventilation, nasotracheal suctioning, neurologic compromise, lying flat, and sepsis (Eglseer et al., 2018).	Identifies patients at high risk so that decision can be made based on safety of gastric versus intestinal feeding (Ukleja et al., 2018).

STEP	RATIONALE
• Perform hand hygiene. Perform physical assessment of abdomen, including auscultation for bowel sounds, before feeding. Report findings to health care provider to determine whether tube feeding can proceed safely (Harding et al., 2020; VanBlarcom and McCoy, 2018).	Objective measures assess potential tolerance to tube feedings, including changes in bowel sounds, expanding girth, tenderness and firmness on palpation, increasing nasogastric output, and vomiting (VanBlarcom and McCoy, 2018).
• Obtain baseline weight and review serum electrolytes and blood glucose measurement. Assess patient for fluid volume excess or deficit, electrolyte abnormalities, and metabolic abnormalities (e.g., hyperglycemia).	Enteral feedings should restore or maintain patient's nutrition status. Measures provide objective baseline to determine selection of formula and measure effectiveness of feedings.

Implementation

STEP	RATIONALE
1 Perform hand hygiene. Apply clean gloves.	Reduces transmission of microorganisms and potential contamination of enteral formula.
2 Reverify correct formula and check expiration date; note integrity of container and appearance of formula.	Ensures that correct therapy is to be administered and checks integrity of formula.
3 Prepare formula for administration, following manufacturer guidelines:	

CLINICAL JUDGMENT *Discard unused reconstituted and refrigerated formula within 24 h of preparation (Boullata et al., 2017).*

STEP	RATIONALE
a Have formula at room temperature.	Cold formula causes gastric cramping and discomfort because liquid is not warmed by mouth and esophagus.

Continued

STEP	RATIONALE
b Use aseptic technique to make all connections, including connection of tubing to enteral feeding container. Use proper ENFit connecter and avoid handling feeding system or touching can tops, container openings, spike, and spike port.	Bag, connections, and tubing must be free of contamination to prevent bacterial growth. The use of a closed system lowers the risk of infections due to bacterial contaminants (Boullata et al., 2017).
c Shake formula container well. Clean top of canned formula with alcohol swab before opening it.	Ensures integrity of formula; prevents transmission of microorganisms.
d For closed systems, connect administration tubing to container. If using open system, pour formula from brick pack or can into administration bag (Fig. 23.1).	Formulas are available in closed-system containers that contain a 24- to 48-h supply of formula, or in an open system in which formula must be transferred from brick packs or cans to a bag before administration.
4 Open roller clamp and allow administration tubing to fill. Clamp off tubing with roller clamp. Hang container on IV pole.	Prevents introduction of air into stomach once feeding begins.
5 Keep patient in high Fowler position or elevate HOB at least 30 degrees (45 degrees is recommended). For patient forced to remain supine, place in reverse Trendelenburg position, which raises head.	Elevated head helps prevent pulmonary aspiration (ASPEN, 2021). Researchers recommend HOB elevation of 45 degrees for patients receiving mechanical ventilation or who are heavily sedated, but lowering the HOB to 30 degrees might be done periodically for patient comfort and for patients at risk for developing pressure injuries (Schallom et al., 2015).

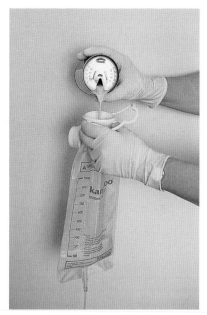

Fig. 23.1 Pour formula into open feeding container.

STEP	RATIONALE
6 Verify tube placement (see Skill 24). Observe appearance of aspirate and note the pH (Fig. 23.2): a Nasoenteric tube: Attach ENFit syringe to end of enteral feeding tube and aspirate gastric or intestinal contents. Observe appearance of aspirate and note pH.	Verifies that tip of tube is in stomach, intestine, or lung based on pH value of less than or equal to 5 (Fan et al., 2017). Gastric fluid in patient who has fasted for at least 4 h usually has pH of 1.0 to 4.0 (unless receiving gastric acid inhibitor, then pH of ≤5) (Fan et al., 2017). If patient is receiving continuous feedings into stomach or intestine, check pH if feedings are held for at least 1 h for diagnostic reasons (stomach pH ≤5, intestinal pH >6) (Fan et al., 2017).

Continued

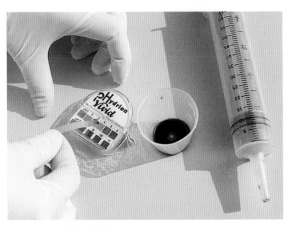

Fig. 23.2 Check pH of gastric aspirate.

STEP	RATIONALE
b Gastrostomy tube: Attach ENFit syringe to end of tube and aspirate gastric contents. Observe appearance of aspirate and note pH.	Gastric fluid in patient who has fasted for at least 4 h usually has pH of 1.0 to 4.0 (unless receiving gastric acid inhibitor, then pH of ≤5) (Fan et al., 2017). If patient is receiving continuous feedings into stomach or intestine, check pH if feedings are held for at least 1 h for diagnostic reasons (stomach pH ≤5, intestinal pH >6) (Fan et al., 2017).
c Jejunostomy tube: Attach ENFit syringe to end of tube and aspirate intestinal secretions. Observe appearance; if significant amounts are returned or resemble gastric secretions, check pH.	Presence of intestinal fluid at pH >6 indicates that end of tube is in small intestine. If fluid tests acidic on pH test or looks like gastric fluid, tube may be displaced into stomach.

STEP	RATIONALE
7 Check GRV per agency policy. Routine use is no longer recommended (Boullata et al., 2017) and should not be used as a single measure of tolerance.	GRV has poor correlation with pneumonia, regurgitation, and aspiration. Frequent checking may delay feeding. However, if other signs (e.g., abdominal distention or pain) of intolerance are present, GRV of 250 to 500 mL may indicate the need to take measures to prevent aspiration or hold feeding completely (Boullata et al., 2017). Determines whether gastric emptying is delayed. Intestinal residual volume is usually very small. If residual volume is >10 mL, displacement of tube into stomach may have occurred.

CLINICAL JUDGMENT *Limit gastric residual checks to recommended standard intervals because acidic gastric contents may cause protein in enteral feeding to precipitate within the lumen of the tube, causing risk for obstruction. Frequent GRV measurements lead to an increased risk of tube occlusion and decreased amount of EN delivered to the patient (Boullata et al., 2017).*

a Draw up 10 to 30 mL air into ENFit syringe and connect to end of feeding tube. Inject air slowly into tube. Pull back slowly and aspirate any available gastric contents.	GRV may not be easy to obtain from small-bore feeding tube owing to smaller tube diameter, which can result in gastric tube collapse (Harding et al., 2020). A 60-mL syringe prevents gastric tube collapse.
b Return aspirated contents to stomach slowly unless volume exceeds 250 mL (see agency policy) (Clore et al., 2019; Metheny, 2016; VanBlarcom and McCoy, 2018).	Prevents loss of nutrients and electrolytes in discarded fluid. Some questions exist regarding safety of returning high volumes of fluid into stomach (Metheny, 2016).

Continued

STEP	RATIONALE
c GRVs in range of 200 to 500 mL should raise concern and lead to implementation of measures to reduce aspiration risk. Automatic cessation of feeding should not occur for GRV less than 500 mL in absence of other signs of intolerance (Metheny et al., 2019; VanBlarcom and McCoy, 2018).	Raising cutoff value for GRV from lower number to higher number does not increase risk for regurgitation, aspiration, or pneumonia. Elevated GRV should raise concern and lead to measures to reduce aspiration risk (Metheny et al., 2019; VanBlarcom and McCoy, 2018).
d Flush feeding tube with 30 mL water.	Prevents tube clogging and ensures that complete feeding is administered.
8 Intermittent feeding (administered at certain times during the day):	
a Pinch proximal end of feeding tube and remove cap. Connect distal end of administration set tubing to ENFit device on feeding tube and release tubing.	Prevents excessive air from entering patient's stomach and leakage of gastric contents. ENFit devices are not compatible with Luer-Lok connections. The use of these devices ensures that feeding will be administered into the correct tubing and prevents administration of enteral feeding or medication by the wrong route, such as IV tubing (Institute for Safe Medication Practices, 2022).

STEP	RATIONALE
b Set rate by adjusting roller clamp on tubing or attach tubing to feeding pump (Fig. 23.3A). Allow bag to empty gradually over 30 to 45 minutes (length of time of a comfortable meal). Label bag with patient identifiers, formula type, enteral delivery site (route and access), administration method and type, and volume and frequency of water flushes (Boullata et al., 2017). Also include label with date, time, and initials when hanging a feeding.	Gradual emptying of tube feeding reduces risk for abdominal discomfort, vomiting, or diarrhea induced by bolus or too-rapid infusion of tube feedings. Critical elements for an EN order should be on EN label (Boullata et al., 2017). Labeling helps to determine when to change administration set and confirms that the right patient is receiving feeding.

CLINICAL JUDGMENT *Use pumps designated for tube feeding, not for IV fluids.*

c Immediately follow feeding with prescribed amount of water (per health care provider's orders or agency policy). Cover end of feeding tube with cap when not in use. Keep bag as clean as possible. Change administration set every 24 h.	Prevents tube from clogging. Prevents air from entering stomach between feedings and limits microbial contamination of system.
9 Continuous infusion method:	Method delivers prescribed hourly rate of feeding and reduces risk for abdominal discomfort.

Continued

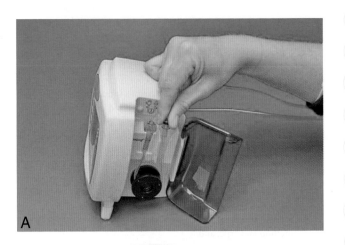

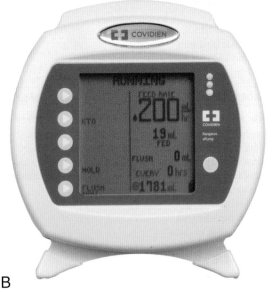

Fig. 23.3 (A) Connect tubing through infusion pump. (B) Set pump as ordered. (Images used with permission of Covidien, Dublin, Ireland. All rights reserved.)

STEP	RATIONALE
a Remove cap on tubing and connect distal end of administration set tubing to feeding tube using ENFit connector as in Step 8a.	Prevents excess air from entering patient's stomach and leakage of gastric contents.
b Thread tubing through feeding pump; open regulator clamp, set rate of infusion on pump, then start pump. (Fig. 23.3A & B).	Delivers continuous feeding at steady rate and pressure. Feeding pump alarms for increased resistance.
c Advance rate of tube feeding (and concentration of feeding) gradually, as ordered.	Tube feeding can usually begin with full-strength formula. Conservative initiation and advancement of EN depend on factors such as patient's age, medical condition, nutrition status, and expected patient tolerance (Boullata et al., 2017; VanBlarcom and McCoy, 2018).

CLINICAL JUDGMENT *Limit infusion time for open EN feeding systems to 4 to 8 h maximum (12 h in the home setting) (Boullata et al., 2017). Follow the manufacturer's recommendations for duration of infusion through an intact closed delivery system (Boullata et al., 2017.)*

10 After feeding, flush tubing with 30 mL water every 4 h during continuous feeding (see agency policy) or before and after an intermittent feeding or medication administration. Have RD recommend total free-water requirement per day and obtain health care provider's order.	Provides patient with source of water to help maintain fluid and electrolyte balance. Clears tubing of formula.
11 Rinse bag and tubing with warm water whenever feedings are interrupted. Use new administration set every 24 h.	Rinsing bag and tubing with warm water clears old tube feedings and reduces bacterial growth.

Continued

STEP	RATIONALE
12 Help patient to assume and remain in comfortable position with HOB elevated at least 30 to 45 degrees.	Promotes patient comfort and reduces risk for aspiration of EN.
13 Perform postprocedure protocol.	
14 Evaluate patient response:	
a Monitor patient's tolerance to feeding by evaluating for abdominal distention, firmness, feeling of fullness, or nausea (Boullata et al., 2017). Measure GRV per agency policy, but measurement frequency should be limited.	Gastrointestinal tolerance of tube feedings must be monitored closely to avoid complications. Excess removal of GRV can cause electrolyte imbalance.
b Monitor intake and output (I&O) at least every 8 h and calculate daily totals every 24 h.	I&O is an indication of fluid balance, which can indicate fluid volume excess or deficit.
c Weigh patient daily until maximum administration rate is reached and maintained for 24 h; then weigh patient three times per week.	Slow weight gain is indicator of improved nutrition status; however, sudden gain of more than 2 lb (0.9 kg) in 24 h usually indicates fluid retention.
d Monitor patient for appropriate tube feeding placement by measuring pH at least every 4 h or per agency policy. Monitor visible length of tubing or marking at tube exit site and check placement when deviation is noted (Boullata et al., 2017).	Accidental displacement of tip of tube could lead to aspiration.

STEP	RATIONALE
e Monitor laboratory values as ordered by health care provider.	Determines correct administration of formula rate and strength.
f Observe patient's respiratory status for coughing, dyspnea, tachypnea, change in oxygen saturation, hoarseness, or crackles in lungs.	Change in respiratory status may indicate aspiration of tube feeding into respiratory tract.
6 Inspect point of tube insertion and securement at least daily for medical device–related pressure injury or MARSI: skin irritation, abrasion, inflammation, tenderness, edema.	Enteral tubes often cause pressure and excoriation at insertion site. If adhesive secures tubing, patient is also at risk for MARSI.

Recording and Reporting

- Record amount and type of feeding, infusion rate (continuous feeding) or time of infusion (bolus method), pH and GRV measurements, feeding tube position, patient's response to tube feeding, tube patency, and skin condition at tube site.
- Document evaluation of patient and family caregiver learning.
- Record volume of formula and any additional water on I&O form.
- Report adverse outcomes to the health care provider.
- During hand-off report, indicate the type of feeding, infusion rate, and patient's tolerance, and trace the administration set tubing to the enteral tube connection point to ensure feeding is being infused enterally (Boullata et al., 2017).

UNEXPECTED OUTCOMES	RELATED INTERVENTIONS
1 Feeding tube becomes clogged.	• Attempt to flush tube with water. • Special products are available for unclogging feeding tubes; **do not** use carbonated beverages and juices. • Hold feeding and notify health care provider. • Maintain patient in semi-Fowler position. • Collaborate with pharmacist and/or health care provider to change medications to liquid form. Flush before and after intermittent feedings and medications (Boullata et al., 2017; Lord, 2018).
2 Patient develops large amount of diarrhea (more than three loose stools in 24 h).	• Notify health care provider. • Consult RD about need to change formula to prevent malabsorption. • Identify and treat underlying medical/surgical issues and infections (Lord, 2018). • Provide perianal skin care after each stool. • Determine other causes of diarrhea (e.g., *Clostridium difficile* infection, contaminated tube feeding, medication containing sorbitol).
3 Patient aspirates formula (auscultation of crackles or wheezes; dyspnea; or fever).	• Immediately report change in condition to health care provider. • Immediately position patient on side with head of bed elevated as tolerated. • Suction nasotracheally or orotracheally.

Enteral Tube Insertion

Small-bore feeding tubes deliver enteral nutrition directly into the stomach (nasogastric [NG] tube) or small intestine (nasointestinal [NI] tube) (Skill 23). The enteral tubes are inserted through either the nose or the mouth. The nose is the most common route. Enteral feeding tubes are soft and flexible and therefore may require a removable guidewire or stylet to provide stiffness during insertion. Some evidence suggests that placing the tip of a feeding tube past the pyloric sphincter (postpyloric feeding) may reduce the risk of aspiration and allow for greater delivery of prescribed nutrition (Seres, 2021).

Placement of a small-bore tube into the intestine can be technically difficult, and assistive devices (electromagnetic tracing, capnography) provide improved safety and success rate of bedside placement (Hodin and Bordeianou, 2019). However, radiographic confirmation remains the gold standard in confirming tube placement (Anderson, 2019; Boullata et al., 2017). In some cases, the health care provider may order a prokinetic agent such as metoclopramide to assist with advancement of a tube beyond the pylorus. Confirmation of the correct position of a newly inserted tube is mandatory via x-ray before any feeding or medication is administered.

Safety Guidelines

- All candidates for NG or NI tube placement require an assessment of their coagulation status. Anticoagulation and bleeding disorders pose a risk for epistaxis during nasal tube placement; the health care provider may order platelet transfusion or other corrective measures before tube insertion.
- Tube placement must be confirmed by x-ray. The most common complication of blindly inserted feeding tubes is improper placement in the esophagus or pulmonary system (Boullata et al., 2017; Irving et al., 2018; Metheny et al., 2019).
- Nasal tubes are associated with sinusitis, otitis, vocal cord paralysis, and medical device–related pressure injuries (MDRPI) to the nose.

Delegation

- The skill of enteral feeding tube insertion cannot be delegated to assistive personnel (AP). However, the AP may help with patient positioning and comfort measures during tube insertion.

Collaboration

- Inserting a nasoenteric feeding tube with a stylet is done in collaboration with an advanced practice nurse or other certified health care provider. Check agency policy.

Equipment

Insertion

Small-bore feeding tube with or without stylet (select the smallest diameter possible to enhance patient comfort)

- 60-mL ENFit syringe
- Stethoscope, pulse oximeter, capnograph *(optional)*
- Hypoallergenic tape, semipermeable (transparent) membrane dressing, or tube fixation device
- Skin barrier protectant
- pH indicator strip (scale 1.0 to 11.0)
- Cup of water and straw or ice chips (for patients able to swallow who are not on nothing by mouth status)
- Water-soluble lubricant
- Emesis basin
- Towel or disposable pad
- Facial tissues
- Clean gloves
- Suction equipment in case of aspiration
- Penlight to check placement in nasopharynx
- Tongue blade
- Oral hygiene supplies

Removal

- Disposable pad
- Tissues
- Clean gloves
- Disposable plastic bag
- Towel

STEP	RATIONALE
1 Perform preprocedure protocol.	
Assessment	
• Verify health care provider's order in electronic health record (EHR) for type of tube and enteric feeding schedule. Assess whether health care provider has requested prokinetic agent (e.g., metoclopramide) to be given before intestinal tube placement.	Health care provider's order is needed to insert feeding tube. Prokinetic agent given before tube placement may help advance tube into intestine.
• Review patient's medical history (e.g., for basilar skull fracture, nasal problems, nosebleeds, facial trauma, nasal-facial surgery, deviated septum, anticoagulant therapy, coagulopathy).	Conditions may contraindicate tube insertion. Consult with health care provider
• Review EHR to determine patient's risk for developing a medical adhesive–related skin injury (MARSI) using adhesive devices or tape: age, dehydration, malnutrition, exposure to radiation therapy, underlying chronic conditions (e.g., diabetes, immunosuppression) and edema of extremity.	Common risk factors for MARSI (Fumarola et al., 2020).

Continued

STEP	RATIONALE
• Ask patient to describe history of allergies: known type(s) of allergies and normal allergic reaction(s). Focus on allergies to foods and adhesives. Check patient's allergy wristband.	Communication of patient allergies is essential for safe patient care. If medical adhesive is used to anchor enteral tube to nose, allergies place patient at risk for MARSI (Fumarola et al., 2020).
• Perform hand hygiene. Have patient close each nostril alternately and breathe. Examine each naris for patency and skin breakdown (apply clean gloves if drainage present).	Reduces transmission of microorganisms. Sometimes nares are obstructed or irritated, or septal defect or facial fractures are present. Place tube in most patent naris.

CLINICAL JUDGMENT *If a patient is at risk for intracranial passage of the tube, avoid the nasal route. Oral placement or placement under medical supervision using fluoroscopic direct visualization is preferable. Insertion of a gastrostomy or jejunostomy tube is another alternative.*

• Assess patient's height, weight, hydration status, electrolyte balance, caloric needs, and intake and output.	Provides baseline information to measure nutritional improvement after enteral feedings.
• Assess patient's mental status (ability to cooperate with procedure), sedation, presence of cough and gag reflex, ability to swallow, critical illness, and presence of artificial airway.	These are risk factors for inadvertent tube placement into tracheobronchial tree (Boullata et al., 2017; Metheny, 2020).

CLINICAL JUDGMENT *Recognize situations in which blind placement of a feeding tube poses an unacceptable risk for placement. Devices designed to detect pulmonary intubation such as CO_2 sensors or electromagnetic tracking devices enhance patient safety. Alternatively, to avoid insertion complications from blind placement in high-risk situations, clinicians trained in the use of visualization or imaging techniques should place tubes (Boullata et al., 2017; Irving et al., 2018).*

STEP	RATIONALE
• Assess the abdomen.	Absence of bowel sounds or presence of abdominal pain, tenderness, or distention may indicate medical problem contraindicating feedings.
• Apply pulse oximeter/ capnograph and measure vital signs. Maintain oximetry or capnography continuously. Remove and dispose of gloves (if worn). Perform hand hygiene.	Provides baseline for objective assessment of respiratory status during tube insertion and throughout time a tube is in place.

Implementation

1 Explain to patient the sensations (e.g., burning in nasal passages) that will be felt during insertion.	Increases patient's cooperation with intubation procedure and helps lessen anxiety.
2 Explain to patient how to communicate during intubation by raising index finger to indicate gagging or discomfort.	Patient must have a way of communicating to alleviate stress and enhance cooperation.
3 Perform hand hygiene. Stand on same side of bed as naris chosen for insertion and position patient upright in high Fowler position (unless contraindicated). If patient is comatose, raise head of bed as tolerated in semi-Fowler position with head tipped forward, using a pillow chin to chest. If necessary, have an AP help with positioning of confused or comatose patients. If patient is forced to lie supine, place in reverse Trendelenburg position.	Reduces transmission of microorganisms. Allows for easier manipulation of tube. Fowler position reduces risk of aspiration and promotes effective swallowing. Forward head position helps with airway closure and tube passing into esophagus.

Continued

STEP	RATIONALE
4 Ensure that pulse oximeter/ capnograph is in place. Maintain oximetry or capnography continuously.	Lowered oxygen saturation or increased end-tidal CO_2 can indicate tube misplacement into the lungs or movement out of the stomach and into the lungs (Hodin and Bordeianou, 2019).

CLINICAL JUDGMENT *If patient has increase in end-tidal CO_2 or decrease in oxygen saturation before or during insertion, tube insertion should be discontinued until patient stability can be determined.*

5 Place bath towel over patient's chest. Keep facial tissues within reach.	Prevents soiling of gown. Tube insertion frequently produces tears.
6 Determine length of tube to be inserted and mark location with tape or indelible ink.	Ensures organized procedure and estimation of the proper length of tube for insertion.
a *Option, adult:* Measure distance from tip of nose to earlobe to xiphoid process of sternum (Fig. 24.1). Mark this distance on tube with tape.	Most traditional method for estimating tube length. Length approximates distance from nose to stomach. Research has shown that this method may be least effective compared with others, although additional research is needed (Hodin and Bordeianou, 2019).
b *Option, adult*: Measure distance from tip of nose to earlobe to midumbilicus (NEMU) for the method to estimate appropriate NG tube placement.	Promotes placement of the tube end closer to the gastric fluid pool (Boullata et al., 2017).
c *Option, adult*: Measure distance from xiphoid process to earlobe to nose + 10 cm.	Technique has been shown to be the most accurate (Hodin and Bordeianou, 2019).

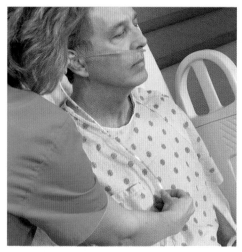

Fig. 24.1 Measurement technique to determine length of tube to insert.

STEP	RATIONALE
d *Option, child*: Use the NEMU option.	Estimates the proper length of tube insertion for pediatric patient.
e Add 20 to 30 cm (8 to 12 inches) for postpyloric tubes.	Length approximates distance from nose to jejunum.

Tip of prepyloric tubes must reach stomach to avoid the risk for pulmonary aspiration, which occurs when tubes terminate in the esophagus.

STEP	RATIONALE
7 Prepare tube for insertion. ***Note:* Do not ice tubes.**	Iced tube becomes stiff and inflexible, causing trauma to nasal mucosa.
a Obtain order for stylet tube and check agency policy for trained clinician to insert tube.	

Continued

STEP	RATIONALE
b If using stylet, make certain that it is positioned securely within tube. Inject 10 mL of water from ENFit syringe into tube.	Activates lubrication to promote smooth passage of tube into gastrointestinal (GI) tract. Improperly positioned stylet can cause tube to kink or injure patient. Ensures that tube is patent and aids in stylet removal. Once tube insertion is confirmed, have trained clinician remove stylet.
8 Prepare tube fixation materials (e.g., membrane, tube fixation device, or a precut piece of hypoallergenic tape, 10 cm (4 inches) long).	Used to secure tubing after insertion. Fixation devices allow tube to float free of nares, thus reducing pressure on nares, preventing medical device–related pressure injury (MDRPI).
9 Apply clean gloves.	Reduces transmission of microorganisms.
10 *Option:* Dip tube with surface lubricant into glass of room-temperature water or apply water-soluble lubricant (see manufacturer directions).	Activates lubricant to facilitate passage of tube into naris and GI tract.
11 Offer an alert patient a cup of water with straw (if able to swallow and not on nothing by mouth status).	Patient is asked to swallow water to facilitate tube passage.
12 Tube insertion.	
a Explain next steps to patient. Gently insert tube through nostril to back of throat (posterior nasopharynx). This may cause patient to gag. Aim back and down toward ear.	Natural contours facilitate passage of tube into GI tract.

STEP	RATIONALE
b Have patient take deep breath, relax, and flex head toward chest after tube has passed through nasopharynx.	Closes off glottis and reduces risk for tube entering trachea.
c Encourage patient to swallow small sips of water. Advance tube as patient swallows. Rotate tube gently 180 degrees while inserting.	Swallowing facilitates passage of tube past oropharynx. Distinct tug may be felt as patient swallows, indicating that tube is following expected path.
d Emphasize need to mouth breathe and swallow during insertion.	Helps facilitate passage of tube and alleviates patient's fears during procedure.
e Do not advance tube during inspiration or coughing because it is more likely to enter respiratory tract. Monitor oximetry and capnography at this time.	Can cause tube to inadvertently enter patient's airway, which will be reflected in changes in oxygen saturation and/or capnography.
f Advance tube each time patient swallows until desired length has been reached (Fig. 24.2).	Reduces discomfort and trauma to patient. Helps facilitate tube passage.

CLINICAL JUDGMENT *Do not force the tube or push against resistance. If patient starts to cough, experiences a drop in oxygen saturation, or shows other signs of respiratory distress, withdraw the tube into the posterior nasopharynx until normal breathing resumes.*

13 Check for position of tube in back of throat using penlight and tongue blade.	Improperly inserted tube may be coiled, kinked, or entering trachea.

Continued

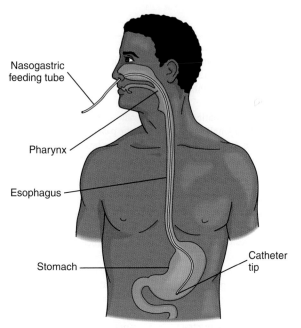

Fig. 24.2   Nasogastric tube inserted through nasopharynx and esophagus into stomach.

STEP	RATIONALE
14 Temporarily anchor tube to nose with small piece of tape.	Movement of tube stimulates gagging. Temporary anchoring of tube allows for assessment of general tube position before anchoring tube more securely.

STEP	RATIONALE
15 Keep tube secure and check its placement by aspirating stomach contents to measure gastric pH. a Attach 60-mL EnFit syringe to end of tube. Draw back on syringe slowly and obtain 5 to 10 mL of gastric aspirate. Observe appearance and color of aspirate. b Gently mix aspirate in syringe. Expel few drops into clean medicine cup. Note color of aspirate. Measure pH of aspirated GI contents by dipping pH strip into fluid or applying few drops of fluid to strip. Compare color of strip with color on pH chart.	Proper tube position is essential before initiating feeding. Mixing ensures equal distribution of contents for testing. Most accurate readings of gastric pH levels are provided by pH paper covering minimal range of 1.0 to 11.0. A pH value of 5.5 or below will exclude 100% of pulmonary placements and more than 93.9% of placements in small intestine (Metheny et al., 2019). Intestinal contents are more basic than stomach contents.

CLINICAL JUDGMENT *Insufflation of air into tube while auscultating abdomen is not a reliable means to determine position of feeding tube tip (Boullata et al., 2017; Irving et al., 2018; Kisting et al., 2019; Metheny, 2016).*

STEP	RATIONALE
16 Anchor tube to patient's nose, avoiding pressure on nares. Ensure that skin over nose is clean and dry. Apply liquid barrier spray or wipe on bridge of patient's nose and allow to dry completely. Select one of the following options for anchoring: a Membrane dressing:	Movement of tube mark can alert nurses to possible displacement of tube. Properly secured tube allows patient more mobility and prevents trauma to nasal mucosa. Skin should be protected with a barrier product before an adhesive medical device is applied (Fumarola et al., 2020). Allows membrane to adhere to skin.

Continued

STEP	RATIONALE
(1) Apply additional skin protectant to patient's cheek and area of tube to be secured.	Reduces risk of MARSI (Fumarola et al., 2020).
(2) Place tube against patient's cheek and secure tube with membrane dressing, out of patient's line of vision.	Eliminates application of tape around naris. Decreases risk for patient's inadvertent extubation.
b Tube fixation device:	Secures tube and reduces friction on naris.
(1) Apply wide end of patch to bridge of nose (Fig. 24.3).	Use of fixation devices on the bridge of a patient's nose reduces inadvertent nasal feeding tube dislodgement (Taylor et al., 2018).
(2) Slip connector around feeding tube as it exits nose (Fig. 24.4).	Secures tube.

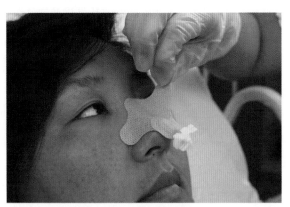

Fig. 24.3 Apply tube fixation device to bridge of nose.

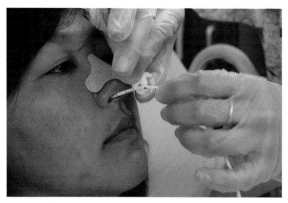

Fig. 24.4 Slip connector around feeding tube.

STEP	RATIONALE
c Apply 4-inch tape:	Prevents pulling of tube. May require frequent change if tape becomes soiled.

CLINICAL JUDGMENT *Adhesive fixation materials create high risk for MARSI (Fumarola et al., 2020). If possible use product with least adhesive content.*

(1) Remove gloves and tear two horizontal slits on each side of tape. Make the tears at locations of one-third and two-thirds down length of tape. Do not split tape. Fold middle sections of tape forward.	Creates a gap in tape that will allow tube to float and exert less pressure on naris.

Continued

STEP	RATIONALE
(2) Next tear a vertical strip at bottom of the 4-inch strip of tape, just below the bottom horizontal tears. Print date and time on top nasal part of tape.	Secures tube firmly and provides date of insertion and subsequent adhesive tape changes.
(3) Place intact end of tape over bridge of patient's nose. Wrap each vertical strip around tube as it exits nose (Fig. 24.5)	Tube is free floating in the naris with this taping method, resulting in movement of tube in pharynx. Securing tape to naris in this method reduces pressure on naris and risk for MDRPI (Zakaria et al., 2018).

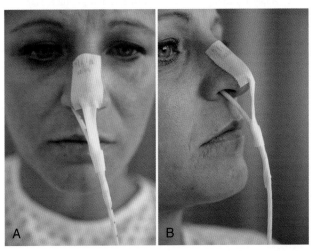

Fig. 24.5   (A) Applying tape to anchor nasoenteral tube. (B) Naris is free of pressure from tape and tube.

STEP	RATIONALE
17 Fasten end of tube to patient's gown using clip or piece of tape. Do not use safety pins to secure tube to gown.	Reduces traction on naris if tube moves, which can cause MDRPI. Safety pins become unfastened and can injure patients.
18 Help patient to comfortable position but keep head of the bed elevated at least 30 degrees (preferably 45 degrees) unless contraindicated (Metheny, 2016; VanBlarcom and McCoy, 2018). For intestinal tube placement, place patient on right side when possible until radiographic confirmation of correct placement is made.	Promotes patient comfort and lowers risk of aspiration should patient receive tube feeding. Placing patient on right side promotes passage of NI tube into small intestine.
19 Remove gloves and perform hand hygiene.	Reduces transmission of microorganisms.

CLINICAL JUDGMENT *Leave stylet in place until correct position is verified by x-ray film. Never try to reinsert a partially or fully removed stylet while feeding tube is in place. This can cause perforation of tube and injure patient.*

20 Contact radiology to obtain x-ray film of chest/abdomen.	Radiographic examination is most accurate method to determine feeding tube placement (Boullata et al., 2017; Irving et al., 2018).
21 Perform hand hygiene and apply clean gloves. Administer oral hygiene. Clean tubing at nostril with washcloth dampened in mild soap and water.	Promotes patient comfort and integrity of oral mucous membranes. Reduces transmission of microorganisms.
22 Perform postprocedure protocol.	

Continued

STEP	RATIONALE
23 Tube removal:	
a Verify health care provider's order for tube removal.	Health care provider's order is needed to remove feeding tube.
b Perform preprocedure protocol.	
c Perform hand hygiene. Apply clean gloves.	Reduces transmission of microorganisms.
d Position patient in high Fowler position unless contraindicated.	Reduces risk for pulmonary aspiration if patient vomits.
e Place disposable pad or towel over patient's chest.	Prevents mucus and gastric secretions from soiling patient's clothing.
f Disconnect tube from enteral feeding administration set (if present) and clamp or cap end.	Prevents formula from spilling from tube as it is removed.
g Gently remove tape or tube fixation device from patient's nose. Unclip tube from patient's gown.	Allows tube to be removed easily.
h Instruct patient to take deep breath and hold it. Then as you kink end of tube securely (folding it over on itself), completely withdraw by pulling it out steadily and smoothly onto towel or disposable bag. Dispose into appropriate receptacle.	Prevents inadvertent aspiration of gastric contents while tube is removed. Kinking prevents leakage of fluid from tube. Promotes patient comfort. Reduces transmission of microorganisms.
i Offer tissues to patient to blow nose.	Clears nasal passages of remaining secretions.
j Offer oral and nasal hygiene.	Promotes patient comfort.
k Perform postprocedure protocol.	

STEP	RATIONALE
24 Evaluate patient response:	
a Observe patient's response to tube placement. Assess lung sounds; have patient speak; check vital signs; note any coughing, dyspnea, cyanosis, or decrease in oxygen saturation or increase in end-tidal CO_2.	Symptoms may indicate placement in respiratory tract. Auscultation of crackles, wheezes, dyspnea, or fever may be delayed response to aspiration. Lowered oxygen saturation or increased end-tidal CO_2 may detect tip of tube in trachea or lung.
b Confirm radiographic film results with health care provider.	Verifies position of tube before initiating enteral feeding.
c Remove stylet (if used) after radiographic film verification of correct placement.	If placement needs adjustment, stylet is still in place.
d Routinely observe condition of nares, location of external exit site marking on tube, and color and pH of fluid aspirated from tube.	Routine evaluation helps to prevent MDRPI and MARSI and verifies correct placement of tube.
e After removal, assess patient's level of comfort.	Provides for continued comfort of patient.

Recording and Reporting

- Record type and size of tube placed, location of distal tip of tube, condition of naris, patient's tolerance to insertion, and confirmation of tube position by radiographic film examination.
- Document evaluation of patient learning.
- Record removal of tube, condition of naris, and patient's tolerance.
- Report to the health care provider any unexpected outcomes and the interventions performed.
- During hand-off, report tube placement, when confirmation of placement was received, and condition of nares.

UNEXPECTED OUTCOMES	RELATED INTERVENTIONS
1 Aspiration of stomach contents into respiratory tract (delayed response or small-volume aspiration), evidenced by auscultation of crackles or wheezes, dyspnea, or fever.	• Report change in patient condition to health care provider; if there has not been a recent chest radiographic film, suggest ordering one. • Position patient on side to protect airway. • Suction nasotracheally and orotracheally. • Prepare for possible initiation of antibiotics.
2 Displacement of feeding tube to another site (e.g., from duodenum to stomach) occurs when patient coughs or vomits.	• Aspirate GI contents and measure pH. • Remove displaced tube and insert and verify placement of new tube. • If there is question of aspiration, obtain chest x-ray film.
3 Erosion of skin at tube exit site or skin tear; blistering and redness around skin of nose.	• Signs of MDRPI or MARSI (Fumarola et al., 2020). • Avoid overwashing the skin. • Use a pH-balanced soap to avoid drying the skin. • Ensure patient is hydrated. • If enteral tube is likely needed long-term, consider reinsertion into opposite naris. Consult with health care provider.

Epidural Analgesia

The administration of analgesics into the epidural space is indicated following chest, abdominal or pelvic trauma (Bos et al., 2017), after major surgery (Hernandez and Singh, 2022) and for chronic cancer pain (Meghani and Vapiwala, 2018). Epidural analgesia leads to statistically significant, but possibly clinically less meaningful, reductions in pain scores compared with intravenous analgesia (Bos et al., 2017).

The spinal cord is approximately 45 cm shorter than the spinal canal in the adult and ends at the first or second lumbar vertebra (Hernandez and Singh, 2022). The spinal cord is suspended in cerebrospinal fluid (CSF) and surrounded by the arachnoid membrane. The arachnoid extends down in the adult to the sacral vertebra S2 to S3 and it is close to the dura mater. The epidural space contains a network of vessels, nerves, and fat located between the vertebral column and the dura mater, the outermost meninges covering the spinal cord (Fig. 25.1). An anesthesia provider, using sterile technique, typically places a temporary short-term or long-term catheter into the epidural space below the second lumbar vertebra, where the spinal cord ends (Fig. 25.2).

Opioids and local anesthetics, separately or in combination, are delivered into the epidural space to block pain transmission through the spinal cord. Reported benefits of epidural analgesia include higher patient satisfaction (Sng and Sia, 2017) and a reduction in complications such as oversedation, nausea and vomiting, and respiratory depression (Bouzat et al., 2017). Common opioids given epidurally include hydromorphone, fentanyl, and sufentanil, which require safe, effective management using a coordinated interprofessional approach. The infusion of both an opioid and a local anesthetic requires careful monitoring because in addition to the risks associated with opioids, there is also risk of local anesthetic toxicity. Morphine is used for inpatient epidural infusions, but is unsuitable when used as an anesthetic (Sivevski et al., 2018) for ambulatory surgery because of its slow onset time (30 to 60 min), dose-related duration of analgesia (13 to 33 h), and side effects, particularly the delayed onset of respiratory depression.

It is recommended that an epidural infusion system use the International Organization for Standardization (ISO) (ISO 80369-6)-compliant connectors, which are incompatible with traditional Luer-Lok systems, thus preventing misconnections with other medical devices (Institute for Safe Medication Practices [ISMP], 2020c). The newest connector designed for neuraxial connections, e.g., epidural infusion,

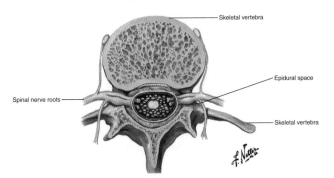

Fig. 25.1 Anatomic drawing of epidural space. (Reprinted from www. netterimages.com, ©Elsevier, Inc. All rights reserved.)

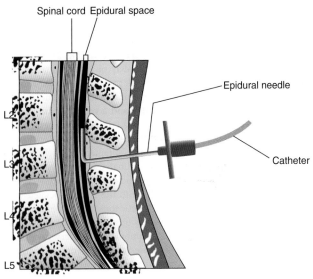

Fig. 25.2 Placement of epidural catheter. *L2–L5*, lumbar vertebrae 2–5.

is called an NRFit. The NRFit connectors were developed because of numerous wrong-route errors (e.g., inappropriate medications, enteral feedings, or air being administered neuraxially), some with fatal outcomes (ISMP, 2020c). Newer NRFit connectors are color-coded yellow (ISMP, 2020c).

Safety Guidelines

- Ensure catheter is labeled as an epidural line.
- If available, use NRFit connectors, which make tubing misconnections unlikely.
- Use strict aseptic technique during any contact with the solution, infusion tubing, dressing, or epidural insertion site to prevent contamination (Brudney and Dunne, 2017).
- Standardize the line reconciliation process as part of hand-off communications. This should involve rechecking tubing connections and tracing all patient tubes and catheters to their source on a patient's arrival in a new setting or service and at staff shift changes.
- Limit access to epidural lines to only health care providers with proper education and training.
- Trace an epidural catheter line from the access site into the patient's body all the way to the end source of an infusion or to a capped access port before you connect or reconnect tubing or administer a medication.

Delegation

The skill of epidural analgesia administration cannot be delegated to assistive personnel (AP). Agencies typically require a RN to be certified in managing and monitoring epidural anesthesia (Sanchez and Perez, 2022). Direct the AP to:

- Observe the dressing over the insertion site when repositioning or ambulating patients to prevent catheter disruption.
- Avoid pulling patient up in bed while lying flat on the back, which can dislodge the epidural catheter.
- Report any catheter disconnection or leakage from dressing immediately.
- Immediately report to the nurse any change in patient status, comfort level, or loss of sensation or movement.

Collaboration

- Consult with anesthesia provider if there are questions about catheter placement, and whether patient may be at risk for unexpected complications.
- Pharmacists are resources for information regarding anesthetic agents.

Equipment

- Clean gloves
- Sterile gloves (if removing epidural dressing)
- Prediluted preservative-free opioid as prescribed by health care provider for use in epidural infusion pump. (This is prepared by pharmacy.)

- Epidural Infusion pump and compatible ISO tubing with NRFit connector. (Do not use Y-ports for infusions; some infusion pumps have color-coded tubing for intraspinal use.)
- 0.2-micron, surfactant-free, particulate-retentive, and air-eliminating filter (INS, 2021).
- Antiseptic wipe: aqueous chlorhexidine solution or povidone iodine solution (INS, 2021)
- Tape
- Label (for injection port)
- Equipment for vital signs and pulse oximetry or capnography (see agency policy)
- Medication administration record (MAR) or computer printout

STEP	RATIONALE
1 Perform preprocedure protocol.	

Assessment

• Before first epidural infusion:	
a Review electronic health record (EHR) to assess patient's medical and medication history (including use of anticoagulants or presence of coagulopathy or raised intracranial pressure in those at risk of cerebral or cerebellar herniation).	Determines need for epidural or possible contraindications. Concurrent use of anticoagulation with epidural anesthesia increases the risk of epidural hematoma, which if left untreated may lead to paralysis (Royal College of Anesthetists, 2020). Recent anticoagulation may contraindicate epidural catheter placement because of inability to apply pressure at insertion site and associated risk for bleeding (Lourens, 2016).
b Assess patient's goal for pain relief (American Nurses' Association, 2018).	Matching management of epidural with patient goal is more likely to improve patient's participation, cooperation, and ownership of pain management.

STEP	RATIONALE
c Assess whether patient has completed informed consent, is aware of risk and benefits of epidural analgesia, and has any questions (see agency policy).	Epidural analgesia is a significant procedure that poses risks of complications ranging from adverse medication reactions to serious neurologic damage (Lourens, 2016; Royal College of Anesthetists, 2020).
d Assess whether patient routinely takes herbal medications; document complete list.	Some herbal medications interfere with the clotting mechanism (e.g., ginkgo biloba, ginseng, ginger). Currently there is no contraindication to their use when receiving epidural medication (Liperoti et al., 2017).
e Ask patient to describe history of allergies: known type of allergies and normal allergic reaction. Be alert for history of reactions to opioids or anesthetics. Check patient's allergy wristband.	Do not administer epidural infusion if there is a known patient allergy. Communication of patient allergies is essential for safe medication administration.

CLINICAL JUDGMENT *Contraindications to epidural analgesia include allergies to anesthetic, hypovolemia, increased intracranial pressure, insertion-site infection or sepsis, thrombocytopenia (<100,000 μL), prior spinal surgery, and spinal instability/abnormalities (Royal College of Anesthetists, 2020; Schreiber, 2015).*

- Before initiating and in ongoing management of epidural:

a Perform hand hygiene and complete a comprehensive pain assessment. Measure pain acuity at rest and during movement (Royal College of Anesthetists, 2020).	Reduces transmission of microorganisms. Assessment data guide safe and effective dosing of pain medication and establish baseline to evaluate epidural efficacy and patient response.

Continued

BOX 25.1   The Pasero Opioid Sedation Scale*

S = Sleep, easy to arouse
1 = Awake and alert
2 = Slightly drowsy, easily aroused
3 = Frequently drowsy, arousable, drifts off to sleep during conversation
4 = Somnolent, minimal or no response to physical stimulation
Remember: sedation precedes respiratory depression.

*Many institutions include within their protocol nursing actions to be taken for each level of sedation.
From Pasero C, McCaffery M: *Pain assessment and pharmacological management*, St Louis, 2011, Mosby.

STEP	RATIONALE
b Assess patient's sedation level by determining level of wakefulness or alertness, ability to follow commands, and drowsiness (Box 25.1).	Establishes baseline before first dose. Assessment of sedation level is more reliable for detecting early opioid-induced respiratory depression than decreased respiratory rate. Sedation always precedes respiratory depression from opioids (Smith et al., 2014).
c Assess rate, pattern, and depth of respirations; pulse oximetry or capnography; blood pressure; and temperature.	Establishes baseline of circulatory and oxygenation status. Capnography measures ventilation. Opioids can cause hypotension. Infection is a complication of an epidural, reflected by fever.
d Assess motor and sensory function of lower extremities. Test sensation to touch in lower extremities. Have patient flex both feet and knees and raise each leg off bed. Pay special attention to patients with preexisting sensory or motor abnormalities.	Establishes baseline. Ongoing monitoring of motor and sensory status ensures that neural blockage is not affecting function (Lourens, 2016).

STEP	RATIONALE
• Remove and dispose of gloves. Perform hand hygiene and reapply clean gloves. Inspect an existing catheter insertion site for redness, warmth, tenderness, swelling, and drainage. Apply sterile gloves when removing occlusive dressing.	Catheter sites are at risk for local infections. Purulent drainage is sign of infection. Clear drainage may indicate cerebrospinal fluid leaking from punctured dura. Bloody drainage may indicate that catheter entered blood vessel (Lourens, 2016).
• Follow catheter tubing and check connection site with epidural IV tubing. Verify that catheter is secured to patient's skin by observing back, side, or front. Be sure that catheter is connected securely to IV tubing with NRFit or similar ISO connector.	Prevents catheter dislodgement or migration. Incidents with catastrophic consequences have been reported due to inappropriate medication, enteral feeding liquid, or air being mistakenly administered into epidural space (ISMP, 2020c; ISO, 2016).
• Patient will usually also have a peripheral IV infusing. Check patency of IV and epidural tubing. Check infusion pumps for flow rate for proper calibration and operation. Remove and dispose of gloves. Perform hand hygiene.	Kinked or clamped tubing interrupts fluid or analgesic infusion; may cause clotting at end of IV catheter and require replacement. A patent IV line allows IV access in case medications are needed to counteract adverse reactions.

CLINICAL JUDGMENT *Epidural Infusion pump should be configured specifically for epidural analgesia with preset limits for maximum infusion rate and bolus size; lockout time should be standardized if used for patient-controlled epidural analgesia (PCEA) (Mattox, 2017).*

Implementation

1 Place patients receiving epidural analgesia close to the nurses' station.	Ensures close supervision during infusion.

Continued

STEP	RATIONALE
2 Provide patient and family caregiver individually tailored education, including information on treatment options for management of postoperative pain with PCEA. If the patient will need opioid therapy at home, a prescription for naloxone along with education and training in the administration of naloxone should be given. Naloxone is available as a nasal spray and auto injector. This is important with patients who have a history of opioid addiction (Kampman and Jarvis, 2015).	It is important that the patient and family caregiver understand pain management with PCEA and establish pain-control goals.
3 Check accuracy and completeness of each MAR or computer printout with health care provider's written medication order. Check patient's name, medication name and dosage, route of administration, and time of administration. Ensure MAR is easy to read and make corrections as necessary.	The order sheet is the most reliable source and only legal record of medications that patient is to receive. Ensures that patient receives the correct medications (Palese et al., 2019). Transcription errors are a source of medication errors (Palese et al., 2019).

CLINICAL JUDGMENT *Note that pharmacies in most health care settings prepare and provide the medication/infusion bags.*

STEP	RATIONALE
4 Prepare infusion without interruptions/distractions. Create a quiet environment. Keep all pages of MARs or computer printouts for one patient separate. Look at only one patient's electronic MAR at a time.	Interruptions contribute to medication errors (Palese et al., 2019).
5 Perform hand hygiene. Prepare infusion for one patient at a time using aseptic technique. Check label of medication carefully with MAR or computer printout when removing from storage and after preparation. Drug cassette or container should be labeled "*for epidural use only*" (Royal College of Anesthetists, 2020). Check drug expiration date.	Reduces transmission of microorganisms. *These are the first and second checks for accuracy* and ensure that correct medication is administered. Dose potency increases or decreases when outdated.
6 Recheck patient's identity at bedside using at least two identifiers (e.g., name and birthday or name and medical record number) according to agency policy. Compare identifiers with information on patient's MAR or medical record.	Ensures correct patient. Complies with The Joint Commission standards and improves patient safety (The Joint Commission, 2022).

Continued

STEP	RATIONALE
7 At the bedside, compare MAR or computer printout with name of medication on drug cassette/container. Perform an independent double check with another qualified RN or healthcare provider (see agency policy) prior to administration (including when syringe/ medication container, rate, and/ or concentration is changed) (INS, 2021).	*This is the third check for accuracy* and ensures that right patient receives right medication.
8 Before initiating analgesia, clarify purpose of epidural. If on-demand setting is ordered, demonstrate how it functions to patient and family caregiver (Cooney, 2016).	Proper explanation enhances patient cooperation with administering an on demand dose and improves likelihood of effective results.
9 Apply clean gloves. Administer infusion: anesthesia provider inserts epidural catheter and typically starts or administers first dose. Thereafter, nurses maintain the infusion.	Prevents transmission of microorganisms.
a Continuous infusion:	
(1) Insert cassette/ container of diluted preservative-free medication into epidural infusion pump. Then connect medication in pump to NRFit infusion tubing. Prime tubing. There should be no injection ports to ensure a closed system (Royal College of Anesthetists, 2020).	Tubing filled with solution and free of air bubbles avoids air embolus. System is closed to prevent entrance of microorganisms.

STEP	RATIONALE
(2) Insert NRFit tubing into infusion pump and attach distal end of tubing to antibacterial filter. Wipe off hub of epidural catheter thoroughly with antiseptic swab, then dry. Using aseptic technique connect end of NRFit tubing to hub of catheter. (Royal College of Anesthetists, 2020).	Filter reduces entrance of microorganisms into closed infusion line.
(3) Check infusion pump for proper calibration, setting, and operation. Many facilities require that two nurses independently check settings.	Ensures that patient is receiving proper dosing.
(4) Tape all tubing and hub connections. Epidural infusion system between pump and patient should be closed with no injection or Y-ports. Epidural infusions should be labeled "For Epidural Use Only." Start infusion.	Taping maintains secure closed system to prevent infection. Labeling helps ensure that analgesic is administered into correct line entering the epidural space (Mattox, 2017).

Continued

STEP	RATIONALE
b Programmed intermittent Bolus dose via infusion pump:	
(1) Prepare pump following steps 9a(1-5) above. Adjust infusion pump setting for preset limit for maximum bolus size. Initiate pump to deliver ordered bolus.	Prevents accidental infusion of an overdose.
c Patient controlled epidural analgesia (PCEA) Dose on demand:	
(1) Prepare pump following steps 9a(1-5) above. Set pump for lockout time (as ordered).	Gives patient control over administration of analgesia. When patient anticipates pain before it becomes severe, analgesic is most effective.
(2) Have patient initiate demand dose as needed to relieve pain.	
10 Explain that nurses will monitor patient's response to epidural analgesic routinely. Also instruct patient on signs or problems to report to nurse (e.g., pruritus, inability to pass urine, change in sensation).	Builds trust and encourages patient to partner with nurse in their care.

CLINICAL JUDGMENT   *For all patients using PCEA, assess for sensory and motor function before ambulation or transfer (Goldberg et al., 2017).*

11 Perform postprocedure protocol.

STEP	RATIONALE
12 Postanalgesia:	
a Keep the IV line patent for 24 h after epidural analgesia has ended.	Provides route for any emergency medications.
b Before removing epidural catheter, check for presence of therapeutic anticoagulation. Check agency policy for removal of epidural catheter and extra precautions if patient is receiving anticoagulation therapy.	Removal of epidural catheter when a patient is receiving anticoagulation therapy increases risk for spinal hematoma due to anticoagulation and inability to compress vessels.
c Assist health care provider as needed in removing catheter. *Note:* Some settings (such as obstetrics) allow trained nurses to remove catheters.	Ensures safe removal of catheter. Patient will require on going analgesia in most cases.
Inform patient that an alternative form of analgesic will continue to be provided as needed/ ordered.	
d Perform postprocedure protocol.	
13 Evaluate patient response	
a Evaluate patient's pain severity using a pain rating scale of 0 to 10. Compare with patient's desired goal. Evaluate character of pain.	Evaluates effectiveness of epidural analgesia.

Continued

STEP	RATIONALE
b Evaluate blood pressure and heart rate; respiratory rate, rhythm, depth, and pattern; pulse oximetry or capnography; and sedation level (using Pasero Opioid Sedation Scale [see Box 25.1]) Evaluate patients after initiating or restarting an epidural infusion for at least the first 24 h; assess every 1 to 2 h until stable, then every 4 h, or with each home visit (INS, 2021). (see agency policy). Minimum frequency after a bolus should be every 5 minutes during the first 30 minutes (Royal College of Anesthetists, 2020). Evaluate after changes made to infusion rate and during periods of cardiovascular or respiratory instability (Nagappa et al., 2017).	Oversedation occurs before respiratory depression; it is the most sensitive indication of opioid-induced respiratory depression (Royal College of Anesthetists, 2020). Postural hypotension, vasodilation, and heart rate changes may occur from pain or medication side effects (Mattox, 2017).

CLINICAL JUDGMENT *Help patient when changing positions. Protect patient who is at risk for postural hypotension.*

STEP	RATIONALE
c Evaluate catheter insertion site every 2 to 4 h for leaking, inflammation, or swelling. Note character of drainage (e.g., bloody, clear, or purulent).	Observations made for intact system and onset of infection at infusion site. Bloody drainage may occur if catheter has migrated into a vessel. Report immediately and treat as emergency (Lourens, 2016).
d Inspect epidural site for disruption or displacement of catheter.	Could lead to infusion of medication into higher level of spinal cord.
e Observe for pruritus, especially of face, head, neck, and torso. Inform patient that this is a common side effect and typically not an allergic response.	Pruritus *alone* rarely indicates an allergy to opioids (Masato et al., 2017).
f Observe for nausea and vomiting and presence of headache. Note any nonverbal signs of headache (grimacing, massaging of head).	Nausea from epidural analgesia worsens by movement. Headache and cerebrospinal fluid leakage may occur from a dural puncture.
g Monitor intake and output. Evaluate for bladder distention and urinary frequency or urgency. Consult with health care provider for possible need for intermittent catheterization.	Prevents urinary retention.
h Evaluate for motor weakness or numbness and tingling of lower extremities (paresthesia).	Reducing epidural dose (per order) may help eliminate unwanted motor and sensory deficits (Goldberg et al., 2017).

Recording and Reporting

- Record drug name, dose, infusion method (bolus, demand, or continuous), and time given (if bolus) or time begun and ended (if continuous or demand infusion) on appropriate MAR. Specify concentration and diluent.
- With continuous or demand infusion, obtain and record pump readout hourly for first 24 h after infusion begins and then every 4 h.
- Record all regular and/or periodic assessment/evaluation measures, appearance of epidural site, presence or absence of side effects or adverse reactions to medication, and presence or absence of complications resulting from placement and maintenance of epidural catheter.
- Document evaluation of patient and family caregiver learning.
- Report the patient's pain management plan, changes, responses, and most recent doses to aid in reducing medication errors (Sadule-Rios et al., 2017).
- The oncoming and outgoing nurse should inspect and agree with PCEA infusion pump programming/settings as a means of medication reconciliation (Kane-Gill et al., 2017).
- Report detailed information regarding vital signs, pulse oximetry and capnography, pain-assessment scores, Pasero Opioid Sedation Scale scores, level of consciousness, anxiety level, and activity level (Cooney, 2016; Meisenberg et al., 2017).

UNEXPECTED OUTCOMES	RELATED INTERVENTIONS
1 Patient states that pain is still present or has increased. Primary cause to look for includes insufficient drug dose delivery.	• Check all tubing for kinking, improper connections, medication dosing, and pump settings. • Confer with health care provider regarding adequacy of medication dose.

UNEXPECTED OUTCOMES	RELATED INTERVENTIONS
2 Patient is sedated or not easily aroused and/or experiences periods of apnea or decreased respirations <8 breaths/min.	• Stop epidural infusion immediately and elevate patient's head of bed 30 degrees (unless contraindicated). *Stay with patient and call for help.* • Notify health care provider and prepare to administer opioid-reversing agent (e.g., naloxone) per health care provider's order (refer to agency protocol). • Monitor all vital signs, pulse oximetry, capnography, and sedation level continuously until patient is easily aroused and respiratory rate is 8 to 10 breaths/min with adequate depth for 2 h.
3 Patient reports sudden headache. Clear drainage is present on epidural dressing, or more than 1 mL of fluid is aspirated from catheter.	• Stop infusion or bolus dosing. Stay with patient and call for help. • Notify health care provider.
4 Patient experiences minimal urinary output, urinary frequency or urgency, bladder distention, pruritus, or nausea and vomiting.	• Consult with health care provider about appropriateness of reducing dose of opioid and/or discuss treatment for side effects.

Eye Irrigation

Chemical injuries to the eye can be work related or can occur at home, caused by accidental exposure to common household cleaning solutions or fumes and aerosols. Burns from acids such as bleach, toilet cleaners, and battery fluid create a haze on the cornea, which often clears, allowing for a good chance of recovery. Burns from alkalis such as lye, ammonia, and dishwasher detergent cause ocular surface damage and vision impairment. Extensive anterior eye injury occurs with alkaline substances with a pH greater than 10 (Ramponi, 2017).

A chemical injury to the eye is an emergency and requires flushing the eye with copious amounts of irrigation fluid. Although irrigating solutions are usually normal saline, cool tap water is recommended during the emergent phase because it is effective, is immediately available for first aid, and initially helps to dilute the concentration of the chemical. Tap water irrigation is also used in emergency situations when a foreign object has entered the eye. If the person wears contact lens and the lens do not wash out with the irrigation, have the person try to remove them. The goal in treating ocular chemical injury is to prevent or reduce visual loss caused by the burn (Ramponi, 2017).

Safety Guidelines

- Instruct patient not to rub the eye; have patient blink several times and allow tears to flush out the irritant (Gudgel, 2019).

Delegation

The skill of eye irrigation cannot be delegated to assistive personnel (AP). Direct the AP to:

- Report any patient reports of discomfort or excess tearing after irrigation.

Collaboration

- Collaborate as needed with the health care provider and optometry services in the care of the patient after eye irrigation.

Equipment

- Emergent: Cool tap water
- Nonemergent: prescribed irrigating solution, volume usually 30 to 180 mL at 32°C to 38°C (90°F to 100°F). (For chemical flushing, use normal saline or lactated Ringer solution in large volume to provide continuous irrigation over 15 to 30 minutes.)

- pH test strip
- Sterile basin or bag of solution
- Curved emesis basin
- Waterproof pad or towel
- 4 × 4-inch gauze pads
- Soft bulb syringe or intravenous (IV) tubing
- Clean gloves, gown
- Penlight
- Medication administration record (MAR)

STEP	RATIONALE

1 Follow preprocedure protocol.

Assessment

- Acute emergent situations (At the scene of injury):

  a Perform hand hygiene and prepare to use copious amounts of clear, cool water (use normal saline or lactated Ringer if quickly available) to flush eyes until secretions are cleared. (*Note:* Use clinical judgment to decide the right amount of time and right amount of irrigation [Marsden, 2016]).

  b Irrigation for at least 15 minutes is recommended; 30 minutes is preferable (Gwenhure, 2020; Stevens, 2016). Follow irrigation steps in Implementation section, below.

Minimizes corneal damage, visual impairment, and permanent loss of vision (Ramponi, 2017). The procedure for irrigation can save eyesight and should be carried out immediately if a patient presents with a chemical injury (Bagheri and Wajda, 2017).

Continued

STEP	RATIONALE
• Nonemergent situations (presented to emergency department):	
a Determine the time the injury occurred, the chemical or substance involved (if known), and action/first aid taken immediately after the injury.	Data aids in selecting ongoing treatment.
• Review health care provider's medication order, including solution to be instilled and affected eye(s) (right, left, or both) to receive irrigation.	Ensures safe and correct administration of irrigant.
• Perform hand hygiene. Apply clean gloves. Determine the patient's ability to open the affected eye. If the patient is unable to open eye, hold eyelids open manually or with an eye speculum (Marsden, 2016).	Reduces transmission of microorganisms. Spasm of the eyelid or pain makes opening the eye difficult. Local anesthetics such as proparacaine or tetracaine cause topical numbness and are used before eye examination procedures.

CLINICAL JUDGMENT *Irrigation should not be delayed for comprehensive eye assessment, nor for acquiring a particular irrigating fluid or administration set. If saline for example is not available, use tap water (Corbett and Bizrah, 2018). Eye irrigation is the immediate treatment for a chemical burn. When possible, determine the chemical. Delays in irrigation have been associated with more severe injury (Ventocilla, 2019).*

• Ask if patient has allergy to local anesthetic. If not, administer local anesthetic eye drops to the eye as ordered (Gwenhure, 2020).	Protects patient from allergic reaction. Anesthetic reduces discomfort during examination and irrigation.

STEP	RATIONALE
• If time permits or after irrigation, perform a complete eye examination.	Provides baseline information and determines continuing presence of any foreign bodies.
a Determine if pupils are equal and round and react to light and accommodation (PERRLA assessment). Have patient look in all directions to determine if there are any visible foreign bodies.	
b Observe eye for redness, excessive tearing, discharge, and swelling. Ask patient about symptoms of itching, burning, pain, blurred vision, or photophobia	
• When chemical contamination of the eye is suspected, assess pH of the patient's tears. *Note:* Do not allow pH measurement to delay irrigation. Insert a folded end of a universal pH indicator strip into the space between the eyelid and eyeball (Fig. 26.1). After about 30 seconds read results (Gwenhure, 2020). Compare pH in both eyes.	pH scale measures how acidic or alkaline a solution is on a scale of 1 (very strong acid) to 14 (very strong alkali), with 7 as neutral. The normal pH of tears is between 7.0 and 7.4 (Corbett and Bizrah, 2018). If one eye is unaffected, pH provides a baseline for normal.
• Ask patient to rate level of eye pain. Use scale of 0 to 10. Remove and dispose of gloves.	Establishes baseline for level of pain. Pain can be severe, requiring management to reduce discomfort and control ciliary spasm (Ramponi, 2017). Reduces transmission of microorganisms.

Continued

Fig. 26.1 Testing pH of eye. (Redrawn from Gwenhure, T: Procedure for eye irrigation to treat ocular chemical injury, *Nursing Times* [online]; 116(2): 46, 2020.)

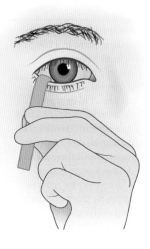

STEP	RATIONALE

CLINICAL JUDGMENT *When eye irrigation is an emergency treatment for a chemical burn, do not stop to obtain a comprehensive assessment of the eye. Perform a brief assessment to ensure the patient does not have a contraindication for eye irrigation. Once the acute phase is over, postexposure management includes artificial tears, topical ophthalmic antibiotic ointment, and topical steroids. Aqueous suppressants and topical cycloplegic agents may also be used (Ramponi, 2017).*

Implementation

1 Carefully explain each step of the procedure to the patient and offer reassurance while the eye is being irrigated, because patient will likely not be able to see what is happening. Explain that eye can be closed periodically and that no object will touch it.	An eye injury can be frightening, and the patient may have concerns about loss of vision.
2 Perform hand hygiene. Apply clean gloves and gown.	Reduces transmission of microorganisms. Personal protective equipment protects you from chemical irritants.

STEP	RATIONALE
3 Remove any contact lens, if possible (Corbett and Bizrah, 2018). Remove gloves after contact lens is removed. Reapply new gloves.	Prompt removal of lenses is needed to safely and completely irrigate foreign substances from patient's eyes. Removing gloves after removing the contact lens prevents reintroduction of chemical transferred from lens to glove.

CLINICAL JUDGMENT *Do not delay treatment* by removing a patient's contact lenses unless rapid swelling is occurring.

---

4 With patient in supine or semi-Fowler position in bed, place towel or waterproof pad under patient's face and curved emesis basin just below patient's cheek on side of affected eye. Turn head toward affected eye. If both eyes are affected, keep patient supine for simultaneous irrigation of both eyes.	Position facilitates flow of solution from inner to outer canthus, preventing contamination of unaffected eye and nasolacrimal duct.
5 Using gauze moistened with prescriber's solution (or normal saline), gently clean visible secretions or foreign material from eyelid margins and eyelashes, wiping from inner to outer canthus.	Minimizes transfer of material into eye during irrigation. Prevents secretions from entering nasolacrimal duct.
6 Explain next steps to patient and encourage relaxation:	
a With gloved finger gently retract upper and lower eyelids to expose conjunctival sacs.	Retraction minimizes blinking and allows irrigation of conjunctiva.
b To hold lids open, apply gentle pressure to lower bony orbit and bony prominence beneath eyebrow. Do not apply pressure over eye.	

Continued

STEP	RATIONALE
7 Hold irrigating syringe or tip of prepared IV fluid tubing approximately 2.5 cm (1 inch) from inner canthus.	Direct contact with irrigation equipment may injure eye.
8 Ask patient to look in all directions while maintaining irrigation. Gently irrigate with steady stream toward lower conjunctival sac, flushing from inner to outer canthus (Gwenhure, 2020) (Fig. 26.2).	Ensures whole eye surface is irrigated (Gwenhure, 2020). Minimizes force of stream on patient's cornea. Flushes irritant out and away from the other eye and nasolacrimal duct, reducing the risk of contaminating the patient's other eye
9 Reinforce importance of procedure and encourage patient by using calm, confident, soft voice.	Reduces anxiety.
10 Allow patient to blink periodically.	Lid closure moves secretions from upper conjunctival sac.

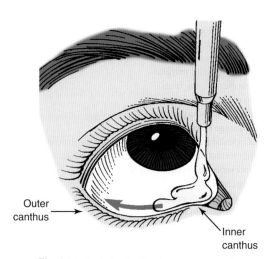

Outer canthus

Inner canthus

Fig. 26.2 Eye irrigation from inner to outer canthus.

STEP	RATIONALE
11 Continue irrigation with prescribed solution volume for 30 minutes (Gwenhure, 2020) or time ordered by health care provider. Irrigate under the upper and lower eyelids. (*Note:* Adequate irrigation is likely achieved more quickly with a liquid chemical injury than a solid chemical injury [Marsden, 2016]).	Eversion removes chemical from lining of eyelid.
12 Blot excess moisture from eyelids and face with cotton swab, gauze, or towel.	Promotes patient comfort.
13 After 5 minutes, retest the pH of the tears. If the pH of the eye is outside the normal range, continue irrigation until a normal pH of 7.0 to 7.4 is achieved (Corbett and Bizrah, 2018).	Determines efficacy of irrigation. Interval measurement ensures irrigation fluid has been cleared from the eyes and the pH will be accurate.
14 Perform postprocedure protocol.	
15 Evaluate patient response.	

CLINICAL JUDGMENT *This may be time to perform a complete eye examination which was deferred due to emergent patient need.*

a Observe for verbal and nonverbal signs of anxiety during irrigation.	Verifies that patient is adequately comforted.
b Assess patient's level of pain on scale of 0 to 10.	Verifies effective removal of irritant.
c Inspect eye for movement and perform PERRLA assessment.	Impaired reaction to light, accommodation, or movement may indicate injury.
d Ask patient about improved visual acuity. Have patient read written material.	Corneal damage from irritant can result in altered visual acuity (e.g., blurred vision, cloudiness).

Recording and Reporting

- Record reason for irrigation, condition of eye before and after irrigation, patient's report of pain and visual symptoms before and after irrigation, type and amount of irrigation solution, and length of time irrigation performed.
- Document evaluation of patient and family caregiver learning.
- Report patient's condition of eye, symptoms, and tolerance of eye irrigation.
- Report immediately to the health care provider patient reports of increased pain, blurred vision, or other visual changes.

UNEXPECTED OUTCOMES	RELATED INTERVENTIONS
1 Patient is anxious.	• Reinforce rationale for irrigation. • Allow patient to close eye periodically during irrigation. • Instruct patient to take slow, deep breaths.
2 Patient reports pain or foreign body sensation, excessive tearing, or photophobia in eye after irrigation.	• Advise patient to close eye and avoid eye movement. • Immediately notify health care provider or eye care practitioner.

Eye Medications

Common eye (ophthalmic) medications are in the form of drops and ointments, including over-the-counter preparations such as artificial tears and vasoconstrictors. However, many patients receive prescribed ophthalmic drugs for eye conditions such as glaucoma and infection and after cataract extraction. A third type of medication delivery system is the intraocular disk. Medications delivered by disk resemble a contact lens, but the disk is placed in the conjunctival sac, not on the cornea, and it remains in place for up to 1 week.

The eye is the most sensitive organ to which you apply medications. The cornea is richly supplied with sensitive nerve fibers. Care must be taken to prevent instilling medication directly onto the cornea. The conjunctival sac is much less sensitive and thus a more appropriate site for medication instillation.

Any patient receiving topical eye medications should learn correct self-administration of the medication, especially patients with glaucoma, who must often undergo lifelong medication administration for control of their disease. You can easily instruct patients and any family caregivers while administering medications.

Safety Guidelines

- Do not allow tip of medication applicator to touch surface of eye.
- Instruct patient to never share eye medications.

Delegation

The skill of administering ophthalmic medications cannot be delegated to assistive personnel (AP). Instruct the AP about:

- The specific potential side effects of medications and to report their occurrence.
- The potential for temporary burning or blurring of vision after administration of eye medications.

Collaboration

- Confer with ophthalmologist if patient's eye condition worsens or different symptoms develop.

Equipment

- Appropriate medication (eyedrops with sterile eyedropper, ointment tube, medicated intraocular disk)
- Clean gloves
- Medication administration record (MAR) (electronic or printed)

291

Eyedrops/ointment

- Cotton ball or tissue
- Wash basin filled with warm water, washcloth
- *Option:* Eye patch and tape

STEP	RATIONALE
1 Perform Preprocedure protocol.	

Assessment

• Check accuracy and completeness of each MAR or computer printout with health care provider's written medication order. Check patient's name, medication name and dosage, route of administration, and time of administration.	Recopy or reprint any part of MAR that is difficult to read. The order sheet is the most reliable source and only legal record of medications that patient is to receive. Ensures that patient receives the correct medications (Palese et al., 2019). Transcription errors are a source of medication errors (Palese et al., 2019).
• Review electronic health record (EHR): assess patient's medical and medication history.	Determines need for medication or possible contraindications for medication administration.
• Review drug reference information for medication action, purpose, normal dose, side effects, time of peak onset, and nursing implications.	Allows you to administer medication safely and monitor patient's response to therapy.
• Ask patient to describe history of allergies: known type of allergies and normal allergic reaction. List drug allergies on each page of MAR. Check patient's allergy wristband. Do not prepare medication if there is a known patient allergy.	Communication of patient allergies is essential part of safe medication administration.
• Determine whether patient has any symptoms of eye discomfort or visual impairment.	Certain eye medications act to either lessen or increase these symptoms.

STEP	RATIONALE
• Perform hand hygiene and assess condition of external eye structures. This may be done just before drug instillation (if drainage is present, apply clean gloves).	Provides baseline to determine whether there is a local response to medications. Also indicates need to clean eye before drug application.
• Assess patient's level of consciousness and ability to follow directions.	If patient becomes restless or combative during procedure, greater risk for accidental eye injury exists.
• Assess patient's ability to manipulate and hold dropper or ocular disk.	Determines whether instruction is needed to prepare patient for self-administering the drug.

Implementation

1	Discuss purpose of each medication, action, indication, and possible adverse effects. Allow sufficient time for patient to ask any questions. Patients who self-instill medications may be allowed to give drops under nurse's supervision (check agency policy).	Makes patient a participant in care, which minimizes anxiety. Patient has the right to be informed, and patient understanding of each medication improves adherence with drug therapy. Prepares patient to self-administer drug, which increases feelings of independence.

CLINICAL JUDGMENT *Tell patients who are receiving eyedrops (mydriatics) that vision will be blurred temporarily and that sensitivity to light may occur.*

2	Prepare medication without interruptions/distractions. Create a quiet environment. Keep all pages of MARs or computer printouts for one patient together or look at only one patient's electronic MAR at a time	Interruptions contribute to medication errors (Palese et al., 2019).

Continued

STEP	RATIONALE
3 Perform hand hygiene. Prepare medications for one patient at a time using aseptic technique. Check label of medication carefully with MAR or computer printout two times when preparing medication.	Ensures that medication is sterile. *These are the first and second checks for accuracy* and ensure that correct medication is administered.
4 Take medication(s) to patient at correct time (see agency policy). Medications that require exact timing include stat, first-time or loading doses, and one-time doses. Give time-critical scheduled medications (e.g., antibiotics, preoperative eye drops) at exact time ordered (no later than 30 minutes before or after scheduled dose). Give non–time-critical scheduled medications within a range of 1 or 2 h of scheduled dose (Institute for Safe Medication Practices [ISMP], 2011). During administration, apply seven rights of medication administration. Perform hand hygiene.	Hospitals must adopt medication administration policy and procedure for timing of medication administration that considers nature of the prescribed medication, specific clinical application, and patient needs (ISMP, 2011; United States Department of Health and Human Services Centers for Medicare & Medicaid [DHHS], 2020). Time-critical scheduled medications are those for which early or delayed administration of maintenance doses of greater than 30 minutes before or after the scheduled dose may cause harm or result in substantial suboptimal therapy or pharmacological effect. Non–time-critical medications are those for which early or delayed administration within a specified range of either 1 or 2 h should not cause harm or result in substantial suboptimal therapy or pharmacological effect (DHHS, 2020; ISMP, 2011).

STEP	RATIONALE
5 Identify patient using at least two identifiers (e.g., name and birthday or name and medical record number) according to agency policy. Compare identifiers with information on patient's MAR or medical record.	Ensures correct patient. Complies with The Joint Commission standards and improves patient safety (The Joint Commission, 2022).
6 At patient's bedside, again compare MAR or computer printout with names of medications on medication labels and patient name. Ask patient if he or she has allergies.	*This is the third check for accuracy* and ensures that patient receives correct medication. Confirms patient's allergy history.

CLINICAL JUDGMENT *Instruct and reinforce to patients receiving eyedrops (mydriatics) that vision will be blurred temporarily and sensitivity to light may occur. Patient should not drive or operate machinery or perform any activity that requires clear vision until vision and sensitivity to light return to normal.*

7 Administer eye medications.	
a Perform hand hygiene. Apply clean gloves. Ask patient to lie supine or sit back in chair with head slightly hyperextended, looking up.	Position provides easy access to eye for medication instillation and minimizes drainage of medication into tear duct.

CLINICAL JUDGMENT *Do not hyperextend the neck of a patient with cervical spine injury.*

b If drainage or crusting is present along eyelid margins or inner canthus, gently wash away. Soak any dried crusts with warm, damp washcloth or cotton ball over eye for several minutes. Always wipe clean from inner to outer canthus (Fig. 27.1). Remove gloves and perform hand hygiene.	Soaking allows easy removal of crusts without applying pressure to eye. Cleaning from inner to outer canthus avoids entrance of microorganisms into lacrimal duct (Burchum and Rosenthal, 2022).

Continued

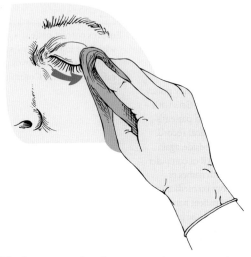

Fig. 27.1 Cleanse eye, washing from inner canthus to outer canthus, before giving eye medication.

STEP	RATIONALE
c Explain that there might be temporary burning sensation from drops.	Corneas are highly sensitive.
d Instill eyedrops.	
(1) *Option:* Apply clean gloves if eye drainage present. **Hold** clean cotton ball or tissue in nondominant hand on patient's cheekbone just below lower eyelid.	Prevents transmission of microorganisms. Cotton or tissue absorbs medication that escapes eye.

STEP	RATIONALE
(2) With tissue or cotton ball resting below lower lid, gently press downward with thumb or forefinger against bony orbit, exposing conjunctival sac. Never press directly against patient's eyeball.	Prevents pressure and trauma to eyeball and prevents fingers from touching eye.
(3) Ask patient to look at ceiling. Rest dominant hand on patient's forehead; hold filled medication eyedropper approximately 1 to 2 cm (¼ to ½ inch) above conjunctival sac.	Action moves cornea up and away from conjunctival sac and reduces blink reflex. Prevents accidental contact of eyedropper with eye and reduces risk of injury and transfer of microorganisms to dropper (ophthalmic medications are sterile).
(4) Drop prescribed number of drops into lower conjunctival sac (Fig. 27.2)	Conjunctival sac normally holds 1 or 2 drops. Provides even distribution of medication across eye.
(5) If patient blinks or closes eye, causing drops to land on outer lid margins, repeat procedure.	Therapeutic effect of drug is obtained only when drops enter conjunctival sac.

Continued

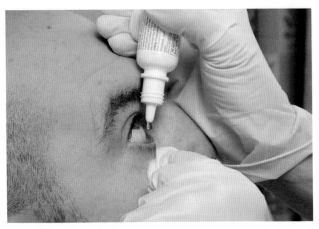

Fig. 27.2 Drop of eye medication drops into conjunctival sac.

STEP	RATIONALE
(6) When administering drops that may cause systemic effects, apply gentle pressure to patient's nasolacrimal duct with clean tissue for 30 to 60 seconds over each eye, one at a time. Avoid pressure directly against patient's eyeball.	Prevents overflow of medication into nasal and pharyngeal passages. Prevents absorption into systemic circulation (Burchum and Rosenthal, 2022; Gudgel, 2018).
(7) After instilling drops, ask patient to close eyes gently.	Helps distribute medication. Squinting or squeezing eyelids forces medication from conjunctival sac (Burchum and Rosenthal, 2022; Gudgel, 2018).

STEP	RATIONALE
e Instill ophthalmic ointment.	
(1) *Option:* Apply clean gloves if eye drainage present.	Reduces transmission of microorganisms.
Ask patient to look at ceiling. Use index finger to retract upper eyelid and thumb of nondominant hand to retract lower lid. Hold ointment applicator above lower lid margin. Apply thin ribbon of ointment evenly along inner edge of lower eyelid on conjunctiva (Fig. 27.3) from inner to outer canthus.	Distributes medication evenly across eye and lid margin.

Continued

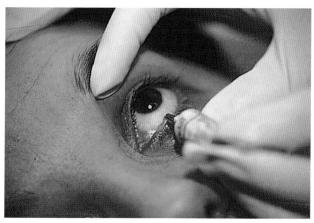

Fig. 27.3 Apply ointment to lower eyelid margin from inner to outer canthus.

STEP	RATIONALE
(2) Have patient close eye and rub lid lightly in circular motion with cotton ball if not contraindicated. Avoid placing pressure directly against patient's eyeball.	Further distributes medication without traumatizing eye.
(3) If excess medication is on eyelid, gently wipe it from inner to outer canthus.	Promotes comfort and prevents trauma to eye.
(4) If patient needs an eye patch, apply clean one by placing it over affected eye so that entire eye is covered. Tape securely without applying pressure to eye.	Clean eye patch reduces risk of infection.
f Insert intraocular disk.	
(1) Apply clean gloves. Open package containing disk. Gently press your fingertip against disk so that it adheres to your finger. It may be necessary to moisten gloved finger with sterile saline. Position convex side of disk on your fingertip.	Allows you to inspect disk for damage or deformity.

STEP	RATIONALE
(2) With your other hand, gently pull patient's lower eyelid away from eye. Ask patient to look up.	Prepares conjunctival sac for receiving medicated disk and moves sensitive cornea away.
(3) Place disk in conjunctival sac so that it floats on sclera between iris and lower eyelid (Fig. 27.4).	Ensures delivery of medication.
(4) Pull patient's lower eyelid out and over disk (Fig. 27.5). You should not be able to see disk at this time. Repeat insertion if you can see disk.	Ensures accurate medication delivery.
8 Perform postprocedure protocol.	
9 Remove intraocular disk.	
a Perform hand hygiene and apply clean gloves. Gently pull downward on lower eyelid using your nondominant hand.	Exposes disk.

Continued

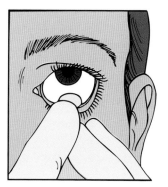

Fig. 27.4 Place intraocular disk in the conjunctival sac between the iris and lower eyelid.

Fig. 27.5 Gently pull the patient's lower eyelid out and over the disk.

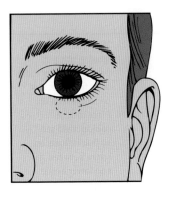

STEP	RATIONALE
b Using forefinger and thumb of your dominant hand, gently pinch disk and lift it out of patient's eye. Remove and discard gloves, perform hand hygiene.	Technique prevents injury to eye. Reduces transmission of microorganisms.
c Perform postprocedure protocol.	
10 Evaluate patient response	
a Observe response to medication by assessing visual changes, asking whether symptoms are relieved, and noting any side effects or discomfort.	Evaluates effects of medication.
b Ask patient to discuss purpose of drug, action, side effects, and demonstrate technique of self-administration.	Determines patient's level of understanding.

Recording and Reporting

- Record drug, concentration, dose or strength, number of drops, application site (left, right, or both eyes), and time of administration on MAR immediately after administration, not before. Include initials or signature.
- Document your evaluation of patient learning.
- Record assessment findings (e.g., redness, drainage, irritation), any subjective data (e.g., pain, itching, altered vision), and patient's response to medications. Note evidence of any side effects.
- Report adverse effects/patient response and/or withheld drugs to nurse in charge or health care provider.

UNEXPECTED OUTCOMES	RELATED INTERVENTIONS
1 Patient complains of burning or pain or experiences local side effects (e.g., headache, bloodshot eyes, eye irritation). Drug concentration and patient's sensitivity both influence chances of side effects developing.	• Eyedrops may have been instilled onto cornea, or dropper touched surface of eye. • Notify health care provider for possible adjustment in medication type and dosage.
2 Patient experiences systemic effects from drops (e.g., increased heart rate and blood pressure from epinephrine, decreased heart rate and blood pressure from timolol).	• Notify health care provider immediately. • Remain with patient. Assess vital signs. • Withhold further doses.
3 Patient is unable to explain drug information or steps for taking medication and/or has trouble manipulating applicator.	• Repeat instructions and include family caregiver as appropriate. Include return demonstration.

Fall Prevention in a Health Care Facility

An estimated 700,000 to 1,000,000 people fall in US hospitals each year (Health Research and Educational Trust [HRET], 2016). Patient falls resulting in injury have remained one of the most frequently reviewed sentinel events by The Joint Commission (TJC, 2021a). A fall may result in fractures, bruises, lacerations, or internal bleeding, leading to increased diagnostic tests and treatments, extended hospital stays, and discharge to rehabilitation or long-term care instead of home. The Centers for Medicare and Medicaid Services (CMS) identifies falls as a preventable or "never" event that should never occur. Therefore the CMS in October 2008 stopped reimbursing hospitals for costs related to patient falls (Fehlberg et al., 2017).

The risk factors for falls include two categories: patient related (intrinsic) and hospital environment and working process related (extrinsic). In research studies examining risk factors for falls, common risks are found for all patients (Berry and Kiel, 2022; HRET, 2016; Severo et al., 2014) (Table 28.1). A validated fall risk assessment tool includes common fall risk factors. The number of risks identified for a specific patient is computed into a fall risk score (e.g., high, medium, and low). The most common risk assessment tools used in hospitals are the Morse Fall Scale, the STRATIFY scale, and the Hendrich II Fall Risk Model (Berry and Kiel, 2022; Severo et al., 2014).

Once a patient's fall risks are identified, it is important to partner with the patient to affirm those risks and to select evidence-based interventions (usually multiple strategies) that appropriately target the patient's risks (Berry and Kiel, 2022). Research by Radecki et al. (2018) was designed to measure patients' perception of fall prevention; they argue that fall prevention programs favor clinician-led plan development and implementation versus patient-led. These researchers recommend that nurses develop relationships with patients to facilitate understanding of their needs. The aim is to reduce overreliance on bed alarms while allowing for implementation of strategies that reduce modifiable risk factors leading to falls (Radecki et al., 2018).

Safety Guidelines

- Fall prevention needs to be individualized because each patient has a different set of fall risk factors. However, **Universal Fall Precautions** are called "universal" because they apply to all patients

TABLE 28.1 Risk Factors for Falls in Hospitalized Patients

Intrinsic Factors	Extrinsic Factors
History of previous fall	Communication issues
Behavioral	Frequency of
Patient does not seek assistance for	rounding
toileting	Inconsistent or
Patient did not know, forgot, or	incomplete
chose not to use call light	communication
Altered cognition	of patient risk
Dementia, sedation, delirium	for falls between
Patient awareness and acknowledgment	caregivers
of own risk for falls	Fall prevention
Altered mobility	education for
Lower extremity weakness	patient and family
Abnormal gait	is not used or is
Shuffling and stumbling	inconsistently used
Requires assistance with mobility	Physical hazards
and/or assistive device	Liquids on floor
Sensory deficit	Electrical cords
Needs corrective lenses	near walking
Wears hearing aids	path
Hard of hearing and does not	Uses IV pole to
wear hearing aids	walk
Medications	Wears compression
Benzodiazepines	stocking with cords
Antipsychotics	Increased use of
Antidepressants	restraints (Miake-
Opiates	Lye et al., 2013)
Barbiturates	Decreased efforts by
Antihistamines	hospital staff to
Anticonvulsants	mobilize patients
Sedatives	(Miake-Lye, 2013)
Antihypertensives	Inappropriate or no
Diuretics	footwear
Issues with toileting	
Use of diuretics	
Bladder urgency or frequency	
Disease conditions causing:	
Dizziness	
Peripheral neuropathy	
Pain (especially in lower extremities)	
Hypotension	

IV, intravenous.

regardless of fall risk (Agency for Healthcare Research and Quality [AHRQ], 2013):

- Familiarize the patient with the environment.
- Have the patient demonstrate call-light use.
- Maintain call light within reach.
- Keep the patient's personal possessions within patient safe reach.
- Have sturdy handrails in patient bathrooms, room, and hallway.
- Place the hospital bed in low position when a patient is resting in bed; raise bed to a comfortable height when the patient is transferring out of bed.
- Keep hospital bed brakes locked.
- Keep wheelchair wheel locks in "locked" position when stationary.
- Keep nonslip, comfortable, well-fitting footwear on the patient.
- Use night-lights or supplemental lighting.
- Keep floor surfaces clean and dry. Clean up all spills promptly.
- Keep patient care areas uncluttered.
- Follow safe patient-handling practices.

Note: There is still no conclusive evidence for any particular set of interventions that will consistently prevent falls, even though numerous individual nursing fall prevention interventions have been tested (Fehlberg et al., 2017). The AHRQ (2013) recommends the following tips:

- **Fall prevention must be balanced with other priorities for the patient.**
- **Fall prevention must be balanced with the need to mobilize patients.**
- **Fall prevention is one of many activities needed to protect patients from harm.**
- **Fall prevention is interdisciplinary.**

Delegation

The skill of assessing and communicating a patient's risks for falls cannot be delegated to assistive personnel (AP). Skills used to prevent falls can be delegated. Direct the AP by:

- Explaining a patient's specific fall risks and associated prevention measures needed to minimize risks.
- Explaining environmental safety precautions to use.
- Explaining specific patient behaviors (e.g., disorientation, wandering) that are precursors to falls and that these should be reported immediately.

Collaboration

- Collaborate with physical therapist for assessment and development of individualized treatment plans including exercises to improve strength, mobility, and balance.
- Occupational therapists assess the patient's normal activity roles and routines, and the home environment to maximize independence while reducing fall risk.

Equipment

- Standardized and valid fall risk assessment tool (HRET, 2016)
- Hospital bed with side rails; *Option:* low bed
- Wedge cushion
- Nurse call system
- Gait belt for assisting with ambulation
- Wheelchair and seat belt (as needed)
- *Optional safety devices:* bed alarm pad, nonslip floor mat, protective head gear, hip protector

STEP	RATIONALE
1 Perform preprocedure protocol.	
Assessment	
• Review electronic health record (EHR) to determine whether patient has a recent history of a fall and risks for injury (ABCDs) (Institute for Healthcare Improvement [IHI], 2017):	These conditions increase likelihood of serious injury from a fall such as fracture or internal hemorrhage.
a Age over 85 years	
b Bone disorders (e.g., metastasis, osteoporosis)	
c Coagulation disorders (e.g.,	
d Leukemia, thrombocytopenia, anticoagulant use)	
e Surgery (specifically thoracic or abdominal surgery or lower limb amputation)	
• Perform hand hygiene. Assess for fall risks using a validated fall risk assessment tool. Compute fall risk score. (Include a cognitive assessment tool and integrate into fall risk assessment tool if cognitive assessment is not included in the fall risk assessment [HRET, 2016]).	Reduces transmission of microorganisms. A variety of intrinsic physiologic factors predispose patients to falls. Fall risk tools based on the risk factors of a population (e.g., elderly, oncologic or neurologic patient) are more likely to be sensitive for predicting falls.

Continued

STEP	RATIONALE

CLINICAL JUDGMENT *Because fall risk assessment is individualized, continue assessment (as appropriate) to include risk factors noted below.*

- Continue with comprehensive individualized patient assessment and consider patient's unique intrinsic fall risks (The Joint Commission [TJC], 2020a) (see Table 28.1). Perform a fall risk assessment in general acute care settings on admission, on transfer from one unit to another, with a significant change in a patient's condition, or after a fall (AHRQ, 2013).

  Reveals all factors placing patient at a fall risk.

- Perform the Banner Mobility Assessment Tool (BMAT) (Boynton, et al., 2014) (see skill 4) or the Timed Up and Go (TUG) test (CDC, 2017; Kiel et al., 2020) if patient is able to ambulate. At a minimum, observe an ambulatory patient walking in room (with or without help).

  The BMAT assesses four functional tasks to identify the level of mobility a patient can achieve, revealing if assistance is needed (Boynton et al., 2014). The TUG test measures the progress of balance, sit to stand, and walking.

CLINICAL JUDGMENT *Do not ask patient to provide a self-report of balance, gait, or ability to ambulate. Subjective report may not be true measure of patient's physical mobility.*

- Assess if patient in pain, assess character and rate severity on scale of 0 to 10.

  Pain, especially when it is associated with lower extremities (e.g., arthritis, injury), is a risk factor for falls.

STEP	RATIONALE
• Ask patient or family caregiver whether patient has a history of recent falls or other injuries within the home. Assess previous falls using the acronym SPLATT (Touhy and Jett, 2020): a) **S**ymptoms at time of fall b) **P**revious fall c) **L**ocation of fall d) **A**ctivity at time of fall e) **T**ime of fall f) **T**rauma after fall	Symptoms are helpful in identifying cause for fall. Onset, location, and activity offer details on how to prevent future falls.
• Review patient's medications (including over-the-counter medications and herbal products) for drugs that create risk for falls (e.g., benzodiazepines, antipsychotics, antidepressants, opioids and barbiturates, anticonvulsants). Compare drugs with those on the Beers Criteria lists (American Geriatrics Society [AGS], 2019).	These are drugs that are associated with drowsiness. The AGS Beers Criteria include lists of certain medications worth reviewing with patients; it lists medications that may not be the safest or most appropriate for older adults (AGS, 2019). The five lists included in the AGS Beers Criteria describe particular medications with scientific evidence suggesting they should be: 1 Avoided by most older people (outside of hospice and palliative care settings). 2 Avoided by older people with specific health conditions. 3 Avoided in combination with other treatments because of the risk for harmful "drug–drug" interactions. 4 Used with caution because of the potential for harmful side effects. 5 Dosed differently or avoided in people with reduced kidney function, which affects how the body processes medicine.

Continued

STEP	RATIONALE
• Assess for polypharmacy (unnecessary use of multiple [five or more] and/or redundant medications in management of the same condition and/or drugs inappropriate for condition).	Over a 2-year period polypharmacy was significantly associated with an increased rate of 21% of falls in a study involving adults older than 60 years (Dhalwani et al., 2017).
• As needed, assess patient's fear of falling. Use the Falls Efficacy Scale (FES-1) or the Activities-specific Balance Confidence (ABC) scale which measures a patient's confidence with doing specific activities of daily living without falling or losing their balance (Soh, 2021).	Fear of falling is significantly associated with falls in community dwelling older adults, especially in individuals with more than 1 fall in the past year (Asai et al., 2022).
• Assess condition of assistive devices or equipment used by patient (e.g., legs on bedside commode, end tips on a walker).	Equipment in poor repair increases risk for fall.
• Discuss results of fall risk assessment with patient and family caregiver and explain significance of risk factors. Explain how a plan for fall prevention will be developed.	Allows determination of content to include in fall prevention education.
• If patient is in a wheelchair, assess level of comfort, fatigue, boredom, mental status, and level of engagement with others.	These factors increase the risk that patient will make an attempt to exit wheelchair without help.

STEP	RATIONALE

Implementation

1 Based on your assessment, if patient is a fall risk, apply color-coded wrist band.(Some agencies also institute fall risk signs on doors, color-coded socks, or gowns.)

Color-coded yellow bands, socks, and gowns are easily recognizable.

2 Explain safety measure to be taken pertaining to patient's specific fall risks. Use patient-centered approach to determine what patient already knows about risks for falling. Explain to patient and family significance of risk factors and plan to modify them.

Clear, concise information with explanations for purpose, benefits, and expectations results in increased patient participation.

Allows you to determine content to include in fall prevention education (Dykes and Hurley, 2021).

3 Conduct hourly purposeful rounds on all patients to determine status of pain and provide pain relief intervention as needed, be proactive in offering assist to toilet, assess comfort of position, and assess need to relocate personal items for easy reach.

Use of purposeful and timely patient rounding has been shown to reduce falls and improve patient satisfaction (Manges et al., 2020). Studies have shown that patients who fall do not seek help while toileting (HRET, 2016).

4 Implement early mobility protocols within health care agency.

A patient's functional decline (loss of the ability to perform self-care activities or activities of daily living) may result from deconditioning, which is associated with inactivity (Gorman et al., 2014; Grass et al., 2018).

Continued

STEP	RATIONALE
5 **Implement Universal Fall Precautions** (AHRQ, 2013). a Adjust bed to low position with wheels locked. Place nonslip padded floor mat at exit side of bed.	Bed height allows ambulatory patient to get in and out of bed easily and safely. Mats provide a nonslip surface for preventing falls and injuries.
b Encourage use of properly fitted skidproof footwear.	Prevents falls resulting from slipping on floor.
c Orient patient to surroundings. Explain nurse call system and routines to expect in plan of care.	Orientation to room and plan of care provides familiarity with environment and activities to anticipate.

CLINICAL JUDGMENT *Agencies with successful fall prevention programs have implemented a patient agreement form to use call light for all ambulation (HRET, 2016). Be sure agreement has been signed.*

---

(1) Provide patient's hearing aid and glasses. Be sure that each is functioning and clean (AHRQ, 2013). If patient complains of visual or hearing problems, refer to appropriate health care provider.	Enables patient to remain alert to conditions in environment.
(2) Place nurse call system in an accessible location within patient's reach. Explain and demonstrate how to use system at bedside and in bathroom. Have patient perform return demonstration.	Knowledge of location and use of call system is essential for patient to be able to call for help quickly. Reaching for an object when in bed can lead to an accidental fall.

STEP	RATIONALE
(3) Explain to patient/ family member when and why to use nurse call system (e.g., reporting pain, requesting assistance to get out of bed or go to bathroom) (HRET, 2016). Provide clear instructions regarding mobility restrictions.	Increases likelihood that patient/ family caregiver will call for help and that hospital personnel will be able to respond to patient's needs in a timely manner.
d Safe use of side rails:	
(1) Explain to patient and family caregiver reason for use of side rails: moving and turning self in bed, comfort and security, (US Food and Drug Administration [FDA], 2017).	Promotes a feeling of comfort and security. Aids in turning and repositioning and provides easy access to bed controls (FDA, 2017).
(2) Check agency policy regarding side rail use.	
i Dependent, less mobile patients: In two–side rail bed, keep both rails up. (*Note:* Rails on newer hospital beds allow for room at foot of bed for patient to safely exit bed.) In four–side rail bed, leave only two upper rails up.	Side rails are restraint devices if they restrict a patient from voluntarily getting out of bed and therefore do not promote individual independent functioning (TJC, 2022).

Continued

STEP	RATIONALE
ii Patient able to get out of bed independently: In four–side rail bed, leave two upper side rails up. In two–side rail bed, keep only one rail up.	Allows for safe exit from bed.
e Ensure a safe patient environment:	
(1) Remove excess equipment, supplies, and furniture from rooms and halls.	Reduces likelihood of falling or tripping over objects.
(2) Keep floors free of clutter and obstacles (e.g., IV pole, electrical cords), particularly path to bathroom (AHRQ, 2013).	Reduces likelihood of falling or tripping over objects.
(3) Coil and secure excess electrical, telephone, and other cords or tubing.	Reduces risk of entanglement.
(4) Clean all spills on floors promptly (AHRQ, 2013). Post sign indicating wet floor. Remove sign when floor is dry (usually done by housekeeping department).	Reduces risk of falling on slippery, wet surfaces.
(5) Ensure adequate glare-free lighting; use a night-light at night.	Glare may be problem for older adults because of vision changes.

STEP	RATIONALE
(6) Have assistive devices (e.g., cane, walker, bedside commode) on exit side of bed. Have chair back of a bedside commode placed against wall of room if possible.	Provides added support when transferring out of bed. Stabilizes commode.
(7) Arrange personal items (e.g., water pitcher, telephone, reading materials, dentures) within patient's easy reach and organized in a logical way (AHRQ, 2013).	Facilitates independence and self-care; prevents falls related to trying to obtain hard-to-reach items.
(8) Secure locks on beds, stretchers, and wheelchairs (AHRQ, 2013).	Prevents accidental movement of devices during patient transfer.
6 Use a mattress properly proportioned to bed size, or mattress with raised foam edges (FDA, 2017).	Prevents patients from being trapped between the mattress and rail.
a Reduce gaps between the mattress and side rails (FDA, 2017).	Prevents patient entrapment.
7 Provide comfort measures; offer ordered analgesics for patients experiencing pain, preferably around-the-clock or prn as ordered.	Pain can cause patients to exit bed and has been associated with an increase in falls (Patel et al., 2014). Be cautious because opioids further increase fall risk.

Continued

STEP	RATIONALE
8 **Interventions for patients at moderate to high risk for falling (based on fall risk assessment):**	
a Prioritize call-light responses to patients at high risk; use a team approach, with all staff knowing responsibility to respond.	Ensures rapid response by care provider when patient calls for help; decreases chance of patient trying to get out of bed on their own.
b Establish elimination schedule, use bedside commode when appropriate.	Proactive toileting keeps patients from being unattended with sudden urge to use toilet.

CLINICAL JUDGMENT *Toileting is a common event leading to a patient's fall (Berry and Kiel, 2018).*

STEP	RATIONALE
c Stay with patient during toileting (standing outside bathroom door). Increase availability and use of raised toilet seats, toilet safety frames/grab bars (VA Healthcare, 2015).	Patients often try to get up to stand and walk back to their beds from the bathroom without help. Raised seats make it easier to sit and then stand up from toilet. Toilet frames and grab bars can be grasped to provide support when standing and sitting.
d Place patient in a geri chair or wheelchair. Use wheelchair only for transport, not for sitting an extended time.	Maintains alignment and comfort.
e Provide hip protectors or padded shorts or underwear that are worn over or in place of underwear (used more often in long-term care settings).	Prevents fractures by distributing the force of a fall on the hip to the softer tissue around the buttocks and thighs (US Department of Veterans Affairs, 2019).

STEP	RATIONALE
f Consider use of a low bed that has lower height than standard hospital bed. Apply nonskid floor mats (US Department of Veterans Affairs, 2019).	Low beds may reduce fall-related injuries by making it difficult for patients with lower extremity weakness or pain in lower joints to exert effort needed to stand. Mats prevent slipping when walking and standing.
g Activate a bed alarm or surveillance system, such as a camera monitoring system (VA Healthcare, 2015).	Alarm activates when patient rises off bed alarm sensor or gets out of bed. Alarm sounds an alert to staff. Camera can detect an unassisted bed exit and alert staff (Jones et al., 2021).

CLINICAL JUDGMENT *Use judgment in choosing use of a bed alarm. Bed and chair alarms can restrict patient activity. Reports have shown that patients perceive that an alarm makes them feel restrained (Growdon et al., 2017). Determine whether use of bed or chair alarm limits frequency of patient getting up and remaining active.*

STEP	RATIONALE
h Confer with physical therapist about gait training, strength and balance training, and regular weight-bearing activities.	Exercise can reduce falls, fall-related fractures, and several risk factors for falls in individuals with low bone density and in older adults. Strength and balance training reduces the rate of injurious falls in older adults (Uusi-Rasi et al., 2015).
i Use sitters or restraints only when alternatives are exhausted.	A sitter is a nonprofessional staff member or volunteer who stays in a patient room to closely observe patients who are at risk for falling. Restraints should be used only as a final option (see Skill 64).
j Consider having patient wear head protective gear (e.g., oncology patient or patients at risk for bleeding).	Contains impact-resistant material within the hat that surrounds the head and protects against head injury.

Continued

STEP	RATIONALE
9 When ambulating a patient, have patient wear a gait belt or use a walking sling and walk along his or her side.	Safe patient-handling techniques allow for safe patient ambulation and prevention of injury to patient and hospital personnel.
10 Safe use of wheelchair:	
a Be sure that wheelchair is correct fit for patient: patient thighs are level while sitting, feet flat on floor; back of chair comes up to midshoulder, elbows rest on armrests without leaning over or tucking arms in, and there are two finger widths of space between patient and side of chair.	Correctly fitted chair promotes comfort, making it less likely for patient to try to exit.
b Transfer patient to wheelchair using safe-handling techniques.	Minimizes fall risk.
c Back wheelchair into and out of elevator or door, leading with large rear wheels first.	Prevents smaller front wheels from catching in crack between elevator and floor, causing chair to tip.
d Manage patient's pain. Refrain from leaving patient sitting in wheelchair for an extended amount of time; provide alternative sitting option.	Reduces restlessness and discomfort that can lead to wheelchair exit.
11 Schedule oral medication administration for at least 2 h before bedtime (HRET, 2016).	Reduces risk created by medications that can cause patients to have to use bathroom during night.

STEP	RATIONALE
12 Perform postprocedure protocol.	
13 Evaluate patient response.	
a Ask patient/family caregiver to identify patient's fall risks.	Demonstrates learning.
b Ask patient/family caregiver to describe fall prevention interventions to implement.	Demonstrates learning.
c Evaluate patient's ability to use assistive devices such as walker or bedside commode at different times during the day.	Adjustments in devices may become necessary. Evaluating at different times can help identify strengths and weaknesses.
d Evaluate for changes in motor, sensory, and cognitive status and review if any falls or injuries have occurred.	May require different interventions to be added. Fall outcomes determine success of plan.
e Evaluate patient's pain level using a pain rating scale.	Determines whether patient's pain is under adequate control.

Recording and Reporting

- Record in the plan of care specific fall prevention interventions. Use whiteboards in patient rooms to communicate patient fall risks to all staff (HRET, 2016).
- Document patient's ability/inability to explain fall risks and interventions taken.
- If fall occurs, complete an agency safety event or incident report, noting objective details of a fall (time, location, patient's condition, treatment, treatment response). Do not place the report in patient's medical record.
- Use a hand-off communication tool that includes specific patient risks for falls and falls with injury between caregivers (include AP). Discuss patient-specific interventions taken (HRET, 2016).
- Report immediately to the health care provider if patient sustains a fall or an injury.

UNEXPECTED OUTCOMES	RELATED INTERVENTIONS
1 Patient/family caregiver unable to identify fall risks or fall prevention strategies.	• Reinforce identified risks and review safety measures with patient and family caregiver. • Consider using other instructional options.
2 Patient found on floor after falling.	• Call for assistance. • Assess for injury and remain with patient until help arrives. • Notify primary health care provider and family caregiver. • Complete an agency occurrence or sentinel event report (see agency policy). • Conduct a post-fall huddle/debrief as soon as possible after the fall. Involve staff at all levels and the patient if possible. Discuss whether appropriate interventions were in place, considerations as to why fall occurred, staffing at time of fall, which environment or care factors were in place, and how care plan will change (HRET, 2016; VA Healthcare, 2015).

Fecal Impaction

Digital Removal

Fecal impaction is the inability to pass a collection of hard stool. This condition occurs in all age groups. Physically and mentally incapacitated individuals and institutionalized older adults are at greatest risk because of conditions that often create poor hydration and nutrition. Patients with acute stroke and spinal cord injuries are at greater risk for fecal impaction due to neurologic injury.

Functional constipation includes a group of disorders associated with persistent, difficult, infrequent, or seemingly incomplete defecation without evidence of an explanation (Sood, 2020). Symptoms of fecal impaction include constipation, rectal discomfort, anorexia, nausea, vomiting, abdominal pain, abdominal bloating, small liquid stools (leaking around the impacted stool), and urinary frequency. Prevention is the best way to manage fecal impaction. With newer bowel-management techniques such as safe long-term use of osmotic laxatives, which pull fluid into the stool and soften it, or transanal irrigation for patients with a neurogenic motility impairment, the need for regular digital removal of fecal material has been reduced. Once fecal impaction has occurred, however, digital removal of stool is the only alternative.

Safety Guidelines

- Use caution and consult with health care provider if patient has active inflammation of the bowel, including Crohn's disease, ulcerative colitis, and diverticulitis; recent radiotherapy to the pelvic area; rectal/anal pain; surgery/trauma to the anal/rectal area; and obvious rectal bleeding.

Delegation

The skill of removing a fecal impaction digitally cannot be delegated to assistive personnel (AP). Instruct the AP to:
- Help position a patient for the procedure.
- Measure heart rate during fecal removal.
- Provide perineal care after each bowel movement.

Collaboration

- Include health care team members in planning a bowel-management program.

Equipment

- Bedpan
- Waterproof pad
- Water-soluble lubricant
- Washcloths, towels, soap
- Bath blanket
- Clean gloves
- Sphygmomanometer and stethoscope

STEPS	RATIONALE
1 Perform preprocedure protocol.	
Assessment	
• Review electronic health record (EHR) and confirm healthcare provider order for removal of impaction.	Order required for procedure.
• Ask patient to describe the usual characteristics of their stools, whether the quality is normally watery or formed, soft or hard, and the typical color.	Baseline to determine fecal characteristics after impaction removal.
• Ask the patient to describe the shape of a normal stool and the number of stools per day. *Option:* Use the Bristol Stool Form Scale (Fig 29.1).	Scale provides an objective measure of stool characteristics.
• Perform hand hygiene. Pull curtains around bed. Obtain patient's heart rate and blood pressure (BP), assess level of comfort, and palpate for abdominal distention.	Reduces transmission of microorganisms. Baseline data used to evaluate patient response to procedure.
Implementation	
1 Offer patient the opportunity to empty their bladder.	A full bladder may cause discomfort during the procedure
2 Help patient lie on left side in Sims position with knees flexed and back facing toward you.	Position aids entry into rectum for stool removal.

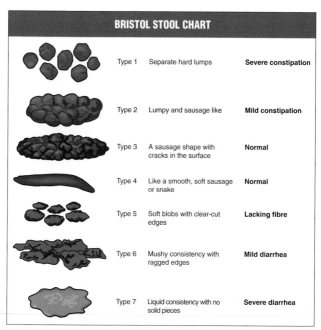

BRISTOL STOOL CHART

	Type 1	Separate hard lumps	**Severe constipation**
	Type 2	Lumpy and sausage like	**Mild constipation**
	Type 3	A sausage shape with cracks in the surface	**Normal**
	Type 4	Like a smooth, soft sausage or snake	**Normal**
	Type 5	Soft blobs with clear-cut edges	**Lacking fibre**
	Type 6	Mushy consistency with ragged edges	**Mild diarrhea**
	Type 7	Liquid consistency with no solid pieces	**Severe diarrhea**

Fig. 29.1 The Bristol Stool Form Scale. (From O'Donnell LJ, Virjee J, Heaton KW: Detection of pseudodiarrhoea by simple clinical assessment of intestinal transit rate, *Br Med J* 300: 439, 1990. Reprinted with permission of the BMJ Publishing Group.)

STEPS	RATIONALE

CLINICAL JUDGMENT *Many older adults are especially prone to dysrhythmias and other problems related to vagal stimulation; monitor heart rate and rhythm closely (Ball et al., 2019).*

3 Drape patient's trunk and lower extremities with a bath blanket and place a waterproof pad under buttocks. Keep a bedpan next to patient.	Provides for patient comfort. Increases cleanliness around patient.
4 Perform hand hygiene and apply clean gloves; lubricate index finger of dominant hand with water-soluble lubricant.	Reduces transmission of microorganisms. Lubricant reduces friction when finger inserted into rectum.

Continued

STEPS	RATIONALE
5 Instruct patient to take slow, deep breaths. Gradually and gently insert index finger into the rectum and advance the finger slowly along the rectal wall.	Relaxes anal sphincter.
6 Gently massage around the fecal mass. Work the finger into the hardened mass.	Loosens feces for removal. Minimizes discomfort.
7 Work the feces downward toward the end of the rectum. Remove small pieces one at a time and discard into bedpan.	
8 Periodically reassess patient's pulse and BP and look for signs of fatigue, headache, flushing, sweating, and hypertension. Stop the procedure if pulse rate or BP drops/rises significantly (check agency policy) or if there are pulse rhythm changes.	Determines patient's tolerance to procedure. Drop in pulse and BP could indicate autonomic dysreflexia (common in spinal cord injury patients).
9 Continue to clear rectum of feces, allowing patient to rest at intervals.	Prevents patient distress.
10 After completion, wash and dry buttocks and anal area.	Promotes comfort and cleanliness.
11 Remove bedpan. Dispose of feces. Remove gloves by turning them inside out and then discard. Perform hand hygiene.	Reduces transmission of microorganisms.
12 Help patient to toilet or onto a bedpan if urge to defecate develops.	

STEPS	RATIONALE
13 Follow procedure with administration of enemas (See skill 22) or cathartics as ordered by health care provider.	Hardened stool is likely to remain in upper descending colon.
14 Perform postprocedure protocol.	
15 Evaluate patient response.	
a Inspect feces for color and consistency.	Determines characteristics of stool.
b Measure patient's vital signs and level of comfort. Observe status of abdominal distention.	Determines tolerance to procedure.

Recording and Reporting

- Record fecal characteristics and amount, patient's tolerance to procedure, vital signs and any adverse effects.
- Report any changes in vital signs and adverse effects to health care provider.

UNEXPECTED OUTCOME	INTERVENTION
1 Patient requires repeated removal of impaction.	• Increase patient's hydration and intake of high fiber foods (if allowed).
	• Consult with registered dietitian regarding ongoing diet for patient.
	• Confer with health care provider regarding appropriate bowel stimulants or laxatives to administer.

Hypothermia and Hyperthermia Blankets

A hypothermia or hyperthermia blanket raises, lowers, or maintains body temperature through conductive heat or cold transfer between the blanket and a patient (Fig. 30.1). When operated manually, a unit is adjusted to reach a desired temperature setting. When operating in the automatic setting, a unit continually monitors a patient's temperature with a thermistor probe (rectal, skin, or esophageal).

Hypothermia blankets are used for patients who have high, prolonged fevers from infectious neurologic diseases, from side effects of anesthesia, and after severe brain injury and myocardial infarction. Research shows that induced hypothermia prevents or moderates neurologic outcomes after neurosurgery, traumatic brain injury, and acute stroke (Rittenberger and Callaway, 2013). In addition, research shows patients who have been successfully resuscitated after cardiac arrest due to ventricular fibrillation benefit from therapeutic mild hypothermia with improved neurologic outcomes and reduced mortality (Soudy, 2018). Mild hypothermia (32°C to 34° C [89.6° F to 93.2° F]) in the first hours after a cardiac ischemic event and for 72 h or until stabilization occurs helps prevent permanent heart damage.

Surgical procedures tend to create hypothermia in patients due to a cold operating room, administration of cool fluids, sedatives, or anesthesia (Soule, 2018). Maintaining normothermia by warming patients who are having major surgery (clean without infection) is recommended to prevent surgical site infections (Berrios-Torres et al., 2017; Ousey and Edward, 2015; Soule, 2018). Forced-air warming devices (most commonly used), circulating water garments, energy transfer pads, and warmed blankets are used intraoperatively to maintain normothermia in patients undergoing major surgery (Koc et al., 2017; Soule, 2018). Continuous use of a warming blanket intraoperatively maintains normothermia.

Safety Guidelines

- Hypothermia devices set too low can cause vasoconstriction, shivering, increased oxygen demand, altered coronary blood flow, cardiac dysrhythmias, acid-base imbalances, and impaired coagulation.
- There is risk of thermal injuries to the skin from warming blankets, thus requiring frequent patient monitoring while these blankets are in use.

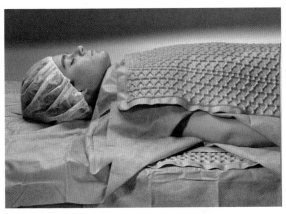

Fig. 30.1 Hypothermia cooling blanket is applied over paper sheet before additional top sheet is applied to bed. (Courtesy Cincinnati Sub-Zero Products, LLC, Cincinnati, OH.)

- Therapeutic hypothermia may have increased risk for patients with (Koyfman et al., 2019):
  - Recent major surgery within 14 days. Hypothermia may increase the risk of infection and bleeding.
  - Systemic infection/sepsis. Hypothermia may inhibit immune function and is associated with a small increase in risk of infection.
  - Coma from other causes (drug intoxication, preexisting coma before cardiac arrest).
  - Known bleeding disorders or with active ongoing bleeding. Hypothermia may impair the clotting system.

Delegation

The skill of applying a hypothermia or hyperthermia blanket can be delegated to assistive personnel (AP) (see agency policy). The nurse is responsible for assessing and evaluating treatment and related patient education. If the patient is unstable and at risk for complications, this skill is not delegated. Direct the AP to:

- Maintain proper temperature of the application throughout the treatment and discontinue the application as specified in the health care provider's order.
- Report any unexpected patient outcomes (e.g., shivering, skin redness).
- Report when treatment is complete so an evaluation of the patient's response can be made.

Equipment

- Forced-air warming device or warming blanket for warming
- Hypothermia device for cooling
- Blanket control panel and rectal probe
- Sheet or thin bath blanket
- Distilled water to fill the units if necessary
- Disposable gloves
- Oral thermometer (for baseline); rectal thermometer (for intraoperative measurement)
- Sphygmomanometer and stethoscope

Implementation

STEP	RATIONALE
1 Complete preprocedure protocol.	
Assessment	
• Review electronic health record (EHR) for healthcare provider's order and temperature setting.	Order required for therapy.
• Review EHR for contraindications to hypothermia (see safety guidelines, above)	
• Perform hand hygiene. Inspect condition of skin over which blanket/ device will be applied and over dependent areas. Assess neurologic and mental status and status of peripheral circulation	Provides baseline for early detection of injuries to skin. Data indicate patient's risks with device. Patients in critical condition or going to operating room are at risk for pressure injury in dependent areas due to immobility.
• Measure patient's vital signs	Provides baseline for subsequent monitoring of patient response to therapy.

SAFETY ALERT *Antipyretic therapy may be used in combination with a cooling blanket. Temperatures greater than 41° C (105.8° F) have detrimental effects in neurologic patients, children, and older adults.*

STEP	RATIONALE

Implementation

1. Prepare blanket according to agency policy and manufacturer's instructions.

   Agencies have specific policies on maintaining equipment in functional order.

2. Perform hand hygiene, and apply clean gloves.

   Reduces transmission of microorganisms.

3. Turn on device and observe that cool or warm light is on. Precool or prewarm device, setting device temperature to desired level. Forced-air warming devices use a hose attached to deliver warm air.

   Verifies that blanket is correctly set to help decrease (cool) or increase (warm) patient's body temperature. Prepares blanket for prescribed therapy.

4. Verify that selected device temperature limits are set at desired safety ranges.

   Safety ranges prevent excessive cooling or warming. The blanket automatically shuts off when preset body temperature is achieved.

5. Cover the hypothermia or hyperthermia device with a thin paper, cloth sheet, or bath blanket.

   Injuries from hot or cold therapies are preventable events (National Quality Forum, 2016). Thin sheet protects patient's skin from direct contact with blanket, thus reducing risk for injury to skin. Sheet or blanket covers plastic and provides insulation between patient and appliance.

6. Position hypothermia or hyperthermia blanket device following manufacturer directions.

   Provides wide distribution of blanket device against patient's skin.

   a. Wrap patient's hands and feet in gauze.

   Reduces risk for thermal injury to body's distal areas.

   b. Wrap scrotum with towels.

   Protects sensitive tissue from direct contact with cold.

Continued

STEP	RATIONALE
7 Lubricate rectal probe, and insert into patient's rectum.	When using hypothermia or hyperthermia blanket, it is imperative that you continuously monitor patient's core interior (rectal) temperature.
8 Turn and position patient regularly to protect from pressure injury development and impaired body alignment. Keep linens free of perspiration and condensation.	Patient has an increased risk for pressure injury development because of skin moisture created by blanket and patient's body temperature.
9 Check condition of patient's skin regularly (see agency protocol)	Ensures early detection of thermal injury to skin.
10 Double-check temperature setting on device at initial setup and before leaving room.	Verifies that pad temperature is maintained at desired level.
11 Complete postprocedure protocol.	
12 Evaluate patient response.	
a Monitor body temperature.	Determines whether excessive warming or cooling develops.
b Inspect skin surfaces.	Prevents development of serious thermal or pressure injury.

Recording and Reporting

▪ Record baseline data: vital signs, neurologic and mental status, status of peripheral circulation, and skin integrity when therapy was initiated. Include type of hyperthermia/hypothermia device used; control settings (manual or automatic and temperature settings); date, time, duration; and patient's tolerance of treatment.

- Record repeated measurements of vital signs on temperature graph to document response to therapy.
- Document your evaluation of patient and family caregiver learning.
- Report any unexpected outcome to health care provider. Further treatment may be needed.

UNEXPECTED OUTCOMES	RELATED INTERVENTIONS
1 Patient's core body temperature decreases or increases rapidly.	• Adjust blanket temperature no more than 1° F (0.6° C) every 15 minutes to avoid complications.
2 Patient's core temperature remains unchanged.	• Patient may need hypothermic or hyperthermic treatment of additional sites, such as axilla, groin, and neck, in addition to those covered by blanket.
	• Discuss use of an antipyretic with health care provider.
3 Patient begins to shiver.	• Adjust temperature to more comfortable range, and assess if shivering decreases.
	• If shivering continues, stop treatment and notify health care provider.

Using Incentive Spirometry

Incentive spirometry helps a patient deep breathe in order to achieve maximum inspiration. Use of the device exercises the lungs and aids in keeping the lungs as healthy as possible (Lung Health Institute, 2017). The devices are commonly used for patient recovery postoperatively. Incentive spirometry works by providing visual feedback that encourages a patient to take long, deep, slow breaths. The use of an incentive spirometer (IS) alone is not recommended to prevent postoperative pulmonary complications. It should be used in combination with other pulmonary maneuvers such as deep breathing and coughing, early mobilization of the patient, and directed coughing (Eltorai et al., 2018b).

The two types of ISs are flow oriented and volume oriented. The flow-oriented IS has one or more plastic chambers with freely movable colored balls. The slow, steady expansion of the lung is an advantage of a flow-oriented IS. As a patient inhales slowly, the balls elevate to a premarked area (based on patient's highest performance) (Fig. 31.1). A patient's goal is to keep the balls elevated for as long as possible to ensure maximal sustained inhalation. Even if a slow inspiration does not elevate the balls, this pattern helps a patient improve lung expansion (Eltorai et al., 2018a).

Volume-oriented devices use a bellows that a patient must raise to a predetermined volume by inhaling slowly (Fig. 31.2). The fact that a patient can achieve a known inspiratory volume and measure it with each breath is an advantage of the volume-oriented IS. This device is also associated with a decreased work of breathing (Eltorai et al., 2018a).

Delegation

The skill of helping a patient to use an IS can be delegated to assistive personnel (AP). The nurse is responsible for assessing and monitoring the patient, evaluating the patient response, educating the patient about the proper use of the IS, and evaluating understanding of the education. Direct the AP by:

- Informing about the patient's target goal for incentive spirometry.
- Instructing to report immediately any unexpected outcomes such as chest pain, excessive sputum production, and fever.

Collaboration

- Respiratory therapists often assess the patient with potential disturbances in oxygenation. Recommendations for alternative respiratory therapy may be given.

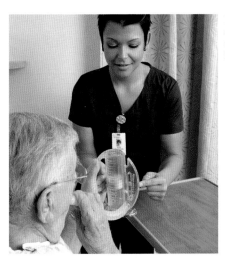

Fig. 31.1 Instructing a patient on how to use a flow-oriented incentive spirometer.

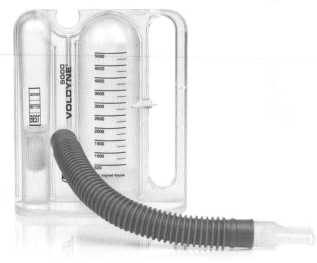

Fig. 31.2 Volume-oriented incentive spirometer.

Equipment

- Flow- or volume-oriented IS
- Stethoscope

- Pulse oximeter monitor, stethoscope
- Personal protective equipment as needed

STEP	RATIONALE
1 Perform preprocedure protocol.	

Assessment

• Review patient's electronic health record (EHR), including health care provider's order and nurses' notes. Review the use of the IS in patients who will benefit from its use (e.g., patients who undergo thoracic or abdominal surgery; patients with a history of chronic obstructive pulmonary disease or cystic fibrosis, rib fractures and patients with sickle cell disease with acute chest syndrome) (Cleveland Clinic, 2022).	Health care agencies often require a medical order for incentive spirometry in order to receive third-party reimbursement. Alerts health care personnel to patients at risk for respiratory complications during illness or after surgery.
• Assess patient for confusion, cognitive impairment, ability to follow directions, age, developmental level, level of consciousness, and decreased necessary motor skills (Restrepo et al., 2011).	Determines risk for difficulty and/or inability to perform incentive spirometry.

CLINICAL JUDGMENT *Patients who are unable to follow directions or who are not developmentally or physically able to perform the actions associated with this skill are not candidates for this intervention. Assessment findings also determine whether to use the flow-oriented versus volume-oriented IS.*

• Perform hand hygiene. Assess patient's respiratory status, including symmetry of chest wall expansion, respiratory rate and depth, sputum production, and lung sounds. Also obtain a pulse oximetry reading.	Reduces transmission of microorganisms. Decreased chest wall movement, crackles or decreased lung sounds, increased respiratory rate, or increased sputum production can indicate a need for incentive spirometry to improve lung expansion.

STEP	RATIONALE
• Assess character of pain at rest and during activity (e.g., coughing) rate severity on a 0-to-10 scale.	Pain decreases effective incentive spirometry by restricting chest expansion. Finding determines whether patient would benefit from analgesic before spirometry.
• Instruct patient about need for IS. Indicate to patient where to find target volume on IS. *Note:* If possible, demonstrate to patient how to use IS.	Education decreases patient anxiety and helps ensure safe and proper use of the equipment. Encourages patients to "do better" with each breath and meet or exceed target volume. When patients have a visual target, they can gauge their improvement.

Implementation

STEP	RATIONALE
1 Perform hand hygiene. Apply personal protective equipment if excess mucous expected.	Reduces transmission of microorganisms.
2 Position patient in most erect/ upright position (e.g., high-Fowler if tolerated) in bed or chair.	Promotes optimal lung expansion during respiratory maneuver.
3 Instruct patient to hold IS upright, exhale normally and completely through mouth, and place lips tightly around mouthpiece.	Allows for proper function of IS (Armstrong, 2017). Showing patient how to correctly place mouthpiece is a reliable technique for teaching psychomotor skill and enables patient to ask questions.
4 Instruct patient to take a slow, deep breath and maintain constant flow, like pulling through a straw. If using a flow-oriented IS, inhalation should raise the ball. If using a volume-oriented IS, inhalation should raise the piston. Remove mouthpiece at point of maximal inhalation, then have patient hold their breath for 3 seconds and exhale normally.	Maintains maximal inspiration; reduces risk for progressive collapse of individual alveoli.

Continued

STEP	RATIONALE

CLINICAL JUDGMENT *Some patients are unable to hold their breath for 3 seconds. Encourage them to do their best and try to extend the duration of breath holding. Allow patients to rest between IS breaths to prevent hyperventilation and fatigue. Remind them it is more important to inhale slowly versus quickly.*

STEP	RATIONALE
5 Have patient repeat maneuver. Offer encouragement to reach prescribed goal.	Ensures correct use of IS and patient's understanding of use.
6 Encourage patient to independently use IS at prescribed frequency. An example of a frequently prescribed timing schedule includes ten attempts every hour while awake (Armstrong, 2017).	Repeated use of IS improves lung expansion and promotes clearing of airways. Encouraging patients to perform independently gives them a sense of control over their care.
7 Encourage patient to cough after cycle of IS breaths.	Helps to clear the airway of secretions. The effects of the IS are augmented when accompanied with coughing (Armstrong, 2017; Eltorai et al., 2018b).
8 Perform postprocedure protocol.	
9 Evaluate patient response.	
a Observe patient's ability to use incentive spirometry by return demonstration.	Determines patient's ability to perform breathing exercise correctly.
b Assess whether patient is able to achieve target volume or frequency.	Measures adherence to therapy and achieved lung expansion.
c Auscultate chest during respiratory cycle and obtain pulse oximeter reading (Armstrong, 2017).	Assesses lung expansion, identifies any abnormal lung sounds, and determines whether airways are clear. Identifies improvement in pulse oximetry readings.

Recording and Reporting

- Record lung sounds, respiratory rate, and pulse oximetry readings before and after incentive spirometry; frequency of use; volumes achieved; patient tolerance of procedure and any adverse effects.
- Document evaluation of patient and/or family caregiver learning.
- Report any unexpected outcome to health care provider or nurse in charge.

UNEXPECTED OUTCOMES	RELATED INTERVENTIONS
1 Patient is unable to achieve incentive spirometry target volume.	• Encourage patient to use IS more frequently, followed by rest periods. • Teach cough-control exercises. • Teach patient how to splint and protect incision sites during deep breathing. • Administer ordered analgesic if acute pain is inhibiting use of IS (Armstrong, 2017).
2 Patient has decreased lung expansion and/or abnormal breath sounds or decreased pulse oximetry readings.	• Teach patient cough-control exercises. • Provide help with suctioning if patient cannot cough up secretions effectively.
3 Patient begins to hyperventilate.	• Encourage longer rest periods between breaths.

Intradermal Injections

Intradermal (ID) injections are administered for skin testing (e.g., tuberculosis [TB] screening and allergy tests). Because such medications are potent, you inject them into the dermis, where blood supply is reduced, and drug absorption occurs slowly. A patient may have an anaphylactic reaction if a medication enters the circulation too rapidly. Skin testing requires you to inspect the ID site visually to determine results. Be sure that ID sites are free of lesions and injuries before giving an injection. The inner forearm and upper back are ideal locations.

Administer an ID injection by using a tuberculin or small syringe with a short (⅜- to ⅝-inch), fine-gauge (25- to 27-gauge) needle. The angle of insertion for an ID injection is 5 to 15 degrees. Inject only small amounts of medication (0.01 to 0.1 mL) intradermally.

Safety Guidelines

- Be vigilant during medication administration. Avoid distractions.
- If a bleb does not appear or if the site bleeds after needle withdrawal, the medication may have entered subcutaneous tissues. Skin test results will not be valid.

Delegation

The skill of administering ID injections cannot be delegated to assistive personnel (AP). Direct the AP to:

- Report side effects or signs and symptoms of allergic response (clarify possible allergic reaction signs).
- Report any change in the patient's vital signs or condition.

Collaboration

- Infection control department is a resource for isolation guidelines if tuberculosis (TB) is expected.

Equipment

- Syringe: 1-mL TB syringe with preattached 25- or 27-gauge needle, ⅜ to ⅝ inch
- Small gauze pad
- Antiseptic swab
- Vial or ampule of medication
- Clean gloves
- Medication administration record (MAR) or computer printout
- Puncture-proof container

STEP	RATIONALE
1 Perform pre-procedure protocol.	

Assessment

- Check accuracy and completeness of MAR or computer printout with health care provider's original medication order. Check patient's name, medication name and dosage, route of administration, and time of administration. Recopy or reprint any part of MAR that is difficult to read.

The order sheet is the most reliable source and only legal record of medications that patient is to receive. Ensures that patient receives the correct medications (Palese et al., 2019). Transcription errors are a source of medication errors (Palese et al., 2019).

- Review drug reference information about expected reaction/anticipated effects of skin test and appropriate time to read site.

Type of reaction depends on patient's ability to mount a cell-mediated immune response. Knowledge of expected and adverse reactions to skin testing helps determine which symptoms to monitor, how frequently, and when to reassess patient.

- Ask patient to describe history of allergies: known types of allergies and normal allergic reaction. Check patient's allergy wristband.

Do not administer any medication for which there is a known patient allergy. Test solutions are potent and can cause severe anaphylaxis.

- Assess for contraindication to ID injections, including reduced local tissue perfusion. Assess for history of severe adverse reactions or necrosis that happened after previous ID injection.

Decreased perfusion reduces absorption of medication. Prior history of severe reactions increases the risk for future severe reactions.

Implementation

- **1** Explain to patient signs and symptoms of expected and unexpected ID reaction.

Lessens patient anxiety and helps patient know what to expect, promoting self-care.

Continued

STEP	RATIONALE
2 Perform preparation to avoid interruptions/distractions. Keep all pages of MARs or computer printouts for one patient together, or look at only one patient's electronic MAR at a time.	Interruptions contribute to medication errors (Palese et al., 2019).
3 Perform hand hygiene. Prepare medications for one patient at a time using aseptic technique. See Skill 48. Check label of medication carefully with MAR or computer printout when removing medication from storage and after preparing medication. Check test solution expiration date.	Ensures that medication is sterile. These are the first and second checks for accuracy and ensure that correct medication is administered. Dose potency increases or decreases when outdated.
4 Take medication(s) to patient at correct time (see agency policy).	Test solutions are usually not ordered for specific times.
5 Identify patient using at least two identifiers (e.g., name and birthday or name and medical record number) according to agency policy. Compare identifiers with information on patient's MAR or medical record.	Ensures correct patient. Complies with The Joint Commission standards and improves patient safety (The Joint Commission, 2022). Some agencies use a barcode system for patient identification.
6 At patient's bedside again compare MAR or computer printout with names of medications on medication labels and patient name. Confirm if patient has allergies.	This is the third check for accuracy and ensures that patient receives correct medication. Confirms patient's allergy history.

STEP	RATIONALE
7 Perform hand hygiene and apply clean gloves. Keep sheet or gown draped over body parts not requiring exposure.	Reduces transmission of infection. Provides privacy to patient.
8 Position patient sitting or lying supine. Have patient extend elbow and support the elbow and forearm on flat surface.	Positions arm for selection of injection site.
9 Select appropriate injection site on inner aspect of forearm. Note lesions or discolorations of skin. If possible, select site three to four finger widths below antecubital space and one hand width above wrist. If you cannot use forearm, inspect upper back. If necessary, use sites appropriate for subcutaneous injections (Fig. 32.1).	The skin of the forearm produces a smaller wheal than using the back (Kowal and DuBuske, 2020).

Continued

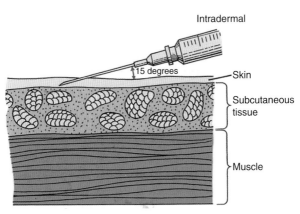

Fig. 32.1 Intradermal needle tip inserted into dermis.

STEP	RATIONALE
10 Instruct patient to keep forearm stable. Clean site with antiseptic swab. Apply swab at center of site and rotate outward in circular direction for about 5 cm (2 inches). *Option:* Use vapocoolant spray (e.g., ethyl chloride) before injection.	Mechanical action of swab removes microorganisms. Decreases pain at injection site.
11 Hold swab or gauze between third and fourth fingers of nondominant hand.	Gauze or swab remains readily accessible when withdrawing needle.
12 Remove needle cap from needle by pulling it straight off.	Preventing needle from touching sides of cap prevents contamination.
13 Hold syringe between thumb and forefinger of dominant hand with bevel of needle pointing up.	Smooth injection requires proper manipulation of syringe parts. Bevel-up position decreases the possibility of depositing medication into tissues below dermis.
14 Administer injection.	
a With nondominant hand, stretch skin over site with forefinger or thumb.	Needle pierces tight skin more easily.
b With needle almost against patient's skin, insert it slowly at 5- to 15-degree angle until resistance is felt. Advance needle through epidermis to approximately 3 mm ($\frac{1}{8}$ inch) below skin surface. You will see bulge of needle tip through skin.	Ensures that needle tip is in dermis. Inaccurate test result occurs if needle not injected at correct angle and depth.

STEP	RATIONALE
c Inject medication slowly. Normally you feel resistance. If not, needle is too deep. Remove the needle and begin again.	Slow injection minimizes discomfort at site. Dermal layer is tight and does not expand easily when you inject solution.

CLINICAL JUDGMENT *It is not necessary to aspirate because dermis is relatively avascular.*

d While injecting medication, note that a small wheal (approximately 6 to 10 mm [¼ to ⅜ inch]) resembling mosquito bite appears on skin surface (see Fig. 32.2)	The wheal should appear as a pale, raised area with distinct edges and an orange-peel appearance that does not disappear immediately.
(1) If no wheal forms, or if the wheal is less than 6 mm of induration, the test should be repeated immediately, approximately 5 cm (2 inches) from original site or on the other arm.	Necessary to obtain accurate test.
e After withdrawing needle, apply antiseptic swab or gauze gently over site.	Do not massage site. Apply bandage if needed.

Continued

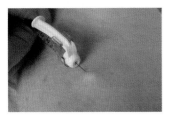

Fig. 32.2 Injection creates small bleb.

STEP	RATIONALE
15 Discard uncapped needle or needle enclosed in safety shield and attached syringe in puncture- and leak-proof receptacle.	Prevents injury to patients and health care personnel. Recapping needles increases risk for a needlestick injury (Occupational Safety and Health Administration, n.d.[a]).
16 Perform postprocedure protocol.	
17 Stay with patient for several minutes and observe for any allergic reactions.	Dyspnea, wheezing, and circulatory collapse are signs of severe anaphylactic reaction and would likely occur immediately after injection.
18 Evaluate patient response:	
a Return to room in 15 to 30 minutes and ask if patient feels any acute pain, burning, numbness, or tingling at injection site.	Continued discomfort could indicate injury to underlying tissues.
b Ask patient to discuss implications of skin testing and signs of hypersensitivity.	Patient's ability to recognize signs of skin testing helps to ensure timely reporting of results.
c Inspect bleb. *Option:* Use skin pencil and draw circle around perimeter of injection site. Read TB test site at 48 to 72 h; look for induration (hard, dense, raised area) of skin around injection site for:	Determines if reaction to antigen occurs. A reaction indicates positive results for TB or tested allergens. Site must be read at various intervals to determine test results. Mark site according to agency policy; this makes site easy to find. Results of skin testing are determined at various times, based on type of medication used or type of skin testing completed. Manufacturer directions determine when to read test results.

STEP	RATIONALE
• 15 mm or more in patients with no known risk factors for TB	Degree of reaction varies based on patient condition.
• 10 mm or more in patients who are recent immigrants; injection drug users; residents and employees of high-risk settings; patients with certain chronic illnesses; children younger than 4 years; and infants, children, and adolescents exposed to high-risk adults (Lewinsohn et al., 2017).	
• 5 mm or more in patients who are HIV-positive, have fibrotic changes on chest x-ray film consistent with previous TB infection, have had organ transplants, or are immunosuppressed.	

Recording and Reporting

- Record drug, dose, route, site, time, and date on MAR in electronic health record (EHR) or chart immediately after administration. Sign MAR according to agency policy.
- Record area of ID injection and appearance of skin.
- Record patient teaching, validation of understanding, and patient's response to medication (including adverse effects).
- Record the location, time, and date on which a final reading for a reaction is required
- Report any undesirable effects from medication to patient's health care provider and document adverse effects according to agency policy.

UNEXPECTED OUTCOMES	RELATED INTERVENTIONS
1 Patient experiences localized pain or continued burning at injection site, indicating potential injury to nerve or vessels.	• Assess injection site. • Notify patient's health care provider.
2 Raised, reddened, or hard zone (induration) forms around ID test site.	• Notify patient's health care provider. • Document sensitivity to injected allergen or positive test result if tuberculin skin testing was completed.
3 Patient has adverse reaction with signs of urticaria, pruritus, wheezing, and dyspnea.	• Notify patient's health care provider. • Follow agency policy for appropriate response to drug reactions (e.g., administration of antihistamine such as diphenhydramine or epinephrine). • Add allergy information to patient's medical record.

Intramuscular Injections

An intramuscular (IM) injection deposits medication into deep muscle tissue, which has a rich blood supply, allowing medication to absorb faster than by the subcutaneous route. Administering medications by the IM route increases the risk for injecting drugs directly into blood vessels. Any factor that interferes with local tissue blood flow affects the rate and extent of drug absorption.

You are responsible for determining the injection site and needle depth and gauge to use for an IM injection and judge whether the volume ordered is appropriate for a single injection. Some medications, such as hepatitis B and tetanus, diphtheria, and pertussis (Tdap) immunizations, are given only IM. A longer and heavier-gauge needle is needed to pass through subcutaneous tissue to penetrate deep muscle tissue. Base your choice of needle length and site of injection on the size of the muscle, the thickness of adipose tissue at the injection site, the volume to be administered, the injection technique, and the depth below the muscle surface to be injected (Centers for Disease Control and Prevention [CDC], 2019a). Investigate other possible medication routes, especially when IM injections are ordered for obese patients (Larkin et al., 2018a). The most common IM injections are immunizations.

Many needles available in health care settings are not long enough to reach the muscle, especially in female patients, or in patients who are obese (Strohfus et al., 2018). Most agencies have needles that range in length from ⅜ to 1½ inches. It may be necessary to choose a different medication route when an IM injection is ordered for these patients.

Muscle is less sensitive to irritating and viscous medications. A normal, well-developed adult patient tolerates 3 mL of medication into a larger muscle without severe discomfort (Lilley et al., 2020). Larger volumes of medication (4 to 5 mL) are unlikely to be absorbed properly. Children, older adults, and thin patients tolerate only 2 mL of an IM injection, depending on the site. Do not give more than 1 mL to small children and older infants, and do not give more than 0.5 mL to smaller infants (Hockenberry et al., 2019).

The angle of insertion for an IM injection is 90 degrees. Rotate IM injection sites to decrease the risk for tissue hypertrophy. Emaciated or atrophied muscles absorb medication poorly so their use should be avoided when possible. The Z-track method, a technique for pulling the skin during an injection, is recommended for IM injections (Strohfus et al., 2018). It prevents leakage of medication into subcutaneous tissues, seals medication in the muscle, and minimizes irritation. To use the Z-track method, apply the appropriate-size needle to the syringe and select an

IM site, preferably in a large, deep muscle such as the ventrogluteal. Pull the overlying skin and subcutaneous tissues approximately 2.5 to 3.5 cm (1 to 1½ inches) laterally to the side with the ulnar side of the nondominant hand. Hold the skin in this position until you have administered the injection (Fig. 33.1). Inject the needle deeply into the muscle. To reduce injection site discomfort, the CDC (2019a) no longer recommends aspiration after the needle is injected *when administering vaccines or toxoids.* Keep the needle inserted for 10 seconds to allow the medication to disperse evenly. Release the skin after withdrawing the needle. This leaves a zigzag path that seals the needle track wherever tissue planes slide across one another (see Fig. 33.2). The medication is sealed in the muscle tissue.

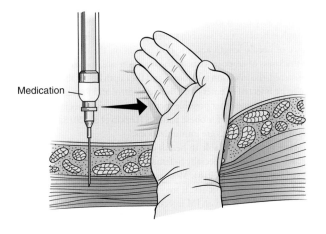

Medication

During injection

Fig. 33.1 Z -track method using hand to pull skill before intramuscular injection.

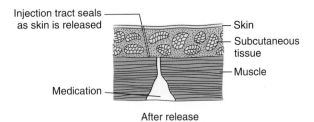

Injection tract seals
as skin is released

Skin

Subcutaneous
tissue

Muscle

Medication

After release

Fig. 33.2 With release of hand after needle removal, tissue slides into place, sealing the needle track.

Injection Sites

Choose an injection site free of pain, infection, necrosis, bruising, and abrasions. Consider the location of underlying bones, nerves, and blood vessels and the volume of medication that you will administer. **Because of the sciatic nerve location, the dorsogluteal muscle is not recommended as an injection site.**

Ventrogluteal Site

The ventrogluteal muscle involves the gluteus medius; it is situated deep and away from major nerves and blood vessels. This site is the preferred and safest site for all adults, children, and infants (Drutz, 2020; Hockenberry et al., 2019; Strohfus et al., 2018). Locate the ventrogluteal muscle by positioning the patient in a supine or lateral position. Using the "V" method position the patient in the lateral position with the knee and hip flexed to relax the muscle. Use your right hand for the left hip and your left hand for the right hip. To administer an injection into the patient's left hip, place the palm of your right hand over the greater trochanter of the patient's hip with your wrist perpendicular to the femur. Then move your thumb toward the patient's groin and your index finger toward the anterior superior iliac spine. Extend or open your middle finger back along the iliac crest toward the patient's buttock. The index finger, middle finger, and iliac crest form a V-shaped triangle, with the injection site in the center of the triangle (Fig. 33.3, A and B) (Larkin et al., 2018a). There is some evidence to suggest that the "V" method is not always reliable because of differences in nurses' hand structure and patients' body structure, especially when a patient is obese (Larkin et al., 2018a). Refer to agency policy as needed.

Vastus Lateralis Muscle

The vastus lateralis muscle is an injection site used in adults and is an alternative site for administering immunizations to infants, toddlers, and children (Hockenberry et al., 2019). The muscle is thick and well developed; it is located on the anterior lateral aspect of the thigh. It extends in an adult from a hand breadth above the knee to a hand breadth below the greater trochanter of the femur (Fig. 33.4A). Use the middle third of the muscle for injection. The width of the muscle usually extends from the midline of the thigh to the midline of the outer side of the thigh. With young children or patients who are thin and have decreased muscle mass, it helps to grasp the body of the muscle during injection to be sure that the medication is deposited in muscle tissue. To help relax the muscle, ask the patient to lie flat with the knee

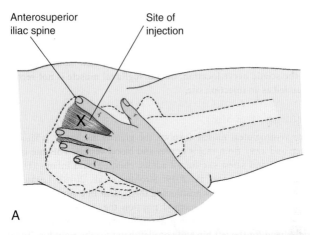

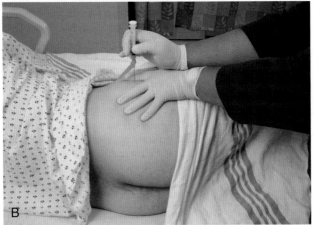

Fig. 33.3 (A), Anatomical view of ventrogluteal site with hand in V position. (B) Injection at ventrogluteal site.

slightly flexed and foot externally rotated or to assume a sitting position (see Fig. 33.4B).

Deltoid Muscle

The deltoid muscle site is easily accessible, but there is potential for injury because the axillary, radial, brachial, and ulnar nerves and the

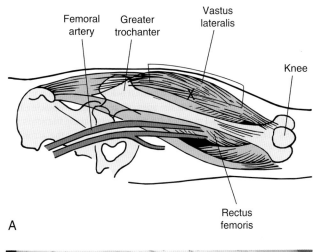

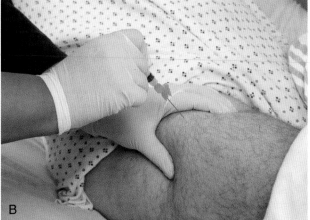

Figure 33.4 (A) Anatomic landmarks for vastus lateralis site. (B) Injection at vastus lateralis site.

brachial artery lie within the upper arm under the triceps and along the humerus. Use this site for small medication volumes (2 mL or less) (CDC, 2019a). *Carefully assess the condition of the deltoid muscle, consult medication references for suitability of medication, and carefully locate the injection site using anatomical landmarks.*

Locate the deltoid muscle by fully exposing the patient's upper arm and shoulder. Have the patient relax the arm at the side or support the arm and flex the elbow. Do not roll up any tight-fitting sleeve. Allow the patient to sit, stand, or lie down. Palpate the lower edge of the acromion process, which forms the base of a triangle in line with the midpoint of the lateral aspect of the upper arm. The injection site is in the center of the triangle, about 3 to 5 cm (1.2–2 inches) below the acromion process (Fig. 33.5, A and B). You locate the apex of the triangle by placing four fingers across the deltoid muscle with the top finger along the acromion process. The injection site is three finger widths below the acromion process.

Safety Guidelines

- Be vigilant during medication administration. Avoid distractions.
- Choose injection sites carefully to avoid injury to underlying bones and nerves.

Delegation

The skill of administering IM injections cannot be delegated to assistive personnel (AP). Direct the AP about:

- Potential medication side effects and to immediately report their occurrence.
- Reporting any change in the patient's condition.

Collaboration

- Agency pharmacist is a resource for determining smallest volume in which the medication for IM injection can be provided.

Equipment

- Proper-size syringe and needle with engineered sharps injury protection needle
- Syringe: 2 to 3 mL for adult, 0.5 to 1 mL for infants and small children
- Antiseptic swab
- Vial or ampule of medication or skin test solution
- Clean gloves
- Medication administration record (MAR) (electronic or printed)
- Puncture-proof container for sharps
- Needle length corresponding to site of injection, age, gender, and body mass index of patient. Refer to the guidelines shown in Table 33.1; length needed may vary outside of these guidelines for patients who are smaller or larger than average.

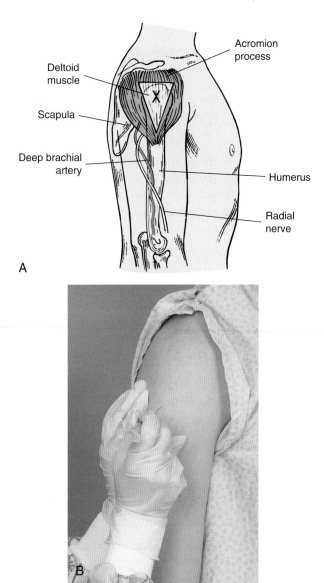

Figure 33.5 (A) Anatomic landmarks for deltoid site. (B) Injection at deltoid site.

TABLE 33.1 Needle Length for Immunizations (Based on 2019 CDC a Guidelines)

Site	Child	Adult
Ventrogluteal	Not recommended	1½ inches (38 mm)
Vastus lateralis	⅝–1¼ inch	⅝–1 inch (16–25 mm)
Deltoid	⅝–1 inch	1½ inches (38 mm)
Gender—Male	**Gender—Female**	**Needle Length**
Less than 130 lb	Less than 130 lb	⅝–1 inch (16–25 mm)
130–152 lb	130–152 lb	1 inch (25 mm)
153–260 lb	153–200 lb	1½ inches (38 mm)
260+ lb	200+ lb	1½ inches (38 mm)
Age-Group	**Needle Length**	**Site**
Infants, 1–12 months	1 inch (25 mm)	Vastus lateralis
Toddlers, 1–2 years	1–1¼ inch (25–32 mm)	Vastus lateralis[b]
	⅝[a]–1 inch (16–25 mm)	Deltoid muscle of arm
Children, 3–10 years	⅝[a]–1 inch (16–25 mm)	Deltoid muscle of arm[b]
	1–1¼ inches (25–32 mm)	Vastus lateralis
Children, 11–18 years	⅝[a]–1 inch (16–25 mm)	Deltoid muscle of arm[b]
	1–1½ inches (25–38 mm)	Vastus lateralis
Men and women, less than 60 kg (130 lb)	1 inch (25 mm)	Deltoid muscle of arm
Men and women, 60–70 kg (130–152 lb)	1 inch (25 mm)	Deltoid muscle of arm
Men, 70–118 kg (152–260 lb)	1–1½ inches (25–38 mm)	Deltoid muscle of arm
Women, 70–90 kg (152–200 lb)	1–1½ inches (25–38 mm)	Deltoid muscle of arm

[a]If skin is stretched tightly and subcutaneous tissues are not bunched.
[b]Preferred site.

Based on Centers for Disease Control and Prevention: *General best practice guidelines for immunization: best practices guidance of the Advisory Committee on Immunization Practices (ACIP)*, 2019a, https://www.cdc.gov/vaccines/hcp/acip-recs/general-recs/administration.html#.

STEP	RATIONALE
1 Perform preprocedure protocol.	

Assessment

STEP	RATIONALE
• Check accuracy and completeness of each MAR or computer printout with health care provider's written medication order. Check patient's name, medication name and dosage, route of administration, and time of administration. Recopy or reprint any part of MAR that is difficult to read.	The order sheet is the most reliable source and only legal record of medications that patient is to receive. Ensures that patient receives the correct medications (Palese et al., 2019). Transcription errors are a source of medication errors (Palese et al., 2019).
• Review electronic health record (EHR): assess patient's medical and medication history.	Determines need for medication or possible contraindications for medication administration.
• Review drug reference information for medication action, purpose, normal dose, side effects, time of peak onset, and nursing implications.	Information allows you to safely administer medication and monitor patient's response to therapy.
• Ask patient to describe history of allergies: known type of allergies and normal allergic reaction. Check patient's allergy wristband.	Do not prepare medication if there is a known patient allergy. Communication of patient allergies is essential for safe medication administration.
• Perform hand hygiene. Assess condition of skin for contraindication to IM injections such as muscle atrophy, reduced blood flow, or circulatory shock. Assess adequacy of adipose tissue.	Atrophied muscle absorbs medication poorly. Factors interfering with blood flow to muscle impairs drug absorption.
• Assess patient's symptoms before initiating medication therapy.	Provides information for you to evaluate desired effects of medication.

Continued

STEP	RATIONALE

CLINICAL JUDGMENT *Because of the documented adverse effects of IM injections, other routes of medication injection are preferred. Consider contacting health care provider for alternative route of medication administration.*

Implementation

1. Explain to patient signs and symptoms to expect from medication. Allow time for patient to ask questions.

   Lessens anxiety by helping patient know what to expect, promoting self-care.

2. Prepare medication without interruptions/distractions. Create a quiet environment. Keep all pages of MARs or computer printouts for one patient together or look at only one patient's electronic MAR at a time.

   Interruptions contribute to medication errors (Palese et al., 2019).

3. Perform hand hygiene. Prepare medications for one patient at a time using aseptic technique (see Skills 48 and 49). Pharmacy may prepare syringe. Check label of medication carefully with MAR or computer printout when removing drug from storage and after preparation. Check drug expiration date.

   Ensures that medication is sterile. *These are the first and second checks for accuracy* and ensure that correct medication is administered.
   Dose potency increases or decreases when outdated.

4. Administer medication at correct time (see agency policy). Give non–time-critical scheduled medications within a range of 1 to 2 h of scheduled dose (Centers for Medicare and Medicaid Services [CMS], 2020). During administration, apply seven rights of medication administration.

   Hospitals must adopt medication administration policy and procedure for timing of medication administration that considers nature of the prescribed medication, specific clinical application, and patient needs (CMS, 2020).

STEP	RATIONALE
5 Identify patient using at least two identifiers (e.g., name and birthday or name and medical record number) according to agency policy. Compare identifiers with information on patient's MAR or medical record.	Ensures correct patient. Complies with The Joint Commission standards and improves patient safety (the Joint Commission, 2022). Some agencies use a barcode system to help with patient identification.
6 At patient's bedside again compare MAR or computer printout with names of medications on medication labels and patient name. Confirm if patient has allergies.	*This is the third check for accuracy* and ensures that patient receives correct medication. Confirms patient's allergy history.
7 Perform hand hygiene and apply clean gloves. Keep sheet or gown draped over body parts not requiring exposure.	Reduces transmission of infection. Respects patient's dignity/privacy while exposing injection site.
8 Position patient comfortably to access site. Select an appropriate site. Note integrity and size of muscle. Palpate for tenderness or hardness. Avoid these areas. If patient receives frequent injections, rotate sites. Use ventrogluteal muscle if possible.	Ventrogluteal is preferred injection site for adults. It is also preferred site for children of all ages (Drutz, 2020; Hockenberry et al., and Wilson, 2019; Strohfus et al., 2018).

CLINICAL JUDGMENT *Ensure that patient's medical condition (e.g., circulatory shock, orthopedic surgery, spinal injury) does not contraindicate the position for injection.*

9 Relocate site using anatomical landmarks (Figs. 33.3–33.5).	Injection into correct anatomical site prevents injury to nerves, bone, and blood vessels.

Continued

STEP	RATIONALE
10 Clean site with antiseptic swab. Apply swab at center of site and rotate outward in circular direction for about 5 cm (2 inches).	Mechanical action of swab removes secretions containing microorganisms.
• *Option:* Apply a eutectic mixture of local anesthetics (EMLA) cream on injection site at least 1 h before IM injection or use vapocoolant spray (e.g., ethyl chloride) just before injection.	Decreases pain at injection site. It has been demonstrated that EMLA does not interfere with response to vaccines (CDC, 2019a).
11 Hold swab or gauze between third and fourth fingers of nondominant hand.	Swab or gauze remains readily accessible for use when withdrawing needle after injection.
12 Remove needle cap or sheath by pulling it straight off.	Preventing needle from touching sides of cap prevents contamination.
13 Hold syringe between thumb and forefinger of dominant hand, as a dart would be held, palm down.	Quick, smooth injection requires proper manipulation of syringe parts.
14 Administer injection using Z-track method:	
a Position ulnar side of nondominant hand just below site and pull skin laterally approximately 2.5 to 3.5 cm (1 to 1½ inches). Hold position while medication is injected. With dominant hand, inject needle quickly at 90-degree angle into muscle (see Fig. 33.1).	The Z-track method creates zigzag path through tissues that seals needle track to avoid tracking medication. A quick dartlike injection reduces discomfort. Use the Z-track method for all IM injections (Strohfus et al., 2018).

STEP	RATIONALE
b *Option*: If patient's muscle mass is small, grasp body of muscle between thumb and forefingers.	Ensures that medication reaches muscle mass (CDC, 2019a; Hockenberry et al., 2019; Strohfus et al., 2018).
c After needle pierces skin, while you are still pulling on skin with nondominant hand, grasp lower end of syringe barrel with fingers of nondominant hand to stabilize it. Move dominant hand to end of plunger. Avoid moving syringe.	Smooth manipulation of syringe reduces discomfort from needle movement. Skin remains pulled until after medication is injected to ensure Z-track administration.
d Pull back on plunger 5 to 10 seconds (except for immunizations). If no blood appears, inject medication slowly at rate of 10 s/mL.	Aspiration of blood into syringe indicates possible placement into a vein. Slow injection rate reduces pain and tissue trauma and reduces chance of leakage of medication back through needle track (Hockenberry et al., 2019). *The CDC (2019a) no longer recommends aspiration when administering an immunization.*

CLINICAL JUDGMENT *If blood appears in syringe, remove needle, dispose of medication and syringe properly, and prepare another dose of medication for injection to prevent injection of medication directly into the bloodstream.*

---

e Once medication is injected, wait 10 seconds, then smoothly and steadily withdraw needle, release the skin, and apply gauze with gentle pressure over site (see Fig. 33.2). If patient is taking anticoagulants, hold alcohol swab or gauze to site for 30 to 60 seconds. Do not massage site.	Allows time for medication to absorb into muscle before removing syringe. Dry gauze minimizes discomfort associated with alcohol on nonintact skin. Massage damages underlying tissue.

Continued

STEP	RATIONALE
15 Dispose of all contaminated supplies in appropriate receptacle, remove and dispose of gloves, and perform hand hygiene.	Reduces transmission of microorganisms. Use appropriate disposal receptacle if patient is receiving hazardous drugs (Oncology Nursing Society, 2018).
16 Perform postprocedure protocol.	
17 Evaluate patient response:	
a Return to room in 15 to 30 minutes and ask if patient feels any acute pain, burning, numbness, or tingling at injection site.	Continued discomfort may indicate injury to underlying bones or nerves.
b Inspect site; note any bruising or induration. *Option:* Apply warm compress to site.	Bruising or induration indicates complication associated with injection. Warm compress promotes comfort and drug absorption. Document findings and notify health care provider.
c Observe patient's response to medication at times that correlate with onset, peak, and duration of medication.	IM medications are absorbed rapidly. Adverse effects of parenteral medications develop rapidly. Evaluate effect of medication based on onset, peak, and duration of actions of medication.

Recording and Reporting

- Immediately after administration, record medication, dose, route, site, time, date given, and any adverse effects in EHR or chart, not before. Correctly sign MAR according to agency policy.
- Record any undesirable effects from the injection.
- Record patient teaching, validation of understanding, and patient's response to medication.
- Report any undesirable effects from medication to patient's health care provider.

UNEXPECTED OUTCOMES	RELATED INTERVENTIONS
1 Patient complains of localized pain or continued burning at injection site, indicating potential injury to nerve or vessels. In addition, if a medication is not injected correctly into a muscle, complications can arise such as abscess, hematoma, ecchymosis, pain, and vascular and nerve injury (Kaya et al., 2016).	• Assess injection site. • Notify patient's health care provider.
2 During injection, blood is aspirated.	• Immediately stop injection and remove needle. • Prepare new syringe of medication for administration.
3 Patient displays adverse reaction with signs of urticaria, eczema, pruritus, wheezing, and dyspnea.	• Follow agency policy or guidelines for appropriate response to allergic reactions (e.g., administration of antihistamine such as diphenhydramine or epinephrine). • Notify patient's health care provider immediately. • Add allergy information to patient's record.

Intravenous Medications by Piggyback and Syringe Pumps

One method of administering intravenous (IV) medications uses small volumes (25 to 250 mL) of compatible IV fluids infused over a desired time frame. This method reduces the risk for rapid dose infusion and provides independence for patients. Patients must have an established IV access site that is kept patent by either a continuous infusion or intermittent flushes of normal saline. You administer intermittent infusion of medication with any of the following methods.

- *Piggyback.* A piggyback is a small (25- to 250-mL) IV bag or bottle connected to a short tubing line that connects to the upper Y-port of a primary infusion line or to an intermittent venous access, such as a saline lock. The IV medication container is labeled following the IV piggyback medication format (The Joint Commission [TJC], 2022). The piggyback tubing is a microdrip or macrodrip system. The set is called a piggyback because the small bag or bottle is set higher than the primary infusion bag or bottle. In the piggyback setup the main line is not infusing while a compatible piggybacked medication is infusing. The port of the primary IV line contains a back-check valve that automatically stops the flow of the primary infusion when a piggyback infusion begins. After the piggyback solution infuses and the solution within the tubing falls below the level of the primary infusion drip chamber, the back-check valve opens, and the primary infusion starts to flow again.

- *Volume-control administration.* Volume-control administration sets (e.g., Volutrol, Buretrol, Pediatrol) are small (50- to 150-mL) containers that attach just below a primary infusion bag or bottle. The set is attached and filled in a manner similar to that used with a regular IV infusion. However, the priming (filling) of the set is different, depending on the type of filter (floating valve or membrane) within the set. Follow package directions for priming sets.

- *Syringe pump.* The mini-infusion pump is battery operated and delivers medication in very small amounts of fluid (5 to 60 mL) within controlled infusion times using standard syringes.

Safety Guidelines

- The Needlestick Safety and Prevention Act of 2001 mandates that health care agencies use safe needle devices and manufactured needleless systems to reduce needlestick injury. Systems with catheter ports or Y-connector sites are designed to contain a needle housed in a protective covering. Needleless infusion lines allow a direct connection with an IV line via a recessed connection port, a blunt-ended cannula, or shielded-needle device, eliminating the risk for exposure to an IV needle (Occupational Safety and Health Administration, nd [a]).
- Be vigilant during IV medication preparation and administration. Avoid distractions (Bravo and Cochran, 2016; Palese et al., 2019).

Delegation

The skill of administering IV medications by piggyback and syringe pumps cannot be delegated to assistive personnel (AP). Direct the AP about:

- Potential medication actions as well as side effects and the need to report them immediately.
- Reporting any patient complaints of moisture or discomfort around IV insertion site.
- Reporting any change in patient's condition or vital signs.

Collaboration

- Agency pharmacists ensure IV medications are properly labeled and dispensed.

Equipment

- Tape (optional): Nonallergenic tape, plastic tape recommended for short-term wear, and paper/cloth tape for long-time wear (Fumarola et al., 2020)
- Antiseptic swab
- Clean gloves
- IV pole
- Medication administration record (MAR) or computer printout
- Puncture-proof container
- Labels for tubing, IV bags, medications

Piggyback or Syringe Pump

- Medication prepared in 5- to 250-mL labeled infusion bag or syringe
- Prefilled syringe of normal saline flush solution (for saline lock only)
- Short microdrip, macrodrip, or mini-infusion IV tubing set with blunt-ended needleless cannula attachment

- Needleless device
- Syringe pump if indicated

Volume-Control Administration Set

- Volutrol or Buretrol
- Infusion tubing with needleless system attachment
- Syringe (1 to 20 mL)
- Vial or ampule of ordered medication Option: pharmacy may prepare medication and deliver in sealed syringe

STEP	RATIONALE
1 Perform preprocedure protocol.	
Assessment	
• Check accuracy and completeness of each MAR or computer printout with health care provider's written medication order. Check patient's name, medication name and dosage, route of administration, and time of administration.	The order sheet is the most reliable source and only legal record of medications that patient is to receive. Ensures that patient receives the correct medications (Palese et al., 2019). Transcription errors are a source of medication errors (Palese et al., 2019).
• Review electronic health record (EHR) to assess patient's medical and medication history.	Determines need for medication or reveals possible contraindications to medication administration.
• Assess relevant laboratory results (e.g., blood urea nitrogen, creatinine, liver function test results).	Provides baseline for measuring response to drug.
• Review medication reference information for medication action, purpose, normal dose, side effects, time and peak of onset, how slowly to give medication, and nursing implications (e.g., need to dilute medication, administer through filter).	Information allows you to safely administer medication and monitor patient's response to therapy.

STEP	RATIONALE
• If you give medication through existing IV line, determine compatibility of medication with existing IV fluids and any additional additives within IV solution.	IV medication is sometimes not compatible with other IV solutions and/or additives.

CLINICAL JUDGMENT *Never administer IV medications through tubing that is infusing blood, blood products, or parenteral nutrition solutions.*

• Ask patient to describe history of allergies: known types of allergies and type of allergic reaction. Check patient's allergy wristband.	IV route delivers medication rapidly. Allergic response is immediate.
• Perform hand hygiene. Assess patency and placement of patient's existing IV infusion line or saline lock.	Do not administer medication if site is edematous or inflamed.

CLINICAL JUDGMENT *If patient's IV site is saline locked, clean the port with alcohol and assess the patency of the IV line by flushing it with 2 to 3 mL of sterile sodium chloride.*

• To reduce the risk for administration set misconnections, trace all catheters/administration sets/add-on devices between the patient and container.	Misconnections can occur when all connections are not checked before initiating or reconnecting infusion/device at each care transition (Infusion Nurses Society [INS], 2021).
• Assess patient's symptoms before initiating medication therapy.	Provides information to evaluate desired effects of medication.

Implementation

1 Explain to patient the signs and symptoms to expect from medication. Discuss how IV piggyback/syringe pump operates.	Reduces anxiety and promotes patient cooperation.

Continued

STEP	RATIONALE
2 Prepare medication without interruptions/distractions. Keep all pages of MARs or computer printouts for one patient together, or look at only one patient's electronic MAR at a time.	Interruptions contribute to medication errors (Palese et al., 2019).
3 Perform hand hygiene. Prepare medications for one patient at a time using aseptic technique (see Skill 48). Pharmacy may prepare medication. Check label of medication carefully with MAR or computer printout when removing medication from storage and after preparation.	Reduces transmission of microorganisms. *These are the first and second checks for accuracy* and ensure that correct medication is administered.
4 Administer medication(s) at correct time (see agency policy). Give non–time-critical scheduled medications within a range of 1 to 2 h of scheduled dose (Centers for Medicare and Medicaid Services [CMS], 2020). During administration, apply seven rights of medication administration.	Hospitals must adopt medication administration policy and procedure for timing of medication administration that considers nature of the prescribed medication, specific clinical application, and patient needs (CMS, 2020).
5 Identify patient using at least two identifiers (e.g., name and birthday or name and medical record number) according to agency policy. Compare identifiers with information on patient's MAR or medical record.	Ensures correct patient. Complies with The Joint Commission standards and improves patient safety (TJC, 2022). Some agencies use a barcode system to help with patient identification.

STEP	RATIONALE
6 At patient's bedside, again compare MAR or computer printout with names of medications on medication labels and patient name. For high alert medications use an independent double-check with another clinician (Gorski, 2023). Ask patient about allergies.	*This is the third check for accuracy* and ensures that patient receives correct medication. Confirms patient's allergy history.
7 Administer infusion. Perform hand hygiene. Apply clean gloves.	Reduces transmission of microorganisms.
a **Piggyback infusion:**	
(1) Connect infusion tubing to piggyback medication bag using sterile technique. Fill tubing by opening regulator flow clamp. Once tubing is full, close clamp and cap end of tubing.	Filling infusion tubing with solution and freeing air bubbles helps prevent air embolus.
(2) Hang piggyback (Fig. 34.1) medication bag above level of primary fluid bag. (*Option:* Use hook to lower main bag.)	Height of fluid bag affects rate of flow to patient.
(3) Wipe IV access port with antiseptic swab and allow to dry. Connect tubing of piggyback infusion to appropriate connector on upper Y-port of primary infusion line:	Connection allows IV medication to enter main IV line.

Continued

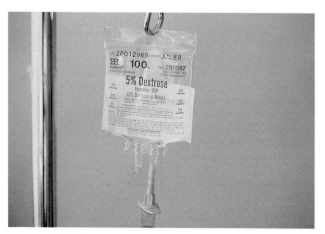

Fig. 34.1 Small-volume minibag for piggyback infusion.

STEP	RATIONALE
b Continuous infusion:	
(1) Wipe off needleless port of primary IV line with antiseptic swab and allow to dry. Then insert needleless cannula tip of piggyback infusion tubing into port (Fig. 34.2a.b).	Use needleless connections to prevent accidental needlestick injuries (INS, 2021; OSHA, nd[a]).

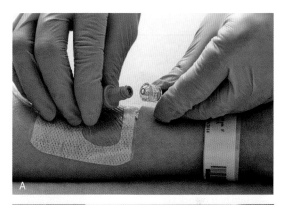

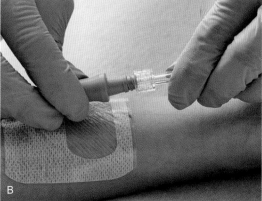

Fig. 34.2 (A) Needleless lock cannula system. (B) Blunt-ended cannula inserts into port and locks.

Continued

STEP	RATIONALE
(2) *Option:* Connect tubing of piggyback infusion to normal saline lock: Follow Steps 9b(1) to (5), in Skill 35 to flush and prepare lock. Wipe off port with alcohol swab, let dry, and insert tip of piggyback infusion tubing into port of lock via needleless access.	Flushing of lock ensures patency.
(3) Regulate flow rate of medication solution by adjusting regulator clamp or IV pump infusion rate. Infusion times vary. Refer to medication reference or agency policy for safe flow rate.	Provides slow, safe, intermittent infusion of medication and maintains therapeutic levels in bloodstream.
(4) Label all tubing, IV bags, and medications with nurse initials, patient initials, date and time the drug was hung, and when it is due to be infused.	Prevents medication errors (Institute for Safe Medication Practices [ISMP], 2018).
(5) Once medication has infused: Check flow rate of primary infusion. Primary infusion automatically begins after piggyback solution is empty.	Back-check valve on piggyback prevents flow of primary infusion until medication infuses. Checking flow rate ensures administration of IV fluids at proper rate.

STEP	RATIONALE
(6) Check normal saline lock: Disconnect piggyback tubing, clean port of lock with antiseptic swab, and flush IV line with 2 to 3 mL of sterile 0.9% sodium chloride. Maintain sterility of IV tubing between intermittent infusions.	Prevents buildup of medication in saline lock device.
(7) Leave IV piggyback and tubing in place for future drug administration (see agency policy) or discard in puncture- and leak-proof container.	Establishing secondary line produces route for microorganisms to enter main line. Repeated changes in tubing increase risk for infection transmission.
c **Volume-control administration set (e.g., Volutrol):**	
(1) Fill Volutrol with desired amount of IV fluid (50 to 100 mL) by opening clamp between Volutrol and main IV bag.	Small volume of fluid dilutes IV medication and reduces risk of fluid infusing too rapidly.
(2) Close clamp and check to be sure that clamp on air vent Volutrol chamber is open.	Prevents additional leakage of fluid into Volutrol. Air vent allows fluid in Volutrol to exit at regulated rate.
(3) Clean injection port on top of Volutrol with antiseptic swab.	Prevents introduction of microorganisms during needle insertion.

Continued

STEP	RATIONALE
(4) Remove needle cap or sheath and insert needleless tip or syringe needle of medication syringe through port and inject medication. Gently rotate Volutrol between hands.	Rotating mixes medication with solution to ensure equal distribution in Volutrol.
(5) Regulate IV infusion rate to allow medication to infuse in time recommended by agency policy, pharmacist, or medication reference manual.	For optimal therapeutic effect, medication should infuse in prescribed time interval.
(6) Label Volutrol with name of medication; dosage and total volume, including diluent; and time of administration, following ISMP (2019) safe-medication label format.	Alerts healthcare team to medication being infused. Prevents other medications from being added to Volutrol.
(7) If patient is receiving continuous IV infusion, check infusion rate after Volutrol infusion is complete.	Ensures appropriate rate of administration.
(8) Dispose of uncapped needle or needle enclosed in safety shield and syringe in puncture- and leak-proof container.	Prevents accidental needlesticks (OSHA, nd[a]). Reduces transmission of microorganisms.

STEP	RATIONALE
c Syringe pump administration:	
(1) Connect prefilled syringe to mini-infusion tubing; remove end cap of tubing.	Special tubing designed to fit syringe delivers medication to main IV line.
(2) Carefully apply pressure to syringe plunger, allowing tubing to fill with medication.	Ensures that tubing is free of air bubbles to prevent air embolus.
(3) Place syringe into mini-infusion pump (follow product directions) and hang on IV pole. Be sure that syringe is secured (Fig. 34.3).	Secure placement is needed for proper infusion.

Continued

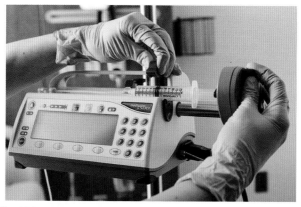

Fig. 34.3 Ensure that syringe is secure after placing it into mini-infusion pump.

STEP	RATIONALE
(4) Connect end of mini-infusion tubing to main IV line or saline lock:	Establishes route for IV medication to enter main IV line.
(a) *Existing IV line:* Wipe off needleless port on main IV line with antiseptic swab, allow to dry, and insert tip of mini-infusion tubing through center of port.	Needleless connections reduce risk for accidental needlestick injuries (OSHA, n.d. (a)).
(b) *Normal saline lock:* Follow Steps 9b(1) to (5), in Skill 35 to flush and prepare lock. Wipe off port with alcohol swab, allow to dry, and insert tip of mini-infusion tubing.	
(5) Set pump to deliver medication within time recommended by agency policy, pharmacist, or medication reference manual. Press button on pump to begin infusion.	Pump automatically delivers medication at safe, constant rate based on volume in syringe.
(6) Once medication has infused:	

STEP	RATIONALE
(a) *Main IV infusion:* Check flow rate. Infusion automatically begins to flow once pump stops. Regulate infusion to desired rate as needed.	Maintains patent primary IV fluids.
(b) *Normal saline lock:* Disconnect tubing, clean port with antiseptic swab, and flush IV line with 2 to 3 mL of sterile 0.9% sodium chloride. Maintain sterility of IV tubing between intermittent infusions.	Prevents buildup of medication in lock device.
8 Stay with patient for several minutes and observe for any allergic reactions.	Dyspnea, wheezing, and circulatory collapse are signs of severe anaphylactic reaction.
9 Perform postprocedure protocol.	
10 Evaluate patient response.	
a Observe patient for signs or symptoms of adverse reaction.	IV medications act rapidly.
b During infusion, periodically check infusion rate and condition of IV site.	IV must remain patent for proper drug administration. Infiltration of IV site requires discontinuing infusion.
c Assess patient ability to explain purpose and side effects of medication.	Evaluates patient's understanding of instruction.

Recording and Reporting

- Immediately after administration record medication, dose, route, infusion rate, and date and time administered in MAR in EHR or chart.
- Record volume of fluid in medication bag or Volutrol on intake and output form.
- Record patient teaching, validation of understanding, and patient's response to medication.
- Report any adverse reactions to patient's health care provider.

UNEXPECTED OUTCOMES	RELATED INTERVENTIONS
1 Patient develops adverse or allergic reaction to medication.	• Stop medication infusion immediately. • Follow agency policy or guidelines for appropriate response to allergic reaction (e.g., administration of antihistamine such as diphenhydramine or epinephrine) and reporting of adverse medication reactions. • Notify patient's health care provider of adverse effects immediately. • Add allergy information to patient record per agency policy.
2 Medication does not infuse over established time frame.	• Determine reason (e.g., improper calculation of flow rate, poor positioning of IV needle at insertion site, infiltration). • Take corrective action to deliver dosage as indicated or notify healthcare provider.

UNEXPECTED OUTCOMES	RELATED INTERVENTIONS
3 IV site shows signs of infiltration or phlebitis (see Skill 54).	• Stop IV infusion and discontinue access device. • Treat IV site as indicated by agency policy. • Insert new IV catheter if continued therapy is needed. • For infiltration, determine how harmful IV medication is to subcutaneous tissue. Provide IV extravasation care (e.g., injecting phentolamine around IV infiltration site) as indicated by agency policy, or consult pharmacist to determine appropriate follow-up care.

Intravenous Medications: Intravenous Bolus

An intravenous (IV) bolus is a method of medication administration involving injection of a concentrated dose of a medication directly into a vein by way of an existing IV access. It is a method for medication administration that poses greater risk to patients because it allows little time to correct errors and drugs act rapidly. An IV bolus or "push" usually requires small volumes of fluid, which is an advantage for patients who are at risk for fluid overload. Refer to agency policies and procedures that identify the medications that nurses can administer by IV bolus. These policies are based on the medication, compatibility with other medications and IV fluids, availability of staff, and type of monitoring equipment available.

Administering an IV push medication too quickly can cause harm to a patient, even death. Use caution when calculating the correct amount of the medication to give and the rate of administration (see agency policy or manufacturer directions). A bolus may cause direct irritation to the lining of blood vessels, so always confirm placement of an IV catheter or needle and monitor for signs of phlebitis. **Never give an IV bolus if the insertion site appears edematous or reddened or if the IV fluids do not flow at the ordered rate**. Accidental injection of some medications into tissues surrounding a vein can cause pain, sloughing of tissues, and abscesses.

Verify the rate of administration of IV push medication using agency guidelines or a medication reference manual. Follow the strategies listed below to reduce harm from rapid IV push medications (Gorski, 2023):

- Use commercially available or pharmacy-prepared IV push medication whenever possible. If mixing is required adhere to safe injection control practices.
- Dilution of IV push medication in ready-to-administer syringes is unsafe and can result in dosage errors, improper labeling and risk for infection.
- Establish vascular access device (VAD) patency by flushing the VAD and aspirating for a blood return before administration.
- Appropriately label syringes clinically prepared by a nurse (see agency policy).
- Determine the appropriate rate and amount of time involved to administer the medication.
- Identify all incompatibilities (i.e., drug or solution) with existing infusions.

- Review the amount of medication that a patient will receive each minute, the recommended concentration, and rate of administration. Most medications are delivered slowly, between 1 and 10 minutes. Example: 6 ml of medication to be given over 3 minutes; thus give 2 mL of IV bolus every minute.

Safety Guidelines

- Be vigilant during IV medication administration and avoid distractions (Bravo and Cochran, 2016; Palese et al., 2019).
- There is higher risk for infusion reactions after IV bolus versus IV medication by intermittent infusion (Skill 34). Some reactions can be severe because the medication reaches peak action quickly.
- Risk for infiltration and phlebitis is increased, especially if a highly concentrated medication, a small peripheral vein, or a short venous access device is used.

Delegation

The skill of administering medications by IV bolus cannot be delegated to assistive personnel (AP). Direct the AP about:

- Potential medication actions and side effects of the medications and to immediately report their occurrence.
- Reporting any moisture or discomfort around IV insertion site noted by the patient.
- Obtaining any required vital signs and reporting any unexpected changes.

Collaboration

- Pharmacist is resource for conferring about incompatibilities of IV medication and any medication in an IV infusion line as well as recommended time for injecting medication.

Equipment

- Watch with second hand
- Clean gloves
- Antiseptic swab
- Medication in pharmacy prepared syringe. (Option: in emergency you may use medication vials or ampules)
- Proper-size syringes for medication (If prepared clinically by nurse) and saline flush, with needleless device or sharp with engineered sharps injury protection (SESIP) needle (21 to 25 gauge)
- IV lock: vial of flush solution (normal saline recommended [Gorski, 2023]); if agency policy indicates use of heparin flush, the most common concentration is 10 units/mL; check agency policy.
- Medication administration record (MAR) or computer printout
- Puncture-proof container

STEP	RATIONALE
1 Perform preprocedure protocol.	

Assessment

- Check accuracy and completeness of each MAR or computer printout with health care provider's written medication order. Check patient's name, medication name and dosage, route of administration, and time of administration. Recopy or reprint any part of MAR that is difficult to read.

The order sheet is the most reliable source and only legal record of medications that patient is to receive. Ensures that patient receives the correct medications (Palese et al., 2019). Transcription errors are a source of medication errors (Palese et al., 2019).

- Review electronic health record (EHR) to assess patient's medical and medication history.

Determines need for medication or reveals possible contraindications to medication administration.

- Assess relevant laboratory results (e.g., blood urea nitrogen, creatinine).

Provides baseline for measuring response to drug.

- Review drug reference information for medication action, purpose, side effects, normal dose, time of peak onset, rate at which to give medication, and nursing implications such as need to dilute medication or administer it through a filter.

Knowledge of medication allows safe administration and monitoring of patient's response to therapy.

- If medication is given through an existing IV line, determine compatibility of medication with IV fluids and any additives within IV solution.

IV medication is not always compatible with IV solution and/or additives, and a new site may need to be initiated (Gorski, 2023).

- Ask patient to describe history of allergies: known type of allergies and type of allergic reaction. Check patient's allergy wristband.

IV bolus delivers medication rapidly. Allergic response is immediate.

- Perform hand hygiene. Assess condition of VAD site for signs of infiltration or phlebitis.

Do not administer medication if site is edematous or inflamed.

STEP	RATIONALE
• Assess patency of patient's existing IV infusion line or saline lock. Perform hand hygiene.	For medication to reach venous circulation effectively, IV line must be patent and fluids must infuse easily.

CLINICAL JUDGMENT *If patient's IV site is saline locked, clean the port with antiseptic swab and assess the patency of the IV line by flushing it with 2 to 3 mL of sterile sodium chloride then check for blood return.*

• To reduce the risks for administration set misconnections, trace all catheters/administration sets/add-on devices between the patient and container.	Misconnections can occur when all connections are not checked before initiating or reconnecting infusion/device at each care transition (Infusion Nurses Society, 2021).
• Assess patient's symptoms before initiating medication therapy.	Provides information to evaluate desired effects of medication.

Implementation

1 Explain to patient signs and symptoms to expect from medications.	Lessens anxiety by helping patient know what to expect, promoting self-care.
2 Prepare medication without interruptions/distractions. Keep all pages of MARs or computer printouts for one patient together, or look at only one patient's electronic MAR at a time.	Interruptions contribute to medication errors (Palese et al., 2019).
3 Perform hand hygiene. Access pharmacy prepared syringe from storage. (If necessary to prepare medication in a syringe follow steps in Skill 48). Check label of medication carefully with MAR or computer printout when removing medication from storage and after preparation.	Reduces transmission of microorganisms. *These are the first and second checks for accuracy* and ensure that correct medication is administered.

Continued

STEP	RATIONALE

CLINICAL JUDGMENT *Some IV medications require dilution before administration. Verify with agency policy or pharmacy if dilution is permitted and follow agency procedure.*

4 Administer medication(s) to patient at correct time (see agency policy). Give non–time-critical scheduled medications within a range of 1 to 2 h of scheduled dose (Institute for Safe Medication Practices (ISMP), 2011). During administration, apply seven rights of medication administration.	Hospitals must adopt medication administration policy and procedure for timing of medication administration that considers nature of the prescribed medication, specific clinical application, and patient needs (ISMP, 2011).
5 Identify patient using at least two identifiers (e.g., name and birthday or name and medical record number) according to agency policy. Compare identifiers with information on patient's MAR or medical record.	Ensures correct patient. Complies with The Joint Commission standards and improves patient safety (The Joint Commission, 2022). Some agencies use a bar-code system to help with patient identification.
6 At patient's bedside again compare MAR or computer printout with names of medications on medication labels and patient name. For high alert medications use an independent double-check with another clinician (Gorski, 2023). Confirm if patient has allergies.	*This is the third check for accuracy* and ensures that patient receives correct medication. Confirms patient's allergy history. Medication label should include rate of IV push).
7 Perform hand hygiene and apply clean gloves.	Reduces transmission of infection.
8 **Administer IV push (existing IV line):**	
a Select injection port of IV tubing closest to patient. Use needleless injection port.	Follows provisions of Needlestick Safety and Prevention Act of 2001 (Occupational Safety and Health Administration [OSHA] n.d.[a]).

STEP	RATIONALE

CLINICAL JUDGMENT *Never administer IV medications through tubing that is infusing blood, blood products, or parenteral nutrition solutions.*

b Clean injection port with antiseptic swab. Allow to dry.

Prevents transfer of microorganisms during blunt cannula insertion.

c Connect syringe to IV line: Insert needleless tip of syringe containing drug through center of port (Fig. 35.1).

Prevents introduction of microorganisms. Prevents damage to port diaphragm and possible leakage from site.

Continued

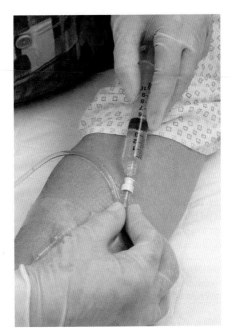

Fig. 35.1 Connect needleless blunt cannula tip to IV port.

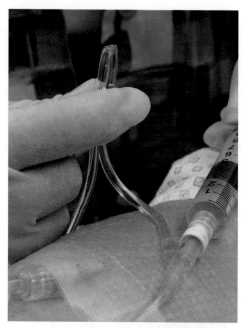

Fig. 35.2   Pinch tubing of IV infusion line.

STEP	RATIONALE
d Occlude IV line by pinching tubing just above injection port (Fig. 35.2). Pull back gently on plunger of syringe to aspirate for blood return.	Final check ensures that medication is being delivered into bloodstream.

CLINICAL JUDGMENT *In the case of smaller-gauge IV needles, blood return sometimes is not aspirated even if IV line is patent. If IV site does not show signs of infiltration and IV fluid is infusing without difficulty, give IV push.*

STEP	RATIONALE
e Release tubing and inject medication within amount of time recommended by agency policy, pharmacist, or medication reference manual. Use watch to time administration. You can pinch IV line while pushing medication, then release it when not pushing medication. Allow IV fluids to infuse at prescribed infusion rate when not pushing medication.	Ensures safe medication infusion. Most medications are delivered slowly, between 1 and 10 minutes; for example, morphine IV push delivery of 15 mg is recommended over 4 to 5 minutes (Gorski, 2023). Rapid injection of IV drug can be fatal. Allowing IV fluids to infuse while not pushing IV drug enables medication to be delivered to patient at prescribed rate.
f After injecting medication, withdraw syringe and recheck IV fluid infusion rate.	Injection of bolus may alter rate of fluid infusion. Rapid fluid infusion can cause circulatory fluid overload.
g *Option:* If IV medication is incompatible with IV fluids, stop IV fluids, clamp IV line, and flush with 10 mL of normal saline or sterile water (see agency policy). Then give IV push medication over appropriate amount of time and flush IV line with another 10 mL of normal saline or sterile water at *same rate* as medication was administered.	Allows IV bolus to be administered without risks associated with IV incompatibilities. Ensure that agency guidelines permit flushing lines with incompatible medications. A new site may need to be initiated.

Continued

STEP	RATIONALE
h *Option:* If the primary IV infusion that is currently hanging is a medication, disconnect it and administer IV push medication as outlined in Step 9, below. Verify agency policy for stopping IV fluids or continuous IV medications. If unable to stop IV infusion, start new IV site and administer medication using IV push (IV lock) method.	Avoids giving patient sudden bolus of medication in existing IV line.
9 Administer IV push (IV saline lock):	
a Prepare flush solutions according to agency policy.	
(1) *Saline flush method (preferred method):* Prepare two syringes filled with 2 to 3 mL of normal saline (0.9%). Many agencies do not provide prefilled normal saline syringes for flushing IV lines. Label syringe so that it does not get confused with the medication that is being administered.	Normal saline is effective in keeping IV locks patent and is compatible with a wide range of medications (Gorski, 2023).

STEP	RATIONALE
(2) Heparin flush method (refer to agency policy).	Many health care agencies no longer use heparin flush for peripheral lines (Gorski, 2018).
b Administer medication:	
(1) Clean injection port with antiseptic swab. Allow to dry. Then release clamp on lock tubing.	Prevents transfer of microorganisms during needle insertion.
(2) Insert needleless tip of syringe containing the normal saline 0.9% through center of injection port of IV lock.	
(3) Pull back gently on syringe plunger and check for blood return.	Indicates whether needle or catheter is in vein.
(4) Flush IV site with normal saline by pushing slowly on plunger.	Clears needle and reservoir of blood. Flushing without difficulty indicates patent IV line.

CLINICAL JUDGMENT *Carefully observe the area of skin above the IV catheter. Note any puffiness or swelling as the IV site is flushed, which could indicate infiltration into the vein, requiring removal of catheter.*

(5) Remove saline-filled syringe.	
(6) Clean injection port with antiseptic swab. Allow to dry.	Prevents transmission of microorganisms.
(7) Insert needleless tip of syringe containing prepared medication through injection port of IV lock.	Allows administration of medication.

Continued

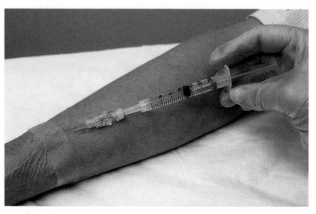

Fig. 35.3 Medication syringe in injection port of intravenous lock.

STEP	RATIONALE
(8) Inject medication within amount of time on medication label (Fig. 35.3). If not labeled confer with pharmacist, or medication reference manual. Use watch to time administration.	Many medication errors are associated with IV pushes being administered too quickly. Following guidelines for IV push rates promotes patient safety.
(9) After administering bolus, withdraw syringe.	
(10) Clean injection port with antiseptic swab. Allow to dry and secure clamp on lock tubing.	Prevents transmission of microorganisms.

STEP	RATIONALE
(11) Flush injection port.	
(a) Attach syringe with normal saline and inject flush at same rate that medication was delivered.	Prevents occlusion of IV access device and ensures that all medication is delivered. Flushing IV site at same rate as medication ensures that any medication remaining within IV needle is delivered at the correct rate.
10 Be sure any continuous IV infusion continues to run at proper hourly rate after administering medication.	Prevents fluid infusion error.
11 Dispose of SESIP covered needles and syringes in puncture- and leak-proof container.	Prevents accidental needlestick injuries and follows Centers for Disease Control and Prevention guidelines for sharps disposal (OSHA, n.d.[a]).
12 Perform postprocedure protocol.	
13 Stay with patient for several minutes and observe for any allergic reactions.	Dyspnea, wheezing, and circulatory collapse are signs of anaphylactic reaction.
14 Evaluate patient response:	
a Observe patient closely for adverse reactions during administration and for several minutes thereafter.	IV medications act rapidly.
b Observe IV site during injection for sudden swelling and for 48 h after IV push; assess for tenderness around IV site.	Swelling indicates infiltration into tissues surrounding vein. Signs of infiltration may not occur for 48 h. Tenderness may indicate phlebitis.
c Assess patient's status after giving medication to evaluate effectiveness of the medication.	Some IV bolus medications can cause rapid changes in patient's physiologic status. Some medications require careful monitoring and assessment and possible future laboratory testing.

Recording and Reporting

- Immediately after administration, record medication administration, including drug, dose, route, time instilled, and date and time administered on MAR, not before. Correctly sign MAR according to agency policy.
- Record patient teaching, validation of understanding, and patient's response to medication.
- Report any adverse reactions to patient's health care provider. Patient's response sometimes indicates need for additional medical therapy.

UNEXPECTED OUTCOMES	RELATED INTERVENTIONS
1 Patient develops adverse reaction to medication.	• Stop delivering medication immediately. Follow agency policy for appropriate response to allergic reaction (e.g., administration of antihistamine such as diphenhydramine or epinephrine) and reporting of adverse drug reactions.
	• Notify patient's health care provider of adverse effects immediately.
	• Add allergy information to patient's record and wristband.
2 IV medication is incompatible with IV fluids (e.g., IV fluid becomes cloudy in tubing) (see agency policy).	• Stop IV fluids and clamp IV line.
	• Flush IV line with 10 mL of 0.9% sodium chloride or sterile water.
	• Give IV bolus over appropriate amount of time.
	• Flush with another 10 mL of 0.9% sodium chloride or sterile water at same rate as medication was administered.
	• Restart IV fluids with new tubing at prescribed rate.
	• If unable to stop IV infusion, start new IV site and administer medication using IV push (IV lock) method.

UNEXPECTED OUTCOMES	RELATED INTERVENTIONS
3 IV site shows symptoms of infiltration or phlebitis.	• Stop IV infusion immediately or discontinue access device and restart in another site. • Determine how much damage IV medication has produced in subcutaneous tissue. • Provide IV extravasation care (e.g., injecting phentolamine around IV infiltration site) as indicated by agency policy, use a medication reference as a guide, and consult pharmacist to determine appropriate follow-up care.

Isolation Precautions

When a patient has a known or suspected source of colonization or infection, specific infection prevention and control practices should be followed to reduce the risk of cross-contamination to other patients (Centers for Disease Control and Prevention [CDC] 2019c, 2020; Marra, 2017).) Standard precautions include infection prevention practices that apply to all patients, regardless of suspected or confirmed infection status, in any setting in which health care is delivered (CDC, 2019c). These include hand hygiene; use of gloves, gown, mask, eye protection, or face shield, depending on the anticipated exposure; and safe injection practices (CDC, 2019c) (see Table 36.1, Tier One). Standard precautions require you to wear clean gloves before coming in contact with mucous membranes, nonintact skin, blood, body fluids, or other infectious material. It is not necessary to wear gloves when simply entering and then leaving a patient room. However, you wear clean gloves routinely when performing a variety of procedures. Masks or face shields are worn when there is risk of splash during a procedure (e.g., suctioning) or when certain sterile procedures (such as changing a central line dressing) are performed. Protective eyewear and masks are important when there is risk for splash of blood or other body fluids to the eyes or mouth. For patients with confirmed or possible SARS-CoV-2 (Covid-19), additional precautions involve the use of N-95 respirators and face shield or goggles (Box 36.1).

Assess the need for personal protective equipment (PPE) for each planned task and for all patients, regardless of their diagnoses. Because of increased attention to the prevention of bloodborne pathogens and tuberculosis (TB) (Box 36.2), the CDC (2019d) and the Occupational Safety and Health Administration (OSHA) (2011) have stressed the importance of barrier protection. The CDC (2019e) published revised guidelines for the routine practices for occupational infection prevention and control. The CDC also published a revised *Guideline for isolation precautions: preventing transmission of infectious agents in health care settings,* important standards that are incorporated into this skill (CDC, 2019c).

When Standard precautions are insufficient the CDC has a Tier Two level of precautions, described as transmission-based precautions, or isolation. The transmission-based precautions are for patients who are known or suspected to be infected or colonized with infectious agents that require additional control measures to effectively prevent transmission (CDC, 2019c). The second tier (Table 36.1) includes

TABLE 36.1 Centers for Disease Control and Prevention Isolation Guidelines

Standard Precautions (Tier One) for Use With All Patients

- Standard precautions apply to blood, blood products, all body fluids, secretions, excretions (except sweat), nonintact skin, and mucous membranes.
- Perform hand hygiene before direct contact with patients; between patient contacts; after touching blood, body fluids, secretions, excretions, or contaminated items; and immediately after removing gloves.
- PPE: Wear gloves for touching blood, body fluids, secretions, excretions, and contaminated items; and for touching mucous membranes and nonintact skin.
- PPE: Wear a gown during procedures and patient-care activities when contact of clothing/exposed skin with blood/body fluids, secretions, and excretions is anticipated.
- PPE: Wear a mask, eye protection (goggles), face shield during procedures and patient-care activities likely to generate splashes or sprays of blood, body fluids, secretions, especially suctioning and endotracheal intubation. During aerosol-generating procedures on patients with suspected or proven infections transmitted by respiratory aerosols (e.g., tuberculosis, SARS-CoV-2 [Covid-19]), wear a fit-tested N95 or higher respirator in addition to gloves, gown, and face/eye protection.
- Soiled patient care environment: Handle in a manner that prevents transfer of microorganisms to others and to the environment; wear gloves if visibly contaminated; perform hand hygiene.
- Environmental control: Develop procedures for routine care, cleaning, and disinfection of environmental surfaces, especially frequently touched surfaces in patient-care areas.
- Bedclothes/linen: Handle in a manner that prevents transfer of microorganisms to others and to the environment (e.g., hold dirty linen away from uniform/gown).
- Handling needles and other sharps: Do not recap, bend, break, or hand-manipulate used needles; if recapping is required, use a one-handed scoop technique only; use safety features when available; place all used sharps in puncture-resistant container.
- Patient resuscitation: Use disposable (when possible) mouthpiece, resuscitation bag, other ventilation devices to prevent contact with mouth and oral secretions.

Continued

TABLE 36.1 Centers for Disease Control and Prevention Isolation Guidelines—cont'd

- Patient placement: Prioritize for single-patient room if patient is at increased risk of transmission, is likely to contaminate the environment, does not maintain appropriate hygiene, or is at increased risk of acquiring infection or developing adverse outcome after infection.
- Respiratory hygiene and cough etiquette: Have patient cover the nose or mouth when sneezing or coughing; use tissues to contain respiratory secretions and dispose in nearest waste container; perform hand hygiene after contact with respiratory secretions and contaminated objects or materials; contain respiratory secretions with procedure or surgical mask; have patient sit at least 3 feet away from others if coughing.
- Safe injection practices: Use a sterile, single-use, disposable needle and syringe for each injection given, and prevent contamination of injection equipment and medication. Whenever possible, use of single-dose vials is preferred over multiple-dose vials, especially when medications will be administered to multiple patients.

Transmission-Based Precautions (Tier Two) for Use With Specific Types of Patients

Category	Infection/Condition	Barrier Protection
Airborne precautions (droplet nuclei smaller than 5 microns)	Measles, chickenpox (varicella), disseminated varicella zoster, pulmonary or laryngeal tuberculosis	Private-room, negative-pressure airflow of at least 6 to 12 exchanges per hour via HEPA filtration; mask or respiratory protection device, N95 respirator (depending on condition)
Droplet precautions (droplets larger than 5 microns; being within 3 feet of patient)	Diphtheria (pharyngeal), rubella, streptococcal pharyngitis, pneumonia or scarlet fever in infants and young children, pertussis, mumps, *Mycoplasma* pneumonia, meningococcal pneumonia or sepsis, pneumonic plague	Private-room or cohort patients; mask or respirator (refer to agency policy)

TABLE 36.1 Centers for Disease Control and Prevention Isolation Guidelines—cont'd

Category	Infection/Condition	Barrier Protection
Contact precautions (direct patient or environmental contact)	Colonization or infection with multidrug-resistant organisms such as VRE and MRSA, *Clostridium difficile*, *Shigella*, and other enteric pathogens; major wound infections; herpes simplex; scabies; disseminated varicella zoster; respiratory syncytial virus in infants, young children, or immunocompromised adults	Private-room or cohort patients (see agency policy), gloves, gowns; patients may leave their room for procedures or therapy if infectious material is contained or covered and placed in a clean gown and hands cleaned
Protective environment	Allogeneic hematopoietic stem cell transplants	Private room; positive airflow with ≥12 air exchanges per hour; HEPA filtration for incoming air; mask to be worn by patient when out of room during times of construction in area

HEPA, High-efficiency particulate air; *MRSA,* methicillin-resistant *Staphylococcus aureus*; *PPE,* personal protective equipment; *VRE,* vancomycin-resistant enterococci.
Adapted from Centers for Disease Control and Prevention (CDC), Siegel JD et al. and the Healthcare Infection Control Practices Advisory Committee: *2007 Guideline for Isolation precautions: preventing transmission of infectious agents in health care settings,* 2007 last update July 2019, 2019c https://www.cdc.gov/infectioncontrol/pdf/guidelines/isolation-guidelines-H.pdf.

precautions designed for care of patients who are known or suspected to be infected, or colonized, with microorganisms transmitted by the contact, droplet, or airborne route (Nulens, 2018) or by contact with contaminated surfaces. The three types of transmission-based precautions—airborne, droplet, and contact precautions—may be combined for diseases that have multiple routes of transmission (e.g., chickenpox). Whether used singly or in combination, use them in addition to standard precautions.

BOX 36.1   Infection Control Precautions for SARS-CoV-2 (Covid-19) Patients

1. Perform hand hygiene
2. **Put on isolation gown.** Tie all of the ties on the gown.
3. **Put on NIOSH-approved N95 filtering facepiece respirator or higher (use a facemask if a respirator is not available).** If the respirator has a nosepiece, it should be fitted to the nose with both hands, not bent or tented. Do not pinch the nosepiece with one hand. Respirator/facemask should be extended under chin. Both your mouth and nose should be protected. Do not wear respirator/facemask under the chin or store in scrubs pocket between patients.[*]
   - **Respirator:** Respirator straps should be placed on crown of head (top strap) and base of neck (bottom strap). Perform a user seal-check each time respirator is applied.
   - **Facemask:** Mask ties should be secured on crown of head (top tie) and base of neck (bottom tie). If mask has loops, hook them appropriately around the ears.
1. **Put on face shield or goggles.** When wearing an N95 respirator or half facepiece elastomeric respirator, select the proper eye protection to ensure that the respirator does not interfere with the correct positioning of the eye protection, and the eye protection does not affect the fit or seal of the respirator. Face shields provide full face coverage. Goggles also provide excellent protection for eyes, but fogging is common.
2. **Put on gloves.** Gloves should cover the cuff (wrist) of gown.

---

[*]Facilities implementing reuse or extended use of personal protective equipment will need to adjust their donning and doffing procedures to accommodate those practices.
NIOSH, National Institute for Occupational Safety and Health.
From Centers for Disease Control and Prevention: *Using personal protective equipment*, 2020, https://public4.pagefreezer.com/browse/CDC%20Covid%20Pages/11-05-2022T12:30/https://www.cdc.gov/coronavirus/2019-ncov/hcp/using-ppe.html. Accessed 12/7/2022.

Multidrug-resistant organisms (MDROs) such as methicillin-resistant *Staphylococcus aureus* (MRSA) and vancomycin-resistant enterococci (VRE) have become increasingly common as a cause of colonization and health care–associated infections (HAIs). VRE poses a greater risk to immune-compromised and debilitated patients and is associated with antibiotic and device use (Davis et al., 2020; Agegne et al., 2018). *Clostridium difficile* infection is one of the most common and costly HAIs. In most instances, patient susceptibility to *C. difficile* infection requires prior treatment with antibiotics. Unlike MRSA and VRE, *C. difficile* is more difficult to eliminate from the environment because it is a spore-forming organism, meaning that it can remain on surfaces in its dormant state for long periods of time. Regardless of the MDRO involved, the most common means of transmission is by way of

BOX 36.2   Special Tuberculosis Precautions

The Centers for Disease Control and Prevention (CDC) published guidelines for preventing tuberculosis (TB) transmission in health care agencies in response to a resurgence of TB in the United States associated with the increasing incidence of HIV infection, TB infection transmission in health care settings, and increasing immigration from countries with a high incidence of TB (CDC, 2019).

- Primary environmental controls consist of controlling the source of infection by using local exhaust ventilation (e.g., hoods, tents, or booths) and diluting and removing contaminated air by using general ventilation.
- Secondary environmental controls consist of controlling the airflow to prevent contamination of air in areas adjacent to the source of airborne infection isolation rooms; and cleaning the air by using high-efficiency particulate air (HEPA) filtration, or ultraviolet germicidal irradiation.
- Current CDC guidelines for preventing and controlling TB focus on early detection of infection, preventing close contact with patients with active TB disease, and applying effective infection control measures in health care settings, including:
- Suspect TB in any patient with respiratory symptoms lasting longer than 3 weeks accompanied by other suspicious symptoms such as unexplained weight loss, night sweats, fever, and a productive cough often streaked with blood.
- Consider the potential for infectious pulmonary or laryngeal TB from documented positive acid-fast bacillus smear or culture, cavitation on chest x-ray film, or history of recent TB exposure.
- Isolation for patients with suspected or confirmed TB includes placing the patient on airborne precautions in a single-patient negative-pressure room.
- Health care workers who care for patients with suspected or confirmed TB must wear special respirators (e.g., N95 or P100). These respirators are high-efficiency particulate masks that have the ability to filter particles at a 95% or better efficiency (OSHA, 2011).
- The CDC now recommends the use of the QuantiFERON-TB Gold test (QFT-GIT) or the T-SPOT (CDC, 2016), a blood test, in place of the traditional TB skin test. The advantages of the QFT-GIT test are that it does not boost responses measured by subsequent tests and the results are not subject to reader bias.

a health care worker's hands. To reduce the risk of cross-contamination among patients, follow contact precautions (see Table 36.1) in addition to standard precautions when caring for these patients.

Safety Guidelines

- Always maintain an infection control conscience. Consider possible exposure and how an organism can be transmitted.
- Monitor health care colleagues and patient visitors in their use of infection control procedures.

Delegation

The skill of caring for patients on isolation precautions can be delegated to assistive personnel (AP). However, nurses must assess patients' isolation status and indications. Instruct the AP about:

- Reason for patient's isolation precautions.
- Precautions to consider when bringing equipment into the patient's room.
- Special precautions regarding individual patient needs such as transportation to diagnostic tests.

Collaboration

- When a patient develops an infection and the causative organism is unclear, collaborate with infection control specialists to determine proper transmission control procedures.
- Communication of isolation precautions is key between all health care workers who come in contact with the isolated patient to avoid a breach in precautions.

Equipment

- PPE for standard and transmission-based precautions: clean gloves, mask, eyewear or goggles, face shield, and gown (gowns may be disposable or reusable, depending on agency policy)
- PPE for patients with probable or confirmed SARS-CoV-2: gown, N95 filtering respirator, face mask if respirator not available, face shield or goggles, clean gloves
- Other patient care equipment as appropriate: hygiene items, medications, dressing supplies, sharps container, disposable blood pressure [BP] cuff
- Soiled linen bag and trash receptacle
- Sign for door indicating type of isolation and/or for visitors to come to the nurses' station before entering room
- TB isolation
  - Room with negative airflow
  - N95 or P100 respirator

STEP	RATIONALE
1 Perform preprocedure protocol.	

Assessment

STEP	RATIONALE
• Assess patient's medical history for possible indications for isolation (e.g., positive test for SARS-CoV-2, risk factors for TB or other communicable disease, major draining wound, or purulent productive cough).	Mode of transmission for infectious microorganism determines type and degree of precautions followed.
• Review laboratory test results (e.g., body fluid/tissue culture, acid-fast bacillus smears, antigen tests and nucleic acid amplification tests for SARS-CoV-2, changes in white blood cell count).	Reveals type of microorganism for which patient is being isolated, body fluid in which it was identified, and whether patient is immunosuppressed.
• Review agency policies and precautions related to specific isolation system needed, including appropriate barriers to apply (see Table 36.1, Box 36.1). Consider the types of care measures to be performed while in patient's room (e.g., medication administration or dressing change).	Allows for organization of care items for procedures and the amount of time to be spent in patient's room. Ensures proper protection.
• Assess whether patient has known latex allergy. If allergy is present, refer to agency policy and resources available to provide full latex-free care.	Protects patient from serious allergic response.

Continued

STEP	RATIONALE
• Review nursing care plan notes or confer with colleagues regarding patient's emotional state and reaction/adjustment to isolation. Assess patient's understanding of purpose of isolation.	Provides opportunity to plan for need to provide patient emotional support and teaching.

Implementation

STEP	RATIONALE
1 Perform hand hygiene.	Reduces transmission of microorganisms.
2 Prepare all equipment to be taken into patient's room. In most cases dedicated equipment such as stethoscopes, BP equipment, and thermometers should remain in room until patient is discharged. If patient is infected or colonized with highly communicable or resistant organism, equipment remains in room and is thoroughly disinfected before removal (see agency policy).	Prevents the need for multiple trips into patient room. The CDC recommends use of dedicated noncritical patient care equipment (CDC, 2019e, CDC, 2019f). Use EPA-registered disinfectants that have microbiocidal (i.e., microbe killing) activity against the pathogens most likely to contaminate the patient care environment (CDC, 2019c).
3 Prepare for entrance into isolation room. Ideally, before applying PPE, step into patient's room and stay by door. Introduce yourself and explain care that will be provided. If this is not possible, or patient is on airborne precautions, apply PPE outside of the room.	Proper preparation ensures protection from microorganism exposure. Allows patient to see you without PPE and without exposing yourself to risk of infection transmission.

STEP	RATIONALE
4 Apply PPE. a Apply gown, being sure that it fully covers torso from neck to knees and from arms to end of wrist and wraps around the back, covering all outer garments (CDC, 2019c). Pull sleeves down to wrist. Tie securely at neck and waist (Fig. 36.1).	Prevents transmission of infection; protects you when patient has excessive drainage or discharges.

Continued

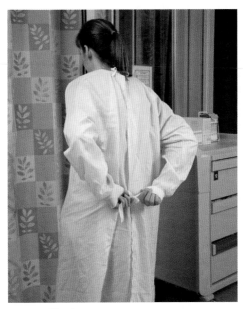

Fig. 36.1 Tie isolation gown at waist.

STEP	RATIONALE
b Apply either surgical mask or fitted N95 respirator. For a mask with ties, secure top tie at back of middle of head, secure bottom tie around back of neck. For a mask with elastic band secure snugly around ears. Next fit flexible band over bridge of nose. Respirator bands fit over back of head and neck. Be sure mask or respirator fits snugly to face and below chin. Fit-check respirator (CDC, 2019c). Type and fit-testing depend on type of isolation and agency policy. You must have a medical evaluation and be fit-tested before using a respirator.	Prevents exposure to airborne microorganisms or microorganisms from splashing fluids.
c If needed, apply eyewear, face shield, or goggles snugly around face and eyes. Side shields may be used for those wearing prescription glasses.	Protects you from exposure to microorganisms that may occur during splashing of fluids.
d Apply clean gloves (select according to hand size). (*Note:* Wear unpowdered, latex-free gloves if you, patient, or another health care worker has latex allergy.) Bring glove cuffs over edge of gown sleeves (Fig. 36.2).	Reduces transmission of microorganisms.

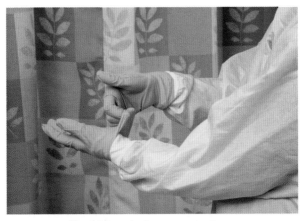

Fig. 36.2 Apply gloves over gown sleeves.

STEP	RATIONALE

CLINICAL JUDGMENT *Keep hands away from face while performing tasks in patient room. Work from clean to dirty surfaces (CDC, 2019c). If gloves become heavily soiled, remove and change to continue care activities.*

5 Enter patient's room. Arrange supplies and equipment. (*Note:* If equipment will be reused, place on clean paper towel.)	Prevents extra trips entering and leaving room. Minimizes contamination of care items.
6 Explain purpose of isolation and precautions that need to be taken by patient and family caregiver. Offer opportunity to ask questions. If patient is on TB precautions, instruct to cover mouth with tissue when coughing and to wear disposable surgical mask when leaving room.	Improves ability of patient and family caregiver to participate in care and minimizes anxiety. Identifies opportunity for planning social interaction and diversional activities. Reduces TB microorganism transmission.

Continued

STEP	RATIONALE

CLINICAL JUDGMENT *In some cases, patients with confirmed SARS-CoV-2 virus will not be allowed visitors (see agency policy). Patients with confirmed or possible SARS-CoV-2 infection should wear a facemask when being evaluated medically (CDC, 2020).*

STEP	RATIONALE
7 Assess vital signs.	
a If patient is infected or colonized with resistant organism, equipment remains in room, including stethoscope and BP cuff (CDC, 2019e).	Decreases risk of infection being transmitted to another patient.
b If stethoscope is to be reused, clean earpieces and diaphragm or bell with 70% alcohol or agency-approved germicide. Set aside on clean surface.	Systematic disinfection of stethoscopes with 70% alcohol or approved germicide minimizes chance of spreading infectious agents between patients (Boulée et al., 2019).
c Use individual or disposable thermometers and BP cuffs when available.	Prevents cross-contamination.

CLINICAL JUDGMENT *If disposable thermometer indicates a fever, assess for other signs/symptoms. Confirm fever using an alternative thermometer. Do not use electronic thermometer if patient is suspected or confirmed to have* C. difficile *infection (McDonald, 2018).*

STEP	RATIONALE
8 Administer medications.	
a Give oral medication in wrapper or cup.	Handle and discard supplies to minimize transfer of microorganisms.
b Dispose of wrapper or cup in plastic-lined receptacle.	
c Continue wearing gloves when administering an injection.	Reduces risk of exposure to blood.
d Discard needleless syringe or safety sheathed needle into designated sharps container.	Needleless devices should be used to reduce risk of needlesticks and sharps injuries to health care workers.

STEP	RATIONALE
9 Provide hygiene care. Encourage patient to ask any questions or express concerns about isolation. Provide informal teaching at this time.	Hygiene practices further minimize transfer of microorganisms. Quality time should be spent with patient when in room.
a Avoid allowing isolation gown to become wet; carry wash basin outward away from gown; avoid leaning against wet tabletop.	Moisture allows organisms to travel through gown to uniform.

CLINICAL JUDGMENT *When there is a risk for excess soiling, wear a gown impervious to moisture.*

STEP	RATIONALE
b Help patient remove own gown; discard in leak-proof linen bag.	Reduces transfer of microorganisms.
c Remove linen from bed; avoid contact with isolation gown. Place in leak-proof linen bag.	Carefully handle linen soiled by patient's body fluids to prevent contact with clean items.
d Provide clean bed linen.	
e Change gloves and perform hand hygiene if gloves become excessively soiled and further care is necessary. Re-glove.	
10 Collect specimens.	
a Place specimen container on clean paper towel in patient's bathroom and follow procedure for collecting specimen of body fluids (see agency policy).	Container will be taken out of patient's room; prevents contamination of outer surface.
b Follow agency procedure for collecting specimen of body fluids.	

Continued

STEP	RATIONALE
c Transfer specimen to container without soiling outside of container. Place container in plastic bag and place label on outside of bag or per agency policy. Label specimen in front of patient (The Joint Commission, 2021b). Perform hand hygiene and re-glove if additional procedures are needed.	Specimens of blood and body fluids are placed in well-constructed containers with secure lids to prevent leaks during transport. Proper labeling prevents diagnostic error.
d Check label on specimen for accuracy. Send to laboratory (warning labels are often used, depending on agency policy). Label containers of blood or body fluids with biohazard sticker.	Ensures that health care providers who transport or handle containers are aware of infectious contents.
11 Dispose of linen, trash, and disposable items.	
a Use sturdy, moisture-impervious bags to contain soiled articles. Double bag if necessary, for heavily soiled linen or heavy wet trash.	Linen or refuse should be entirely contained to prevent exposure of personnel to infectious material.
b Tie bags securely at top in knot.	
12 Remove all reusable pieces of equipment. Clean any contaminated surfaces with hospital-approved disinfectant (Marra, 2017) (see agency policy).	All items must be properly cleaned, disinfected, or sterilized for reuse.

STEP	RATIONALE
13 Resupply room as needed. Have staff colleague hand new supplies into room.	Limiting trips by personnel into and out of room reduces patient and health care staff exposure to microorganisms.
14 Leave isolation room. Order of removal of PPE depends on what was worn/required for specific isolation system. The sequence that follows describes an approach for removing all barriers worn. PPE worn in room must be removed before leaving room.	Order of removal minimizes exposure to any infectious material on barriers.
a Remove gloves. *Remember:* outside of gloves is contaminated. Remove one glove by grasping cuff and pulling glove inside out over hand. Hold removed glove in gloved hand (Fig. 36.3) while sliding fingers of ungloved hand under remaining glove at wrist. Peel glove off over first glove. Discard gloves in proper waste container.	Technique prevents contact with outer contaminated surface of glove. Change gloves between exposures to body sites and patient equipment. Inadequate glove changes and subsequent hand hygiene can lead to contamination, increasing the risk of HAIs (CDC, 2019e).
b Remove eyewear, face shield, or goggles. Handle by headband or earpieces. Discard in proper waste container.	Outside of goggles/eyewear is contaminated. Hands have not been soiled.

Continued

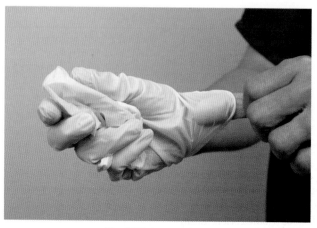

Fig. 36.3 Remove gloves.

STEP	RATIONALE
c Remove gown. Untie neck strings and then untie back strings of gown. Allow gown to fall from shoulders (Fig. 36.4); touch inside of gown only. Remove hands from sleeves without touching outside of gown. Hold gown inside at shoulder seams and fold inside out into bundle; discard in proper waste container.	Hands do not come in contact with soiled front of gown.

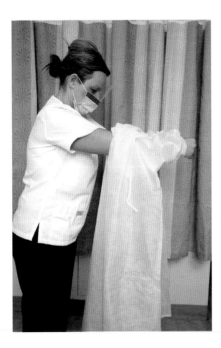

Fig. 36.4 Remove gown by allowing it to fall from shoulders.

STEP	RATIONALE
d Remove mask. If mask secures over ears, remove elastic from ears and pull mask away from face. For tie-on mask, untie *bottom* mask string and then top strings, pull mask away from face (Fig. 36.5A), and drop into proper waste container (Fig. 36.5B). Do not touch outer surface of mask.	Ungloved hands are not contaminated by touching only elastic or mask strings. Prevents top part of mask from falling down over uniform.

Continued

Fig. 36.5 (A) Pull
mask away from face.
(B) Drop into trash
receptacle.

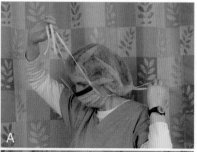

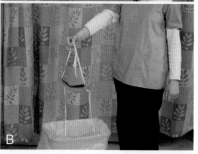

STEP	RATIONALE

CLINICAL JUDGMENT *The CDC (2020) offers these steps removing PPE when caring for SARS-CoV-2 patients:*
- *Remove gloves.*
- *Remove gown. Untie all ties (or unsnap all buttons). Some gown ties can be broken rather than untied. Do so in gentle manner, avoiding a forceful movement. Dispose in trash receptacle.*
- *Healthcare personnel may now exit patient room.*
- *Perform hand hygiene.*
- *Remove face shield or goggles. Carefully remove face shield or goggles by grabbing the strap and pulling upward and away from head. Do not touch the front of face shield or goggles.*
- *Remove and discard respirator (or facemask if used instead of respirator). Do not touch the front of the respirator or facemask.*
- *Respirator: Remove the bottom strap by touching only the strap and bring it carefully over the head. Grasp the top strap and bring it carefully over the head, and then pull the respirator away from the face without touching the front of the respirator.*
- *Facemask: Carefully untie (or unhook from the ears) and pull away from face without touching the front.*
- *Perform hand hygiene.*

STEP	RATIONALE

CLINICAL JUDGMENT *If patient is on TB precautions, place reusable mask in labeled paper bag for storage, being careful not to crush mask (check agency policy for number of times reusable masks can be used).*

e	Perform hand hygiene.	Reduces transmission of microorganisms.
f	Retrieve wristwatch and stethoscope (unless items must remain in room).	
g	Explain to patient when you plan to return to room. Ask whether patient requires any personal care items. Offer books, magazines, audiotapes.	Diversions can help to minimize boredom and feeling of social isolation.
15	Perform postprocedure protocol.	
16	Evaluate patient response:	
a	Observe other health care providers, or patient's and family caregiver's use of isolation precautions when visiting.	Promptly identifies any improper use of a precaution.
b	While in room, ask whether patient has had sufficient chance to discuss health problems, course of treatment, or other topics of personal importance.	Measures patient's perception of adequacy of discussions with caregivers.

Recording and Reporting

- Document procedures performed and patient's response to social isolation. Also document any patient or family education performed and reinforced.
- Document type of isolation in use and the microorganisms (if known).
- During hand-off report share type of isolation precautions, any infectious disease testing results, and how patient has been responding to social isolation.

UNEXPECTED OUTCOMES	RELATED INTERVENTIONS
1 Patient avoids social and therapeutic discussions.	• Confer with family caregiver and/or significant other and determine best approach to reduce patient's sense of loneliness and depression.
2 Patient or health care worker may have an allergic response to wearing latex gloves.	• Notify health care provider/ employee health and treat sensitivity or allergic reaction appropriately. • Use latex-free gloves for future care activities.

Mechanical Lifts: Transfer Skills

Safe patient handling and mobility (SPHM) involves the use of assistive devices (e.g., mechanical lifts) to ensure that patients can be moved and mobilized safely and that care providers avoid performing high-risk manual patient handling tasks (US Department of Veterans Affairs, 2016). Using principles of SPHM during patient transfer and positioning decreases work effort and places less strain on musculoskeletal structures. Key principles in determining the SPHM techniques and technology used for patients are knowing whether a patient is weight-bearing, and the patient's weight, height, strength, and ability to cooperate and provide help (Matz, 2019). Patients who are at high risk for complications from improper positioning and injury during transfer include those with poor nutrition, poor circulation, loss of sensation, alterations in bone formation or joint mobility, and impaired muscle development.

The variety of mechanical lifts available for patient transfer include mechanical, hydraulic, and ceiling lifts. Lifts provide varying levels of support including total lifts and sit-to-stand lifts. Analyze patients' assessment data and refer to their mobility status and safe-handling algorithms (e.g., Veterans Affairs Safe Patient Handling app) available in most agencies, to determine whether a lift device or mechanical transfer device is needed, the proper device to use, and the number of people needed to help with transfer. This skill covers use of lifts to transfer a patient to a chair.

Safety Guidelines

- Follow the principles of proper body mechanics when lifting a patient or using any patient care equipment.
- Do not start procedure until all required caregivers are available.

Delegation

The skill of effective transfer techniques using mechanical lifts can be delegated to trained assistive personnel (AP). The nurse is responsible for initially assessing a patient's readiness and functional ability to transfer. Direct the AP by:

- Assisting and supervising how to move patients who are transferred for the first time after prolonged bed rest, extensive surgery, critical illness, or spinal cord trauma.

- Explaining the patient's mobility restrictions, changes in blood pressure to look for, or sensory or neurologic alterations that may affect safe transfer.
- Explaining observations to report such as patient's dizziness or the ability/inability to assist.

Collaboration

- Physical therapy can conduct a functional assessment and suggest best transfer method for patient.

Equipment

- Gait belt, sling, or lapboard (as needed)
- Nonskid shoes, bath blankets, and pillows
- Chair with arms or wheelchair (position chair at 45- to 60-degree angle to bed, remove footrests on wheelchair, and lock both bed and chair brakes)
- Stretcher (position next to bed, lock brakes on both stretcher and bed)
- Mechanical/hydraulic/ceiling lift (use frame, canvas strips or chains, and hammock or canvas strips) (Fig. 37.1A & B).
- *Option:* Stand-assist lift device
- *Option:* Clean gloves (if risk of contact with soiled linen)
- *Option:* Lateral transfer device

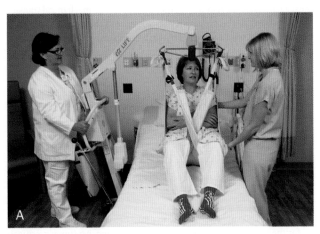

Fig. 37.1 (A) Hydraulic lift raises patient off bed mattress.

(Continued)

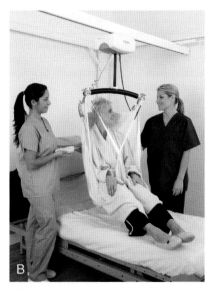

Fig. 37.1, cont'd (B) Electric control raises patient in ceiling lift. (Image B courtesy Handicare USA, St Louis, MO.)

STEP	RATIONALE
1 Perform preprocedure protocol.	
Assessment	
• Refer to electronic health record (EHR) for most recent recorded weight and height for patient. If no recorded data, obtain height and weight measurements.	Determines whether mechanical transfer device or friction-reducing device is needed for transfer.
• Review history for previous fall and/or if patient has a fear of falling.	Previous fall history is one of the significant fall risk factors. Fear of falling is related to a patient's physical performance, such as balance, gait and security in walking (Schoene et al., 2019; Liu et al, 2021).
• Assess previous mode of transferring to bed or chair (if applicable).	Ensures consistency in assisting with transfer.

Continued

STEP	RATIONALE
• Assess patient's cognitive status: ability to follow verbal instructions, short-term memory, motor strength and coordination, recognition of physical deficits, and limitations to movement.	Determines patient's ability to follow directions and participate in transfer techniques.
• Perform hand hygiene.	Reduces transmission of microorganisms.
• Obtain assistance from AP to assist with patient handling. Assess the patient's mobility by administering the Banner Mobility Assessment Tool (BMAT) (Matz, 2019):	The BMAT is a tool that assesses four functional tasks to identify the level of mobility a patient can achieve (Matz, 2019). The assessment aids in determining a patient's level of mobility and recommends assistive devices needed to safely lift, transfer, and mobilize a patient.
a Sit and Shake: From a semireclined position, ask patient to sit upright and rotate to a seated position at the side of the bed; patient may use the bed rail to assist. Note patient's ability to maintain bedside position. Ask patient to reach out and grab your hand and shake, making sure patient reaches across their midline.	
If patient fails to sit and shake: Use a total lift with sling and/or positioning sheet and/or straps; and/or use lateral transfer devices such as a rollboard or friction-reducing (slide sheets/tube) or air-assisted device to transfer patient.	

STEP	RATIONALE
b Stretch and point: Have patient assume a seated position at the side of the bed and then place both feet on the floor (or stool) with knees no higher than hips. Ask patient to extend one leg and straighten the knee, and then bend the ankle and point the toes. Repeat with the other leg.	
If patient fails to stretch and point: Use a total lift for patient unable to bear weight on at least one leg; use sit-to-stand lift for patient who can bear weight on at least one leg.	
c Stand: Ask patient to elevate off the bed or chair (seated to standing) using an assistive device (walker, cane, bed rail). Patient should be able to raise buttocks off bed and hold for a count of five. May repeat once. Note patient's proprioception (awareness of position of body) and balance.	
If patient fails to stand: Use nonpowered/powered raising/stand aid (sit-to-stand lift if no stand aid available) or use total lift with ambulation accessories or assistive device (cane, walker, crutches) to transfer patient.	

Continued

STEP	RATIONALE
d Walk (march in place and advance step): Ask patient to march in place at bedside, and then ask patient to step forward and back with each foot. Patient should display stability while performing tasks. Assess for stability and safety awareness.	
If patient cannot walk: Use nonpowered raising/stand aid (default to powered sit-to-stand lift if no stand aid available) or use total lift with ambulation accessories or assistive device (cane, walker, crutches).	

CLINICAL JUDGMENT *An objective assessment is needed to accurately determine a patient's ability to sit, stand, or ambulate. Avoid gathering a self-report from patient or family caregiver as to patient's ability to sit, stand, or ambulate as sole source of information.*

• While assessing mobility, note any weakness, dizziness, or risk for orthostatic hypotension (OH) (e.g., previously on bed rest, first time arising from supine position after surgical procedure, history of dizziness when arising).	Determines risk of fainting or falling during transfer. Immobilized patients have decreased ability of autonomic nervous system to equalize blood supply. Specifically, after 3 minutes of standing (or 3 minutes of sitting upright), a decrease of ≥20 mm Hg in systolic BP or a decrease of ≥10 mm Hg in diastolic BP indicates that a patient has OH (Biswas et al., 2019).
• Assess activity tolerance, noting fatigue during sitting/standing.	Determines ability of patient to participate in transfer.

STEP	RATIONALE
• Assess sensory status: central and peripheral vision, hearing adequacy, and presence of peripheral sensation loss.	Visual field loss decreases patient's ability to see in direction of transfer and may impact balance. Peripheral sensation loss decreases proprioception. Patients with visual and hearing losses need transfer techniques and communication methods adapted to their deficits.

CLINICAL JUDGMENT *Patients with hemiplegia may "neglect" one side of the body (inattention to or unawareness of one side of body or environment), which distorts perception of the visual field. If patients experience neglect of one side, instruct them to scan all visual fields when transferring.*

STEP	RATIONALE
• Assess level of comfort (e.g., joint discomfort, muscle spasm) and rate severity on scale of 0 to 10. Offer prescribed analgesic 30 minutes before transfer.	Pain reduces patient's motivation and ability to be mobile. Pain relief before a transfer enhances ability to participate.
• Assess patient's level of motivation, such as eagerness versus unwillingness to be mobile and perceived value of exercise.	Affects patient's desire to engage in activity.
• Assess patient's vital signs just before transfer.	Baseline measures determine whether vital sign changes occur during activity, indicating activity intolerance.
• Analyze assessment data and refer to mobility status and safe-handling algorithms (e.g., Veterans Affairs Safe Patient Handling app) available in most agencies, to determine whether a lift device or mechanical transfer device is needed and the number of people needed to help with transfer. **Do not start procedure until all required caregivers are available.**	Ensures safe patient handling, reducing risk of injury to patient and caregivers.

Continued

STEP	RATIONALE

Implementation

1 Explain to patient the preparation needed for application of lift and transfer technique and the safety precautions to be used.

Provides for clearer understanding by patient. Motivates patient to be involved in transfer.

2 Perform hand hygiene. Position patient supine in bed. Raise bed level with your hips. Raise upper side rail on side where patient will exit bed. Be sure to lock bed brakes.

Reduces transmission of microorganisms. Minimizes strain on your back during patient transfer. Patient can use side rails for lifting upward into sitting position.

3 Transfer patient from bed to chair using lift (*Option:* apply clean gloves if bed linen soiled):

   a If patient is limited cognitively, is uncooperative, has weight-bearing precautions with upper body strength, or caregiver must lift more than 15.9 kg (35 lb), use a full-body sling lift with minimum of two or three caregivers (Matz, 2019; Nelson, 2008). Follow manufacturer lift guidelines to apply correctly.

Research supports use of mechanical lifts to prevent musculoskeletal injuries (American Nurses Association, 2013; Occupational Safety and Health Administration [OSHA], nd[b]). Use of ceiling-mounted lifts is a popular choice (when available) because of location in patient rooms.

CLINICAL JUDGMENT *Hoyer lifts should not be used for patients with recent hip replacements who have hip precaution orders because it may promote hip flexion >90 degrees, which is contraindicated for patients with posterior hip precautions.*

   b Bring mechanical floor lift to bedside, or lower ceiling lift and position properly.

Ensures safe elevation of patient off bed.

STEP	RATIONALE
c Ensure chair is positioned along one side of bed, facing foot of bed. Allow adequate space to maneuver the lift.	Prepares environment for safe use of lift and subsequent transfer of patient into chair.
d Raise bed to safe working height with mattress flat. Lower side rail on side near chair.	Allows you to use proper body mechanics.
e Have second caregiver positioned at opposite side of bed.	Maintains patient safety, preventing fall from bed.
f Roll patient to opposite side from where you are standing.	Positions patient for placement of lift sling.
g Place hammock or canvas strips under patient to form sling. With two canvas pieces, lower edge fits under patient's knees (wide piece) and upper edge fits under patient's shoulders (narrow piece).	Two types of seats are supplied with mechanical/hydraulic lift: hammock style is better for patients who are flaccid or are weak and need support; canvas strips can be used for patients with normal muscle tone. Ensure hooks face away from patient's skin. Place sling under patient's center of gravity and greatest part of body weight.
h Roll patient back toward you as second nurse pulls hammock (straps) through.	Ensures that sling is in proper position before lift.
i Return patient to supine position. Be sure that hammock or straps are smooth over bed surface. Sling should extend from shoulders to knees (hammock) to support patient's body weight equally.	Completes positioning of patient on mechanical/hydraulic sling.

Continued

STEP	RATIONALE
j Remove patient's glasses, if worn.	Swivel bar is close to patient's head and could break eyeglasses.
k Roll the horseshoe base of floor lift under patient's bed (on side with chair).	Positions lift efficiently and promotes smooth transfer.
l Lower horizontal bar to sling level by following manufacturer directions. Lock valve if required.	Positions hydraulic lift close to patient. Locking valve prevents injury to patient.
m Attach hooks on strap (chain) to holes in sling. Short chains or straps hook to top holes of sling; longer chains hook to bottom of sling (see manufacturer directions).	Secures hydraulic lift to sling.
n Elevate head of bed to Fowler position. Have patient fold arms over chest.	Positions patient in sitting position. Prevents injury to patient's arms during transfer.
o If the lift is electric, push the button to raise the patient off the bed. If the lift is a nonelectric lift, pump the hydraulic handle using long, slow, even strokes until patient is raised off bed (Fig. 37.1A). For ceiling lift turn on control device to move lift (Fig. 37.1B).	Ensures safe support of patient during elevation.
p Use lift to raise patient off bed and use steering handle to pull hydraulic lift from bed as you and another caregiver maneuver patient to chair. With ceiling lift move patient along ceiling tract towards chair. Have second caregiver remain alongside patient.	Lifts patient off the bed safely; second caregiver's position reduces any risk of patient falling from sling.

STEP	RATIONALE
q Roll base of hydraulic lift around chair. Release check valve slowly or push the button down and lower patient into chair (see manufacturer directions) (Fig. 37.2).	Positions lift in front of the chair into which patient is to be transferred. Safely guides patient into back of chair as seat descends.
r Close check valve, if needed, as soon as patient is fully down in chair and straps can be released. Newer lifts may not need this step (see manufacturer directions).	If valve is left open, boom may continue to lower and injure patient.
s Remove straps and roll mechanical/hydraulic lift out of patient's path.	Prevents damage to skin and underlying tissues.
t Check patient's sitting alignment and correct if necessary.	Prevents injury from poor posture.

Continued

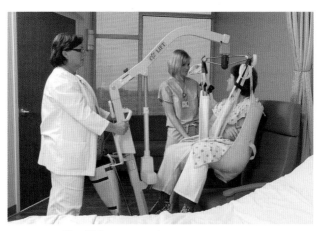

Fig. 37.2 Hydraulic lift lowers patient into chair.

STEP	RATIONALE
4 Perform lateral transfer from bed to stretcher using lift.	
a If patient is partially or not at all able to assist and is >91 kg (200 lb), use a ceiling lift with supine sling and three caregivers. *Options:* Use a lateral transfer device or air-assisted device with three caregivers (Nelson and Baptiste, 2006).	Prevents the need for nurse to lift patient. During any patient-transferring task, if any caregiver is required to lift more than 35 lb (15.8 kg) of a patient's weight, the patient should be considered to be fully dependent and assistive devices should be used for the transfer (Matz, 2019; OSHA, nd[b]).
b Position a caregiver at head of patient's bed	Protects and supports head if neck is weak or patient is unable to assist.
c Apply clean gloves if there is risk of soiling. Lower head of bed to supine position if patient can tolerate, and then raise bed to comfortable working height. Be sure to lock bed brakes.	Reduces transmission of microorganisms. Eases positioning on lift sling. Prevents accidental patient fall during transfer.
d Have second caregiver go to opposite side of bed.	Assists with turning and positioning patient onto lift sling.
e Follow Steps 3 e-j for turning and positioning patient onto the lift sling.	Assures correct position of sling to support patient's body weight.
f Have patient cross arms on chest.	Prevents injury to arms during transfer.
g Bring stretcher along one side of bed. Have one caregiver remain on opposite side at all times. Be sure stretcher brakes are locked.	Prevents patient fall

STEP	RATIONALE
h Turn on powered lift or activate hydraulic or ceiling lift, raise patient straight off bed (additional caregiver assists in guiding patient), and then slowly position patient over center of stretcher. Lower patient onto center of stretcher. Raise head of stretcher if not contraindicated. Raise stretcher side rails. Cover patient with blanket.	Provides for patient comfort and safety.
5 After transferring patient to bed, chair, or stretcher, be sure patient is positioned comfortably.	Restores comfort and sense of well-being.
6 Perform postprocedure protocol.	
7 Evaluate patient response:	
a Monitor vital signs. Ask if patient feels dizzy or tired and rate any existing pain using an appropriate pain scale.	Evaluates patient's response to postural changes and activity.
b Note patient's behavioral response to transfer.	Reveals level of motivation and self-care potential.
c Be sure to check condition of patient's skin after next transfer.	Determines whether injury to skin has occurred.

Recording and Reporting

- Record procedure, including pertinent observations: weakness, pain level, ability to follow directions, number of personnel used to assist, type of lift device used, and patient's response in.
- Document evaluation of patient and family caregiver learning.

- Report transfer ability and help needed to next shift or other caregivers.
- Report progress or remission to rehabilitation staff (physical therapist, occupational therapist).

UNEXPECTED OUTCOMES	RELATED INTERVENTIONS
1 Patient is unable to comprehend or is unwilling to follow directions for transfer.	• Reassess continuity and simplicity of instruction. • If patient is tired or in pain, allow for rest period before transferring. • Consider medicating for pain (if indicated).
2 Patient sustains injury on transfer.	• Evaluate incident that led to injury (e.g., inadequate assessment, improper use of equipment). • Complete incident report according to agency policy.

Metered-Dose Inhalers

Medications administered with handheld inhalers are dispersed through an aerosol spray, mist, or powder that penetrates the airways. Pressurized metered-dose inhalers (MDIs), breath-actuated metered-dose inhalers (BAIs), and dry powder inhalers (DPIs) deliver medications that produce localized respiratory effects, such as bronchodilation. Some of these medications are absorbed rapidly through the pulmonary circulation and can cause systemic side effects (e.g., albuterol may cause palpitations, tremors, tachycardia). Drugs administered by inhalation provide control of airway hyperactivity or bronchial constriction, common in patients with asthma. Because patients depend on these medications for disease control, patient teaching is vital for correct use of inhalers and to ensure effectiveness of inhaled medications.

An MDI is a small handheld device that requires coordination during the breathing cycle. Many patients spray only the back of their throats and fail to receive a full dose. The inhaler must be depressed to expel medication just as the patient inhales. This ensures that medication reaches the lower airways. Children or patients with decreased coordination may need to use a spacer device or a BAI to administer the medication properly. A spacer device decreases the amount of medication deposited into the oropharyngeal mucosa. Some spacers have a one-way valve that activates on inhalation, thereby removing the need for good hand-breath coordination (Burchum and Rosenthal, 2022).

Safety Guidelines

- Common problems in using inhalers include the following:
  - Not taking a medication as prescribed: Taking either too much or too little. (A normal dose is two puffs).
  - Incorrect activation: Occurs through pressing the canister before taking a breath. Taking a breath at the same time as activation carries the medication down to the lungs with the breath.
  - Forgetting to shake an inhaler: The medication is contained within a suspension.
  - Not waiting long enough between puffs: A delay between puffs is needed before taking a second puff; otherwise, an incorrect dose may be delivered or the medication may not penetrate airways.
  - Failure to clean the valve: Particles may jam the valve in the mouthpiece unless it is cleaned occasionally.
  - Failure to observe whether an inhaler is actually releasing a spray.
  - Failure to recognize when a canister is empty.

Delegation

The skill of administering MDIs cannot be delegated to assistive personnel (AP). Instruct AP about:

- Potential side effects of medications and to report their occurrence.
- Reporting breathing difficulty (e.g., paroxysmal or sustained coughing, audible wheezing).

Collaboration

- Check with pharmacist if inhaler does not work correctly.
- Respiratory therapists are able to assist patients who have difficulty using an MDI.

Equipment

- Inhaler device with medication canister (MDI, BAI or DPI)
- Facial tissues
- Stethoscope
- Medication administration record (MAR) (electronic or printed)
- *Option:* Spacer device such as AeroChamber or InspirEase
- *Option:* Peak flowmeter

STEPS	RATIONALE
1 Perform preprocedure protocol.	
Assessment	
• Check accuracy and completeness of each MAR or computer printout with health care provider's written medication order. Check patient's name, medication name and dosage, route of administration, and time of administration.	The order sheet is the most reliable source and only legal record of medications that patient is to receive. Ensures that patient receives the correct medications (Palese et al., 2019). Transcription errors are a source of medication errors (Zhu and Weingart, 2022).
• Review electronic health record (EHR) for patient's medical and medication history. Note history of cardiopulmonary disease.	Determines need for medication or possible contraindications for medication administration.

STEPS	RATIONALE
• Ask patient to describe history of allergies: known types of allergies and normal allergic reaction. Check patient's allergy wristband.	Communication of allergies is essential for safe and effective care. Do not prepare medication if there is a known patient allergy.
• Review drug reference information regarding medication action, purpose, normal dose, side effects, time of peak onset, and nursing implications.	Knowledge of expected and adverse reactions helps in determining responses to monitor.
• Perform hand hygiene. Assess respiratory pattern and auscultate breath sounds. (*Option:* Measure peak flow.) Assess exercise tolerance; does patient develop shortness of breath easily?	Establishes baseline of airway status for comparison during and after treatment.
• Assess patient's learning ability and ability to hold, manipulate, and depress canister and inhaler.	Any grasp impairment or presence of hand tremors interferes with patient's ability to depress canister within inhaler. Spacer device is often necessary.
• If patient was previously instructed in self-administration, review knowledge regarding device and ask patient to demonstrate use of device.	Ongoing assessment of inhaler technique identifies areas for further education and reinforcement (Ari, 2015).

Implementation

1	Explain to patient signs and symptoms to expect from medication.	Lessens anxiety by helping patient know what to expect, promoting self-care.

Continued

STEPS	RATIONALE
2 Prepare medication without interruptions/distractions. Create a quiet environment. Keep all pages of MARs or computer printouts for one patient together or look at only one patient's electronic MAR at a time.	Interruptions contribute to medication errors (Palese et al., 2019).
3 Perform hand hygiene. Prepare medications for one patient at a time using aseptic technique (see Skill 49). Check medication label carefully with MAR or computer printout when removing drug from storage and after preparation. Check expiration date.	Ensures that medication is sterile. These are the *first and second checks for accuracy* and ensure that correct medication is administered. Dose potency increases or decreases when outdated.
4 Take medication(s) to patient at correct time (see agency policy). Give non–time-critical scheduled medications within a range of 1 to 2 h of scheduled dose (Institute for Safe Medication Practice [ISMP], 2011). During administration, apply seven rights of medication administration.	Hospitals must adopt medication administration policy and procedure for timing of medication administration that considers nature of the prescribed medication, specific clinical application, and patient needs (ISMP, 2011; US Department of Health and Human Services, 2011).
5 Identify patient using at least two identifiers (e.g., name and birthday or name and medical record number) according to agency policy. Compare identifiers with information on patient's MAR or medical record.	Ensures correct patient. Complies with The Joint Commission standards and improves patient safety (The Joint Commission, 2023).

STEPS	RATIONALE
6 At patient's bedside, again compare MAR or computer printout with names of medications on medication labels and patient name. Ask patient again if an allergy exists.	This is the *third check for accuracy* and ensures that patient receives correct medication. Confirms patient's allergy history.
7 Allow adequate time for patient to manipulate inhaler, canister, and spacer device (if provided). Explain and demonstrate how canister fits into inhaler.	Ensures patient is familiar with how to use equipment.

CLINICAL JUDGMENT *If using an MDI that is new or has not been used for several days, push a "test spray" into the air to prime the device before using. This ensures that the MDI is patent and the metal canister is positioned properly.*

STEPS	RATIONALE
8 Explain and demonstrate steps for administering an MDI without spacer.	Simple one-on-one instruction and demonstration of step-by-step administration allows patient to ask questions during procedure and increases patient adherence to inhaler use (Ari, 2015; Shealy et al., 2017).
a Remove mouthpiece cover from inhaler after inserting MDI canister into holder.	
b Shake inhaler well for 2 to 5 seconds (five or six shakes).	Ensures mixing of medication in canister.
c Hold inhaler in dominant hand.	Ensures firmer grip and better manipulation of device.
d Have patient stand or sit and instruct on positioning of inhaler (Step f). Have patient demonstrate positioning.	Position ensures accurate delivery of medication.

Continued

STEPS	RATIONALE
e While holding the mouthpiece have patient take deep breath and exhale completely.	Empties lung volume and prepares airway to receive medication.
f Have patient place the mouthpiece in the mouth between the teeth and over the tongue, pointing toward back of throat, with lips closed tightly around it. Do not block the mouthpiece with the teeth or tongue (Fig. 38.1).	Ensures proper fit to inhale medication.
g With inhaler positioned, have patient hold with thumb at mouthpiece and index and middle fingers at top. This is a three-point or bilateral hand position.	Hand position ensures proper activation of MDI and distribution of dosage (Burchum and Rosenthal, 2022).

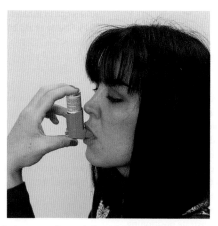

Fig. 38.1 Patient opens lips and places the inhaler in the mouth with the opening toward the back of throat.

STEPS	RATIONALE
h Instruct patient to tilt head back slightly and inhale slowly and deeply through mouth for 3 to 5 seconds while depressing canister fully. This is one puff.	Medication is distributed to airways during inhalation.
i Have patient hold breath for about 10 seconds.	Allows tiny drops of aerosol spray to reach deeper branches of airways.
j Remove MDI from mouth before exhaling and exhale slowly through nose or pursed lips.	Keeps small airways open during exhalation.
9 Explain and demonstrate steps to administer MDI using spacer device.	Simple one-on-one instruction and demonstration of step-by-step administration allows patient to ask questions during procedure and increases patient adherence to inhaler use (Ari, 2015; Schmitz et al., 2019).
a Remove mouthpiece cover from MDI and mouthpiece of spacer device.	Inhaler fits into end of spacer device.
b Shake inhaler well for 2 to 5 seconds (five or six shakes).	Ensures mixing of medication in canister.
c Insert MDI into end of spacer device.	Spacer device traps medication released from MDI; patient then inhales medication from device. These devices improve delivery of correct dose of inhaled medication (Burchum and Rosenthal, 2022).

Continued

STEPS	RATIONALE
d Instruct patient to place spacer device mouthpiece in mouth and close lips. Do not insert beyond raised lip on mouthpiece. Avoid covering small exhalation slots with lips.	Medication should not escape through mouth.
e Have patient breathe normally through spacer device mouthpiece (Fig. 38.2).	Allows patient to relax before delivering medication.
f Instruct patient to depress medication canister, spraying one puff into spacer device.	Spacer contains fine spray and allows patient to inhale more medication. The spacer increases drug delivery and deposition of the medication on the oropharyngeal mucosa (Burchum and Rosenthal, 2022).
g Have patient breathe in slowly and fully for 5 seconds.	Ensures that particles of medication are distributed to deeper airways.

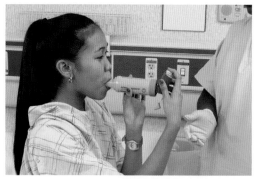

Fig. 38.2 Placement of spacer device.

STEPS	RATIONALE
h Instruct patient to hold full breath for 10 seconds.	Ensures full drug distribution.
10 Instruct patient to wait 20 to 30 seconds between inhalations (if same medication) or 2 to 5 minutes between inhalations (if different medications).	Medications must be inhaled sequentially. Always administer bronchodilators before steroids so that dilators can open airway passages (Burchum and Rosenthal, 2022).
11 Instruct patient not to repeat inhalations before next scheduled dose. (Beta-adrenergic medications are used either "as needed" or regularly every 4 to 6 h.)	Medications are prescribed at intervals during day to provide constant drug levels, and to minimize side effects.
12 Warn patients that they may feel gagging sensation in throat caused by droplets of medication on pharynx or tongue.	This occurs when medication is sprayed and inhaled incorrectly.
13 About 2 minutes after last dose, instruct patient to rinse mouth with warm water and spit water out.	Steroids may alter normal flora of oral mucosa and lead to fungal infection. Rinsing reduces risk of fungal infection (Ari, 2015).
14 Clean the MDI.	Removes residual medication and reduces spread of microorganisms. Water damages valve mechanism of canister.
a For daily cleaning, instruct patient to remove medication canister, rinse inhaler and cap with warm running water, and ensure that inhaler is completely dry before reuse. Do not get valve mechanism of canister wet.	

Continued

STEPS	RATIONALE
b Instruct patient to clean mouthpiece twice a week with a mild dishwashing soap, rinse thoroughly, and dry completely before storage.	
15 Ask whether patient has any questions.	Clarifies misconceptions or misunderstanding and provides opportunity for further patient teaching (Ari, 2015).
16 Perform postprocedure protocol.	
17 Evaluate patient response:	
a Auscultate patient lungs, listen for abnormal breath sounds, and obtain peak flow measures if ordered.	Determines patient response to medication.
b Have patient explain and demonstrate steps in use and cleaning of inhaler.	Return demonstration evaluates patient learning and allows for reinforcement as needed.
c Ask patient to explain medication schedule and dose of medication, possible side effects, and criteria for contacting health care provider.	Improves adherence to therapy. Enables patient to recognize signs of overuse and when to seek medical support.

Recording and Reporting

- Immediately record medication, dose or strength, number of inhalations, and time given after administration (not before) in MAR. Include initials or signature in MAR.
- Record patient's response to MDI (e.g., respiratory rate and pattern, peak expiratory flow rate, breath sounds), evidence of side effects (e.g., arrhythmia, patient's feelings of anxiety), and patient's ability to use MDI.
- Document evaluation of patient learning.
- Report any adverse effects/patient response to nurse in charge or health care provider.

UNEXPECTED OUTCOMES	RELATED INTERVENTIONS
1 Patient's respirations are rapid and shallow; breath sounds indicate wheezing.	• Evaluate vital signs and respiratory status. • Notify health care provider. • Reassess type of medication and/or delivery method.
2 Patient needs bronchodilator more than every 4 h (may indicate respiratory problem).	• Reassess type of medication and delivery methods needed. • Notify health care provider.
3 Patient experiences cardiac dysrhythmias (light-headedness, syncope), especially if receiving beta-adrenergic medications.	• Withhold further doses of medication. • Evaluate cardiac and pulmonary status. • Notify health care provider for reassessment of type of medication and delivery method.

Moist Heat Applications (Compress and Sitz Bath)

Moist heat applications are beneficial in increasing skeletal muscle and ligament relaxation and flexibility; promoting healing; and relieving spasm, joint stiffness, and pain (Table 39.1). Because there is poor skin penetration (less than 1 cm [<½ inch]), superficial heat generally only affects cutaneous blood flow and cutaneous nerve receptors (Chen, 2021). In addition to increasing local blood flow by applying heat, the higher cutaneous temperature also has an analgesic effect. Moist heat is most commonly used after the acute phase of a musculoskeletal injury and during and after childbirth, surgery, and superficial thrombophlebitis (Petrofsky et al., 2017a; Szekeres et al., 2017). Moist local heat applications include warm compresses and commercial moist heat packs. Immersing in moist heat involve uses of warm baths, soaks, and sitz baths. Sitz baths are commonly used for anal fissures, or small tears in the skin lining the opening of the anus, irritation associated with constipation or diarrhea, hemorrhoids, prostatitis, and after a vaginal delivery. Newer electronic digital moist heat packs allow patients to control the temperature of the heat application. Dry heat is also used to reduce pain and increase healing by increasing blood flow to tissues and can be used at a lower level for a longer period of time with little chance of tissue injury (Petrofsky et al., 2016) (Skill 2).

TABLE 39.1 Physiologic Effects of Heat Applications

	Heat
Pain	↓
Spasm	↓
Metabolism	↑
Blood flow	↑
Inflammation	↑
Edema	↑
Extensibility	↑

Safety Guidelines

- Your primary patient care responsibility is to know whether a patient is at risk for injury from a heat application, and how to apply heat safely.
- Older adults, or patients who have diabetes mellitus, vascular diseases, paralysis, peripheral neuropathy, rheumatoid arthritis, or those taking certain cardiovascular medications are at greater risk for thermal injury (Ratliff, 2017).

Delegation

The skill of applying dry or moist heat can be delegated to assistive personnel (AP), after you assess the condition of skin and tissues. However, in most settings a nurse applies sterile applications. If there are risks or expected complications, this skill should not be delegated. Instruct the AP about:

- Purpose and proper temperature of the application.
- Skin changes to immediately report (e.g., pain, burning, blistering, or excessive redness).
- Specific patient complaints and changes in vital signs to report immediately (e.g., dizziness or light-headedness, increased or decreased pulse, decreased blood pressure).
- Specific requirements for positioning and application time based on agency policy and manufacturer instructions.
- Reporting when treatment is complete so that patient's response to treatment can be evaluated.

Collaboration

- Therapists often use heat as a form of treatment combined with exercise for patients who undergo outpatient physical therapy.

Equipment

- Prescribed analgesia (if ordered)
- Dry bath towel, bath blanket
- Warmed prescribed solution (i.e., normal saline) or commercially prepared compress
- Biohazard waste bag
- Clean gloves
- Compress
- Clean basin
- Waterproof pad

- Ties or nonallergenic cloth tape
- Clean gauze or towel
- Equipment for measuring blood pressure
- Options for moist heat application, depending on health care provider's order:
  - Sterile compress, sterile basin, sterile gauze, and sterile gloves
  - Disposable sitz bath: prescribed solution and any topical medication to be applied after the soak

STEP	RATIONALE
1 Perform preprocedure protocol.	

Assessment

• Refer to health care provider's order for type of heat application, location and duration of application, and desired temperature. Check agency policies regarding temperature.	Ensures safe practice by verifying specific location for therapy and type and duration of heat application.
• Refer to patient's electronic health record (EHR) to identify any contraindications to moist heat application: unstable cardiac conditions, active bleeding, nitroglycerin or other therapeutic medicinal patch, acute inflammatory reactions, recent (<72 h) musculoskeletal injury, persons with multiple sclerosis sensitive to heat, and skin conditions such as eczema.	Patients with certain cardiovascular conditions and those who exhibit side effects of certain medications may be at risk for sudden changes in blood pressure and blood flow caused by vasodilation. Heat increases vasodilation, which aggravates active bleeding, increasing hemorrhage or bleeding into soft tissues adjacent to musculoskeletal injury (Petrofsky et al., 2017b). Vasodilation increases rate of medication absorption when direct heat is applied over a medication patch.

STEP	RATIONALE
• Perform hand hygiene, apply gloves, and assess condition of skin around area to be treated. Perform neurovascular assessments for sensitivity to temperature and pain by measuring light touch, pinprick, and temperature sensation.	Certain conditions alter conduction of sensory impulses that transmit temperature and pain, predisposing patients to injury from heat applications. Patients with diminished sensation to heat or cold should be monitored closely during treatment.

CLINICAL JUDGMENT *When conducting assessment related to temperature sensitivity, consider those patients most at risk (see safety guidelines above) (Ratliff, 2017).*

• Assess patient's blood pressure and pulse.	Establishes baseline to determine response to therapy.
• When treating a wound (see implementation, Step 5c), assess for size, color, drainage volume, pain (using pain scale), and odor (this assessment may be deferred until dressing is removed and heat is applied). Remove and discard gloves; perform hand hygiene.	Provides baseline to determine change in wound after heat application. Provides baseline for patient's comfort level.
• Assess patient's level of consciousness and responsiveness (e.g., confusion, disorientation, dementia).	Patients with reduced level of consciousness are unable to recognize or report reduced sensation or discomfort from therapy, which may necessitate more frequent monitoring.
• Ask patient to describe pain character and intensity on pain scale of 0 to 10. If patient is having extremity treated, assess range of motion (ROM).	Provides baseline to determine whether pain relief or improved ROM is achieved after heat therapy.

Continued

STEP	RATIONALE
• Assess patient's mobility (e.g., ROM): ability to align extremity for moist compress and ability to position self in sitz bath and sit up from bath.	Determines level of help patient requires for treatment.

CLINICAL JUDGMENT *Note that in some situations, applying heat can override pain signals and decrease pain perception in the cerebral cortex (Wu et al., 2017).*

Implementation

1 Perform hand hygiene and apply clean gloves.	Reduces transmission of microorganisms.
2 Position patient in bed, keeping affected body part in proper alignment. Expose body part to be covered with heat application and drape patient with bath blanket or towel as needed.	Limited mobility in uncomfortable position causes muscular stress. Draping prevents cooling.
3 Place waterproof pad under patient (exception: do not do this with sitz bath).	Protects bed linen from moisture and soiling.
4 Describe expected sensations to patient, such as warmth and wetness. Explain precautions to prevent burning.	Minimizes patient's anxiety and promotes relaxation during procedure.
5 Apply moist sterile compress:	
a Heat prescribed solution to desired temperature by immersing closed bottle of solution in basin of warm water. **DO NOT USE A MICROWAVE TO WARM SOLUTION.**	Prevents burns by ensuring proper temperature of solution.

STEP	RATIONALE
b Prepare aquathermia pad if it is to be placed over compress (Skill 2). Temperature is usually preset by manufacturer or bioengineering. **If** using a commercially prepared compress, follow manufacturer's instructions for warming.	Using proper temperature prevents accidental burning.
c Remove any existing dressing covering wound. Inspect condition of wound and surrounding skin. Inflamed wound appears reddened, but surrounding skin is less red in color. Remove and place gloves and soiled dressing in biohazard bag and dispose per agency policy.	Reduces transmission of microorganisms. Provides baseline to measure wound healing.

CLINICAL JUDGMENT *If skin surrounding wound is inflamed or reddened or has active bleeding or drainage, moist heat application may be contraindicated. Verify with health care provider.*

d Perform hand hygiene.	Reduces transmission of microorganisms.
e Moisten gauze for the compress.	Use of appropriate aseptic technique keeps gauze compress clean or sterile. Sterile compress is needed when applied to open wound.
(1) Pour warmed solution into container. **If sterile asepsis is required**, use sterile container.	Reduces transmission of microorganisms.

Continued

STEP	RATIONALE
(2) Open gauze. **If applying sterile technique,** open and lay on sterile wrapper. Then immerse sterile gauze into sterile solution (See skill 68).	Sterile compress is needed when applied to open wound.
(3) **If sterile technique is NOT required**, immerse gauze into container of solution using clean aseptic technique.	

CLINICAL JUDGMENT *To avoid injury to patient, test temperature of sterile solution by applying a drop to your inner forearm (without contaminating solution). It should feel warm to the skin without burning.*

---

f Apply sterile gloves if compress is sterile; otherwise apply clean gloves.	Allows manipulation of sterile dressing and touching of open wound as needed.
g Pick up one layer of immersed gauze, wring out any excess solution, and apply lightly to wound; avoid surrounding unaffected skin. *Option:* Apply commercial compress or heat pack over wound only; use only with clean wounds.	Excess moisture macerates skin and increases risk for burns and infection. Skin is sensitive to sudden change in temperature.
h After a few seconds, lift edge of gauze to assess for skin redness or other injuries.	Increased redness indicates burn. Burns and injuries from warm therapies are preventable events.

STEP	RATIONALE
i If patient tolerates compress, pack gauze snugly against wound. Be sure to cover all wound surfaces with warm compress.	Packing compress prevents rapid cooling from ambient air currents.
j Cover moist compress with dry sterile dressing and bath towel. If necessary, pin or tie in place. Remove and dispose of gloves and perform hand hygiene.	Dry sterile dressing prevents transfer of microorganisms to wound via capillary action caused by moist compress. Towel insulates compress to prevent heat loss.
k *Option:* Apply aquathermia or commercial heat pack (Skill 2). Keep it in place for desired duration of application.	Provides constant temperature to compress.
l Leave compress in place for 15 to 20 minutes or less (per order or agency policy) and change warm compress using appropriate aseptic technique every 5 to 10 minutes (observing condition of skin) or as ordered during duration of therapy.	Maintains constant temperature for best therapeutic benefit. Moist heat promotes transfer of heat to underlying subcutaneous tissues, which helps reduce thermal injury to skin (Petrofsky et al., 2017b). Time limits when using higher temperatures prevent risk of overexposure and injury to underlying skin.
m After prescribed time, perform hand hygiene and apply clean gloves. Remove pad, towel, and compress. Evaluate wound and condition of skin and replace dry sterile dressing (using sterile gloves) as ordered.	Continued exposure to moisture macerates skin. Dressing prevents entrance of microorganisms into wound site.

Continued

STEP	RATIONALE
6 Apply sitz bath or warm soak to intact skin or wound:	
a Remove any existing dressing covering a perineal wound. Remove and dispose of gloves and dressings in proper receptacle and perform hand hygiene.	Reduces transmission of microorganisms.
b Inspect condition of wound and surrounding skin. Pay particular attention to suture line as applicable.	Provides baseline to determine response to warm soak.
c When exudate or drainage is present, apply a new pair of clean gloves and clean the intact skin around open area with clean cloth and soap and water. Sterile gloves and gauze may be needed to clean open wound (check agency policy). Remove and dispose of gloves and perform hand hygiene.	Cleaning removes organisms so that bath solution does not spread infection.
d Fill sitz bath or bathtub in bathroom with warmed solution (Fig. 39.1). Check temperature (check agency policy). *Option:* If using bag of normal saline, warm per agency policy.	Ensures proper temperature and reduces risk for burns.

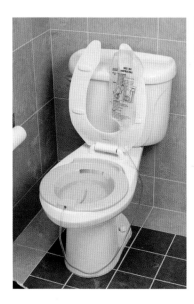

Fig. 39.1 Disposable sitz bath. (Image used with permission, Briggs Healthcare, Clive, IA.)

STEP	RATIONALE
e Assist patient to bathroom to immerse body part being treated in sitz bath, bathtub, or basin. Cover patient with bath blanket or towel once position is achieved.	Prevents falls. Covering patient prevents heat loss through evaporation, maintains constant temperature, and provides for privacy.
f Assess heart rate. Observe that patient does not feel light-headed or dizzy and that nurse call system is within reach. Check every 5 minutes for patient tolerance to treatment.	Provides baseline to determine whether vascular response to vasodilation occurs during treatment. Prevents injury.
g After 15 to 20 minutes remove patient from soak or bath; dry body thoroughly. (Wear clean gloves.)	Avoids chilling. Enhances patient's comfort.

Continued

STEP	RATIONALE
h Assist patient to preferred comfortable position.	Maintains patient's comfort.
i Drain solution from basin or tub. Clean and place in proper storage area according to agency policy. Dispose of soiled linen.	Reduces transmission of microorganisms.
7 Perform postprocedure protocol.	
8 Evaluate patient response:	
a Inspect condition of body part or wound; observe skin integrity, color, and temperature, and note any dryness, edema, blistering, drainage, or sensitivity to touch. After a sitz bath, inspect perineal or rectal area.	Evaluates effectiveness of heat application and whether injury has occurred.
b Obtain blood pressure and pulse; compare with baseline.	Determines whether systemic vascular response to vasodilation has occurred.
c Ask patient to describe character of pain and severity on pain scale of 0 to 10. Ask about any sensation of burning after treatment.	Determines whether patient was exposed to temperature extreme, resulting in burn. Evaluates patient's subjective response to therapy.
d Evaluate ROM of affected body part.	Determines whether edema or muscle spasm is relieved.

CLINICAL JUDGMENT *Avoid immediate exercise of muscle by patient to evaluate results of therapy. Active exercise can aggravate muscle strain. Heat in conjunction with exercise as a form of therapy is beneficial.*

Recording and Reporting

- Record type of application (solution, compress); location and duration of application; condition of body part, wound, or skin before and after treatment; and patient's response to therapy.
- Document evaluation of patient and family caregiver learning.

- During hand-off to next shift, report the location and type of heat therapy, duration and time of therapy, skin assessment, vital signs, pain assessment before and after therapy, and patient response to therapy.
- Report any worsening condition of treated wound to health care provider.

UNEXPECTED OUTCOMES	RELATED INTERVENTIONS
1 Patient's skin is reddened, tender, swollen, and sensitive to touch during/after moist heat application, or patient complains of burning.	• Discontinue moist application immediately. • Verify proper temperature or check aquathermia device for proper functioning. • Notify health care provider and, if there is a burn, complete an incident or adverse event report (see agency policy).
2 Body part remains painful and is difficult to move after heat application.	• Discontinue aquathermia pad, compress, or heat pack use. • Observe for localized swelling or skin breakdown. • Notify health care provider.
3 Patient or family caregiver applies heat incorrectly or is unable to explain precautions.	• Reinstruct patient or family caregiver as needed. Consider possible home health referral (if patient is eligible).

Mouth Care for an Unconscious or Debilitated Patient

Special oral care is recommended for unconscious or debilitated patients (e.g., stroke patients), who are more susceptible to infection due to the change in normal flora of the oral cavity. There is an increase in plaque formation from dryness of the mouth and decreased salivation. Dryness of the oral mucosa is also caused by mouth breathing and oxygen therapy. Respiratory secretions are often thick and place patients at risk for ineffective airway clearance, requiring oral suction. Secretions in the oral cavity may change from gram-positive to gram-negative pneumonia-producing bacteria if aspiration occurs.

Because many debilitated patients have either a reduced or absent gag reflex as a result of change in consciousness or a neurologic injury, providing oral care requires safeguarding patients from choking and aspiration during the procedure (Skill 3). The safest technique is to have two nurses or assistive personnel (AP) provide care. One provides oral care while the other suctions oral secretions as needed with a Yankauer suction tip (Skill 71). When delegating oral care to AP, provide them appropriate instructions. Evaluate the patient's need for level and frequency of oral care on a daily basis during assessment of the oral cavity.

Safety Guidelines

- Routine suctioning of the mouth and pharynx is required to manage oral secretions and reduce the risk for aspiration.

Delegation

The skill of providing oral hygiene to an unconscious or debilitated patient can be delegated to AP. Nurses are responsible for assessing patients' gag reflex. Instruct the AP to:

- Obtain assistance from a second AP and properly position patient for mouth care.
- Be aware of aspiration precautions.
- Use an oral suction catheter for clearing oral secretions.
- Report signs of impaired integrity of oral mucosa, bleeding, or excessive coughing or choking.

Collaboration

- It is safer if two nurses and/or AP provide oral care to unconscious patients.

Equipment

- Small pediatric, soft-bristled toothbrush, toothette sponges, or suction toothbrushes (for patients for whom brushing is contraindicated)
- Antibacterial solution per agency policy (e.g., chlorhexidine gluconate [CHG])
- Fluoride toothpaste
- Water-based mouth moisturizer
- Tongue blade
- Penlight
- Oral suction equipment
- Oral airway device (for use with an uncooperative patient or patient who shows bite reflex)
- Water-soluble lip lubricant
- Water glass with cool water
- Face and bath towel
- Emesis basin
- Clean gloves

STEP	RATIONALE
1 Perform preprocedure protocol.	
Assessment	
• Review patient's electronic health record (EHR), including health care provider's order and nurses' notes. Note previous suctioning and antiseptic solutions used.	Health care provider's order is needed for any special antiseptic solutions used for mouth care. (CHG does not require an order.)
• Review patient's EHR to assess patient's risk for oral hygiene problems (e.g., dental caries; gingivitis; receding gum lines; halitosis; dry, cracked lips).	Certain conditions increase likelihood of alterations in integrity of oral cavity mucosa and structures, necessitating more frequent care.

Continued

STEP	RATIONALE
• Perform hand hygiene and apply clean gloves.	Reduces transmission of microorganisms in blood or saliva.
• Assess for presence of gag reflex by placing tongue blade on back half of tongue.	Helps in determining aspiration risk.

CLINICAL JUDGMENT *Patients with impaired gag reflex still require oral care; however, they have a higher risk for aspiration. Keep suction equipment available when caring for patients who are at risk for aspiration.*

• Inspect condition of oral cavity. Inspect lips, teeth, gums, buccal mucosa, palate, and tongue using tongue depressor and penlight if necessary. Observe for color, moisture, lesions, injury, ulcers, and condition of teeth or dentures.	Determines need for oral hygiene. Establishes baseline to show improvement after oral care.

CLINICAL JUDGMENT *The critically ill patient with an artificial airway and who is on mechanical ventilation is at risk for ventilator-associated pneumonia, which significantly increases risk of mortality and, at a minimum, increases ventilator time and length of stay in critical care (Institute for Healthcare Improvement, 2021). Once intubated, the artificial airway bypasses normal airway defenses, which causes a rapid change in the normal oral flora. Some patients require mouth care as often as every 1 to 2 h until the mucosa returns to normal.*

• Assess patient's respirations or oxygen saturation.	Assists in early recognition of aspiration.
• Remove gloves. Perform hand hygiene.	Prevents transmission of infection.

Implementation

1 Apply clean gloves.	Reduces transfer of microorganisms.

STEP	RATIONALE
2 Place towel on overbed table and arrange equipment. If needed, turn on suction machine and connect tubing to suction catheter.	Prevents soiling of tabletop. Equipment prepared in advance ensures smooth, safe procedure. Supplies within reach create organized workspace.
3 Raise bed to appropriate working height; lower side rail.	Use of good body mechanics with bed in high position prevents injury.
4 Unless contraindicated (e.g., head injury, neck trauma), position patient in Sims or side-lying position. Turn patient's head toward mattress in dependent position with head of bed elevated at least 30 degrees.	Allows secretions to drain from mouth instead of collecting in back of pharynx. Prevents aspiration. If patient is overweight, follow safe handling techniques for positioning.
5 Place towel under patient's head and emesis basin under chin.	Prevents soiling of bed linen.
6 Remove dentures or partial plates if present.	Allows for thorough cleaning of prosthetics later. Provides clearer access to oral cavity.
7 If patient is uncooperative or having difficulty keeping mouth open, insert an oral airway. Insert airway upside down and turn sideways and over tongue to keep teeth apart. Insert when patient is relaxed if possible. Do not use force.	Prevents patient from biting down on nurse/AP fingers and provides access to oral cavity.

CLINICAL JUDGMENT *Never place fingers into the mouth of an unconscious or debilitated patient. This could occlude the airway. Also, the normal patient response is to bite down.*

Continued

STEP	RATIONALE
8 Clean mouth using brush moistened in water. Apply toothpaste or use antibacterial solution first to loosen crusts. Hold toothbrush bristles at 45-degree angle to gum line. Be sure that tips of bristles rest against and penetrate under gum line. a Brush inner and outer surfaces of upper and lower teeth by brushing upward from gum to crown of each tooth (Fig. 40.1A) b Clean biting surfaces of teeth by holding top of bristles parallel with teeth and brushing gently back and forth (Fig. 40.1B). c Brush sides of teeth by moving bristles back and forth (Fig. 40.1C). Use a toothette sponge if patient has bleeding tendency or if the use of a toothbrush is contraindicated. Suction any accumulated secretions.	Brushing action removes food particles between teeth, along chewing surfaces, and crusts for mucosa. The use of a CHG oral hygiene protocol as part of daily oral care reduces the incidence of ventilator-associated pneumonia (Jackson and Owens, 2019). The Institute for Healthcare Improvement (2021) recommends the use of 0.12% CHG as part of daily oral care in critically ill patients.

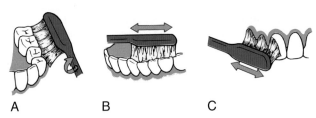

A   B   C

Figure 40.1 (A)–(C) Directions of toothbrush for brushing teeth.

STEP	RATIONALE
9 Moisten brush with clear water or CHG solution to rinse. Clean lips and mucosa with toothette. Use brush or toothette to clean roof of mouth, gums, and inside cheeks. Gently brush tongue but avoid stimulating gag reflex (if present). Repeat rinsing several times and use oral Yankauer tip suction to remove secretions. Apply suction intermittently while removing secretions. Use towel to dry off lips.	Repeated rinsing removes all debris and aids in moistening mucosa. Suction removes secretions and fluids that collect in posterior pharynx, thus reducing aspiration risk. Intermittent suction reduces mucosal injury.
10 Apply thin layer of water-soluble moisturizer to lips.	Lubricates lips to prevent drying and cracking.
11 Inform patient when procedure is completed. Help patient to a comfortable side-lying position with head of bed elevated.	Provides meaningful stimulation to unconscious or less responsive patient. Position reduces aspiration.
12 When suction equipment is used, be sure to have a clean suction catheter ready and attached to the suction source.	In case of an emergency, suction equipment is clean and ready to use to clear patient's airway.
13 Perform postprocedure protocol.	
14 Evaluate patient response: a Apply clean gloves and use tongue blade and penlight to inspect oral cavity.	Determines efficacy of cleaning. Once thick secretions are removed, underlying inflammation or lesions may be revealed.
b Ask debilitated patient if mouth feels clean.	Evaluates level of comfort.

Recording and Reporting

- Record procedure, appearance of oral cavity, presence of gag reflex, and patient's response to procedure.
- Document evaluation of patient and family caregiver learning.
- Report any unusual findings (e.g., bleeding, ulceration, choking response) to nurse in charge or health care provider.

UNEXPECTED OUTCOMES	RELATED INTERVENTIONS
1 Secretions or crusts remain on mucosa, tongue, or gums.	• Provide more frequent oral hygiene.
2 Localized inflammation or bleeding of gums or mucosa is present.	• Provide more frequent oral hygiene with toothette sponges.
	• Apply water-based mouth moisturizer to provide moisture and maintain integrity of oral mucosa.
	• Chemotherapy and radiation can cause mucositis (inflammation of mucous membranes in mouth) because of sloughing of epithelial tissue. Room-temperature saline rinses, bicarbonate and sterile water rinses, and oral care with a soft-bristled toothbrush decrease severity and duration of mucositis.
3 Lips are cracked or inflamed.	• Increase frequency of moisturizing gel or water-soluble lubricant application to lips.

UNEXPECTED OUTCOMES	RELATED INTERVENTIONS
4 Patient aspirates secretions.	• Suction oral airway as secretions accumulate to maintain airway patency (see Skill 71). • Elevate patient's head of bed to facilitate breathing. • If aspiration is suspected, notify health care provider. Prepare patient for chest x-ray film examination.

Nail and Foot Care

The best time to provide nail and foot care is during a patient's daily bath. Feet and nails often require special care to prevent infection, odors, pain, and injury to soft tissues. Patients are often unaware of foot or nail problems until discomfort or pain occurs. Instruct patients on how to protect their feet from injury: keep feet and toes clean and dry, wear moisture-wicking socks, wear shoes that fit well and do not rub feet, and keep toenails trimmed (American Diabetes Association [ADA], 2021). Instruct patients on how to properly inspect all surfaces of the feet for lesions, dryness, or signs of infection.

Patients most at risk for developing serious foot problems are those with peripheral neuropathy and peripheral vascular disease (PVD), disorders commonly found in patients with diabetes mellitus. The condition causes a reduction in blood flow to the extremities and a loss of sensory, motor, and autonomic nerve function. As a result, a patient is unable to feel heat, cold, pain, pressure, and/or problematic positioning of the foot or feet. The reduction in blood flow creates the risk for foot ulcers and infection. If foot ulcers do not heal, they can become infected quickly and lead to gangrene and subsequent amputation.

Safety Guidelines

- Consult agency policy regarding nail trimming. In many cases, nurses are prohibited from trimming due to risk of accidental cuts, which can become infectious.

Delegation

The skill of nail and foot care and cleansing for patients *without diabetes mellitus or circulatory compromise* can be delegated to assistive personnel (AP). Nail trimming cannot be delegated. Instruct the AP about:
- Avoiding trimming of patient's nails (see agency policy).
- Special considerations for patient positioning.
- Reporting any breaks in skin, redness, numbness, swelling, or pain.

Collaboration

- Collaborate with a podiatrist or foot care specialist to identify specific procedure for foot care for patients with PVD, diabetes mellitus, and foot ulcers (American Podiatric Medical Association, 2022).

Equipment

- Washbasin (emesis basin can be utilized)
- Washcloth and towel
- Nail clippers (check agency policy)
- Soft nail or cuticle brush
- Plastic applicator stick
- Emery board or nail file
- Body lotion
- Disposable bathmat
- Clean gloves

STEP	RATIONALE
1 Perform preprocedure protocol.	
Assessment	
• Review patient's electronic health record (EHR), including health care provider's order and nurses' notes. Verify health care provider's order for trimming nails (check agency policy).	Many agencies require a health care provider's order before nails can be trimmed. A podiatrist should assess and develop a regular schedule for nail care for patients with vascular insufficiency or peripheral neuropathy.
• Review EHR for patient's risk for foot or nail problems.	Certain conditions (e.g., diabetes mellitus, immunocompromised individuals) increase the likelihood of foot or nail problems.
a Older adult	Normal physiologic changes such as vision changes, decreased coordination, and/or inability to bend as far from the waist contribute to difficulty in performing foot and nail care (Touhy and Jett, 2020). Normal physiologic changes of aging can result in brittle nails. Discolored, extremely thickened, and deformed nails can indicate infection, fungus, or disease (Bryant and Nix, 2016)

Continued

STEP	RATIONALE
b Diabetes mellitus	Vascular changes reduce blood flow to peripheral tissues. Break in skin integrity places patient at high risk for skin infection.
c Heart failure, renal disease	Both conditions increase tissue edema, particularly in dependent areas (e.g., feet). Edema reduces blood flow to neighboring tissues.
d Cerebrovascular accident (stroke)	Presence of residual foot or leg weakness or paralysis results in altered gait patterns, which can cause increased friction and pressure on feet.
e History of leg pain	Claudication (pain in thigh, calf, or buttocks when walking) is related to ischemia with diabetic and neuropathic disorders.
• Assess patient's foot and nail care practices for existing foot problems. During assessment instruct patients about foot care:	Identifies self-care practices that place patient at risk for foot injuries. Certain preparations or applications cause more injury to soft tissue than initial foot problem.
a Over-the-counter liquid preparations to remove corns.	Liquid preparations cause burns and ulcerations.
b Cutting corns or calluses with razor blade or scissors.	Can result in infection caused by a break in skin integrity. The patient with diabetes or any patient with decreased peripheral circulation has an increased risk for infection secondary to a break in skin integrity.
c Use of oval corn pads.	Oval pads exert pressure on toes, thereby decreasing circulation to surrounding tissues.

STEP	RATIONALE
d Application of adhesive tape.	Skin of older adult is thin and delicate and prone to tearing when adhesive tape is removed.
• Ask patients whether they use nail polish and polish remover frequently.	Chemicals in these products cause excessive dryness.
• Assess type of footwear utilized by patient: Does patient wear socks? Compression hose? Are shoes tight or ill-fitting? Are garters or knee-high nylons worn? Is footwear clean?	Certain types of shoes and footwear predispose patients to foot and nail problems (e.g., infection, areas of friction, ulcerations). These conditions decrease mobility and increase risk for amputation in patients with diabetes (Chapman, 2017).
• If possible, observe patients walking to assess their gait.	Alterations in bony structures of the foot or sores often cause pain, imbalance, and unsteady gait.
• Perform hand hygiene. Apply clean gloves if drainage present. Inspect all surfaces of fingers, toes, feet, and nails. Pay particular attention to areas of dryness, inflammation, or cracking. Also inspect areas between toes, heels, and soles of feet. Instruct patient on self-examination of feet.	Integrity of feet and nails determines frequency and level of hygiene required. Heels, soles, and sides of feet are prone to irritation from ill-fitting shoes.
• Assess color and temperature of toes, feet, and fingers. Assess capillary refill of nails. Palpate radial and ulnar pulse of each hand and dorsalis pedis pulse of foot, noting character of pulses.	Assesses adequacy of blood flow to extremities. Circulatory alterations often change integrity of nails and increase patient's chance of localized infection when break in skin integrity occurs.

CLINICAL JUDGMENT *Patients with PVDs or diabetes mellitus, older adults, and patients whose immune system is suppressed should have nail care deferred (other than washing the feet) until podiatrist or foot care specialist has consulted.*

Continued

STEP	RATIONALE
• Assess patient and/or family caregiver's ability to care for nails or feet. Observe patient for visual alterations, fatigue, and musculoskeletal weakness. Remove gloves and perform hand hygiene.	Extent of patient's ability to perform self-care determines degree of help required from nurse, and the need for family caregiver education.

Implementation

STEP	RATIONALE
1 Explain to patient that proper soaking of nails on hands requires several minutes in warm water. *Exception: Patients with diabetes mellitus do not soak hands or feet (ADA, 2021).*	Patient must be willing to place fingers in basin up to 10 minutes. Patient may become anxious or tired.
2 Help ambulatory patient sit in chair and place disposable bathmat on floor under patient's feet. Help bedfast patient to supine position with head of bed elevated 45 degrees and place waterproof pad on mattress (keep side rail up until ready to begin).	Sitting in chair facilitates immersing feet in basin. Bathmat protects feet from exposure to soil or debris.
3 Fill washbasin with warm water. Test water temperature. Place basin on floor, or lower side rail and place basin on waterproof pad on mattress. Have patient immerse feet. If patient has diabetes mellitus, peripheral neuropathy, or PVD, proceed to Step 11 to begin foot care.	Prevents accidental burns to patient's skin.

CLINICAL JUDGMENT *Soaking the feet of patients with diabetes mellitus or PVD is not recommended. Soaking may lead to maceration (excessive softening of the skin) and drying of the skin (ADA, 2021), leading to tissue breakdown and infection.*

STEP	RATIONALE
4 Adjust overbed table to low position and place it over patient's lap. Instruct patient to place fingers in basin and to relax arms into a comfortable position.	Easy access prevents accidental spills. Prolonged positioning causes discomfort unless normal anatomical alignment is maintained.
5 Allow feet and fingernails to soak 5 to 10 minutes. If patient has diabetes mellitus, peripheral neuropathy, or PVD, skip this step and go straight to Step 11.	Goal is to soften debris beneath nails so that it can be removed easily.
6 Perform hand hygiene and apply clean gloves. Clean gently under fingernails with end of plastic applicator stick while fingers are immersed.	Reduces transmission of microorganisms. Removes debris under nails that harbors microorganisms.

CLINICAL JUDGMENT *Check agency policy for appropriate process for cleaning beneath nails. Do not use an orange stick or end of cotton swab as these can splinter and cause injury.*

STEP	RATIONALE
7 Use soft cuticle brush or nailbrush to clean around cuticles to decrease overgrowth.	Nailbrush helps to prevent inflammation and injury to cuticles. The cuticle slowly grows over the nail and must be pushed back with a soft nail brush regularly.
8 Remove basin and dry fingers thoroughly.	Thorough drying impedes fungal growth and prevents maceration of tissues.

Continued

STEP	RATIONALE
9 *Check agency policy on nail care regarding filing and trimming.* File fingernails straight across and even with tops of fingers. If permitted by agency policy, use nail clippers and clip fingernails straight across and even with tops of fingers (Fig. 41.1) and then smooth nail using file. Use disposable emery board and file nail to ensure that there are no sharp corners. Remove and dispose of gloves.	Filing nail straight across to eliminate sharp nail edges minimizes risk that nail can injure the adjacent tissue (Bryant and Nix, 2016) Shaping corners of toenails damages tissues, which increases the risk for infection (Jeffcoate et al., 2018).
10 Move overbed table away from patient.	

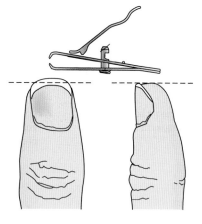

Fig. 41.1 Trim nails straight across when using nail clipper.

STEP	RATIONALE
11 Perform hand hygiene and apply new clean gloves. Continue foot care by scrubbing callused areas of feet with washcloth. Clean between toes with washcloth.	Provides easier access to feet. Friction removes dead skin layers.
12 Dry feet thoroughly and clean under toenails.	Nails harbor debris and dirt and are a source of potential infection from ineffective hygiene practices (Ball et al., 2019).
13 Apply lotion to feet and hands. Rub in thoroughly. Do not leave excess lotion between toes. Sanitize equipment according to organizational policy and return equipment to proper place.	Lotion lubricates dry skin by helping to retain moisture.
14 Perform postprocedure protocol.	
15 Evaluate patient response	
a Inspect nails, areas between fingers and toes, and surrounding skin surfaces.	Allows you to evaluate condition of skin and nails and note if there are any remaining rough nail edges.
b If possible, have patient stand and walk. Observe gait and determine whether any foot pain noted (have patient rate level of pain).	Evaluates whether nail care removed excess skin or uneven nail surfaces that can cause discomfort. Pain causes unsteady gait

Recording and Reporting

- Record procedure and assessment of condition of nails and skin around nails.
- Document evaluation of patient and family caregiver learning.
- Report areas of discomfort, breaks in skin, ulcerations, or signs of infection to charge nurse or health care provider.

UNEXPECTED OUTCOMES	RELATED INTERVENTIONS
1 Cuticles and surrounding tissues are inflamed and tender to touch.	• Repeat nail care. • Evaluate need for antifungal cream.
2 Localized areas of tenderness occur on feet with calluses or corns at point of friction.	• Change in footwear or corrective foot surgery may be needed for permanent improvement in calluses or corns. • Refer patient to podiatrist.
3 Ulcerations involving toes or feet may remain.	• Institute wound care policies. • Consult with wound care specialist and/or podiatrist. • Increase frequency of assessment and hygiene.

Nasogastric Tube Insertion for Gastric Decompression: Maintenance and Removal

There are times after major surgery, or with conditions affecting the gastrointestinal (GI) tract, when normal peristalsis is altered temporarily. Because peristalsis is slowed or absent, a patient cannot eat or drink fluids without developing abdominal distention. The temporary insertion of a nasogastric (NG) tube into the stomach decompresses the stomach, keeping it empty until normal peristalsis returns.

An NG tube is a hollow, pliable tube inserted through a patient's nasopharynx into the stomach. It removes gastric secretions and can be used to introduce solutions into the stomach. Sometimes an NG tube is used for enteral feedings, but a softer, small-bore feeding tube is preferred for feeding purposes (see Skill 23). The Salem sump tube is most commonly used for stomach decompression. The tube has two lumens: one for removal of gastric contents and one to provide an air vent, which prevents suctioning of gastric mucosa into eyelets at the distal tip of a tube. A blue "pigtail" is the air vent that connects with the second lumen (Fig. 42.1). When the main lumen of the sump tube is connected to suction, the air vent permits free, continuous drainage of secretions. ***Never clamp off the air vent, connect to suction, or use for irrigation.***

Safety Guidelines

- Nasogastric tubes cause irritation to mucous membranes lining the nares. Adhesive products are often used to secure tubes. Patients are therefore at risk for developing medical device--related pressure injuries (MDRPI) and medical adhesive related--pressure injuries (MARSI). Routine and ongoing assessment of nares and secondary pressure sites underlying medical devices, and implementing skin-care practices such as proper taping methods can reduce the risk for MDRPI and MARSI (Fumarola et al, 2020; Stellar et al., 2020).
- Follow agency policies to verify correct placement of NG tubes, which includes radiographic verification after insertion and

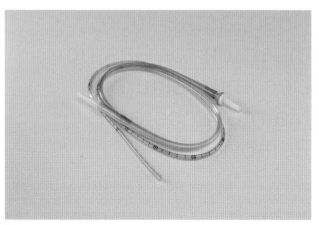

Fig. 42.1 Salem sump tube. (Courtesy Covidien, Mansfield, MA.)

subsequent pH verification. Gastric pH usually has a range of 1 to 5 (Fan et al., 2017; Judd, 2020).
- When a patient with an NG tube experiences nausea and/or vomiting, assess both placement and patency of tube, because these symptoms indicate an increased risk of aspiration. Reposition and irrigate tube as needed.

Delegation

The skill of inserting and maintaining an NG tube cannot be delegated to assistive personnel (AP). Instruct the AP to:
- Measure and record the drainage from an NG tube.
- Provide oral and nasal hygiene measures.
- Perform selected comfort measures, such as positioning or offering ice chips if not contraindicated.
- Anchor the tube to patient's gown during routine care to prevent accidental displacement.
- Immediately report any signs or symptoms of burning, redness or irritation to nares.

Equipment

- 14 Fr or 16 Fr NG tube (smaller lumen catheters are not used for decompression in adults because they must be able to remove thick secretions)
- Water-soluble lubricating jelly
- pH test strips 1.0 to 11.0 or higher (measure gastric aspirate acidity)

- Tongue blade
- Clean gloves
- Flashlight
- Emesis basin
- Asepto bulb or catheter-tipped syringe
- 2.5 cm (1 inch) Hypoallergenic tape, semipermeable (transparent) membrane dressing, or tube fixation device
- Skin barrier protectant
- Rubber band and plastic clip or tape to attach tube to gown
- Clamp, drainage bag, or suction machine or pressure gauge if wall suction is to be used
- Towel
- Glass of water with straw
- Facial tissues
- Normal saline
- Gastric suction equipment
- Stethoscope
- Pulse oximeter

STEP	RATIONALE
1 Perform preprocedure protocol.	

Assessment

• Verify health care provider order for type of NG tube to be placed and whether tube is to be attached to suction or drainage bag.	Requires order from health care provider. Adequate decompression depends on NG suction.
• Perform hand hygiene (apply clean gloves if risk of body fluid exposure). Inspect condition of skin integrity around patient's nares and nasal and oral cavity.	Provides baseline data on the condition of the patient's skin before NG tube insertion. All patients with any medical device are at risk for MDRPI (Delmore and Ayello, 2017).
• Ask if patient has history of nasal surgery or congestion and note if deviated nasal septum is present.	Alerts nurse to potential obstruction. Insert tube into uninvolved nasal passage. Procedure may be contraindicated if surgery is recent.

Continued

STEP	RATIONALE
• Assess patient's age and presence of dry skin, dehydration, malnutrition, certain medications (e.g. long-term use of corticosteroids, chemotherapeutic agents, anti-inflammatory agents and anticoagulants), dermatological conditions, radiation therapy, medical conditions (e.g. diabetes, Infection, immunosuppression, chronic venous insufficiency), and edema.	Risk factors for developing MARSI (Fumarola et al., 2020).
• Assess history of allergies: known type(s) of allergies and normal allergic reaction(s). Compare information with health history. Focus on allergies to latex, adhesive, or skin preparations.	Prevents exposure to allergic agent and anticipates possible reactions.
• Auscultate for bowel sounds. Palpate patient's abdomen for distention, pain, and rigidity. Remove and discard gloves if applied and perform hand hygiene.	In presence of diminished or absent bowel sounds, auscultate abdomen in all four quadrants (Ball et al., 2019). Documents baseline for abdominal distention, GI ileus, and general GI function, which later serves as comparison once tube is inserted. Reduces transmission of microorganisms.
• Assess patient's level of consciousness and ability to follow instructions.	Determines patient's ability to cooperate during procedure.

CLINICAL JUDGMENT *If patient is confused, disoriented, or unable to follow commands, get help from another staff member to insert the tube.*

• Determine whether patient had previous NG tube and, if so, which naris was used.	Alternate naris should be used if tube insertion was recent. Patient's previous experience complements any explanations you give about insertion.

STEP	RATIONALE

Implementation

1 Explain procedure. Inform patient that procedure may elicit gagging, and that there will be a burning sensation in nasopharynx as tube is passed. Develop hand signal with patient to aid in communication during procedure.

Increases patient's cooperation and ability to anticipate your actions. Use of hand signal will alert you if patient is unable to tolerate procedure.

2 Perform hand hygiene. Raise the bed to working height. Position patient upright in high Fowler position unless contraindicated. If patient is comatose, raise head of bed as tolerated in semi-Fowler position with head tipped forward, chin to chest.

Reduces transmission of microorganisms. Promotes patient's ability to swallow during procedure. Good body mechanics prevent injury to patient as well as health care staff.

3 Place bath towel over patient's chest and supply facial tissues. Have patient blow nose if needed. Place emesis basin within reach.

Prevents soiling of patient's gown. Tube insertion through nasal passages may produce tears and induce coughing with increased salivation.

4 Wash bridge of nose with soap and water. Dry thoroughly.

Removes oils from nose to allow fixation device to adhere.

CLINICAL JUDGMENT *Avoid preparing nose by using alcohol-based skin preparation products that can cause excessive dryness of the skin (Fumarola et al., 2020).*

5 **Insert NG tube.** Stand on the side of the patient that corresponds with your dominant hand. Lower side rail.

Allows easiest manipulation of tubing.

Continued

STEP	RATIONALE
6 Instruct patient to relax and breathe normally while occluding one naris. Repeat this action for other naris. Select nostril for insertion that has greatest airflow.	Tube passes more easily through naris that is more patent.

CLINICAL JUDGMENT *Insertion of an NG tube is a painful procedure. Research provides evidence that in some instances, topical lidocaine, either as a gel or a spray, significantly reduces pain (Boullata et al., 2017).*

7 Determine length of tube to be inserted and mark location with tape or indelible ink.	Ensures organized procedure and estimation of the proper length of tube to be inserted into patient.
a *Option, adult:* Measure distance from tip of nose to earlobe to xiphoid process (NEX) of sternum (Fig. 42.2). Mark this distance on tube with tape.	Most traditional method. Length approximates distance from nose to stomach. Research has shown that this method may be least effective compared with others, although more research is needed (Santos et al., 2016).

Fig. 42.2 Determine length of nasogastric tube to be inserted.

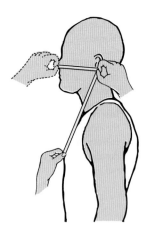

STEP	RATIONALE
b *Option, adult:* Measure distance from tip of nose to earlobe to midumbilicus (NEMU).	Promotes placement of the tube end holes in or closer to the gastric fluid pool (Boullata et al., 2017).
c *Option, adult:* Measure distance from xiphoid process to earlobe to nose + 10 cm.	Shown to be more accurate than NEX method.
d Option, child: Use the NEMU method.	Estimates proper length of tube insertion for the pediatric patient.

CLINICAL JUDGMENT *Tip of NG tube must reach stomach to avoid the risk for pulmonary aspiration, which occurs when tube terminates in the esophagus. Research has revealed mixed findings with regard to the best technique for estimating tube length (Santos et al., 2016). Confirmation of placement via x-ray immediately after completed insertion is required regardless of method used.*

---

8 With small piece of tape placed around tube, mark length indicating point to which tube will be inserted.	Indicates length of tube that you will insert.
9 Prepare materials for tube fixation: open membrane dressing or another fixation device, or tear off a 7.5- to 10-cm (3- to 4-inch) length of hypoallergenic tape.	Fixation devices allow tube to float free of nares, thus reducing pressure on nares and preventing MDRPIs.
10 Perform hand hygiene and apply clean gloves.	Reduces transmission of infection.
11 Apply pulse oximetry/ capnography device and measure vital signs. Monitor oximetry/ capnography during insertion.	Provides objective assessment of respiratory status before and during tube insertion.

Continued

STEP	RATIONALE
12 Option: Dip tube with surface lubricant into glass of room-temperature water or lubricate 7.5 to 10 cm (3 to 4 inches) of end of tube with water-soluble lubricant (see manufacturer directions).	Water activates lubricant, minimizes friction against nasal mucosa, and aids in insertion of tube. If aspirated, water-soluble lubricant is less toxic than oil-based lubricant.
13 If patient is alert, able to hold a cup, and swallow, provide a cup of water. Explain that tube insertion is about to begin.	Swallowing water facilitates tube passage through esophagus. Explanation decreases patient anxiety and increases cooperation.
14 Tube insertion. Explain next steps. Insert tube gently and slowly through naris to back of throat (posterior nasopharynx). Aim back and down toward patient's ear.	Natural contour facilitates passage of tube into GI tract and reduces gagging.
15 Have patient relax and flex head toward chest after tube is passed through nasopharynx.	Closes off glottis and reduces risk of tube entering trachea.
16 Encourage patient to swallow by taking small sips of water when possible. Advance tube as patient swallows. Rotate tube gently 180 degrees while inserting.	Swallowing facilitates passage of tube past oropharynx. A tug may be felt as patient swallows, indicating that tube is following desired path.
17 Emphasize need to mouth-breathe during procedure.	Helps facilitate passage of tube and alleviates patient's anxiety and fear during procedure.
18 Do not advance tube during inspiration or coughing because it will likely enter respiratory tract. Monitor oximetry/capnography.	When tube inadvertently enters airway, changes in oxygen saturation or end-tidal CO_2 (capnography) occur.

STEP	RATIONALE
19 Advance tube each time patient swallows until length previously marked has been reached.	Reduces discomfort and trauma to patient.

CLINICAL JUDGMENT *Do not force NG tube. If patient starts to cough or has a drop in O_2 saturation or an increased CO_2 level, withdraw tube into the posterior nasopharynx until normal breathing resumes.*

---

20 Using penlight and tongue blade, check to be sure that tube is not positioned in back of throat.	Tube could become coiled or kinked or could enter trachea.
21 Temporarily anchor tube to nose with small piece of tape.	Securing tube momentarily prevents movement of tube and subsequent gagging. Allows for verification of tube placement.
22 Verify tube placement. Check agency policy for recommended methods of verifying tube placement.	
a Follow order for bedside x-ray study and notify radiology department for examination of chest and abdomen.	Radiography remains the gold standard for verification of initial placement of tube (Boullata et al., 2017; McFarland, 2017). This must be done before any medication or liquid is administered.
b While waiting for x-ray results, follow these procedures: Attach Asepto or catheter-tipped syringe to end of tube. Aspirate gently back on syringe to obtain gastric contents, observing amount, color, and quality of return (Fig. 42.3).	Observation of gastric contents is useful to determine initial tube placement. Gastric contents are usually green but are sometimes off-white, tan, bloody, or brown. Other common aspirate colors include yellow or bile-stained (duodenal placement), or saliva-like (esophagus).

Continued

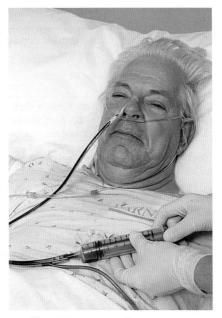

Fig. 42.3 Aspiration of gastric contents.

STEP	RATIONALE
c Use color-coded pH test paper to measure aspirate for pH. Be sure that the paper range of pH is at least 1.0 to 11.0.	Most accurate readings of gastric pH levels are provided by pH paper covering minimal range of 1.0 to 11.0. A pH value of 5.5 or below will exclude 100% of pulmonary placements and more than 93.9% of placements in small intestine (Metheny et al., 2019). Intestinal contents are more basic than stomach contents.

STEP	RATIONALE
23 After tube is confirmed to be properly inserted and positioned, either clamp end or connect it to drainage bag or suction source. Remove strip of tape temporarily holding tube but use nondominant hand to hold tube.	Drainage bag is used for gravity drainage. Intermittent low suction is most effective for decompression. Proper anchoring and marking of tube helps prevent migration of tube and pressure injury formation.
24 Anchor tube to patient's nose, avoiding pressure on nares. Be sure skin over nose is clean and dry. Apply liquid skin barrier spray or wipe on bridge of patient's nose and allow to dry completely. Select one of the following options for anchoring:	Movement of tube mark can alert nurses to possible displacement of tube. Properly secured tube allows for greater patient mobility and prevents trauma to nasal mucosa. Skin should be protected with a barrier product before an adhesive medical device is applied (Fumarola et al., 2020).
a Membrane dressing:	Allows membrane to adhere to skin.
(1) Apply additional skin protectant to patient's cheek and area of tube to be secured.	Reduces risk of MARSI (Fumarola et al., 2020).
(2) Place tube against patient's cheek and secure tube with membrane dressing, out of patient's line of vision.	Eliminates application of tape around naris. Decreases risk for patient's inadvertent dislodgement of tube.
b Tube fixation device:	Secures tube and reduces friction on naris.
(1) Apply wide end of patch to bridge of nose (see Fig. 42.4).	Use of fixation device on the bridge of a patient's nose reduces inadvertent nasal feeding tube dislodgement (Taylor et al., 2018)
(2) Slip connector around feeding tube as it exits nose (Fig. 42.5).	Secures tube.

Continued

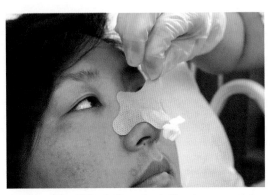

Fig. 42.4 Apply patch to bridge of nose.

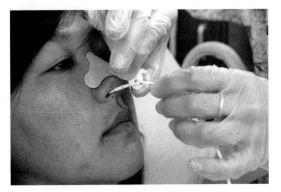

Fig. 42.5 Slip connector around nasogastric tube.

STEP	RATIONALE
c Apply 4 inch tape:	Prevents pulling of tube. May require frequent change if tape becomes soiled.

CLINICAL JUDGMENT *Adhesive fixation materials create high risk for MARSI (Fumarola et al., 2020). If possible use product with least adhesive content.*

STEP	RATIONALE
(1) Remove gloves and tear two horizontal slits on each side of tape. Make the tears at locations of one-third and two-thirds down length of tape. Do not split tape. Fold middle sections of tape forward.	Creates a gap in tape that will allow tube to float and exert less pressure on naris.
(2) Next tear a vertical strip at bottom of the 4-inch strip of tape, just below the bottom horizontal tears. Print date and time on top nasal part of tape.	Secures tube firmly and provides date of insertion and subsequent adhesive tape changes.
(3) Place intact end of tape over bridge of patient's nose. Wrap each vertical strip around tube as it exits nose (Skill 24)	Tube is free-floating in the naris with this taping method, resulting in movement of tube in pharynx. Securing tape to naris in this method reduces pressure on naris and risk for MDRPI (Zakaria et al., 2018).

CLINICAL JUDGMENT *Assess the condition of the naris and mucosa for inflammation, blistering, excoriation, or any type of skin or tissue injury at least twice daily. Injury can develop for many reasons: rigidity of device rubbing against mucosa, sensitivity to device adhesive, difficulty in securing or adjusting the device to the body, increased moisture surrounding the tubing, tight securement of the device, and poor positioning or fixation of the device (Delmore and Ayello, 2017; Fumarola et al., 2020).*

25 Fasten end of NG tube to patient's gown with piece of tape or clip. Do not use safety pins to fasten tube to gown.	Anchors tubing to prevent pulling on nose. Safety pins can accidentally open and injure patient.

Continued

STEP	RATIONALE
26 Keep head of bed elevated 30 to 45 degrees (preferably 45 degrees) unless contraindicated (Wound, Ostomy and Continence Nurses Society, 2016b).	Patients receiving NG tube feedings have an increased risk for aspiration. Head-of-bed elevation reduces risk for aspiration of stomach contents.

CLINICAL JUDGMENT *If inserting a Salem sump tube, keep the blue "pigtail" of the tube above level of the stomach. This prevents a siphoning action that clogs the tube. The blue pigtail is the air vent that connects with the second lumen When the main lumen of the sump tube is connected to suction, the air vent permits free, continuous drainage of secretions.* **Never clamp off the air vent, connect to suction, or use for irrigation.**

STEP	RATIONALE
27 Remove gloves, perform hand hygiene, and help patient to comfortable position.	Reduces transmission of microorganisms. Restores comfort and sense of well-being.
28 Once placement is confirmed, measure amount of tube that is external and mark exit of tube at nares with indelible marker as guide for any tube displacement. Record this information in electronic health record (EHR) or chart.	The mark alerts health care team to possible tube displacement, which will require reconfirmation of tube placement.

CLINICAL JUDGMENT *Never reposition an NG tube of a gastric surgical patient, because positioning can rupture the suture line.*

STEP	RATIONALE
29 Attach NG tube to suction as ordered. Suction settings should be confirmed any time the patient is disconnected or at the beginning of each nursing shift.	Suction setting is usually ordered at low intermittent setting, which decreases gastric irritation from NG tube.
30 Explain that it is normal if patient feels sore throat or irritation in pharynx.	Result of tube irritation.

STEP	RATIONALE
31 Perform postprocedure protocol.	

CLINICAL JUDGMENT *If lumen of tube is narrow and secretions are thick, NG tube will not drain as desired. Irrigate tube (see Step 32, below). Consult with health care provider for higher suction setting if unable to irrigate tube because of thick secretions.*

STEP	RATIONALE
32 NG tube irrigation:	
a Obtain and organize supplies. Perform hand hygiene and apply clean gloves.	Reduces transmission of microorganisms.
b Verify tube placement in stomach by disconnecting NG tube, connecting irrigating syringe, and aspirating contents (see Step 22b). Temporarily clamp NG tube or reconnect to connecting tube and remove syringe.	pH of gastric aspirate must measure below 5.5 to ensure that NG tube is in the stomach (Metheny et al., 2019; Judd, 2020). Prevents accidental entrance of irrigating solution into lungs.
c Empty syringe of aspirate and use syringe to draw up 30 mL of normal saline.	Use of saline minimizes loss of electrolytes from stomach fluids.
d Disconnect NG tube from connecting tubing and lay end of connection tubing on towel.	Reduces soiling of patient's gown and bed linen.
e Insert tip of irrigating syringe into end of NG tube. Remove clamp. Hold syringe with tip pointed at floor and inject saline slowly and evenly. Do not force solution.	Position of syringe prevents introduction of air into vent tubing, which causes gastric distention. Solution introduced under pressure causes gastric trauma.

CLINICAL JUDGMENT *Do not introduce saline through blue pigtail air vent of Salem sump tube.*

Continued

STEP	RATIONALE
f If resistance occurs, check for kinks in tubing. Turn patient onto left side. Repeated resistance should be reported to health care provider.	Tip of tube may lie against stomach lining. Repositioning on left side may dislodge tube away from stomach lining. Buildup of secretions causes distention.
g After instilling saline, immediately aspirate or pull back slowly on syringe to withdraw fluid. If amount aspirated is greater than amount instilled, record difference as output. If amount aspirated is less than amount instilled, record difference as intake.	Irrigation clears tubing, so stomach should remain empty. Measure and document amount of irrigant fluid inserted in tube as intake.
h Use an Asepto syringe to inject 10 mL of air into blue pigtail.	Ensures patency of air vent.
i Reconnect NG tube to drainage or suction. (Repeat irrigation if solution does not return.)	Reestablishes drainage collection; may repeat irrigation or repositioning of tube until NG tube drains properly.
j Perform postprocedure protocol.	
33 Removing NG tube:	
a Verify order to remove NG tube.	A health care provider order is required for procedure.
b Per agency policy, auscultate abdomen for presence of bowel sounds or clamp the tube for a short period of time assessing for nausea or discomfort.	Verifies return of peristalsis. Early removal of the NG tube helps to restore normal anatomy and physiology of the GI system (Goudar et al., 2017).

STEP	RATIONALE
c Explain procedure to patient and reassure that removal is less distressing than insertion.	Minimizes anxiety and increases cooperation. Tube passes out smoothly.
d Perform hand hygiene and apply clean gloves.	Reduces transmission of microorganisms.
e Turn off suction and disconnect NG tube from drainage bag or suction. With irrigating syringe, insert 20 mL of air into lumen of NG tube. Remove tape or fixation device from bridge of nose and patient's gown.	Ensure tube is free of connections before removal. Clears gastric fluids from tube to prevent aspiration of contents or soiling of clothing and bedding.
f Provide patient with facial tissue; place clean towel across chest.	Some patients wish to blow nose after tube is removed. Towel keeps gown from soiling.
Instruct patient to take a breath and hold as tube is removed.	Temporary airway obstruction occurs during tube removal.
g Clamp or kink tubing securely and pull tube out steadily and smoothly into towel held in other hand while patient holds breath.	Clamping prevents tube contents from draining into oropharynx. Reduces trauma to mucosa, and minimizes patient's discomfort. Towel covers tube, which can be unpleasant for patient to view. Holding breath helps to prevent aspiration.
h Inspect intactness of tube.	
i Measure amount of drainage and note character of content. Dispose of tube and drainage equipment into proper container.	Provides accurate measure of fluid output. Reduces transfer of microorganisms.

Continued

STEP	RATIONALE
j Clean nares and provide mouth care.	Promotes comfort.
k Position patient comfortably and explain procedure for drinking fluids if not contraindicated. Instruct patient to report if nausea occurs.	Sometimes patients are not allowed anything by mouth for up to 24 h. When fluids are allowed, orders usually begin with small amount of ice chips each hour and increase as patient is able to tolerate more.
34 Perform postprocedure protocol.	
35 Evaluate patient response:	
a Observe amount and character of contents draining from NG tube. Ask whether patient feels nauseous.	Determines whether tube is decompressing stomach of contents.
b Turn off suction and auscultate for presence of bowel sounds. If tube is clamped for short trial period, assess for nausea and patient discomfort.	Sound of suction apparatus is sometimes misinterpreted as bowel sounds. Nausea and discomfort will occur if peristalsis has not returned.
c Palpate patient's abdomen periodically. Note any distention, pain, and rigidity.	Determines success of abdominal decompression and return of peristalsis.
d Inspect condition of nares, nose, and skin and tissue around NG tubing as per agency policy.	Evaluates onset of skin and tissue irritation, including early detection of MARSI.
e Observe position of tubing.	Prevents tension applied to nasal structures.

Recording and Reporting

- Record length, size, and type of gastric tube inserted, and the naris in which tube was introduced. Also record condition of naris, patient tolerance of procedure, confirmation of tube placement by X-ray, character and pH of gastric contents, whether the tube is clamped or connected to drainage bag or to suction, and amount of suction supplied.
- Document evaluation of patient learning.
- When irrigating NG tube, record difference between amount of normal saline instilled and amount of gastric aspirate removed on intake and output sheet. Record amount and character of contents draining from NG tube every shift.
- Record removal of "intact" tube, patient's tolerance of procedure, condition of naris, and final amount and character of drainage.
- Report occurrence of abdominal distention, unexpected increase or sudden cessation of gastric drainage, and patient complaint of gastric distress to health care provider.

UNEXPECTED OUTCOMES	RELATED INTERVENTIONS
1 Patient experiences nausea, or abdomen is distended and painful.	• Assess patency of tube. NG tube may be occluded or no longer in stomach. Verify placement. • Irrigate tube. • Verify that suction is on as ordered. • Notify health care provider if distention is unrelieved.
2 Patient develops irritation or erosion of skin around naris.	• Provide frequent skin care to area. • Use taping method designed to reduce MDRPI (see taping methods [Step 22]). • Consider switching tube to other naris.
3 Patient develops signs and symptoms of pulmonary aspiration: fever, shortness of breath, or pulmonary congestion.	• Perform complete respiratory assessment. • Notify health care provider. • Obtain chest x-ray examination as ordered.

Negative-Pressure Wound Therapy

Negative-pressure wound therapy (NPWT) or vacuum-assisted closure (VAC), is the application of subatmospheric (negative) pressure to a wound through suction to facilitate healing and collect wound fluid (Netsch et al., 2016). NPWT (Figs. 43.1 and 43.2) supports wound healing by removing wound exudates and reducing edema, macrodeformation and wound contraction, and microdeformation and mechanical stretch perfusion. Secondary effects include angiogenesis, granulation tissue formation, and reduction in bacterial bioburden (Netsch et al., 2016). The VAC instill system allows intermittent instillation of fluids into a wound and liquefies infectious material and wound debris, especially in wounds not responding to traditional NPWT (Fernandez et al., 2019).

Indications for NPWT include chronic, acute, traumatic, subacute, and dehisced wounds; partial-thickness burns; injuries (e.g., diabetic and pressure); flaps and grafts (once nonviable tissue has been removed); and select high-risk postoperative surgical incisions (e.g., orthopedic, sternal). NPWT is also used in wounds with tunnels, undermining, or sinus tracts as long as the wound filler can fill the dead space and is easily retrieved (Netsch et al., 2016). Research also supports the instillation of wound-rinsing agents to facilitate healing in some chronic wounds (Matiasek et al., 2018).

There are several different NPWT systems. Some are gauze or foam based; some are designed for acute care settings or for outpatient care (Netsch et al., 2016). NPWT can be delivered intermittently or continuously. Review of evidence shows improved microvascular blood flow and granulation tissue formation with intermittent versus continuous therapy delivered at 125 mm Hg (Wound, Ostomy and Continence Nurses Society (WOCN), 2016a). However, for patients with severe pain, lower levels of pressure (75 to 80 mm Hg) can be used to reduce pain and discomfort without compromising effectiveness (European Pressure Ulcer Advisory Panel and National Pressure Injury Advisory Panel, and Pan Pacific Pressure Injury Alliance [EPUAP/NPIAP/ PPPIA], 2019a, 2019b; Netsch et al., 2016).

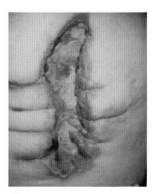

Fig. 43.1 Dehisced wound before negative-pressure wound therapy. (Courtesy KCI USA, San Antonio, TX.).

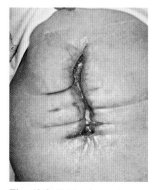

Fig. 43.2 Dehisced wound after negative-pressure wound therapy. (Courtesy KCI USA, San Antonio, TX.).

Safety Guidelines

- Contraindications to NPWT include necrotic tissue with eschar present; untreated osteomyelitis; nonenteric and unexplored fistulas; malignancy in the wound; exposed vasculature; and exposed nerves, anastomotic sites, or organs.
- Other safety precautions to consider are patients at high risk for bleeding or hemorrhage; patients taking anticoagulants; and patients requiring magnetic resonance imaging, hyperbaric chamber, or defibrillation (Netsch et al., 2016).
- Provide analgesia as ordered 30 minutes before a dressing change.

Delegation

The skill of NPWT cannot be delegated to assistive personnel (AP). Direct the AP to:

- Use caution in positioning or turning patient to avoid tubing displacement.
- Report any change in dressing shape or integrity.
- Report any change in patient's temperature or comfort level.
- Report any wound fluid leakage around the edges of the adhesive drape and any activation of alarms on the NPWT system.

Collaboration

- Collaborate with wound care specialists when needed if there is difficulty applying the NPWT dressing or in maintaining an airtight seal on larger or more complex wounds.

Equipment

- NPWT unit (requires health care provider's order). The VAC unit is provided as illustration for this skill; several other systems are available, and their applications may differ. (See manufacturer instructions.)
- NPWT dressing (gauze or foam, see manufacturer recommendations transparent dressing; adhesive drape)
- NPWT suction device
- Supplies for wound irrigation if needed
- Tubing for connection between NPWT unit and NPWT dressing
- Three pairs of gloves, clean and sterile (as needed)
- Scissors, sterile
- Skin preparation/skin barrier protectant/hydrocolloid dressing/skin barrier
- Adhesive remover
- Personal protective equipment: gown, mask, goggles (worn when splashing from wound is a risk)
- Waterproof biohazard bag for disposal

STEP	RATIONALE
1 Perform preprocedure protocol.	
Assessment	
• Review patient's electronic health record (EHR), including health care provider's order and nurses' notes, for frequency of dressing change, amount of negative pressure, type of foam or gauze to use, and pressure cycle (intermittent or continuous).	Determines frequency of dressing change, negative-pressure setting, and special instructions. Health care provider's order is also necessary for insurance reimbursement.

STEP	RATIONALE
• Review EHR for signs and symptoms of complications and/or wound condition from previous wound assessments.	Provides baseline to compare current findings with previous dressing change assessments, and reflects wound-healing progress.
• Assess character of patient's pain and rate severity on pain scale of 0 to 10.	Serves as baseline to measure patient's comfort level during and after wound therapy.
• Perform hand hygiene. Apply clean gloves. Assess condition of wound and status of NPWT dressing without disrupting NPWT. Remove and dispose of gloves. Perform hand hygiene.	Provides information regarding condition of skin around wound and existing dressing, presence of complications, and proper type of supplies and help needed for procedure.

Implementation

STEP	RATIONALE
1 Administer prescribed analgesic (as needed) 30 minutes before dressing change.	Comfortable patient will be less likely to make sudden movements, causing wound or supply contamination.
2 Explain procedure to patient and family caregiver, instructing patient not to touch wound or sterile supplies. Discuss whether the patient or caregiver will be participating in changing the NPWT dressing in the home	Relieves anxiety and promotes understanding of healing process. Prevents contamination of sterile supplies.
3 Cuff top of disposable waterproof biohazard bag and place within reach of work area.	Cuff prevents accidental contamination of top of outer bag.
4 Perform hand hygiene and apply clean gloves. If risk for spray exists, apply protective gown, goggles, and mask.	Reduces transmission of infectious organisms.

Continued

STEP	RATIONALE
5 Follow manufacturer directions for removal and replacement as instructions vary slightly for each NPWT unit. Turn off NPWT unit by pushing therapy on/off button.	Deactivates therapy and allows for proper drainage of fluid in drainage tubing.
6 Keeping tube connectors attached to NPWT unit, raise tubing connectors; disconnect tubes from one another and drain fluids into drainage collector.	Prevents backflow of drainage in tubing back into wound.
7 Before draining, tighten clamp on canister tube and disconnect canister and dressing tubing at connection points.	Prevents drainage from exiting tubing when removed.
8 Remove old transparent membrane dressing by loosening a corner of the dressing and stretching it horizontally in the opposite direction of the wound (stretch and relax technique). Walk fingers under the dressing to continue stretching it. Use one hand to continuously support the skin adhered to the dressing. The process can be repeated around the dressing. Discard in bag.	Stretching action gently breaks dressing seal (Bryant and Nix, 2016). Reduces excoriation, tearing, or irritation of skin during dressing removal (Fumarola et al., 2020).

STEP	RATIONALE
9 Remove old dressing one layer at a time and discard in bag. Observe drainage on dressing. Prevent patient from seeing old dressing because sight of wound drainage may be upsetting. Use caution to avoid tension on any drains that are present near the wound or surrounding area. Remove and dispose of gloves.	Determines type and amount of dressings needed for replacement. Lessens patient anxiety. Prevents accidental removal of drains.
10 Perform hand hygiene, apply clean gloves and conduct a wound assessment. Observe surface area and tissue type, color, odor, and drainage within wound. Measure length, width, and depth of wound as ordered.	Wound measurement is necessary to assess wound-healing progression and justify continuation of NPWT for third-party payers (Netsch et al., 2016). Determines condition of wound and need for replacement of dressing.

CLINICAL JUDGMENT *A wound care nurse or physician might be needed to debride the wound at this point in the process. Debridement of eschar or slough, if present, removes devitalized tissue to prepare the wound bed (Netsch, 2016).*

STEP	RATIONALE
11 Remove and discard gloves in biohazard bag.	Reduces transmission of microorganisms.
12 Clean wound per order or recommendations of wound care specialist.	Cleaning periwound is essential for airtight seal.
a Perform hand hygiene. Apply sterile or clean gloves, depending on agency policy and wound status.	Reduces transmission of infectious organisms.

Continued

STEP	RATIONALE
b If ordered, irrigate wound with normal saline or other solution ordered by health care provider (see Skill 83). Gently blot periwound with gauze to dry thoroughly.	Irrigation removes wound debris and cleans wound bed. Cleaning and removal of infectious material reduces infection and improves healing (EPUAP/NPIAP/PPPIA, 2019b; Fernandez et al., 2019).

CLINICAL JUDGMENT *Health care providers may order wound cultures routinely. However, when drainage is more copious, looks purulent, or has a foul odor, a wound culture should be obtained. This may be an indication that NPWT may need to be discontinued.*

CLINICAL JUDGMENT *Health care providers may use normal saline instillation with large, complex wounds. NPWT with instillation in wounds needing cleaning and removal of infectious material reduces infection and improves wound healing (Fernandez et al., 2019).*

13 Apply skin protectant, barrier film, solid skin barrier sheet, or hydrocolloid dressing to periwound skin.	Provides surface to maintain airtight seal needed for NPWT wound therapy (Netsch et al., 2016). Skin barrier protects periwound skin from moisture-associated skin damage and medical adhesive related skin injury (Fumarola et al., 2020).
14 Fill any uneven skin surfaces (e.g., creases, scars, and skinfolds) with skin-barrier product (e.g., paste, strip).	Further helps to maintain airtight seal (Netsch et al., 2016).
15 Remove and discard gloves. Perform hand hygiene.	Prevents transmission of microorganisms.
16 Depending on type of wound, apply sterile or new clean gloves (see agency policy).	Fresh sterile wounds require sterile gloves. Chronic wounds require clean technique (WOCN, 2016a).

STEP	RATIONALE
17 Apply NPWT:	
a Prepare NPWT filler dressing. Consult with wound care expert for appropriate type.	Filler dressing depends on NPWT used and can include foam or gauze dressings with or without antimicrobials (such as silver). Type of dressing may be adjusted based on undermining, tunneling, or sinus tracts present (Netsch et al., 2016).
(1) Measure clean wound and select appropriate-size dressing.	Establishes baseline for wound size. Black polyurethane foam has larger pores and is most effective in stimulating granulation tissue and wound contraction. White soft foam is denser with smaller pores and used when growth of granulation tissue needs to be restricted (Netsch et al., 2016; Panayi et al., 2017).
(2) Using sterile scissors, cut filler dressing foam to wound size, making sure to fit exact size and shape of wound, including tunnels and undermined areas.	Proper size of foam dressing maintains negative pressure to entire wound (Netsch et al., 2016).

CLINICAL JUDGMENT *In some instances an antimicrobial product such as silver-impregnated gauze or topical antibiotic is indicated. These products help reduce the bioburden of the wound.*

Continued

STEP	RATIONALE
b Place filler dressing in wound following manufacturer instructions. Be sure that filler dressing is in contact with entire wound base, margins, and tunneled and undermined areas. Count number of filler dressings and document in patient's chart.	Maintains negative pressure to entire wound. Edges of foam dressing must be in direct contact with patient's skin. Dressing count provides nurse who removes dressing with number of filler dressings that should be removed.
c Place suction device near bedside per manufacturer instructions.	Prepares for assembly
d Apply NPWT transparent dressing over foam wound dressing.	
(1) Trim transparent dressing to cover wound and dressing so it will extend onto periwound skin approximately 2.5 to 5 cm (1 to 2 inches).	Prepares dressing of appropriate size for wound.
(2) Apply transparent dressing, keeping it wrinkle-free (Fig. 43.3).	Dressing should be airtight with no wrinkles or tunnels to maintain a negative-pressure environment. A snug and tight application of the dressing must be applied to ensure an airtight seal (Box 43.1).
(3) Secure drainage tubing to transparent film, aligning drainage holes to ensure occlusive seal. Do not apply tension.	Excessive tension may compress foam dressing and impede wound healing. It also produces shear force on periwound area (Netsch, 2016).

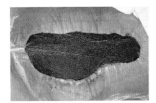

Fig. 43.3 Foam wound filler; transparent dressing over existing wound. (Courtesy KCI USA, San Antonio, TX.)

BOX 43.1 Maintaining an Airtight Seal with Negative-Pressure Wound Therapy

To avoid loss of suction (negative pressure), the wound and dressing must stay sealed after therapy is initiated. Problem seal areas include wounds around joints, near skin creases and folds, and near moisture such as diaphoresis, wound drainage, and urine or stool. The following suggestions may help to maintain an airtight seal:

- Clip hair on skin around wound (check agency policy).
- Fill uneven skin surfaces with a skin-barrier product such as paste or strips.
- Ensure the periwound skin surface is dry.
- Cut transparent film to extend 2.5 to 5 cm (1 to 2 inches) beyond wound perimeter.
- Frame periwound area with skin sealant, solid skin barrier, hydrocolloid, or transparent film dressing.
- Cut or mold transparent dressing to fit wound.
- Avoid wrinkles when applying transparent film.
- Identify air leaks with a stethoscope and repair with a sealant dressing (e.g., transparent dressing). Use only one or two additional layers for large leaks. Multiple layers reduce moisture vapor transmission and cause maceration of wound.
- If an adhesive remover is used, be sure to cleanse periwound well because it leaves a residue that can hinder film adherence.

Data from Netsch DS: Refractory wounds. In *Wound, Ostomy and Continence Nurses Society Core Curriculum: wound management*, Philadelphia, 2016, Wolters Kluwer, and Netsch DS, et al: Negative-pressure wound therapy. In Bryant RA, Nix DP, editors: *Acute and chronic wounds: current management concepts*, ed 5, St Louis, 2016, Mosby.

STEP	RATIONALE
(4) Secure tubing several centimeters away from dressing, avoiding pressure points.	Drainage tubes over bony pressure prominences can cause medical device–related pressure injuries (Netsch, 2016; Netsch et al., 2016).

Continued

STEP	RATIONALE
18 After wound is completely covered, connect tubing from dressing to tubing from canister and NPWT unit. Then set NPWT system to ordered suction level.	Intermittent or continuous negative pressure varies from 75 mm Hg to 125 mm Hg, depending on the device and the characteristics of the wound (Netsch et al., 2016; WOCN, 2016a).

   a Remove canister from sterile packing and push unit until you hear a click. *Note:* An alarm sounds if canister is not properly engaged.

   b Connect dressing tubing to canister tubing, ensuring that both clamps are open.

   c Place on level surface or hang from foot of bed. *Note:* Unit alarms and deactivates therapy if tilted beyond 45 degrees.

   d Press power button (commonly this is a green-lit button) and set pressure as ordered.

STEP	RATIONALE
19 Remove and dispose of gloves. Perform hand hygiene.	Reduces transmission of microorganisms.

20 Inspect NPWT system:

   a Verify that the system is on. *Note:* This is different for each type of NPWT unit. For example, on some units the display screen shows "Therapy On." Check agency policy and procedure for specific information.

STEP	RATIONALE
b Verify that all clamps are open and all tubing is patent.	
c Examine system to be sure that seal is intact and therapy is working.	Negative pressure is achieved when a tight seal is present (Netsch et al., 2016).
d If a leak is present, use strips of transparent film to patch areas around edges of wound.	
21 Record your initials, date, and time on new dressing.	Provides reference for next dressing change.
22 Dispose of sharps (scissors) in designated sharps disposal bin.	Prevents exposure of patient or heath care worker to contaminated sharps.
23 Perform postprocedure protocol.	
24 Evaluate patient response:	
a Inspect condition of wound and wound bed on an ongoing basis; note drainage and odor.	Determines status of wound healing.
b Ask patient to describe pain and rate severity on scale of 0 to 10.	Determines patient's level of comfort after the procedure.
c Verify airtight dressing seal and correct negative-pressure setting.	Determines effective negative pressure being applied.
d Measure wound drainage output in canister on regular basis.	Monitors fluid balance and wound drainage.

Recording and Reporting

- Record appearance of wound, characteristics of drainage, placement of NPWT (time and type of dressing, pressure mode and setting), and patient response to dressing change.

- Document evaluation of patient and family caregiver learning.
- Report brisk, bright-red bleeding, evidence of poor wound healing, evisceration or dehiscence, and possible wound infection to health care provider immediately.

UNEXPECTED OUTCOMES	RELATED INTERVENTIONS
1 Wound appears inflamed and tender, drainage has increased, and odor is present.	• Notify health care provider and wound care specialist. • Obtain wound culture if ordered. • Increase frequency of dressing changes.
2 Patient reports increase in pain.	• Consult with health care provider about need for change in analgesia. • Instill normal saline to moisten foam and other filler dressings to allow for increased loosening from granulation tissue. • Decrease pressure setting. • Change from intermittent to continuous cycling. • Change type of NPWT system.
3 Negative-pressure seal has broken.	• Take preventive measures (see Box 43.1).
4 Wound hemorrhages.	• Stop NPWT immediately and notify health care provider.
5 Patient or family caregiver is unable to perform dressing change.	• Provide additional teaching and support. • Obtain services of home care agency.

Oral Medications

Patients are usually able to ingest or self-administer oral medications with few problems. The form and/or preparation of an oral medication affects how well it is absorbed after it is ingested. Liquids are absorbed faster than tablets or capsules and are usually absorbed in the stomach. Give an oral medication with a meal if its absorption is enhanced by food in the stomach. Some medications must be taken between meals, 2 to 3 h after eating a meal (Burchum and Rosenthal, 2022).

Some oral medications are absorbed in the intestinal tract. Enteric-coated preparations resist being dissolved by gastric juices. The enteric coating protects the stomach lining from irritation by the medication. These preparations are absorbed in the small intestine. *Never crush or split an enteric-coated medication.* Crushing or splitting these preparations causes the medication to be released too early and the medication may become inactive in the stomach or fail to reach the intended site of action (Institute for Safe Medication Practices [ISMP], 2020b).

Safety Guidelines

- If oral medications are contraindicated (e.g., inability to swallow, gastric suction), take precautions to protect patients from aspiration (see Skill 3).
- Always follow the seven rights of medication administration when administering oral medications.
- Be vigilant during preparation and administration of oral medications.

Delegation

The skill of administering oral medications cannot be delegated to assistive personnel (AP) *Note:* Medication technicians who are certified nursing assistants may be qualified to administer select medications in long-term care. Instruct the AP about:

- Potential side effects of medications and to report their occurrence.
- Reporting if patient condition changes or worsens (e.g., pain, itching, or rash) after medication administration.

Collaboration

- Collaborate with pharmacist to obtain liquid preparations for patients with impaired swallowing.

Equipment

- Automated, computer-controlled drug-dispensing system or medication cart

- Disposable medication cups (milliliter-only cups)
- Glass of water, juice, or preferred liquid and drinking straw
- Pill-crushing device *(optional)*
- Paper towels
- Medication administration record (MAR) (electronic or printed)
- Clean gloves (if handling an oral medication) *Note:* Gloves must be worn when administering an oral chemotherapy drug.

STEP	RATIONALE
1 Perform preprocedure protocol.	

Assessment

• Verify accuracy and completeness of each MAR or computer printout with health care provider's written medication order. Verify patient's name, medication name and dosage, route of administration, and time of administration. Clarify incomplete or unclear orders with health care provider before administration.	The order sheet is the most reliable source and only legal record of medications that patient is to receive. Ensures that patient receives the correct medications (Palese et al., 2019). Transcription errors are a source of medication errors (Zhu and Weingart, 2022).
• Review drug reference information for medication action, purpose, normal dose and route, side effects, time of onset and peak action, indication, and nursing implications.	Allows for anticipation of medication effects and observation of patient response.
• Ask patient to describe history of allergies: known type of allergies and normal allergic reaction. Enter medication allergies and prominently display on patient MAR and medical record. When indicated, patient should wear an allergy bracelet. Check patient's allergy wristband before medication administration.	Do not prepare medication if there is a known patient allergy. Communication of patient allergies is essential for safe medication administration.

STEP	RATIONALE
• Perform hand hygiene and assess for NPO (nothing by mouth) status, inability to swallow, nausea/vomiting, bowel inflammation, reduced peristalsis, recent gastrointestinal (GI) surgery, gastric suction, and decreased level of consciousness (LOC). Notify health care provider if any contraindications are present.	Contraindications for oral medication. Alterations in GI function can interfere with drug absorption, distribution, and excretion. Giving oral medications to patients with impaired swallowing, impaired cognition, or decreased LOC increases their risk for aspiration. Patients on GI suction do not receive actions of oral medications because medications are suctioned from the GI tract before they are absorbed.
• Assess risk for aspiration using a dysphagia screening tool if available (see Skill 3).	Aspiration occurs when food, fluid, or medication intended for GI administration is inadvertently administered into the respiratory tract. Patients with difficulty swallowing are at higher risk for aspiration pneumonia (Bartlett, 2021).
• Obtain current, nurse-measured (actual) patient weight.	Used to calculate certain medication doses. Actual weight is more accurate than self-report by patient or taken from previous recorded visit (ISMP, 2021).
• Gather and review physical assessment findings and laboratory data related to medication administration, e.g., vital signs and results of renal and liver function studies.	Data may reveal contraindication to medication administration. Renal and liver function status affects metabolism and excretion of medications (Burchum and Rosenthal, 2022).

Continued

STEP	RATIONALE
• Assess patient's preference for fluids and determine whether medications are compatible. Maintain fluid restrictions as prescribed.	Some fluids interfere with medication absorption (e.g., dairy products affect tetracycline). Offering fluids during drug administration is an excellent way to increase patient's fluid intake. Fluids ease swallowing and facilitate absorption from the GI tract. However, with fluid restrictions, skillful planning of fluid intake must coordinate with timing and types of ordered medications.

Implementation

STEP	RATIONALE
1 Explain to patient signs and symptoms to expect from medication. Allow time for patient to ask questions.	Lessens anxiety by helping patient know what to expect, promoting self-care.
2 Prepare medication without interruptions/distractions. Create a quiet environment. Keep all pages of MARs or computer printouts for one patient together or look at only one patient's electronic MAR at a time.	Interruptions contribute to medication errors (Palese et al., 2019).
3 Perform hand hygiene. Prepare medications for one patient at a time using aseptic technique. a Arrange medication tray and cups in medication preparation area or move medication cart to position outside patient's room.	Ensures that medications are sterile and correctly prepared. Organization of equipment saves time and reduces error.

STEP	RATIONALE
b Select correct medication from automated drug-dispensing unit, unit-dose drawer, or stock supply. Check label of medication carefully with MAR or computer printout *when removing drug from storage and after preparation.* Check drug expiration date. Return expired drugs to pharmacy.	*These are the first and second checks for accuracy* and ensure that correct medication is administered. Dose potency increases or decreases when outdated. Expired medications may be harmful to patient.
c Verify or calculate medication dose as needed. Double-check any calculation.	Double-checking pharmacy calculations reduces risk for error. Agency policy may require verification of calculations for certain medications such as insulin with another nurse (ISMP, 2018).
d If preparing a controlled substance, verify previous medication count and compare current count with available supply. Controlled medications are stored in a computerized locked cart/system.	Controlled substance laws require nurses to carefully monitor and count dispensed narcotics.
e Prepare solid forms of oral medications:	
(1) To prepare unit-dose tablets or capsules, place packaged tablet or capsule directly into medication cup without removing wrapper. Administer medications only from containers with clearly marked labels.	Wrappers maintain cleanliness and identify medication name and dose, which can also facilitate patient teaching.

Continued

STEP	RATIONALE
(2) When using a blister pack, "pop" medications through foil or paper backing into a medication cup.	Packs provide a 1-month supply, with each "blister" usually containing a single dose.
(3) When preparing tablet or capsule from a floor stock bottle, pour required number into bottle cap and transfer to medication cup. Do not touch medication with fingers. Return unused medication to container.	Avoids contamination and waste of medication.
(4) If it is necessary to give half the dose of a medication, pharmacy should split, label, package, and send medication to unit.	Reduces contamination of tablet.
(5) Place all tablets or capsules enclosed in unit-dose individual packets in one medicine cup, except for those requiring preadministration assessments (e.g., pulse rate or blood pressure). Separate those medications into an additional cup with wrappers intact.	Keeping medications that require preadministration assessments separate from others serves as reminder and makes it easier to withhold drugs if indicated.

STEP	RATIONALE
(6) If patient has difficulty swallowing and liquid medications are not an option, use a pill-crushing device. Clean device before using. Place medicine into device and grind and crush. Mix ground tablet in small amount (teaspoon) of soft food according to patient preference (e.g., custard or applesauce).	Large tablets are often difficult to swallow. Ground tablet mixed with palatable soft food is usually easier to swallow.

CLINICAL JUDGMENT *Not all medications can be crushed safely. Consult with a pharmacist or the ISMP Do Not Crush List (ISMP, 2020b).*

f Prepare liquids: (1) Use unit-dose container with correct amount of medication. Gently shake container. Administer medication packaged in a single-dose cup directly from the single-dose cup. Do not pour medicine into another cup.	Using unit-dose container with correct dosage of medication provides most accurate dose of medication. Shaking container ensures that medication is mixed before administration.

CLINICAL JUDGMENT *According to current best practice (ISMP, 2021), liquid medications that are not available or are not in correct dose in a unit-dose container should be dispensed by the pharmacy in special oral syringes marked "Oral Use Only." These syringes do not connect to any type of parenteral (e.g., intravenous) tubing. In addition, current evidence shows that liquid measuring devices on patient care units result in inaccurate dosing. Having oral medications prepared in the pharmacy ensures that you give the most accurate dose of a medication possible and prevents parenteral administration of oral medications.*

Continued

STEP	RATIONALE
(2) Administer medications in oral syringe or enteral syringe (e.g., ENFit) prepared by pharmacy (see Fig. 44.1) and labeled Oral Use Only. *Do not use hypodermic syringe or syringe with needle or syringe cap).*	If using hypodermic syringes, the medication may be accidentally administered parenterally; or the syringe cap or needle, if not removed from the syringe before administration, may become dislodged and accidentally aspirated during administration of oral medications (ISMP, 2021).
g Return unused unit-dose medications to shelf or drawer. Label medication cups and poured medications with patient's name before leaving medication preparation area. Do not leave drugs unattended.	Allows more accurate measurement of small amounts. Ensures that correct medications are prepared for correct patient.

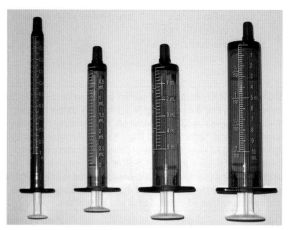

Fig. 44.1 Use special oral medication syringes to prepare small amounts of liquid medications.

STEP	RATIONALE

4 Administer medications:

a Take medication(s) to patient at correct time (see agency policy). Medications that require exact timing include STAT doses, first-time or loading doses, and one-time doses. Give time-critical scheduled medications (e.g., antibiotics, anticoagulants, insulin) at exact time ordered (no more than 30 minutes before or after scheduled dose). Give non–time-critical scheduled medications within a range of 1 or 2 h of scheduled dose (CMS, 2020). During administration, apply seven rights of medication administration.

Hospitals must adopt medication administration policy and procedure for timing of medication administration that considers nature of the prescribed medication, specific clinical application, and patient needs (US Department of Health and Human Services, 2020; CMS, 2020).

b Identify patient using at least two identifiers (e.g., name and birthday or name and medical record number) according to agency policy. Compare identifiers with information on patient's MAR or medical record.

Ensures correct patient. Complies with The Joint Commission standards and improves patient safety (The Joint Commission, 2023).
Some agencies use a barcode system to help with patient identification.

c At patient's bedside, again compare MAR or computer printout with names of medications on medication labels and patient name. Ask whether patient has any allergies.

This is the third check for accuracy and ensures that patient receives correct medication.
Confirms patient's allergy history.

Continued

STEP	RATIONALE
d Perform necessary preadministration assessment (e.g., blood pressure, pulse) for specific medications.	Determines whether specific medications should be withheld at that time.
e Help patient to sitting or semi/high-Fowler position. Use side-lying position if patients are unable to sit. Have a patient remain in this position for 30 minutes after administration.	Decreases risk for aspiration during swallowing.
f *For tablets:* Patient may wish to hold solid medications in hand or cup before placing in mouth. Offer water or preferred liquid to help patient swallow medications.	Patient can become familiar with medications by seeing each drug. Choice of fluid can improve fluid intake.

CLINICAL JUDGMENT *If administering an oral chemotherapy pill or tablet, it can be administered from the cup directly into the patient's mouth, or if there is a need to handle the medication, apply clean gloves. Never use bare hands to touch a chemotherapy medication because residue can be absorbed through the skin (Occupational Safety and Health Administration, nd[c]).*

---

g *For orally disintegrating formulations (tablets or strips):* Remove medication from packet just before use. Do not push tablet through foil. Place medication on top of patient's tongue. Caution against chewing it.	Formulations begin to dissolve when placed on tongue. Water is not needed. Careful removal from packaging is necessary because tablets and strips are thin and fragile.

STEP	RATIONALE
h *For sublingually administered medications:* Have patient place medication under tongue and allow it to dissolve completely (see Fig. 44.2). Caution patient against swallowing tablet.	Drug is absorbed through blood vessels of undersurface of tongue. If swallowed, it is destroyed by gastric juices or rapidly detoxified by liver, preventing therapeutic blood level.
i *For buccal-administered medications:* Have patient place medication in mouth against mucous membranes of cheek and gums until it dissolves (see Fig. 44.3)	Buccal medications act locally or systemically as they are swallowed in saliva.

CLINICAL JUDGMENT *Avoid administering anything by mouth until orally disintegrating buccal or sublingual medications are completely dissolved.*

j *For powdered medications:* Mix with liquids at bedside and give to patient to drink.	When prepared in advance, powdered drugs thicken; some even harden, making swallowing difficult.
k *For crushed medications mixed with food:* Give each medication separately in teaspoon of soft food according to patient preference.	Ensures that patient swallows all of medicine.

Continued

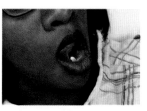

Fig. 44.2 Proper placement of sublingual tablet in sublingual pocket.

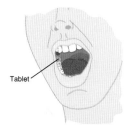

Tablet

Fig. 44.3 Buccal administration of tablet.

STEP	RATIONALE
l *For lozenge:* Caution patient against chewing or swallowing lozenges.	Lozenges act through slow absorption through oral, not gastric, mucosa.
m *For effervescent medication:* Add tablet or powder to glass of water. Administer immediately after dissolving.	Effervescence improves unpleasant taste and often relieves GI problems.
n If patient is unable to hold medications, place medication cup or syringe to lips and gently introduce each medication into mouth one at a time. A spoon can also be used to place pill in patient's mouth. Do not rush or force medications.	Administering a single tablet or capsule eases swallowing and decreases risk for aspiration.

CLINICAL JUDGMENT *If tablet or capsule falls to the floor, discard it and repeat preparation because that medication has become contaminated.*

o Stay until patient swallows each medication completely or takes it by the prescribed route. Ask patient to open mouth if uncertain whether medication has been swallowed.	Ensures that patient receives ordered dose. If left unattended, patient may not take dose or may save medications, causing health risks.
p For highly acidic medications (e.g., aspirin), offer patient a nonfat snack (e.g., crackers) if not contraindicated by condition.	Reduces gastric irritation. Fat content of foods may delay drug absorption.

STEP	RATIONALE
5 Dispose of all contaminated supplies in appropriate receptacle, remove and dispose of gloves, and perform hand hygiene.	Reduces transmission of microorganisms. Use appropriate disposal receptacle if patient is receiving hazardous medications (Oncology Nursing Society, 2018).
6 Perform postprocedure protocol.	
7 Replenish stock such as cups and straws, return cart to medication room, and clean work area.	Enhances efficiency and reduced transfer of microorganisms.
8 Evaluate patient response.	
a Return to bedside to evaluate patient's response to medications at times that correlate with onset, peak, and duration of the medication.	Evaluates therapeutic benefit of medication and helps to detect onset of side effects or allergic reactions. Sublingual medications act in 15 minutes; most oral medications act in 30 to 60 minutes.
b Ask patient or family caregiver to identify medication name and explain purpose, action, dose schedule, and potential side effects.	Determines level of knowledge gained by patient and family caregiver.

Recording and Reporting

- Record drug, dose, route, and time administered on patient's MAR immediately after administration. Include initials or signature.
- Record patient's response to medication.
- Document evaluation of patient learning.
- If medication is withheld, record reason on flow sheet or in EHR and follow agency policy for noting withheld doses.
- Report adverse effects/patient response and/or withheld critical drugs to nurse in charge or health care provider.

UNEXPECTED OUTCOMES	RELATED INTERVENTIONS
1 Patient exhibits adverse effects (e.g., side effect, toxic effect, allergic reaction).	• Notify health care provider and pharmacy. • Withhold further doses. • Assess vital signs. • Symptoms such as urticaria, rash, pruritus, rhinitis, and wheezing may indicate an allergic reaction and need for emergency medications or medical response. • Add allergy information to patient's medical record.
2 Patient refuses medication.	• Assess why patient is refusing medication. • Provide further instruction. • Do not force patient to take medications. • Notify health care provider.
3 Patient is unable to explain drug information.	• Further assess patient or family caregiver knowledge of medications and guidelines for drug safety. • Further instruction or different approach to instruction may be necessary.

Oral Medications Administered Through a Feeding Tube

Patients who have enteral feeding tubes are unable to receive food or medications by mouth. Nasogastric feeding tubes generally are small-bore tubes that are inserted into the stomach via one of the nares (see Skill 24). For long-term enteral feedings, a percutaneous endoscopic gastrostomy tube or a jejunostomy tube may be inserted surgically. ***Never administer medications into nasogastric tubes that are inserted for the purpose of decompression.***

To administer oral medications safely via the enteral route, ensure the enteral access connector is an ENFit connector. The International Organization for Standardization recommended the ISO 80369 series connector (trademarked ENFit) to avoid misconnection between two unrelated delivery systems (e.g., enteral syringe connected to an intravenous catheter), which can cause patient injuries or deaths (Institute for Safe Medication Practices [ISMP], 2020c). To address patient safety issues, The Joint Commission (TJC) and the American Society for Parenteral and Enteral Nutrition have strongly recommended widespread implementation of ENFit. The ENFit has a reverse Luer-Lok connector with twist-in functionality compared with traditional friction-held connectors (Medline, 2022).

Medications administered by enteral tubes should preferably be in liquid form. However, when the liquid form of the medication is not available, check with a pharmacist to determine whether an oral medication tablet or capsule can be crushed or dissolved for medication administration. Hospital pharmacies may be able to provide the prescribed medication in a liquid suspension, which does not affect its effectiveness (ISMP, 2020a). However, *do not crush* sublingual, sustained-release, chewable, long-acting, or enteric-coated medications.

Safety Guidelines

- Always verify correct placement of a nasogastric tube before administering oral medications by enteral route (refer to agency policy) (see Skill 24).
- Always follow the seven rights of medication administration when administering a medication via an enteral feeding tube.
- Be vigilant during preparation and administration of oral medications.

513

Delegation

The skill of administering oral medications by enteral feeding tubes cannot be delegated to assistive personnel (AP). Instruct the AP to:

- Keep the head of the bed elevated a minimum of 30 degrees (preferably 45 degrees) for 1 h after medication administration (follow agency policy).
- Immediately report coughing, choking, gagging, or drooling of liquid.
- Report the occurrence of possible medication side effects (specific to medication).

Collaboration

- Consult with the hospital pharmacist about whether certain medications can be crushed or dissolved.

Equipment

- Medication administration record (MAR) (electronic or printed)
- Appropriate medication syringe or 60-mL Asepto syringe for large-bore tubes only
- Enteral-only connector (ENFit) designed to fit the specific enteral tube (TJC, 2018) (Fig. 45.1)
- Gastric pH test strip (scale of 1.0 to 11.0)
- Graduated container
- Medication to be administered (usually pre-prepared in the medication syringe)
- Pill crusher if medication in tablet form (if indicated)
- Water or sterile water for immunocompromised patients
- Tongue blade or straw to stir dissolved medication
- Clean gloves
- Stethoscope and pulse oximeter (for evaluation)

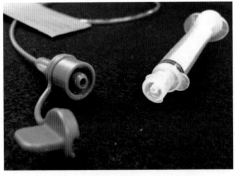

Fig. 45.1 ENFit connector and syringe.

STEP	RATIONALE

1 Perform preprocedure protocol.

Assessment

- Check accuracy and completeness of MAR or computer printout with health care provider's original medication order. Check patient's name, medication name and dosage, route of administration, and time of administration. Clarify incomplete or unclear orders with health care provider before administration.

The order sheet is the most reliable source and only legal record of medications that patient is to receive. Ensures that patient receives the correct medications (Palese et al., 2019). Transcription errors are a source of medication errors (Zhu and Weingart, 2022).

- Review medication reference information for action, purpose, normal dose and route, side effects, time of onset and peak action, indications, and nursing implications.

Allows for anticipation of medication effects and observation of patient response.

- Ask patient to describe history of allergies: known type(s) of allergies and normal allergic reaction(s). Enter medication allergies and prominently display on patient MAR and/or medical record. When indicated, patient should wear an allergy bracelet. Check patient's allergy wristband before medication administration.

Do not prepare medication if there is a known patient allergy. Communication of patient allergies is essential for safe medication administration.

- Review electronic health record (EHR) and assess for contraindications to receiving enteral medications, including presence of bowel inflammation, reduced peristalsis, recent gastrointestinal (GI) surgery, and gastric suction that cannot be temporarily turned off.

Alterations in GI function can interfere with drug absorption, distribution, and excretion. Patients with GI suction do not benefit from medication because it may be suctioned from the GI tract before it is absorbed.

Continued

STEP	RATIONALE
• For postoperative patient, review postoperative orders for type of enteral tube care.	Manipulation and irrigation of tube or instillation of medications may be contraindicated.
• Perform hand hygiene. Gather and review physical assessment data (e.g., bowel sounds, abdominal distention) and laboratory data (e.g., renal and liver function) that may influence medication administration.	Reduces transmission of microorganisms. Physical examination findings or laboratory data may contraindicate drug administration.
• Check with pharmacy for availability of liquid preparation for patient's medications. Prescriber may need to change dosage form.	When possible, liquid formulation of the medication is the best option. The agency pharmacy may have the ability to provide a liquid preparation that is compatible with the enteral nutrition formula (Boullata et al., 2017).
• Avoid complicated medication schedule that interrupts enteral feedings. Check with health care provider and use alternative medication route when possible.	Ensures proper medication administration route. Avoids medication interactions.
• Assess where medication is absorbed and ensure that point of absorption is not bypassed by feeding tube. For example, some antacids are absorbed in the stomach. If the enteral tube is placed in the intestine, medication may not be absorbed.	Proper administration will ensure absorption of medication.
• Determine whether medication interacts with enteral feedings. If there is a risk of interaction, stop feeding for at least 20 minutes before administering medication (check agency policy).	Interaction can cause feeding to congeal and clog feeding tube.

STEP	RATIONALE

Implementation

1 Explain to patient signs and symptoms to expect from medication. Allow time for patient to ask questions.

Lessens anxiety by helping patient know what to expect, promoting self-care.

2 Prepare medication without interruptions/distractions. Create a quiet environment. Keep all pages of MAR or computer printouts for one patient together or look at only one patient's electronic MAR at a time.

Interruptions contribute to medication errors (Palese et al., 2019).

3 Perform hand hygiene. Prepare medications for one patient at a time using aseptic technique. Check label of medication carefully with MAR or computer printout when removing medication from storage and after preparation. Check expiration date. Return expired medications to pharmacy. Prepare medications for instillation into feeding tube (see Skill 44). Fill graduated container with 50 to 100 mL of tepid water. Use sterile water for immunocompromised or critically ill patients (Boullata et al., 2017).

Reduces transmission of microorganisms. *These are the first and second checks for accuracy.* Preparation process ensures that right patient receives right medication. Tepid water prevents abdominal cramping, which can occur with cold water.

CLINICAL JUDGMENT *Whenever possible, use liquid medications instead of crushed tablets. If crushed tablets must be used, flush the tubing before and after the medication administration to prevent the medication from adhering to the inside of the tube. In addition, make sure that concentrated medications are thoroughly diluted. Never add crushed medications directly to a tube feeding (Boullata et al., 2017; Lord, 2018).*

Continued

STEP	RATIONALE

CLINICAL JUDGMENT *There is limited data surrounding enteral tube administration of most oral chemotherapies (Spencer et al., 2020). Check pharmacist for safe administration.*

a	*Tablets:* Crush each tablet into a fine powder, using pill-crushing device. Dissolve each tablet in separate cup of 30 mL of warm water.	Fine powder dissolves more easily, reducing chance of occluding feeding tube.
b	*Capsules:* Ensure that contents of capsule (granules or gelatin) can be expressed from covering (consult with pharmacist). Apply gloves, and open capsule or pierce gel cap with sterile needle and empty contents into 30 mL of warm water (or solution designated by pharmaceutical company). Gel caps dissolve in warm water, but this may take 15 to 20 minutes.	Ensures that contents of capsules are in solution to prevent occlusion of tube.
c	Prepare liquid medication according to Skill 44.	
4	Never add medications directly to a container or bag of tube feeding. Sometimes stopping or holding of tube feeding may be required during medication administration. Verify this and the amount of holding time needed with agency policy.	Prevents feeding tube occlusion and ensures timely administration of full dose.

STEP	RATIONALE
5 Take medication(s) to patient at correct time (see agency policy). Medications that require exact timing include stat, first-time or loading doses, and one-time doses. Give time-critical scheduled medications (e.g., antibiotics, anticoagulants, insulin, anticonvulsants, immunosuppressive agents) at exact time ordered (no later than 30 minutes before or after scheduled dose). Give non–time-critical scheduled medications within a range of 1 or 2 h of scheduled dose (CMS, 2020). During administration, apply seven rights of medication administration. Perform hand hygiene.	Hospitals must adopt medication administration policy and procedure for timing of medication administration that considers nature of the prescribed medication, specific clinical application, and patient needs (ISMP, 2011; US Department of Health and Human Services, 2020). Time-critical scheduled medications are those for which early or delayed administration greater than 30 minutes before or after the scheduled dose may cause harm or result in substantial suboptimal therapy or pharmacological effect. Non–time-critical medications are those for which early or delayed administration within a specified range of either 1 or 2 h should not cause harm or result in substantial suboptimal therapy or pharmacologic effect (US Department of Health and Human Services, 2020; CMS, 2020).
6 Identify patient using at least two identifiers (e.g., name and birthday or name and medical record number) according to agency policy. Compare identifiers with information on patient's MAR or medical record.	Ensures correct patient. Complies with The Joint Commission standards and improves patient safety (TJC, 2023).

Continued

STEP	RATIONALE
7 At patient's bedside again compare MAR or computer printout with names of medications on medication labels and patient name. Ask patient again about allergies.	*This is the third check for accuracy* and ensures that patient receives correct medication. Confirms patient's allergy history.
8 Assist patient to sitting position. Elevate head of bed to minimum of 30 degrees and preferably 45 degrees (unless contraindicated) or sit patient up in a chair (Boullata et al., 2017).	Keeping head above stomach reduces risk for aspiration..
9 If continuous enteral tube feeding is infusing, adjust infusion pump setting to hold tube feeding.	Feeding solution should not infuse while residuals are checked or medications are administered. The presence of a feeding solution may impede drug absorption (Boullata, 2017).
10 Apply clean gloves. Auscultate for presence of bowel sounds. Verify placement of feeding tube (see Skill 24) by observing gastric contents and checking pH of aspirate contents. *Gastric pH less than 5.5 is a good indicator that tip of tube is correctly placed in stomach* (Boullata et al., 2017; Metheny et al., 2019).	Presence of bowel sounds indicates gastric peristalsis. Verification of feeding tube ensures proper tube placement and reduces risk of introducing fluids into respiratory tract and subsequent aspiration.

STEP	RATIONALE
11 Check for gastric residual volume (GRV). Draw up 10 to 30 mL of air into a 60-mL syringe and connect syringe to ENFit connector on feeding tube. Flush tube with air and pull back slowly to aspirate gastric contents. Determine GRV using either scale on syringe or a graduate container. Return aspirated contents to stomach unless a single GRV exceeds 250 mL (see agency policy). When GRV is excessive, hold medication and contact health care provider (Boullata et al., 2017).	GRV categories have been identified in studies as significant when patients have two or more GRVs exceeding 500 mL (Boullata et al., 2017). Large residuals indicate delayed gastric emptying and put patient at increased risk for aspiration (Boullata et al., 2017; Burcham and Rosenthal, 2022).

CLINICAL JUDGMENT *Standards (Boullata et al., 2017; IOS, 2020). Do not attach the enteral tubing to a standardized Luer syringe or needleless device (IOS, 2020).*

STEP	RATIONALE
12 Irrigate the tubing. Pinch or clamp enteral tube and remove syringe. Draw up 30 mL of water into syringe. Reinsert tip of syringe onto connector of tube, release clamp, and flush tubing. Clamp tube again and remove syringe.	Pinching or clamping tubing prevents leakage or spillage of stomach contents. Flushing ensures that tube is patent.

Continued

STEP	RATIONALE
13 Administer medication: a Attach medication syringe to connector port on the enteral feeding tube. Ensure there is an airtight connection between the syringe and enteral tube and administer medication slowly.	Ensures delivery of medications.

CLINICAL JUDGMENT *If oral medication comes in a bulk container or if dose is small, pharmacy should prepare the patient-specific dose in an oral or enteral syringe (ISMP, 2021).*

STEP	RATIONALE
b After giving only one dose of medication, flush tubing with 30 to 60 mL of water after administration.	Maintains patency of enteral tube and ensures that medication passes through tube to stomach (Boullata et al., 2017).
c To administer more than one medication, give each separately and flush between medications with 15 to 30 mL of water.	Allows for accurate identification of medication if dose is spilled. In addition, some medications may be incompatible, and giving medication separately followed by a flush solution decreases the risk for medication incompatibilities (Boullata et al., 2017).
d Follow last dose of medication with 30 to 60 mL of water.	Maintains patency of enteral tube and ensures passage of medication into stomach (Boullata et al., 2017).
14 Clamp proximal end of feeding tube (if tube feeding is not being administered) and cap end of tube.	Prevents air from entering stomach between medication doses.

STEP	RATIONALE
15 When continuous tube feeding is being administered by infusion pump, disconnect infusion pump and administer medication as ordered, followed by at least 15 mL of water, and then immediately reattach infusion pump. If medications are not compatible with feeding solution, hold feeding for additional 30 to 60 minutes (Boullata et al., 2017; Burchum and Rosenthal, 2022).	Allows for adequate absorption of medication and avoids potential drug-food interaction between medication and enteral feeding (Boullata et al., 2017).
16 Dispose of all contaminated supplies in appropriate receptacle, remove and dispose of gloves, and perform hand hygiene.	Reduces transmission of microorganisms. Use appropriate disposal receptacle if patient is receiving hazardous medications (Oncology Nursing Society, 2018).
17 Perform postprocedure protocol.	
18 Evaluate patient response:	
a Observe patient for signs of aspiration, such as choking, gurgling, garbled speech, breath sounds, and difficulty breathing.	Provides for prompt intervention if aspiration has occurred.
b Return within 30 minutes to evaluate patient's response to medications.	Monitoring patient's response evaluates therapeutic benefit of medication and helps detect onset of side effects or allergic reactions.

Recording and Reporting

- Record method used to check for tube placement, GRV, and pH of aspirate. Record drug, dose, route, and time administered immediately on MAR after administration.
- Document evaluation of patient learning.

- Record total amount of water used for medication administration on intake and output form.
- Report adverse effects/patient response and withheld drugs to nurse in charge or health care provider.

UNEXPECTED OUTCOMES	RELATED INTERVENTIONS
1 Patient exhibits signs of aspiration, including respiratory distress, changes in vital signs, or changes in oxygen saturation.	• Stop all medications/fluids through feeding tube. • Elevate head of bed and stay with patient. • Assess vital signs and breath sounds while another staff member notifies health care provider.
2 Patient does not receive medication because of blocked enteral tube.	• For newly inserted tube, notify health care provider and obtain x-ray film confirmation of placement. • Requires interventions to unclog tube to ensure drug delivery (Box 45.1).

BOX 45.1   Unclogging a Blocked Feeding Tube

- Prevent tube from becoming blocked by flushing it with at least 15 to 30 mL of tepid water before and after administering each dose of medication (30 to 60 mL after last dose of medication), before and after checking gastric residual volumes, and every 4 to 12 h around the clock (refer to agency policy).
- Gently flush tube with large-bore syringe and warm water. Do not use small-bore syringe because this exerts too much pressure and may rupture tube.
- If irrigation with water is not effective, obtain an order for a pancrelipase tablet and follow manufacturer guidelines for tube irrigation. In addition, a declogging stylus may be used (see agency policy).
- If urgent medication administration is required, the tube may have to be removed and a new one inserted.

Data from Boullata J, et al: ASPEN safe practices for enteral nutrition therapy, *JPEN J Parenter Enteral Nutr* 41(1):15, 2017.

UNEXPECTED OUTCOMES	RELATED INTERVENTIONS
3 Patient exhibits adverse effects (side effect, toxic effect, allergic reaction).	• Withhold further doses. • Always notify health care provider and pharmacy when patient exhibits adverse effects. • Symptoms such as urticaria, rash, pruritus, rhinitis, and wheezing indicate allergic reaction. • Enter patient allergy in medical record.

Ostomy Care (Colostomy and Ileostomy Pouching)

Immediately after a fecal surgical diversion, it is necessary to place a pouch over a newly created stoma (an artificial opening into the colon or small intestine) on the abdomen to contain effluent when the stoma begins to function. The pouch keeps a patient clean and dry, protects the skin from damage, and provides a barrier against odor. A cut-to-fit, transparent pouching system is preferred because it protects the peristomal skin, allows the stoma to be visualized, and adapts to changes in stoma size as swelling decreases after surgery.

A stoma may be budded (lining of the intestine appears on surface of abdomen) (Fig. 46.1) or a stoma may be flush or retracted (lining of intestine not visible, stoma is flat). Immediately after surgery, a stoma may be edematous, and the abdomen distended. These symptoms will resolve over a 4- to 6-week period after surgery, but during this time it will be necessary to revise the pouching system to meet the changing size of the stoma and the changes in body contours (Colwell and Goldberg, 2021).

There are many types of pouching systems. All have a protective layer that adheres to the skin (a *skin barrier* or *wafer)* and a pouch. The wafer is a solid skin barrier that creates an adhesive seal and protects the skin around the stoma (Wound, Ostomy, and Continence Nurses Society, [WOCN] 2018). A one-piece pouching system has two parts integrated together. A two-piece system has a separate skin barrier and pouch. The flush or retracted stoma may require a convex wafer for successful placement of a pouch. This type of wafer provides gentle pressure on the peristomal skin to push the stoma through the opening in the wafer. You apply the pouch to the skin barrier by attaching it to a flange (a plastic ring) on the wafer. Use the skin barrier with a flange that fits the corresponding size pouch from the same manufacturer to avoid leakage between the skin barrier and the pouch. Some pouching systems have precut openings in the barrier for the stoma, whereas others need to be custom cut to size for a patient's stoma measurement. Be sure you understand how to use each of these different pouching systems before applying them to patients (Colwell and Goldberg, 2021).

The risk of medical adhesive related skin injury (MARSI) is low when ostomy pouches are applied and removed correctly. Most ostomy products have wafers that do not require additional skin barrier.

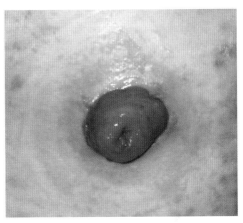

Fig. 46.1 Budded stoma. (Courtesy Jane Fellows.)

Safety Guidelines

- Empty ostomy pouches when they are one-third to one-half full to avoid leakage, which can lead to chemical or enzymatic injury to the skin.
- Know the signs/appearance of a healthy stoma and surrounding skin:
  - Color/moisture: Stoma should be red or pink and moist. Report a gray, purple, black, or very dry stoma to the health care provider immediately.
  - Size: In the 4 to 6 weeks after surgery, the stoma will likely decrease in size as postoperative edema and abdominal distention decrease.
  - Peristomal skin: Skin is normally intact with some reddening after the adhesive wafer is removed. Presence of blisters, a rash, or excoriated skin is abnormal and could indicate maceration or medical adhesive--related skin injury (MARSI) (Fumarola et al., 2020).
- Wear gloves during pouch and stoma care to reduce exposure to and transmission of infectious microorganisms.

Delegation

The skill of pouching a new ostomy should not be delegated to assistive personnel (AP). In some agencies care of an established ostomy (2 to 3 weeks or more after surgery) can be delegated to AP. Direct the AP about:

- The expected amount, color, and consistency of drainage from patient's ostomy.
- The expected appearance of the stoma.

- Special equipment needed to complete pouching.
- Changes in a patient's stoma and surrounding skin integrity that should be reported.

Collaboration

- Refer to a wound, ostomy, continence nurse (WOCN), when available, for postsurgical assessment, selection of proper barrier and pouch, and patient education regarding self-care.

Equipment

- Skin barrier/pouch: clear, drainable one-piece or two-piece, cut-to-fit or precut size
- Pouch closure device such as a clip, if needed
- Ostomy measuring guide
- Adhesive remover
- Clean gloves
- Washcloth
- Towel or disposable waterproof barrier
- Basin with warm tap water
- Scissors
- Waterproof bag for disposal of pouch
- Gown or goggles (optional if there is any risk of splashing when emptying pouch)

STEP	RATIONALE
1 Perform preprocedure protocol.	
Assessment	
• Review patient's electronic health record (EHR), including nurse's notes for type of intestinal diversion, type of pouching system used, and whether patient has any problems related to stoma.	Allows for anticipation of supplies needed and if special skin care is required.
• Ask patient to describe history of allergies: known type(s) of allergies and normal allergic reaction(s). Check patient's allergy wristband. Focus on adhesive and latex.	Reduces risk for exposing patient to allergens that can cause localized or systemic allergic reactions. Presence of an allergy affects your choice of a skin barrier and whether use of latex should be avoided.

STEP	RATIONALE
• Identify patient's history: age, dehydration, malnutrition, exposure to radiation therapy, underlying chronic conditions (e.g., diabetes, immunosuppression) and edema of skin.	Common risk factors for MARSI (Fumarola et al., 2020). Factors raise level of observation if patient has a pouching system with adhesive.
• Perform hand hygiene and apply clean gloves.	Reduces transmission of microorganisms.
• Note: Inspection of pouch and stoma can be deferred until just before pouch change. With patient lying supine or semi-reclining, observe existing skin barrier and pouch system for leakage and check EHR for length of time in place. Pouch should be changed every 3 to 7 days (Colwell and Goldberg, 2021). If an opaque pouch is being used, remove it to fully observe stoma.	Assesses effectiveness of pouching system and detects potential for problems. To minimize skin irritation and MARSI, avoid unnecessary changing of entire pouching system. When pouch leaks, skin damage from effluent causes more skin trauma than early removal of wafer (Colwell and Goldberg, 2021).

CLINICAL JUDGMENT *Repeated leaking may indicate need for different type of pouch or addition of products such as stoma paste or seal. If the pouch is leaking, change it. Taping or patching it to contain effluent leaves the skin exposed to chemical or enzymatic irritation.*

• Observe and measure amount of effluent in pouch and empty it before it is 1/3 to 1/2 full (WOCN, 2018) by opening the pouch and draining it into a container for measurement of output. Note consistency of effluent and record intake and output.	Weight of pouch may disrupt seal of adhesive on skin. Monitors fluid balance and bowel function after surgery. Normal colostomy effluent is soft or formed stool, whereas normal ileostomy effluent is liquid.

Continued

STEP	RATIONALE
• Remove used pouch and skin barrier gently by pushing skin away from barrier in direction of hair growth (WOCN, 2018). Loosen and lift the edge with one hand and press down on the skin near the sticky backing with the other hand. It may be helpful to start at the top and work down to the bottom for better visualization of removal. This also allows the pouch to catch any urine or stool the stoma produces (WOCN, 2018). Use adhesive remover to facilitate removal of skin barrier. With stoma exposed, observe type, location, color, swelling, presence of sutures, trauma, and healing or irritation of peristomal skin.	Method reduces risk of skin stripping or tears. Stoma characteristics influence selection of an appropriate pouching system. Convexity in skin barrier is often necessary with a flush or retracted stoma (Colwell and Goldberg, 2021).
• Assess peristomal skin for temperature, color, moisture level, turgor, fragility, and integrity. Observe for local signs of irritation or skin damage, e.g., stripping or blisters, where any adhesive has been or will be applied.	Signs and symptoms of MARSI (Fumarola et al., 2020).
• Inspect area, noting location of stoma in relation to abdominal contours and presence of scars or incisions. Remove and dispose of gloves; perform hand hygiene.	Determines whether current pouching system is effective or whether new selection is needed. Abdominal contours, scars, or incisions affect type of system and adhesion to skin surface. Reduces transmission of microorganisms.

STEP	RATIONALE
• Explore patient's attitudes, perceptions, knowledge of stoma and ostomy care, and acceptance of stoma and change in functioning. Discuss interest in learning self-care. Identify others who will be helping patient after leaving hospital.	Determines patient's willingness to learn. Assesses patient's body image. Facilitates teaching plan and timing of care to coincide with availability of family caregivers (Goldberg et al, 2018).

Implementation

STEP	RATIONALE
1 Have patient stay in semi-reclining or supine position. (*Note:* Some patients with established ostomies prefer to stand.) If possible, provide patient with mirror for observation.	When patient is semi-reclining, there are fewer skinfolds, which allows for ease of application of pouching system.
2 Perform hand hygiene and apply clean gloves.	Reduces transmission of microorganisms.
3 Place towel or disposable waterproof barrier under patient and across patient's lower abdomen.	Protects bed linen; maintains patient's dignity.
4 If not done during assessment, remove used pouch and skin barrier at this time, inspect stoma and peristomal skin, and empty pouch. Dispose of pouch in an appropriate receptacle. Measure output if needed. *Note:* There may be no output at time of first pouch change.	Reduces skin trauma. Improper removal of pouch and barrier can cause peristomal skin irritation or breakdown. A patient with new stoma may not yet have normal peristalsis. Use of adhesive releaser reduces risk of MARSI (Fumarola et al, 2020).

Continued

STEP	RATIONALE
5 Clean peristomal skin gently with warm tap water using washcloth; do not scrub skin. Minor bleeding is normal when touching stoma. Pat skin dry. Have washcloth handy for additional cleaning if there is output from the stoma while preparing pouch.	Soap leaves residue on skin, which may irritate skin. Pouch does not adhere to wet skin. Ileostomies have frequent output, especially after eating.
6 Measure stoma (Fig. 46.2) by placing measuring guide over stoma. Expect size of stoma to change for first 4 to 6 weeks after surgery.	Allows for proper fit of pouch that will protect peristomal skin. Swelling is related to normal postoperative response.
7 Trace pattern of stoma measurement on pouch backing or skin wafer (Fig. 46.3).	Prepares for cutting opening in pouch.

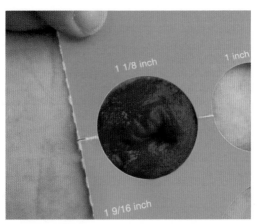

Fig. 46.2 Measure stoma. (Courtesy Coloplast, Minneapolis, MN.)

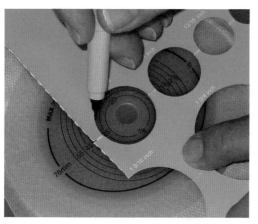

Fig. 46.3 Trace measurement on pouch backing. (Courtesy Coloplast, Minneapolis, MN.)

STEP	RATIONALE
8 Cut opening on pouch wafer or skin barrier wafer (Fig. 46.4). If using a moldable or shape-to-fit barrier, use fingers to mold barrier over stoma.	Customizes pouch to provide appropriate fit over stoma.

CLINICAL JUDGMENT *Instruct patients to remeasure stomas occasionally if they notice that the stoma has changed shape or size (Colwell and Goldberg, 2021).*

STEP	RATIONALE
9 Remove protective backing from adhesive backing or wafer (Fig. 46.5).	Prepares skin barrier for placement on skin over stoma.
10 Apply pouch over stoma (Fig. 46.6). Press firmly into place around stoma and outside edges. Have patient hold hand over pouch to apply heat to secure seal.	Pouch adhesives are heat- and pressure-sensitive and hold more securely at body temperature.

Continued

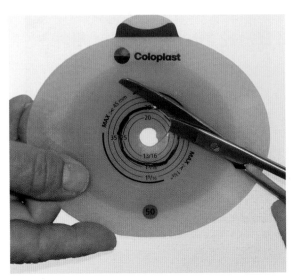

Fig. 46.4 Cut opening in protective wafer. (Courtesy Coloplast, Minneapolis, MN.)

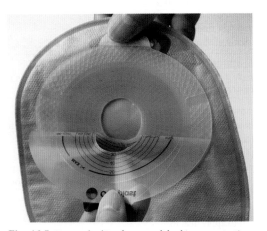

Fig. 46.5 Remove backing from pouch backing or protective wafer. (Courtesy Coloplast, Minneapolis, MN.)

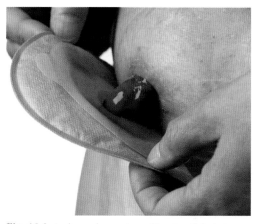

Fig. 46.6 Apply pouch over stoma. (Courtesy Coloplast, Minneapolis, MN.)

STEP	RATIONALE
11 Close end of pouch with clip or integrated closure. Remove drape from patient.	Ensures that pouch is secure. Contains effluent.
12 Perform postprocedure protocol.	
13 Evaluate patient response:	
a Observe condition of skin barrier and adherence of pouch to abdominal surface.	Determines presence of leaks.
b Observe appearance of stoma, peristomal skin, abdominal contours, and suture line during pouch change.	Determines condition of stoma and peristomal skin and progress of wound healing.
c Note whether there is flatus during pouch change.	Determines whether peristalsis is returning.

Continued

STEP	RATIONALE
d Observe patient's and family caregiver's willingness to view stoma and ask questions about procedure.	Determines level of adjustment and understanding of stoma care and pouch application. Allows planning for future education needs and progress toward acceptance of altered body image (Colwell and Goldberg, 2018).

Recording and Reporting

- Record type of pouch and skin barrier applied, time of procedure, amount and appearance of effluent in pouch, location, size and appearance of stoma, and condition of peristomal skin.
- Record patient and family caregiver's level of participation, teaching performed, and evaluation of learning.
- Report any of the following to nurse and/or health care provider: abnormal appearance of stoma, suture line, peristomal skin, or character of output.

UNEXPECTED OUTCOMES	RELATED INTERVENTIONS
1 Skin around stoma is irritated, blistered, or bleeding or a rash is noted. May be caused by undermining of pouch seal by fecal contents, causing irritant dermatitis, or by adhesive removal causing skin stripping, or by MARSI.	• Remove pouch more carefully. • Change pouch more frequently or use different type of pouching system. • Consult WOCN. • Avoid use of alcohol or acetone-based products. • Follow skin care guidelines for MARSI (Fumarola et al., 2020). • Avoid excessively washing the skin and use a pH-balanced soap or plain water to avoid drying the skin. Handle skin with care.

UNEXPECTED OUTCOMES	RELATED INTERVENTIONS
2 Necrotic stoma manifesting with purple or black color, dry instead of moist texture, failure to bleed when washed gently, or tissue sloughing.	• Report to nurse in charge or health care provider immediately. • Document appearance.
3 Patient refuses to view stoma or participate in care.	• Obtain referral for ostomy care nurse. • Allow patient to express feelings. • Encourage family support.

Oxygen Therapy

Various pulmonary diseases (e.g., pneumonia, chronic lung diseases) require the use of oxygen therapy. Pneumonia is the inflammation of lung tissue with buildup of mucous in the alveoli. This pathological process impairs gas exchange, decreasing the diffusion of oxygen from the lungs to the arterial blood supply. Patients with chronic lung disease such as emphysema suffer enlargement of alveoli, a decrease in gas exchange surface area, and loss of lung elasticity. These patients may require home oxygen therapy 24 h a day; therefore, care is taken to plan administration around patient needs (ATS, 2020; Huether et al., 2020).

Oxygen therapy is inexpensive, widely available, and used in a variety of settings. The type of oxygen-delivery system selected is based on a patient's need for oxygen support, the severity of the hypoxia/hypoxemia, and the disease process. Consider other factors such as the patient's age and developmental level, health status and orientation, presence of an artificial airway, the setting (home or hospital), type of home environment when applicable, and type of support and care needed after discharge.

Oxygen-delivery devices are classified into either high-flow or low-flow devices, depending on how much oxygen they deliver to the patient. Health care providers consider how much oxygen a device delivers as well as its effects on the patient's respiratory pattern when choosing an oxygen-delivery device. High-flow devices include Venturi mask (Fig. 47.1), large-volume nebulizers, and blender masks. A newer type of high-flow device is the high-flow nasal cannula (Fig. 47.2). Low-flow devices include the traditional nasal cannula and simple face mask, nonrebreather, and partial rebreather masks (Fig. 47.3). These devices deliver fixed percentages of oxygen, and each one has advantages and disadvantages. You can estimate an approximate fraction of inspired oxygen (FiO_2) by the flow rate. Collaborate with a respiratory therapist.

An oxygen flowmeter connects to an oxygen source to regulate the flow rate in liters per minute. A variety of oxygen sources are used in health care facilities ranging from wall connections at patient's bedsides or cylinders or oxygen tanks. In addition, smaller, easily transported cylinders are available for home oxygen therapy. Patients requiring home oxygen commonly use concentrators, some of which are portable.

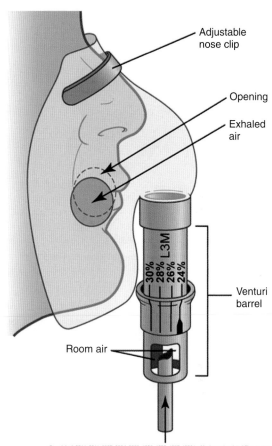

24% **26%** **28%** **30%** L3M

Labels: Adjustable nose clip, Opening, Exhaled air, Venturi barrel, Room air

Fig. 47.1 Venturi mask.

Safety Guidelines

- Supplemental oxygen therapy is treated as a medication. Obtain patient's most recent hemoglobin values and past and current arterial blood gas (ABG) values to assess oxygenation.
- Place an "Oxygen in Use" sign on the door of patient's hospital room or residence. Keep oxygen-delivery systems at least 1.5 meters (5 feet) from any heat source. Oxygen supports combustion, but

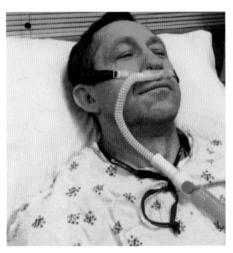

Fig. 47.2   High-flow nasal cannula. (Courtesy Fisher & Paykel Healthcare, Irvine, CA.)

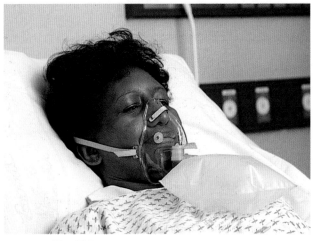

Fig. 47.3   Partial rebreather mask with reservoir bag.

will not explode. Caution visitors or family caregivers that smoking is not allowed when oxygen is in use.
- When using oxygen cylinders, secure them so they will not fall over. Store oxygen cylinders upright, chained, or in appropriate holders.
- Patients infected with Covid-19 can develop worsening "silent" atelectasis and decline rather abruptly, even without numerous symptoms. Covid-19 may cause hypoxemia with relatively little respiratory distress ("silent hypoxemia") Therefore, work of breathing cannot be relied upon to detect patients who are developing respiratory failure (Internet Book of Critical Care, 2020).

Delegation

Certain agencies allow delegation of the skill of applying a nasal cannula or oxygen mask to assistive personnel (AP) (check agency policy). The nurse is responsible for assessing patient's respiratory system, response to oxygen therapy, and setup of oxygen therapy, including adjustment of oxygen flow rate. Direct the AP by:
- Informing how to safely adjust the device (e.g., loosening the strap on the oxygen cannula or mask) and clarifying correct placement and positioning.
- Instructing to report immediately any changes in vital signs or respiratory symptoms; skin irritation from the cannula, mask, or straps; or patient reports of pain or breathlessness.
- Instructing when to provide extra skin care around patient's ears and nose to prevent skin breakdown.

Collaboration

- Health care providers are responsible for prescribing the oxygen-delivery device, the flow rate, and the amount of oxygen to deliver.
- Respiratory therapists are usually responsible for setup of oxygen-delivery devices.
- Physical therapists, occupational therapists, and speech therapists should be informed of patient pulmonary status, oxygen requirements, and tolerance to activity to accurately and safely perform prescribed therapies.

Equipment

- Oxygen-delivery device (as ordered)
- Oxygen tubing (consider extension tubing)

- Humidifier, if indicated
- Sterile water for humidifier
- Clean gloves and other personal protective equipment (PPE) as patient condition warrants
- Oxygen source
- Oxygen flowmeter
- Appropriate "Oxygen in Use" sign (as required by health care agency)
- Pulse oximeter
- Stethoscope
- *Option:* gauze pads as needed for padding device around ear, skin
  Note: If device is used in the home, the home care equipment vendor provides the equipment.

STEP	RATIONALE
1 Perform preprocedure protocol.	

Assessment

• Review patient's electronic health record (EHR), including health care provider's order and nurses' notes. Include patient's vital signs, pulse oximetry values, baseline and trends in respiratory rate and effort of breathing, medical history, past oxygen requirements, and most recent ABG results.	Information helps to explain the amount of oxygen to deliver, patient's past responses to oxygen, and patient's trends in breathing rate and effort. Ensures safe and accurate oxygen administration. Safe oxygen delivery includes the seven rights of medication administration.
• Review patient's EHR for order for oxygen, noting delivery method, flow rate, duration of oxygen therapy, and parameters for titrating oxygen settings.	Ensures safe and accurate oxygen administration.
• Perform hand hygiene and apply clean gloves.	Reduces transmission of microorganisms.

STEP	RATIONALE
• Perform respiratory assessment, including symmetry of chest wall expansion, chest wall abnormalities (e.g., kyphosis), temporary conditions (e.g., pregnancy, trauma) affecting ventilation, respiratory rate and depth, sputum production, and lung sounds.	Changes in ventilation and gas exchange resulting in hypoxia require oxygen therapy. Signs of hypoxia: Apprehension, anxiety, behavioral changes Decreased level of consciousness, confusion, drowsiness Increased pulse rate (Note: In late-stage cardiac disease, the pulse rate may not increase.) Cardiac dysrhythmias Elevated blood pressure, evolving to decreased blood pressure Increased rate and depth of respiration or irregular respiratory patterns Decreased lung sounds, adventitious lung sounds (e.g., crackles, wheezes) Pulse oximetry (SpO2) less than 90% Dyspnea
• Observe for cognitive and behavioral changes, fatigue, and dizziness.	Decreased levels of oxygen (hypoxia) or increased levels of carbon dioxide (hypercapnia) affect a person's cognitive abilities, interpersonal interactions, and mood (Harding et al., 2020).

CLINICAL JUDGMENT *Patients with sudden changes in vital signs, level of consciousness, or behavior may be experiencing profound hypoxia. Patients who show subtle changes over time may have worsening of a chronic or existing condition or a new medical condition (Harding et al., 2020).*

Continued

STEP	RATIONALE
• Assess airway patency and remove airway secretions by having patient cough and expectorate mucus or by suctioning (see Skill 71). Auscultate lung sounds. *Note:* Remove and dispose of gloves and perform hand hygiene if there is contact with mucus. Reapply gloves if further contact with mucus is likely.	Secretions obstruct the airway, decreasing amount of oxygen that is available for gas exchange in lungs.

CLINICAL JUDGMENT *Excessive amounts of secretions, signs of respiratory distress (increased work of breathing, increased respiratory rate), presence of rhonchi on auscultation, excessive coughing, or decrease in patient oxygen saturation indicate need for suctioning.*

STEP	RATIONALE
• Inspect condition of skin around nose and ears. Note whether patient has history of impaired sensation, poor perfusion, altered tissue tolerance, poor nutrition, edema, and the tendency for moisture to develop under device.	Provides baseline for monitoring development of a medical device–related pressure injury (MDRPI). Risk factors for MDRPI (The Joint Commission [TJC], 2018).
• Remove and discard gloves as indicated; perform hand hygiene.	Prevents transmission of organisms.
• If patient will require home oxygen therapy, assess knowledge and experience of patient and family caregiver with oxygen administration.	Helps to determine teaching needed for patient and family caregiver as well as opportunity to correct any misinformation. Helps to identify comfort level with the skill.

STEP	RATIONALE
Implementation	
1 Instruct patient and/or family caregiver about need for oxygen. If the oxygen is for home use, educate patient about oxygen safety in the home and the equipment that will be used.	Education decreases patient and caregiver anxiety. Proper education about the use of and need for oxygen equipment helps to ensure safe and proper use of the equipment.
2 Perform hand hygiene. Apply PPE: a Face shield if risk of exposure to splashing mucus exists. b Gloves if patient has oral or nasal secretions. c Gown if agency policy requires or if there is risk of excessive splashing of secretions.	Reduces transmission of microorganisms.
3 Position patient comfortably in semi-Fowler position.	Minimizes caregiver's muscle strain and prevents injury. Position promotes ventilation.
4 Connect oxygen-delivery device (e.g., cannula, mask) to oxygen tubing and attach end of tubing to humidified (if needed) oxygen source. Adjust to prescribed flow rate.	Humidity prevents drying of nasal and oral mucous membranes and airway secretions. Flowmeters with smaller calibrations may be required for patients requiring low-dose oxygen such as pediatric patients or patients with chronic obstructive pulmonary disease (Hockenberry et al., 2019; Walsh and Smallwood, 2017).
5 Apply oxygen device as ordered. Ensure that the patient receives the proper size and type of device; that the device is secure, to decrease movement or slippage; and that the skin is padded, to reduce friction (TJC, 2018).	Correct selection and fit of device reduces occurrence of MDRPI.

Continued

STEP	RATIONALE
a Place tips of the nasal cannula into patient's nares. If tips are curved, they should point downward inside nostrils. Next, loop cannula tubing up and over patient's ears. Adjust lanyard so cannula fits snugly (but not too tightly) without pressure to patient nares and ears.	Tips of cannula direct flow of oxygen into patient's upper respiratory tract.
b Apply oxygen mask by placing over patient's mouth and nose. Bring straps over patient's head and adjust to form a comfortable but tight seal (see Fig. 47.1).	A properly fitting device is one that does not create pressure on nares or ears and is comfortable. Patient is more likely to keep it in place and risk for MDRPI is reduced (Barakat-Johnson et al., 2019).
6 Maintain sufficient slack on oxygen tubing.	Allows patient to turn head without causing mask to shift position or dislodge nasal cannula.
7 Observe for proper function of oxygen-delivery device:	Ensures patency of delivery device and accuracy of prescribed oxygen flow rate.
a *Nasal* cannula: Positioned properly in nares; oxygen flows through tips.	Provides prescribed oxygen rate and reduces pressure on tips of nares.
b *Oxygen-conserving cannula:* Fit same as for nasal cannula. Reservoir is located under patient's nose or worn as a pendant.	Delivers higher flow of oxygen than with nasal cannula. Delivers 2:1 ratio (e.g., 6 L/min nasal cannula is approximately equivalent to 3.5 L/min with oxygen-conserving cannula device).

STEP	RATIONALE
c *Nonrebreather mask:* Application same as regular mask. Contains one-way valves with reservoir; exhaled air does not enter reservoir bag. Can be combined with nasal cannula to provide higherFiO$_2$.	Device of choice for short-term high FiO$_2$ delivery. Valves on mask side ports permit exhalation but close during inhalation to prevent inhaling of room air.
d *Simple face mask:* Select appropriate flow rate.	Used for short-term oxygen therapy.
e *Venturi mask* (see Fig. 47.1): Select appropriate flow rate.	Used when high-flow device is desired.
f *High-flow nasal cannula* (see Fig.47.2): Fit same as for nasal cannula.	Provides adjustable O$_2$ delivery and flow rates that assist in reducing the work of breathing while increasing oxygen delivery (Drake, 2018).

CLINICAL JUDGMENT *Changing gloves and performing hand hygiene may need to be performed more often than indicated with these steps. If the gloves become contaminated with secretions while applying the delivery device, they should be changed before touching flowmeters or side rails to prevent transmission of organisms.*

8 Verify setting on flowmeter and oxygen source for proper setup and prescribed flow rate.	Ensures delivery of prescribed oxygen therapy in conjunction with specific cannula/mask.
9 Check cannula/mask and humidity device (if used) and condition of underlying skin every 4 to 8 h or as agency policy indicates. Ensure that humidity container is filled at all times.	Ensures patency of cannula and oxygen flow. Prevents MDRPI. Oxygen is a dry gas; you must add humidification to prevent thickening of secretions, minimize atelectasis, and prevent heat loss.

Continued

STEP	RATIONALE
10 Post "Oxygen in Use" signs on wall behind bed and at entrance to room (check agency policy).	Alerts visitors and care providers that oxygen is in use. No smoking allowed.
11 Perform postprocedure protocol.	
12 Evaluate patient response:	
a Monitor patient's response to changes in oxygen flow rate with SpO$_2$. *Note:* Monitor ABGs when ordered; however, ABG measurement is an invasive procedure, and ABGs are not measured frequently.	Continual monitoring with SpO$_2$ is required for patients on oxygen therapy. Changes in supplemental oxygen should be based on individual patient's oxygen saturation levels.
b Perform respiratory assessment: auscultate lung sounds; palpate chest excursion; inspect color and condition of skin; and observe for decreased anxiety, improved level of consciousness and cognitive abilities, decreased fatigue, and absence of dizziness. Obtain vital signs.	Evaluates patient's response to supplemental oxygen. As patient's oxygen level improves, physical signs and symptoms should improve.
c Assess adequacy of oxygen flow each shift or as agency policy dictates.	Ensures patency of oxygen-delivery device.
d Observe patient's external ears, bridge of nose, nares, and nasal mucous membranes for inflammation, skin tears, ulcers, or edema.	Oxygen therapy sometimes dries out nasal mucosa. The oxygen-delivery device can cause MDRPI where device contacts patient's face, neck, and ears (Barakat-Johnson et al., 2019).

Recording and Reporting

- Record the respiratory assessment findings, method of oxygen delivery, oxygen flow rate, skin integrity and patient's response to intervention, and any adverse reactions or side effects.
- Document evaluation of patient and family caregiver learning.
- Report patient status, including recent assessment findings, ongoing oxygen flow rate, vital signs, SpO2, and skin integrity before and after oxygen administration.
- Include patient response to the flow rate adjustments and effectiveness of interventions.
- Report any unexpected outcome to health care provider or nurse in charge.

UNEXPECTED OUTCOMES	RELATED INTERVENTIONS
1 Patient experiences skin irritation or breakdown (e.g., at ears, bridge of nose, nares, other pressure areas), sinus pain, or epistaxis.	• Increase humidification to oxygen-delivery system for epistaxis and sinus pain. • Provide appropriate skin/wound care (keep skin dry, do not use alcohol-containing soaps). Do not use petroleum-based gel around oxygen because it is flammable.
2 Patient experiences continued hypoxia.	• Notify health care provider: Obtain order for follow-up SpO_2 monitoring or ABG determinations. • Consider measures to improve airway patency, including but not limited to coughing techniques and oropharyngeal or orotracheal suctioning.

Continued

UNEXPECTED OUTCOMES	RELATED INTERVENTIONS
3 Patient experiences nasal and upper airway mucosa drying.	• If oxygen flow rate is greater than 4 L/min, use humidification. At rates greater than 5 L/min, dry nasal mucous membranes, and pain in frontal sinuses may develop (Harding et al., 2020). • Assess patient's fluid status and increase fluids if appropriate. • Provide frequent oral care.

Parenteral Medication Preparation: Ampules and Vials

Preparing parenteral injections requires drawing up single doses of medication from either ampules or vials. Using aseptic technique during preparation ensures a sterile medication dose will be administered to a patient.

Ampules are available in single-dose sizes containing from 1 to 10 mL or more. They are made of glass with a constricted, prescored neck that is snapped off to allow access to medication. A colored ring around the neck indicates where the ampule is prescored to be broken easily.

Vials are available in single-dose or multidose plastic or glass container with a rubber seal at the top. A single-dose vial should be discarded after opening, regardless of the amount of medication used. A multidose vial contains several doses of a medication and thus can be used several times. Vials contain liquid or dry forms of medications; medications that are unstable in solution are packaged in dry form. The vial label specifies the solvent or diluents used to dissolve the medication and the amount needed to prepare a desired medication concentration. Normal saline and sterile distilled water are the most common solutions.

Two-chambered vials have two chambers separated by a rubber stopper. One chamber contains the diluent solution; the other contains the dry medication. Before preparing the medication, push on the upper chamber to dislodge the rubber stopper and allow the powder and the diluent to mix. Gently roll the vial to mix the diluent and medication powder; do not shake.

Safety Guidelines

- Use filter needles when preparing medication from a glass ampule to prevent glass particles from being drawn into the syringe (Painchart et al., 2018). Do not use the filter needle to administer the medication. Place an appropriate-size needle on the syringe after withdrawing the medication.
- In perioperative and other procedural settings both on and off a sterile field, label medications and solutions that *are not immediately* administered. This applies even if there is only one medication being used (The Joint Commission [TJC], 2021b).

- In perioperative or procedural settings, labeling a medication is not necessary if it is immediately administered. An immediately administered medication is one that an authorized staff member prepares or obtains, takes directly to a patient, and administers to that patient with no break in the process (TJC, 2023).

Delegation

- The skill of preparing injections from ampules and vials cannot be delegated to assistive personnel.

Collaboration

- Agency pharmacist is a resource for safe medication administration.

Equipment

Medication in an Ampule

- Syringe, sharps with engineered sharps injury protections (SESIP) needle, and filter needle
- Small sterile gauze pad or unopened antiseptic swab

Medication in a Vial

- Syringe and two needles
- Needles:
  - SESIP needle with safety sheath or needleless blunt-tip vial access cannula (Fig. 48.1) for drawing up medication (if needed). Note: Needleless blunt-tip access cannulas are used for preparing and administering medications intravenously (IV) (see Skill 35).
  - Filter needle, if indicated
- Small, sterile gauze pad or antiseptic swab
- Diluent (e.g., 0.9% sodium chloride or sterile water if indicated)

Both

- Medication administration record (MAR) or computer printout
- SESIP safety needle for injection
- Medication in vial or ampule
- Puncture-proof container for disposing of syringes, needles, and glass

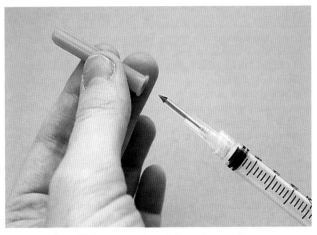

Fig. 48.1 Syringe with needleless vial access adapter.

STEP	RATIONALE

Assessment

- Check accuracy and completeness of each MAR or computer printout with health care provider's written medication order. Check patient's name, medication name and dosage, route of administration, and time of administration. Clarify incomplete or unclear orders with health care provider before administration.

  The order sheet is the most reliable source and only legal record of medications that patient is to receive. Ensures that patient receives the correct medications (Palese et al., 2019). Transcription errors are a source of medication errors (Palese et al., 2019).

- Review medication reference for medication action, purpose, normal dose and route, side effects, time of onset and peak action, indication, and nursing implications.

  Allows anticipation of effects of medication while observing patient response.

Continued

STEP	RATIONALE
• Assess patient's medical and medication history and history of allergies. List medication allergies on each page of the MAR and prominently display on patient's medical record. When allergies are present, patient should wear an allergy bracelet.	Factors influence actions of certain medications. Reveals patient's need for medication. Allergy alert helps prevent adverse effects.
• Perform hand hygiene.	Prevents transmission of microorganisms. Determines type and size of syringe and needle for injection. Some doses based on patient weight.
• Assess patient's body build, muscle size, and weight if giving subcutaneous or intramuscular (IM) medication. Confirm patient's weight.	

Implementation

STEP	RATIONALE
1 Plan medication preparation to avoid interruptions/distractions. Keep all pages of MARs or computer printouts for one patient together, or look at only one patient's electronic MAR at a time.	Interruptions contribute to medication errors (Palese et al., 2019).
2 Prepare medications.	
a If using a medication cart, move it outside patient's room.	Organizing equipment saves time and reduces error.
b Unlock medication drawer or cart or log onto automated dispensing machine (ADM).	Medications are safeguarded when locked in cabinet, cart, or ADM.
c Select correct medication from stock supply or unit-dose drawer. Compare label of medication with MAR computer printout or computer screen.	*This is the first check for accuracy.*

STEP	RATIONALE
d Check expiration date on each medication separately.	Expired medications are often inactive, less effective, or harmful to patients.
e Calculate medication dose as necessary. Double-check your calculations. For high-risk medications, have another nurse independently double-check dosage (see agency policy).	Double-checking reduces error. Independent double checks should be used only for very selective high-alert medications that require this safeguard (Institute for Safe Medication Practices [ISMP], 2020a).
f Do not leave medications unattended.	Nurse is responsible for safekeeping of medications.
3 Preparing ampule.	
a Tap top of ampule lightly and quickly with finger until fluid moves from its neck (Fig 48.2)	
b Place small gauze pad around neck of ampule (Fig. 48.2).	Protects fingers from trauma as glass tip is broken off. Do not use opened antiseptic swab to wrap around top of ampule because antiseptic may leak into ampule.
c Snap neck of ampule quickly and firmly away from hands (see Fig. 48.3).	Protects your fingers and face from shattering glass.
d Ampule is an open system. Draw up medication quickly, using a filter needle long enough to reach bottom of ampule to access medication.	System is open to airborne contaminants. Filter needles filter out any fragments of glass (Painchart et al., 2018).
e Hold ampule upside down or set it on flat surface. Insert filter needle into center of ampule opening. Do not allow needle tip or shaft to touch rim of ampule.	Broken rim of ampule is considered contaminated. When ampule is inverted, solution dribbles out if needle tip or shaft touches rim of ampule.

Continued

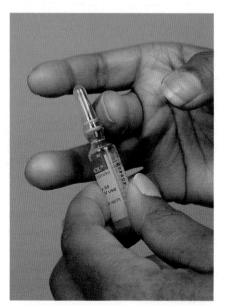

Fig. 48.2 Tapping moves fluid down ampule neck.

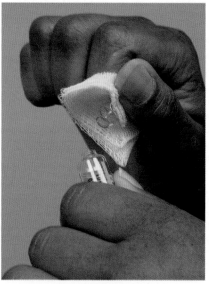

Fig. 48.3 Neck snapped away from hands.

STEP	RATIONALE
f Gently pull back on syringe plunger to aspirate medication into syringe (Fig. 48.4).	Withdrawing plunger creates negative pressure within syringe barrel, which pulls fluid into syringe.
g Keep needle tip under surface of liquid. Tip ampule to bring all fluid within reach of needle.	Prevents aspiration of air bubbles.
h If aspiration of air bubbles occurs, do not expel air into ampule.	Air pressure forces fluid out of ampule, and medication will be lost.

Continued

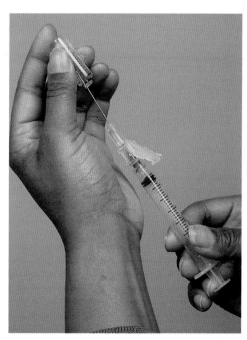

Fig. 48.4 Medication aspirated with ampule inverted.

STEP	RATIONALE
i To expel excess air bubbles, remove needle from ampule. Hold syringe vertically with needle pointing up. Tap side of syringe to cause bubbles to rise toward needle. Draw back slightly on plunger and push plunger upward to eject air. Do not eject fluid.	Withdrawing plunger too far removes it from barrel. Holding syringe vertically allows fluid to settle in bottom of barrel. Pulling back on plunger allows fluid within needle to enter barrel so fluid is not expelled. You then expel air at top of barrel and within needle.
j If syringe contains excess fluid, use sink for disposal. Hold syringe vertically with needle tip up and slanted slightly toward sink. Slowly eject excess fluid into sink. Recheck fluid level in syringe by holding it vertically.	Safely disperses excess medication into sink. Position of needle allows expelling of medication without having it flow down needle shaft. Rechecking fluid level ensures proper dose.
k Cover needle with safety sheath or cap. Replace filter needle with regular SESIP needle.	Minimizes needlesticks. Filter needles cannot be used for injection.
4 Preparing vial	
a Remove cap covering top of unused vial to expose sterile rubber seal. If a multidose vial has been used before, cap is already removed. Firmly and briskly wipe surface of rubber seal with antiseptic swab and allow it to dry.	Vial is packaged with cap that cannot be replaced after seal removal. Not all drug manufacturers guarantee that rubber seals of unused vials are sterile. Swabbing with antiseptic reduces transmission of microorganisms. Drying the antiseptic prevents antiseptic from coating needle and mixing with medication.

STEP	RATIONALE
b A vial is a closed system requiring injection of air. Pick up safety syringe and remove needle cap or cap covering needleless access device. Pull back on plunger to draw amount of air into syringe equivalent to volume of medication to be aspirated from vial.	Injecting air into vial prevents buildup of negative pressure in vial when aspirating medication.

CLINICAL JUDGMENT *Some medications and/or agencies require use of a filter needle when preparing medications from vials. Check agency policy or medication reference. After preparing medication with filter needle, replace with a regular SESIP needle of the appropriate size to administer medication (Antoszyk et al., 2018).*

c With vial on flat surface, insert tip of safety needle or needleless device through center of rubber seal (Fig. 48.5). Apply pressure to tip of needle during insertion.	Center of seal is thinner and easier to penetrate. Using firm pressure prevents dislodging rubber particles that could enter vial or needle.
d Inject air into air space of vial, holding onto plunger. Hold plunger firmly; plunger is sometimes forced backward by air pressure within vial.	Injection of air creates vacuum needed for medication to flow into syringe. Injecting into air space of vial prevents formation of bubbles and an inaccurate dose.
e Invert vial while keeping firm hold on syringe and plunger. Hold vial between thumb and middle fingers of nondominant hand (Fig. 48.6). Grasp end of syringe barrel and plunger with thumb and forefinger of dominant hand to counteract pressure in vial.	Inverting vial allows fluid to settle in lower half of container. Position of hands prevents forceful movement of plunger and permits easy manipulation of syringe.

Continued

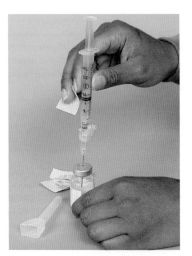

Fig. 48.5 Insert safety needle through center of vial diaphragm (with vial flat on table).

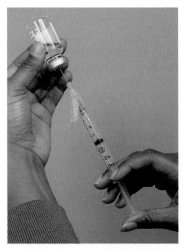

Fig. 48.6 Withdraw fluid with vial inverted.

STEP	RATIONALE
f Keep tip of SESIP needle, or needleless device below fluid level.	Prevents aspiration of air.
g Allow air pressure from vial to fill syringe gradually with medication. If necessary, pull back slightly on plunger to obtain correct amount of medication.	Positive pressure within vial forces fluid into syringe.
h When you obtain desired volume, position SESIP needle or needleless device into air space of vial; tap side of syringe barrel gently to dislodge any air bubbles. Eject any air remaining at top of syringe into vial.	Forcefully striking barrel while needle is inserted in vial may bend needle. Accumulation of air displaces medication and causes dose errors.
i Remove needle or needleless access device from vial by pulling back on barrel of syringe.	Pulling plunger rather than barrel causes plunger to separate from barrel, resulting in loss of medication.
j Hold syringe at eye level at 90-degree angle to ensure correct volume and absence of air bubbles. Tap barrel to dislodge any remaining air/bubbles (Fig. 48.7). Draw back slightly on plunger; then push it upward to eject air. Do not eject fluid. Recheck volume of medication.	Holding syringe vertically allows fluid to settle in bottom of barrel. Tapping dislodges bubbles to top of barrel. Pulling back on plunger allows fluid within needle to enter barrel so fluid is not expelled. You then expel air at top of barrel and within needle.

CLINICAL JUDGMENT *When preparing medication from single-dose vial, do not assume that volume listed on label is the same as total volume in vial. Some manufacturers provide small amount of extra liquid, expecting loss during preparation. Be sure to draw up correct volume.*

Continued

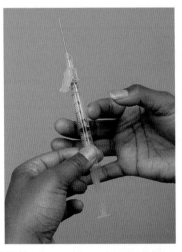

Fig. 48.7 Hold syringe upright; tap barrel to dislodge air bubbles.

STEP	RATIONALE
k Before injecting medication into patient's tissue, change needle with regular SESIP to appropriate gauge and length according to route of medication administration. (*Exception:* If giving IV, blunt-tip device can remain on syringe.)	Inserting needle through rubber stopper dulls beveled tip. New needle is sharper and, because no fluid is along shaft, does not track medication through tissues. Filter needles cannot be used for injection.
l Cover needle with safety sheath or cap.	Minimizes needlesticks.
m Label multidose vial with date of opening, concentration of drug per milliliter, and your initials.	Ensures that information is available for future doses to be prepared correctly. Some drugs are discarded within a certain time frame after mixing.

STEP	RATIONALE
5 Prepare vial containing powder:	
a Remove cap covering vial of powdered medication and cap covering vial of appropriate diluent. Firmly swab both rubber seals with antiseptic swab and allow antiseptic to dry.	Reconstituting medication prevents antiseptic from coating needle and mixing with medication.
b Draw up volume and diluent type suggested by medication manufacturer into syringe following Steps 4b through 4l.	Prepares diluent in syringe for injection into vial containing powdered medication.
c Next, insert tip of needle or needleless device through center of rubber seal of vial of powdered medication. Inject diluent into vial. Remove needle.	Diluent begins to dissolve and reconstitute medication.
d Mix medication thoroughly by rolling side to side between palms of your hands. *Do not shake.*	Ensures proper dispersal of medication throughout solution and prevents formation of air bubbles.
e Reconstituted medication in vial is now ready to be drawn into new syringe for administration. Read label carefully to determine dose after reconstitution.	Once you add diluent, concentration of medication (mg/mL) determines dose to be given. Reading medication label carefully decreases medication errors.
f Draw up reconstituted medication into new syringe. Insert SESIP needle or needleless device into vial. *Do not add air.* Then follow Steps 4b through 4l.	Prepares medication for administration.

CLINICAL JUDGMENT *Some agencies require that doses of certain medications (e.g., insulin and heparin) be checked using an independent double check by another nurse (ISMP, 2020a). Check policies and procedures before administering medication.*

Continued

STEP	RATIONALE
6 Compare medication label against MAR, computer screen, or computer printout.	*This is the second check for accuracy.*
7 Vials and/or ampules and the syringe may contain barcodes. Both will go to the bedside and the barcodes are scanned before administration.	Prevents medication errors.
8 Dispose of soiled supplies. Place broken ampule and/or used vials and used SESIP needle or needleless device in puncture- and leak-proof container. Clean work area and perform hand hygiene.	Controls transmission of infection. Proper disposal of glass and needle prevents accidental injury to staff.
9 Take prepared medication to bedside. Just before administering drug to patient, compare MAR with label of prepared drug and compare dose in syringe with desired dose.	Ensures that dose is accurate. This is the *third check for accuracy.*

UNEXPECTED OUTCOMES	RELATED INTERVENTIONS
1 Air bubbles remain in syringe.	• Expel air from syringe and add medication, if needed, until you prepare correct dose.
2 Incorrect dose of medication is prepared.	• Discard prepared dose and prepare new dose.

Parenteral Medication Preparation: Mixing Medications in One Syringe

Some medications require preparation that involves mixing from two vials or from a vial and an ampule. Mixing compatible medications avoids the need to give a patient more than one injection. Most patient care facilities have medication compatibility resources (charts or internet/intranet databases). Contact a pharmacist with questions about medication compatibility. When mixing medications, correctly aspirate fluid from each type of container. When using multidose vials, do not contaminate the contents of the vial with medication from another vial or ampule.

Prepare medications from a vial first if mixing an ampule and vial. Then withdraw medication from the ampule using the same syringe and a filter needle. When mixing medications from two vials, do not contaminate one medication with another. Be sure the final dose is accurate, and maintain aseptic technique.

In some situations, for patients who are ordered to receive a combination of different types of insulin, mixing of insulins from two different vials may be required. Although this is becoming less common, it is important to understand how to mix insulins properly. Before drawing up insulin doses, gently roll a cloudy insulin preparation between the palms of the hands to resuspend the insulin. Do not shake insulin vials because this causes bubbles to form. Bubbles take up space in a syringe and alter the dose (Burchum and Rosenthal, 2022). Always prepare the short- or rapid-acting insulin first to prevent it from being contaminated with the longer-acting insulin (Burchum and Rosenthal, 2022).

Safety Guidelines

- Confirmation of accurate insulin preparation requires a second nurse to verify accurate insulin type and accurate dose.
- Do not mix insulin with any other medications or diluents unless approved by the health care provider.
- Never mix insulin glargine or insulin detemir with other types of insulin.
- Inject rapid-acting insulins mixed with NPH insulin within 15 minutes before a meal.

Delegation
- Mixing of two medications in a syringe cannot be delegated to AP.

Collaboration
- Agency pharmacist has information about insulin onset, peak, and duration if not readily available through other sources.

Equipment
- Single-dose or multidose vials and ampules containing medication
- Syringe and two needles: (needleless blunt-tip vial access cannula or engineered sharps injury protection (SESIP) needle), filter needle if indicated
- Antiseptic swab
- Puncture-proof container for disposing of syringes, needles, and glass
- Medication administration record (MAR) or computer printout
- Medication label

STEP	RATIONALE
Assessment	
• Check accuracy and completeness of MAR or computer printout with health care provider's written medication order. Check patient's name, medication name and dosage, route of administration, and time of administration. Recopy or reprint any part of MAR that is difficult to read.	The order sheet is the most reliable source and only legal record of medications that patient is to receive. Ensures that patient receives the correct medications (Palese et al., 2019). Transcription errors are a source of medication errors (Palese et al., 2019).
• Review medication reference for medication action, purpose, side effects, and nursing implications	Allows for safe medication administration and monitoring of patient response to therapy.
• Consider compatibility of medications to be mixed, and type of injection.	

STEP	RATIONALE
• Assess electronic health record (EHR) for medical and medication history and history of allergies. List medication allergies on each page of the MAR and prominently display on the patient's medical record. When allergies are present, patient should wear an allergy bracelet.	Knowing patient's condition allows you to monitor patient response. Reduces risk of allergic reaction.
• Perform hand hygiene.	Reduces transmission of microorganisms.
• Assess patient body build, muscle size, and weight if giving subcutaneous or intramuscular medication. Confirm patient weight.	Many medication doses are based on accurate weight, calculated by health care provider or pharmacist.

Implementation

1 Plan preparation to avoid interruptions/distractions. Keep all pages of MARs or computer printouts for one patient together, or look at only one patient's electronic MAR at a time.	Interruptions contribute to medication errors (Palese et al., 2019).
2 Prepare medications:	
a If using a medication cart, move it outside patient's room. Unlock medication drawer or cart or log onto automated dispensing machine (ADM).	Organization of equipment saves time and reduces error. Medications are safeguarded when locked in cabinet, cart, or ADM.
b Select correct medication from stock supply or unit-dose drawer. Compare medication label with MAR computer printout or computer screen.	*This is the first check for accuracy.*

Continued

STEP	RATIONALE
c Check expiration date separately for each medication.	Expired medications are often inactive, less effective, or harmful to patients.
d Calculate medication dose as necessary. Double-check calculations. For high-risk medications (e.g., insulin), ask another nurse to perform an independent double check of dosage (see agency policy).	Double-checking reduces error. Independent double checks should be used only for very selective high-alert medications that require this safeguard (Institute for Safe Medication Practices [ISMP], 2020a).
e Do not leave medication dose unattended.	Principle of medication safety.
3 Mixing medications from two vials: (Fig. 49.1)	
a Take syringe with needleless device or filter needle and aspirate volume of air equivalent to first medication dose (vial A).	Ensures dose accuracy.

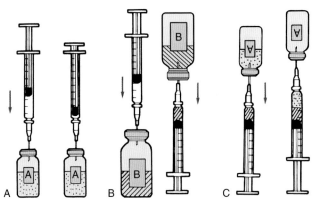

Fig. 49.1 (A) Injecting air into vial A. (B) Injecting air into vial B and withdrawing dose. (C) Withdrawing medication from vial A; medications are now mixed.

STEP	RATIONALE
b Inject air into vial A, making sure that needle or needleless device does not touch solution (Fig. 49.1A).	Especially important with multidose vials so that needle does not contaminate medication in vial B during insertion.
c Holding onto plunger, withdraw needle or needleless device and syringe from vial A. Aspirate air equivalent to second medication dose (vial B) into syringe.	
d Insert needle or needleless device into vial B, inject volume of air into vial B, and withdraw medication from vial B into syringe (Fig. 49.1B).	
e Withdraw needle or needleless device and syringe from vial B. Ensure that proper volume from vial B has been obtained.	Ensures correct dose from vial B.
f Using syringe markings, determine the appropriate combined volume of medications that should be measured and administered.	Ensures accurate total dose.
g Insert needle or needleless device into vial A, being careful not to push plunger and expel medication within syringe into vial. Invert vial and carefully withdraw the desired amount of medication from vial A into syringe (Fig. 49.1C).	Air previously injected with medication into vial A allows for easy removal of dose.

Continued

STEP	RATIONALE
h Withdraw needle or needleless device and expel any excess air from syringe. Check fluid level in syringe for proper total dose. Medications are now mixed.	Final check for dosage.

CLINICAL JUDGMENT *If too much medication is withdrawn from second vial, discard syringe and start over. Do not push medication back into either vial.*

i Change needle or needleless device to the appropriate-size SESIP needle to be used for medication injection. Keep needle or needleless device capped until administration time.	
4 Mixing insulins:	
a Mixing insulins is less common. When ordered, follow medication guidelines for appropriate vial to prepare first. If administering insulin that is cloudy, roll bottle of insulin between hands to resuspend preparation. Follow actions in Step 3, above, for mixing medications from two vials.	Mixing insulins does not ensure the total dose accuracy that a combination insulin provides.
5 Mixing medications from a vial and an ampule:	
a Prepare medication from vial first, following Skill 48.	

STEP	RATIONALE
b Utilizing syringe markings, determine the appropriate combined volume needed for both medications.	Ensures accurate total dosage.

CLINICAL JUDGMENT *If needleless access device was used in preparing medication from vial, change needleless system to a filter needle to remove medication from ampule.*

---

c Next, using the same syringe, prepare second medication from ampule, following Skill 48.	
d Withdraw filter needle from ampule and verify fluid level in syringe. Once dose confirmed, change filter needle to appropriate SESIP needle. Cap device or needle until ready to administer medication.	SESIP needle used for injections. *Exception:* If intravenous push medication is to be given, blunt cannula can be used.
c Check syringe carefully for total combined dose of medications. Label syringe.	Ensures correct dose. Labelling prevents administration to wrong patient.
6 Compare MAR, computer screen, or computer printout with prepared medication and labels on vials/ampules.	*This is the second check for accuracy.*
7 The vial and/or ampules and syringes must be saved if barcode scanning is required (ISMP, 2018). The labeled syringe is placed next to the vial and both barcodes are scanned at the bedside.	Used for patient identification and financial tracking of medications.

Continued

STEP	RATIONALE
8 Dispose of soiled supplies. Place used ampules and/ or vials and needle or needleless device in puncture- and leak-proof container.	Reduces transmission of microorganisms.
9 Take prepared medication to bedside. Just before administering medication to patient, compare MAR with label of prepared medication and compare dose in syringe with desired dose.	*This is the third check for accuracy.*

UNEXPECTED OUTCOMES	RELATED INTERVENTIONS
1 Air bubbles remain in syringe.	• Expel air from syringe and add medication until correct dose is prepared.
2 Incorrect dose of medication is prepared.	• Discard prepared dose and prepare new dose.

Patient-Controlled Analgesia

Patient-controlled analgesia (PCA) is an interactive method of pain management that gives patients pain control through self-administration of analgesics. PCA is typically administered intravenously (IV), through an epidural catheter, or a peripheral nerve catheter (Pastino and Lakra, 2022). PCA offers safe analgesic administration for acute and chronic pain, including pain that is postoperative, or related to trauma, labor and delivery, sickle cell crisis, myocardial infarction, cancer, and end of life (Pastino and Lakra, 2022). Research comparing use of subcutaneous versus IV opioids via PCA for cancer patients found that significant adverse effects were rarely observed (Nijland et al., 2019). Patients receive analgesic doses as needed by using a small, computerized pump to deliver a prescribed dose of medication with the push of a button. The three most common medications used in PCA are the opioids morphine, hydromorphone, and fentanyl.

Because patients depress a button on a PCA device to deliver a regulated dose of analgesic, they must be able to understand how, why, and when to self-administer medication and physically be able to depress the device. Family members must understand the purpose of the PCA, and the reason why they cannot push the PCA button for a patient. The exception is in the care of children, where some hospitals allow parents to press the device; this is called *authorized agent-controlled analgesia* (American Society of Pain Management Nursing, 2016). Nurses must advise patients, family, and other visitors that **PCA is for patient use only**. PCA is not recommended in situations in which oral analgesics could easily manage pain.

Safety Guidelines

- Patient safety is critical during PCA administration. Patient risk factors for oversedation and respiratory depression when using PCA include an opioid-naïve status; obesity; age (infants and small children or older adults); confusion; obstructive sleep apnea syndrome (OSAS); multiple co-morbid conditions such as lung, renal, heart and hepatic diseases; smoking; and dependence on medications (e.g., opioids, muscle relaxants, sleeping medications) (Gupta et al., 2018).
- Excess sedation (difficulty arousing) precedes respiratory depression, especially in opioid-naïve patients (i.e., patients who are not chronically receiving opioid analgesics on a daily basis) (Rosenquist, 2022). Using standardized sedation scales can prevent respiratory depression by observing and intervening for oversedation (Hall and Stanley, 2019).

573

Delegation

The skill of PCA administration cannot be delegated to assistive personnel (AP). Direct the AP to:

- Report if the patient complains of change in status, including unrelieved pain or difficulty awaking.
- Report if the patient has questions about the PCA process or equipment.
- Report if anyone other than the patient is observed administering a PCA dose.

Collaboration

- Nurses, health care providers, and pharmacists should collaborate to ensure appropriate PCA to oral or IV conversion, adjuvant medications, opioid reversal, and management of adverse effects.

Equipment

- PCA pump system and tubing
- Analgesic cartridge or syringe with identification label and time tape (may already be attached and completed by pharmacy)
- Needleless connector
- Antiseptic swab
- Nonallergenic tape
- Clean gloves (when applicable)
- Opioid-reversal agent (e.g., naloxone)
- Equipment for vital signs, pulse oximetry, and capnography
- Medication administration record (MAR)

STEP	RATIONALE
1 Perform preprocedure protocol.	
Assessment	
• Check accuracy and completeness of each MAR or computer printout with health care provider's written medication order. Check patient's name, medication name and dosage, route of administration, lockout period, and frequency of medication (demand, continuous, or both).	The order sheet is the most reliable source and only legal record of medications that patient is to receive. Ensures that patient receives the correct medications (Palese et al., 2019).

STEP	RATIONALE
• Review electronic health record (EHR) to assess patient's medical and medication history, including risk factors for opioid-induced respiratory depression (see safety guidelines).	Determines need for medication or possible contraindications for medication administration. In patients with underlying risk factors the dose of opioids should be carefully titrated.
• Review medication reference information for medication action, purpose, normal dose, side effects, time of peak onset, and nursing implications.	Allows safe medication administration and monitoring of patient response to therapy.
• Ask patient to describe history of allergies: known type(s) of allergies (including medications, latex, and adhesives) and normal allergic reaction(s). Check patient's allergy wristband.	Do not prepare medication if there is a known patient allergy. Communication of patient allergies is essential for safe medication administration.

CLINICAL JUDGMENT *When assessing allergies, be aware that nausea is not an allergic reaction, but a typical side effect that can be treated; likewise, pruritus alone is not an allergic reaction and is common to opioid use. Pruritus is treatable and does not contraindicate the use of PCA (Masato et al., 2017).*

STEP	RATIONALE
• Identify patient using at least two identifiers (e.g., name and birthday or name and medical record number) according to agency policy. Compare identifiers with information on patient's MAR or medical record.	Ensures correct patient. Complies with The Joint Commission (TJC) standards and improves patient safety (TJC, 2023).
• Assess patient's or family caregiver's knowledge and experience with PCA use. Review the importance of patient being only one to initiate PCA. Assess patient goal for pain relief.	Determines level of information patient will require to administer PCA safely.

Continued

STEP	RATIONALE
• Assess patient's current pain acuity and character of pain. Use appropriate pain scale of 0 to 10.	Provides baseline for patient response to PCA.
• Assess patient's vital signs and SpO_2. (*Option:* Assess capnography)	Baseline vital signs can provide early warning signs of respiratory depression.
• Assess patient's ability to manipulate PCA control, and cognitive status for ability to understand purpose of PCA and how to use control device.	Determines patient's ability to use PCA safely and correctly.
• Assess environment for factors that could contribute to pain (e.g., noise, room temperature).	Elimination of irritating stimuli may help to reduce pain perception.
• Assess for presence of known, untreated, or unknown obstructive sleep apnea syndrome (OSAS); condition poses risk for respiratory depression (Olson et al., 2022). Use the STOP-Bang questionnaire to assess the patient for OSAS (see agency policy (Olson et al., 2022).	Identifies patient risk for oversedation (should be completed before surgery by anesthesia or nursing). Identification allows health care providers to take appropriate precautions, such as providing continuous positive airway pressure (CPAP) or bi-level positive airway pressure (BiPAP) ventilation devices.
• Apply clean gloves. Assess patency of IV access and surrounding tissue for inflammation or swelling.	IV line needs to be patent for safe administration of pain medication.
• If patient has had surgery, don clean gloves and inspect incision. Gently palpate around area for tenderness. Use sterile gloves, if necessary, to place hand directly on incision. Remove and dispose of gloves and perform hand hygiene.	Status of incision influences level of patient discomfort. Unusual incisional pain, swelling, redness, and/or discharge may indicate infection. Reduces transmission of infection.

STEP	RATIONALE
Implementation	
1 Provide patient and family caregiver with individually tailored education, including information on procedure for administration and treatment options for management of postoperative pain with PCA. If the patient will need opioid therapy at home, a prescription for naloxone and training in the administration of naloxone should be given. Naloxone is available as a nasal spray and auto-injector (CDC, 2022). This is particularly important with patients who have a history of opioid addiction (Kampman and Jarvis, 2015).	It is important that the patient and family caregiver understand pain management with PCA, know how to administer it safely, and have realistic pain-control goals.
2 Perform hand hygiene. Eliminate any distractions during preparation of PCA. Follow the seven rights for medication administration. Obtain PCA analgesic in module prepared by pharmacy. Check label of medication two times: first when removed from storage, and second when preparing for assembly.	Reduces transmission of microorganisms. Ensures safe and appropriate medication administration. *These are the first and second check for accuracy.*
3 Recheck patient's identity at bedside, using at least two identifiers (e.g., name and birthday or name and medical record number) according to agency policy. Compare identifiers with information on patient's MAR or medical record.	Ensures correct patient. Complies with TJC standards and improves patient safety (TJC, 2023).

Continued

STEP	RATIONALE
4 At bedside, compare MAR or computer printout with name of medication on drug cartridge. Have second registered nurse (RN) confirm health care provider's order and correct setup of PCA. Second RN should perform an independent check of the order and the device, not just a verification of existing setup.	Ensures that correct patient receives right medication. *This is the third check for accuracy.*
5 Before initiating analgesia, reiterate the purpose of PCA and demonstrate function of PCA to patient and family caregiver:	It is important that the patient and family members understand how to use PCA safely. Allows for patient-centered care and improved patient outcomes with pain control (Shindul-Rothschild et al., 2017).
a Explain type of medication and method of delivery.	Informs patient of therapy to be received.

CLINICAL JUDGMENT *Background basal infusion of opioids has been associated with increased risk of nausea, vomiting, and respiratory depression. However, in opioid-tolerant patients, a background basal infusion may be necessary due to the potential for undertreatment and possible opioid withdrawal (Chou et al., 2016).*

---

b If a background basal rate is used, explain that device safely administers continuous medication, but self-initiated small, frequent amounts of medication can be administered for unrelieved pain by using the PCA button.	A background basal infusion delivers a continuous dose of analgesic medication. The PCA pump is programmed to allow additional patient-controlled doses for pain that is not relieved by the continuous infusion (breakthrough pain) (Stewart, 2017).

STEP	RATIONALE
c Explain that self-dosing is desirable because it aids patient in repositioning, walking, and coughing or deep breathing.	Promotes patient's participation in care; pain relief encourages early ambulation.

CLINICAL JUDGMENT *A patient using PCA who ambulates should have a nurse assist to decrease risk for falls.*

---

d Explain that device is programmed to deliver ordered type and dose of pain medication, lockout interval, and 1- to 4-h dosage limits. Explain how lockout time prevents overdose.	Relieves anxiety in patients who might be concerned about overdosing.
e Demonstrate to patient how to push medication demand button. Instruct family members not to push PCA button to give medication.	Administration by proxy is not recommended in adults (Chou et al., 2016).
f Instruct patient to notify nurse if experiencing side effects, if pain is not relieved, any changes in severity or location of pain, PCA pump alarm sounding, or questions about pump.	Engages patient as partner in care.
6 Apply clean gloves. Check infuser and patient-control module for accurate labeling or evidence of leaking.	Reduces transmission of infection. Avoids medication error and injury to patient.
7 Position patient to ensure that venipuncture or central-line site is accessible.	Ensures unimpeded flow of infusion.

Continued

STEP	RATIONALE
8 Insert drug cartridge into infusion device (see manufacturer's directions) and prime infusion tubing.	Locks system and prevents air from infusing into IV tubing.
9 Attach needleless adapter to tubing adapter of patient-controlled module.	Needed to connect with IV line.
10 Wipe injection port of maintenance IV line vigorously with antiseptic swab for 15 seconds and allow to dry.	Minimizes entry of surface microorganisms during needle insertion, reducing risk of catheter-related bloodstream infection.
11 Insert needleless adapter into injection port nearest patient. PCA tubing should not be available for administering IV push of other medications.	Establishes route for medication to enter main IV line. Needleless systems prevent needlestick injuries. Prevents medication interaction and incompatibility.
12 Secure connection and anchor PCA tubing onto patient's arm with tape. Label PCA tubing.	Prevents dislodging of needleless adapter from port. Facilitates patient's ability to ambulate. Label prevents error from connecting tubing from different device to PCA.
13 Program computerized PCA pump as ordered to deliver prescribed medication dose and lockout interval. Have second nurse check setting. (*Note:* Recheck with oncoming RN during shift hand-off to ensure line reconciliation.)	Ensures safe, therapeutic drug administration. With appropriate dose intervals (e.g., 10 minutes), an appreciable analgesic effect and/or mild sedation is typically achieved before patient can access the next dose; thus there is lower chance for oversedation and respiratory depression. A second nurse check reduces risk for medication error (Kane-Gill et al., 2017).
14 Administer loading dose of analgesia as prescribed. Manually give one-time dose or turn on pump and program dose into pump.	Establishes initial level of analgesia.

STEP	RATIONALE
15 Remove and discard gloves and used supplies in appropriate containers. Dispose of empty cassette or syringe in compliance with institutional policy. Perform hand hygiene.	Reduces transmission of microorganisms. The federal Controlled Substances Act regulates control and dispensation of opioids for all institutions.
16 If experiencing pain, have patient demonstrate use of PCA system; if not, have patient repeat instructions given earlier.	Repeating instructions reinforces learning. Checking patient's understanding through return demonstration helps determine patient's level of understanding and ability to manipulate device.
17 Be sure that venipuncture or central-line site is protected, and recheck infusion rate before leaving patient.	Ensures patency of IV line.
18 Perform postprocedure protocol.	
19 To discontinue PCA:	
a Check health care provider order for discontinuation. Obtain necessary PCA information from pump for documentation; note date, time, amount of medication infused, amount (if any) wasted and reason for wastage.	Ensures correct documentation of a Schedule II drug. Two RNs must witness wastage of opioids (narcotics) and sign record to meet requirements of the Controlled Substances Act for scheduled drugs.
b Perform hand hygiene and apply clean gloves. Turn off pump. Disconnect PCA tubing from primary IV line but maintain IV access.	Reduces transmission of microorganisms. Follow health care provider order for maintenance of IV site.

Continued

STEP	RATIONALE
c Dispose of empty cartridge, tubing, and soiled supplies according to agency policy. Remove and dispose of gloves and perform hand hygiene.	Reduces transmission of microorganisms.
20 Evaluate patient response:	
a Ask patient whether pain is relieved. Then use pain rating scale to evaluate patient's pain intensity after ambulation, treatments, and procedures according to agency policy.	Determines subjectively and objectively patient's response to PCA dosing. Documenting "PCA in use" or "PCA effective" is not an adequate record of patient's pain level.
b Observe patient for nausea or pruritus.	Common treatable side effects of opioids.
c Monitor patient's vital signs and level of sedation. It is recommended that the Pasero Opioid-Induced Sedation Scale (POSS) (see Box 24.1) be used to monitor for unintended patient sedation (Davis et al., 2017; Hall and Stanley, 2019). Monitoring should be frequent per agency policy and health care provider order (e.g., every 1 to 2 h for first 12 h for the first 24-h period after surgery). Monitor more often at start, during first 24 h, and at night when hypoventilation and hypoxia tend to occur during sleep.	Patient is at highest risk for oversedation and respiratory distress (OSRD) during the first 24 h of PCA administration. Although there is low sensitivity for detecting hypoventilation with pulse oximetry when supplemental oxygen is used, and evidence is insufficient to firmly recommend capnography (Chou et al., 2016), these interventions are used in monitoring for OSRD and provide important clinical information in your assessment.

STEP	RATIONALE
d Have patient demonstrate dose delivery.	Confirms skill in use of PCA.
e According to agency policy, evaluate number of attempts (number of times patient pushed button), delivery of demand doses (number of times drug actually given and total amount of medication delivered in particular time frame), and basal dose if ordered.	Helps evaluate effectiveness of PCA dose and frequency in relieving pain. Maintains compliance with Controlled Substances Act.
f Observe patient initiate self-care and deep breathing exercises.	Demonstrates pain relief.

Recording and Reporting

- Record on MAR appropriate medication, concentration, dose (basal and demand), time started, lockout time, and amount of solution infused and remaining per agency policy.
- Record assessment of patient's response to analgesic on PCA medication form, narrative notes, or patient assignment flow sheet (see agency policy), including vital signs, oximetry and capnography results, sedation status, pain rating, and status of vascular access device.
- Calculate infused dose: add demand and continuous doses together. Enter on appropriate flow sheet.
- Document evaluation of patient learning.
- Include in hand-off report detailed information regarding vital signs, pulse oximetry and capnography, pain-assessment scores, STOP-Bang score for OSAS if done, POSS sedation scores, level of consciousness, and activity level (Cooney, 2016; Meisenberg et al., 2017).
- During a hand-off report, the oncoming and outgoing nurse should inspect and agree with PCA pump programming as a means of medication reconciliation (Kane-Gill et al., 2017).
- Report signs of oversedation to health care provider immediately.

UNEXPECTED OUTCOMES	RELATED INTERVENTIONS
1 Patient verbalizes continued or worsening discomfort and/or displays nonverbal behaviors indicative of pain.	• Perform complete pain reassessment. • Assess for possible complications other than pain. • Inspect IV site for possible catheter occlusion or infiltration. • Evaluate number of attempts and deliveries initiated by patient and whether pump has operational problems. • Consult with health care provider.
2 Patient is sedated and not easily aroused.	• Stop PCA immediately. • Notify health care provider immediately. • Elevate head of bed 30 degrees unless contraindicated and instruct patient to take deep breaths (if able). • Apply oxygen at 2 liters/min per nasal cannula (if ordered). • Assess vital signs, oxygen saturation, and/or capnography. • Evaluate amount of opioid delivered within past 4 to 8 h. • Ask family members if they pressed button without patient's knowledge. • Review MAR for other possible sedating drugs. • Prepare to administer an opioid-reversing agent (e.g., naloxone). • Continue frequent observations.

UNEXPECTED OUTCOMES	RELATED INTERVENTIONS
3 Patient unable to manipulate PCA device to maintain pain control.	• Consult with health care provider regarding alternative medication route or the possibility of a basal (continuous) dose.

Peak Flowmeter

For patients who have changes in the flow of air through their airways, such as patients with asthma or reactive airway disease, peak expiratory flow rate (PEFR) measurements are useful. The PEFR is the maximum flow that a patient forces out during one quick, forced expiration. It is measured in liters per minute. Peak flow measures are an objective indicator of a patient's current airway status or the effectiveness of a treatment, e.g., bronchodilator or anti-inflammatory medication. Normal PEFR values vary according to a person's age, gender, and size (American Lung Association [ALA], 2020).

Patients with asthma perform PEFR measures in the home to monitor the status of their airways. Health care providers usually recommend that patients measure and record their PEFR preferably at the following times: same time every day (values are lowest in the morning and typically highest between noon and 5 p.m..), before taking asthma medicines, during asthma symptoms or an asthma attack, after taking medicine for an asthma attack, and at other times recommended by the health care provider (ALA, 2020).

Safety guidelines

- Recognizing changes from "normal" is important. A patient's health care provider will suggest the target zone to follow; however, the following are general guidelines (ALA, 2020):

Green Zone:

A reading of 80% to 100% of a patient's usual or "normal" PEFR signals all clear. A reading in this zone means asthma is under reasonably good control.

Yellow Zone:

A reading of 50% to 80% of a patient's usual or "normal" PEFR signals caution. Airways are narrowing and may require extra treatment. Refer to health care provider for a plan to adjust treatments for yellow zone readings.

Red Zone:

Less than 50% of a patient's usual or "normal" PEFR signals a medical alert. Severe airway narrowing may be occurring. Contact health care provider immediately.

Delegation

Initial assessment of a patient's condition is a nursing responsibility and cannot be delegated. The skills of follow-up PEFR measurements in a stable patient can be delegated to assistive personnel (AP). Instruct the AP to:

- Report immediately patient's difficulty breathing or a decrease (compared with normal readings) in PEFR measurement.

Collaboration

- Health care providers are responsible for prescribing any changes in medications/therapy based on PEFR measurements.
- Respiratory therapists are often responsible for administering nebulized medications necessitated by PEFR measurements.

Equipment

- Peak flowmeter (Fig. 51.1)
- Stethoscope
- Patient diary/action plan (if appropriate)
- Clean gloves (optional)

STEPS	RATIONALE
1 Perform preprocedure protocol.	
Assessment	
• Review electronic health record (EHR) for medical condition and baseline PEFR readings (if available).	Reveals need for PEFR and provides baseline to evaluate efficacy of treatments.
• Assess the target zone set by patient's health care provider.	Baseline to determine patient's ongoing clinical status.
• Perform hand hygiene. Assess lung sounds, respirations, and character of respirations.	Reduces transmission of microorganisms. Provides baseline data on clinical status.
• Observe patient manipulating PEFR device.	Determines whether patient has the manual dexterity to correctly measure PEFR.
• Confirm patient's knowledge of rationale for measurement of PEFR and frequency of measurement.	Determines whether there is a need for reinforcement or new instruction.

Continued

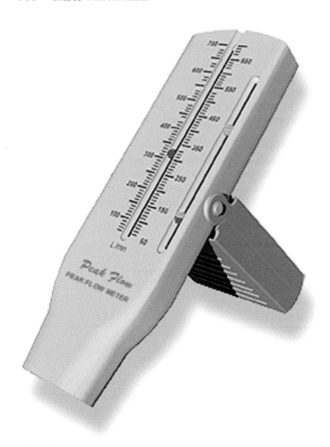

Fig. 51.1 Peak flowmeter. (Courtesy Philips Respironics, Murrysville, PA.)

STEPS	RATIONALE

Implementation

1 Perform hand hygiene. Apply clean gloves if exposure to mucus is likely.
    Reduces transmission of microorganisms.

STEPS	RATIONALE
2 Help patient to stand or to assume a high-Fowler position (or any other position that promotes optimum lung expansion). Have patient remove gum or food from mouth if applicable.	Promotes lung expansion and ability to exhale.
3 Instruct patient on proper use of device: a Slide the marker on the peak flowmeter to the bottom of the scale.	
b Slide clean mouthpiece into base of the numbered scale. Instruct patient on how to place mouthpiece in mouth and close lips, making a firm seal. Instruct patient to keep tongue away from mouthpiece.	Mouth position affects accuracy of measurement.
c Instruct patient to take a deep breath and blow out. Then have patient take another deep breath and hold. Have patient quickly place meter mouthpiece in mouth, close lips firmly, and blow out as hard and fast as possible through mouth only. Note the number on scale and record on a piece of paper.	Goal is to have patient exhale a maximum expiratory flow.
4 Have patient repeat maneuver two more times.	

Continued

STEPS	RATIONALE
5 Record the highest of the three values.	Patient will have done the routine correctly when the numbers from all three tries are very close together. Highest reading is highest flow patient can exert.
6 Inform patient of their individualized acceptable range and mark on meter.	Supports patient's autonomy in self-care.
7 Demonstrate for patient how to record PEFR accurately at home on a chart using "traffic light" pattern with the three target zones: green, yellow, and red (see Safety Guidelines, above).	Confirms understanding of instructions.
8 Instruct patient to measure PEFR every day, close to the same time every day. Have patient keep a chart of daily peak flow values that can be shared with health care provider.	PEFR measures are more comparable over time using this method.
9 Instruct patient to clean unit weekly, following manufacturer instructions.	Prevents contamination of device. Sediment collected in the meter may make PEFR measurements inaccurate (ALA, 2020).
10 Perform postprocedure protocol.	

11 Evaluate patient response:
  a Compare patient's PEFR with personal best.
  b Compare respirations and lung sounds with patient's baseline.
	Determines progress of lung disease and response to treatments.

Recording and Reporting

- Record PEFR measurement before and after therapy and patient's ability and effort to perform PEFR.
- Report to health care provider if patient is in yellow or red zone.
- Report to nurses/respiratory therapists the patient's PEFR values and tolerance of performance of peak flow measurements.

UNEXPECTED OUTCOMES	RELATED INTERVENTIONS
1 Patient's PEFR reading is less than targeted zone.	• Ensure that three consecutive readings are collected. • Report finding to health care provider.

Peripheral Intravenous Care: Dressing Change and Discontinuation

Administration of intravenous (IV) solutions can result in systemic or local complications (Gorski, 2023). Systemic complications (e.g., septicemia, circulatory overload)occur within the vascular system and are usually remote from the primary infusion site. Local complications result from trauma to the inner layer of a vein as a direct result of many factors, such as poor insertion technique, inappropriate size of short peripheral device, inadequate catheter stabilization, fluid osmolarity, poor assessment, and incorrect technique or frequency of short peripheral catheter dressing changes.

Another complication directly related to an IV site dressing is medical adhesive–related skin injuries (MARSIs). Such injuries can occur from any adhesive (e.g., tape, device adhesive) that results in mechanical injury (skin stripping, blistering, skin tears), dermatitis (irritation in response to the adhesive), and other complications (maceration and folliculitis) (Fumarola et al., 2020). Use of skin barriers during application of any adhesive device and the use of sterile adhesive removers is recommended to prevent MARSI (Fumarola et al., 2020).

The skin insertion site of a peripheral IV is the most common source of catheter-related infections (Gorski, 2023). Short peripheral catheter transparent semipermeable membrane (TSM) dressing changes should be performed every 5 to 7 days, and gauze dressings every 2 days (Gorski et al., 2021). If a gauze dressing is underneath a TSM, it should be changed every 2 days unless the dressing becomes soiled sooner (Gorski et al., 2021). Stabilizing short peripheral catheters decreases risk of catheter-related complications and premature loss of access. Preferred options for stabilization include an adhesive engineered stabilization device or an integrated feature on the IV catheter with use of a bordered polyurethane dressing (Gorski et al., 2021). Although sterile tape or surgical strips can be used, they are not as effective as an engineered stabilization device (Gorski, 2023; Gorski et al., 2021). The INS (2021) has new standards for hand hygiene when handling IV sites and equipment and for infusion management, Aseptic Non Touch Technique (ANTT). It is achieved by integrating standard precautions including hand hygiene, use of personal protective equipment (PPE) with appropriate aseptic field management, non-touch technique of an IV site, and sterile supplies.

Discontinue a short peripheral IV catheter when the prescribed length of therapy is completed or when a complication occurs (e.g., phlebitis, infiltration, or catheter occlusion). The technique for discontinuing a short peripheral IV catheter follows infection-prevention guidelines to minimize the chance of the patient acquiring an infection

Safety Guidelines

- Short peripheral IV catheters require strict adherence to infection-prevention measures to avoid systemic and local complications.
- Apply IV catheter dressings securely and change any dressing immediately if it becomes wet, soiled, or loosened or if the integrity of the dressing is compromised (Gorski et al., 2021).

Delegation

The skill of changing a short peripheral IV dressing cannot be delegated to assistive personnel (AP). Instruct the AP to:

- Report if a patient complains of moistness or loosening of an IV dressing.
- Protect the IV dressing during hygiene and activities of daily living.

Collaboration

- Consult with wound care nurse if patient develops MARSI from any adhesive used for dressing.

Equipment

- Clean gloves
- Antiseptic swabs (chlorhexidine gluconate [CHG]) solution preferred, povidone-iodine, or 70% alcohol)

Dressing Change

- Sterile adhesive remover
- Skin barrier protectant (film, cream, swab, or wipe)
- Engineered stabilization device or precut strips of sterile tape
- Commercially available IV site protection device (optional)
- Sterile TSM dressing or sterile 2 × 2 or 4 × 4 inch gauze pad

Discontinuation

- Sterile 2 × 2 inch or 4 × 4 inch gauze sponge
- Nonallergenic tape

STEP	RATIONALE
1 Perform preprocedure protocol.	

Assessment

• Refer to electronic health record (EHR) to determine when dressing was last changed. Dressing should also be labeled with date and time dressing applied, size and type of vascular access device (VAD), and insertion date.	Provides information regarding length of time that present dressing has been in place and allows planning for dressing change.
• For discontinuation of IV, check EHR for medical order.	Order is required.
• Review EHR to determine patient's risk for developing a MARSI using adhesive devices or tape: age, dehydration, malnutrition, exposure to radiation therapy, underlying chronic conditions (e.g., diabetes, immunosuppression), and edema of extremity.	Common risk factors for MARSI (Fumarola et al., 2020).
• For discontinuation, assess whether patient is receiving an anticoagulant or has a history of a bleeding disorder.	Factors can increase bleeding at IV site once catheter is removed.
• Perform hand hygiene using ANTT and apply clean gloves. Observe present IV dressing for moisture and adherence. If moisture present, determine whether it is from site leakage or external source.	Nonadhering dressing must be changed because it increases risk for insertion site infection or VAD dislodgement. Moisture causes skin maceration.

STEP	RATIONALE
• Inspect and palpate VAD site for patency of IV and signs and symptoms of IV site–related complications (e.g., VAD occlusion, inflammation, swelling around IV site, patient complaints of tenderness or pain, and drainage or leaking under dressing).	Identifies signs and symptoms of complications (e.g., phlebitis, infiltration, infection) that compromise VAD integrity and may necessitate its replacement.
• Assess skin around dressing for temperature, color, moisture level, turgor, fragility, and integrity.	Signs and symptoms of MARSI (Fumarola et al., 2020).
• Observe for local signs of irritation or skin damage at the site where any adhesive has been or will be applied.	
• Remove and discard gloves in appropriate receptacle and perform hand hygiene.	Using ANTT Reduces transmission of microorganisms.
• Ask patient to describe history of allergies: known type(s) of allergies and normal allergic reaction(s). Focus on latex, antiseptics, and adhesives. Check patient's allergy wristband.	Prevents exposure to allergen. Communication of patient allergies is essential for safe patient care.

Implementation

STEP	RATIONALE
1 Explain that patient will need to hold affected extremity still. Explain how long procedure will take.	Decreases anxiety, promotes cooperation, and gives patient time frame around which to plan personal activities.
2 Dressing change (Use ANTT). Apply clean gloves. Remove existing dressing:	Reduces transmission of microorganisms.

Continued

STEP	RATIONALE
a For TSM dressing: (1) Stabilize catheter with nondominant hand. (2) Loosen the edges of the TSM dressing with the fingers of the dominant hand by pushing the skin down and away from the TSM dressing. (3) With fingers of the dominant hand, loosen a corner of the dressing and stretch it horizontally in the opposite direction of the IV site (stretch-and-relax technique) (Fig. 52.1). Walk fingers under the dressing to continue stretching. One hand should continuously support the skin adhered to the TSM dressing. (4) This process can be repeated around the dressing. Use medical adhesive remover if needed to loosen the adhesive bond. Follow the manufacturer's instructions for use.	Technique minimizes discomfort during removal. Use of sterile adhesive remover on TSM dressing next to patient's skin loosens dressing without excessive pulling (Fumarola et al., 2020).

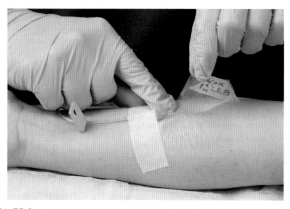

Fig. 52.1 Remove transparent semipermeable membrane dressing by pulling in the opposite direction of IV site.

STEP	RATIONALE

b For gauze dressing:
  (1) Stabilize catheter hub.
  (2) Remove tape strips by slowly lifting and removing each side toward the center of dressing. When both sides are completely loosened, lift the strip up from the center of the dressing.
  (3) Remove old dressing one layer at a time by pulling toward insertion site. Be cautious if tubing becomes tangled between two layers of dressing. Use medical adhesive remover if needed to loosen the adhesive bond of tape.
	Guidelines for MARSI prevention (Fumarola et al., 2020).

Continued

STEP	RATIONALE
3 Assess exposed VAD insertion site for signs and symptoms of IV site–related complications. If complication exists, determine whether VAD requires removal. Remove catheter if ordered by health care provider.	Presence of complication may necessitate VAD removal.
4 If catheter is to remain in place, assess integrity of engineered stabilization device. Continue to stabilize catheter and remove as recommended by manufacturer directions for use. Inspect for signs of MARSI from adhesive-based engineered stabilization devices. *Note:* Some stabilization devices are designed to remain in place for length of time VAD is in place as long as adequate stabilization is evident.	Removing stabilization device allows for appropriate skin antisepsis before applying dressing and new stabilization device (Gorski et al., 2021). Stabilization prevents accidental dislodgement of VAD.

CLINICAL JUDGMENT *Always keep one finger over catheter until dressing secures catheter hub. If patient is restless or uncooperative, it is helpful to have another staff member help with procedure.*

5 While stabilizing IV line, perform skin antisepsis around insertion site with CHG swab using friction in back-and-forth motion for 30 seconds. If using alcohol or povidone-iodine, clean in concentric circle, moving from insertion site outward with the swab. Allow any antiseptic solution to dry completely.	Reduces incidence of catheter-related infections (Gorski, 2023). Drying of antiseptic agent is necessary for complete antisepsis (Gorski et al., 2021).

STEP	RATIONALE
6 *Optional:* Apply skin barrier protectant to area where tape, dressing, or engineered stabilization device will be reapplied (Fumarola et al., 2020). Allow to dry.	Coats skin with protective solution to maintain skin integrity, prevents irritation from adhesive, and promotes adhesion of dressing.
7 While stabilizing catheter, apply sterile dressing over site (procedures may differ, follow agency policy). Ensure skin surface is dry.	Moisture reduces effectiveness of adhesion.
a *TSM dressing:* Apply TSM dressing as directed in Skill 18 using ANTT.	Protects catheter insertion site and minimizes risk for infection (Gorski, 2023). Dressing allows visual assessment of insertion site and surrounding area Gorski et al., 2021).
b *Sterile gauze dressing:* Apply sterile gauze dressing as directed in Skill 16 using ANTT. Use only sterile tape (plastic preferred for short-term use) (Fumarola et al., 2020).	Gauze dressing obscures observation of insertion site and is changed every 2 days (Gorski et al., 2021).
8 If new engineered catheter stabilization device is needed, apply device as directed in Skill 54.	Device can reduce risk for VAD complications and unintentional loss of access (Gorski et al., 2021).

CLINICAL JUDGMENT *Because Band-Aid brand adhesive bandages are not occlusive and nonsterile tape increases the risk for insertion site infection, do not use either over catheter insertion points.*

STEP	RATIONALE
9 *Optional:* Apply site protection device.	Reduces risk of VAD dislodgement (Gorski et al., 2021).
10 Anchor extension tubing or IV tubing alongside dressing on patient arm and secure with tape directly over tubing. When using TSM dressing, avoid placing tape over dressing.	Prevents accidental dislodgement of VAD tubing.

Continued

STEP	RATIONALE
11 Label dressing per agency policy. Information on label includes date and time of IV insertion, VAD gauge size and length, and your initials.	Communicates type of device and time interval for dressing change and site rotation.
12 Perform postprocedure protocol.	
13 Discontinuation of peripheral IV:	
a Perform preprocedure protocol.	
b Turn IV tubing roller clamp to "off" position or (when indicated) turn electronic infusion device off and roller clamp to "off." position.	Prevents leakage of solution.
c Carefully remove VAD or gauze dressing, tape, and engineered stabilization device.	Prevents pulling and lessens risk of MARSI.
d Stabilize IV catheter hub with middle finger of nondominant hand.	Minimizes local discomfort.

CLINICAL JUDGMENT *Never use scissors to remove the tape or dressing because the catheter may accidentally be cut.*

e Place sterile gauze pad above insertion site and, using dominant hand, withdraw catheter using a slow, steady motion, keeping the hub parallel to skin (Fig. 52.2).	Prevents catheter from breaking and reduces microorganism transmission.

CLINICAL JUDGMENT *To avoid trauma or hematoma formation, do not raise or lift catheter before it is completely out of the vein.*

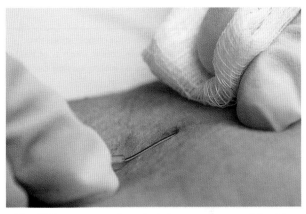

Fig. 52.2 Remove IV catheter slowly, keeping catheter parallel to skin.

STEP	RATIONALE
f Use gauze to apply pressure to IV site for a minimum of 30 seconds or until bleeding has stopped. *Note:* Apply pressure for at least 5 to 10 minutes if patient is receiving anticoagulants. Inspect catheter for intactness after removal; note tip integrity and length.	Promotes hemostasis. Retained portion of catheter can lead to infection.
g Apply clean, folded gauze dressing over insertion site and secure firmly with plastic tape.	Prevents bleeding from insertion site
h Perform postprocedure protocol.	
14 Evaluate patient response:	
a Evaluate function, patency of IV system, and flow rate after changing dressing.	Validates that IV line is patent and functioning correctly. Manipulation of catheter and tubing will affect rate of infusion.

Continued

STEP	RATIONALE
b Evaluate patient at established intervals (per agency policy and procedure) for signs and symptoms of IV site–related complications.	Identifies complications that compromise integrity of VAD or cause inaccurate flow rate of IV solution.
c Monitor IV site for 24 to 48 h after discontinuation/removal.	Postinfusion phlebitis can develop.

Recording and Reporting

- Record the time short peripheral dressing was changed, reason for change, type of dressing material used, patency of system, description of VAD site, any complications, interventions performed, and patient response to treatment.
- Record patient's and family caregiver's understanding of IV problems to report.
- Record discontinuation of IV, confirm catheter intact, and record appearance of IV site.
- Report to oncoming nursing staff dressing changes, whether IV is discontinued, and significant information about condition of IV site.
- Report to health care provider any IV-related complications, interventions, and response to treatment.

UNEXPECTED OUTCOMES	RELATED INTERVENTIONS
1 IV catheter is accidentally dislodged.	• Restart new short peripheral IV line in other extremity or above previous insertion site if continued therapy is needed/ordered.

UNEXPECTED OUTCOMES	RELATED INTERVENTIONS
2 IV solution is not infusing or runs more slowly than ordered.	• Check IV catheter for bending, kinking, or dislodgement (catheter may require replacement). • Check for positional IV site and reposition catheter, applying new dressing if necessary. • Check and adjust height of IV container, and for kinking or obstruction of IV tubing.
3 Site of discontinued IV develops inflammation, edema, and localized tenderness.	• Report to health care provider. • Consult on use of heat to reduce inflammation.

Peripheral Intravenous Care: Regulating Intravenous Flow Rates and Changing Solutions

Appropriate regulation of intravenous (IV) infusion rates reduces complications (e.g., phlebitis, infiltration) associated with IV therapy (Gorski, 2023; Gorski et al., 2021). Infusion rates can be altered by changes in patient position, flexion of the IV site extremity, occlusion or manipulation of the IV device, and vein trauma. **Frequent monitoring is essential**.

Electronic infusion devices (EIDs) maintain correct flow rates and catheter patency and prevent an unexpected bolus of IV infusion (Gorski et al., 2021). Many EIDs provide a record of the volume infused while delivering a measured amount of fluid over a period of time (e.g., 100 mL/h) using positive pressure. An electronic sensor signals an alarm if the pressure in the system changes and the desired flow rate alters. Even with an EID you are responsible for regularly checking to ensure that a pump is functioning and infusing at the prescribed rate or to detect infiltration or extravasation at an IV site (Gorski et al., 2021). Multifunctional EIDs or "smart pumps" have an embedded computer system with built-in software that is programmed from health care pharmacy databases with medication and patient unit-specific profiles. The pump has an audible and visual alert when the setting does not match the preselected dose or volume limits, helping to prevent infusion errors.

Manual flow-control devices (i.e., dial or barrel-shaped) and mechanical infusion devices without a power source (i.e., elastomeric devices, piston-driven pumps) may be used when control of flow rate is not critical (Gorski, 2023). They are not recommended for use in infants and children, since accuracy is not guaranteed (Gorski, 2023).

Flow regulators, such as volume-control devices, deliver small volumes of fluid with the aid of gravity. Mechanical factors (e.g., height of the IV container, IV tubing size, or fluid viscosity) affect an IV gravity controller. A small volume of IV solution (usually limited to 2 h of ordered solution) is placed in the chamber and regulated for administration. The advantage of this system is that, if the rate of the IV is inadvertently increased, only a limited amount of solution will infuse.

Patients receiving IV therapy periodically require changes of IV solutions at the end of an infusion, to avoid exceeding hang time of an existing solution, or in the middle of an infusion when orders for the type of solution changes (Gorski, 2023). You change a container when there is an order for a new solution or when it becomes necessary to add a sequential container to avoid exceeding hang time (Gorski, 2023). The maximum hang time for routine replacement of IV containers is established by agency policy and procedure (Gorski, 2023; Gorski et al., 2021). Maximum hang time is based on maintenance of strict aseptic technique, whether the system remains closed without injection ports or add-on tubing, stability of the solution or medication being infused, and how long the solution in the IV container will last (Gorski, 2023).

An important component of IV therapy is maintaining the integrity of the IV system through the conscientious use of infection-prevention principles during tubing changes using Aseptic Non Touch Technique (ANTT) (See skill, 52). Administration sets are the primary method of delivering IV solutions to patients. In addition, patients may have add-on devices (e.g., filters, extension sets), which are connected to the primary administration set as indicated by the prescribed therapy. Secondary sets may be used as a method to administer medications in conjunction with the primary infusion (e.g., antibiotics). Luer-Lok connections should be used to prevent accidental tubing disconnection (Gorski et al., 2021). Follow agency policy and procedures for specific requirements. Policies for changing tubing for parenteral nutrition and blood or blood products have separate, specific criteria (See skill 6).

Safety Guidelines

- Use strict aseptic technique using ANTT recommended by INS (2021) when changing an IV solution or tubing.
- Administer IV solutions carefully. Isotonic solutions can cause increased risk for fluid overload in patients with renal or cardiac disease, hypotonic solutions can worsen a hypotensive state, and hypertonic solutions irritate veins and can increase the risk of heart failure and pulmonary edema.
- Whenever possible, schedule IV tubing changes when it is time to hang a new IV container to minimize opening within the system.

- If IV tubing and/or IV bag becomes damaged, is leaking, or becomes contaminated, it should be changed, regardless of the solution or tubing change schedule.

Delegation

The skill of regulating IV flow rates and changing solutions/tubing cannot be delegated to assistive personnel (AP). Delegation to licensed practical nurses varies by state Nurse Practice Act. Instruct AP to:

- Report when the EID alarm signals or an IV container is near completion.
- Report any indications from patient of discomfort related to infusion such as pain, burning, bleeding, or swelling.
- Report any cloudiness or precipitate in the IV solution.
- Report any leakage from or around the IV tubing.
- Report if tubing has become contaminated (lying on the floor).

Equipment

- Tape
- Label for solution and/or tubing
- Clean gloves
- IV solution bag and appropriate administration set

Regulating infusion rate

- Watch with digital display or second hand
- Calculator, paper, and pencil
- EID or flow regulator

Changing IV solution

- IV solution as ordered

Changing IV tubing

- Antiseptic swabs (chlorhexidine gluconate) solution preferred, or 70% alcohol)
- Microdrip or macrodrip administration set of IV tubing as appropriate
- Add-on device as needed (e.g., filters, extension set, needleless connector)
- For intermittent infusions: intermittent extension set, 3- to 5-mL syringe filled with preservative-free 0.9% sodium chloride (normal saline) and short extension tubing (if needed), injection cap

STEP	RATIONALE
1 Perform preprocedure protocol.	

Assessment

- Review patient's electronic health record (EHR) for accuracy and completeness of health care provider order, including patient name and correct solution, and type, volume, additives, infusion rate, and duration of IV therapy. Follow seven rights of medication administration.

Ensures delivery of correct IV solution and prescribed volume over prescribed time.

- Determine compatibility of all IV solutions and additives by consulting approved online database, drug reference, or pharmacist.

Incompatibilities cause physical, chemical, and therapeutic changes, which can contribute to adverse patient outcomes (Gorski, 2023).

- Check pertinent laboratory data (such as potassium level).

Compare data with baseline to determine ongoing response to IV solution administration.

- For IV tubing or solution change, note date and time when last changed.

Ensures correct timing of solution and tubing changes.

- Review EHR and identify patient's risk for fluid and electrolyte imbalances related to ordered IV solution (e.g., neonate, older adult, history of cardiac or renal disease).

Helps prioritize assessments. Volume control needs to be strict. Guides choice of infusion device.

- Perform hand hygiene and apply clean gloves; Use ANTT to inspect and gently palpate skin around and above IV site and over dressing. Assess vascular access device (VAD) for patency and signs and symptoms of IV site–related complications (e.g., infiltration, VAD occlusion, phlebitis, infection, patient reports of pain, or leaking under dressing).

Identifies complications that compromise integrity of VAD and ability to regulate infusion.

Continued

STEP	RATIONALE
• Check infusion system from solution container down to VAD insertion site for fluid discoloration or cloudiness, leakage of solution, punctured or leaking tubing, or occluded tubing. Note expiration date of solution.	A break in integrity of solution container necessitates a container change (Gorski, 2023). Compromised tubing results in fluid leakage and bacterial contamination, requiring a tubing change.
• Remove and discard gloves and perform hand hygiene.	Reduces transmission of microorganisms.
• Calculate flow rate:	Calculating hourly flow rates ensures that the prescribed amount of fluid to be infused over the prescribed time frame is correct.
a Have paper and pencil or calculator to calculate flow rate.	
b Check order for length of time each liter of fluid should infuse. If hourly rate (mL/h) is not provided in health care provider order, calculate it by dividing total volume in infusion container by hours of infusion, for example:	Basis of calculation to ensure infusion of solution over prescribed hourly rate.

$$mL / h = \frac{\text{Total infusion} \, (mL)}{\text{House of infusion}}$$

$$1000 \ mL / 8h = 125 \ mL / h$$

or if 3 L is ordered for 24 h:

$$3000 \ mL/24h = 125 \ mL/h$$

CLINICAL JUDGMENT *It is common for health care providers to write an abbreviated IV order such as "D_5W with 20 mEq KCl 125 mL/h continuous." This order implies that the IV should be maintained at this rate until an order has been written for the IV to be discontinued or changed to another order.*

STEP	RATIONALE
c If a keep vein open (KVO) rate is ordered, check agency policy regarding flow rate of KVO. Rates may vary from 0.5 mL/h to 30 mL/h based on the type of VAD, patient specific therapy, and method of infusion (gravity or EID).	Prevents catheter clotting, thus preserving venous access while infusing a minimal amount of fluid. An order for KVO rate must specify an infusion rate as required by the seven rights of medication administration.
d Use hourly rate to program EID or, if gravity-flow infusion, use the hourly rate to calculate the minute flow rate (gtt/mL).	EID automatically delivers correct minute flow rate. Gravity infusion requires calculation of drops per milliliter.
e Verify the calibration (drop factor), in drops per milliliter (gtt/mL), of infusion set used by agency:	
(1) Microdrip: 60 gtt/mL: Used to deliver rates less than 100 mL/h.	Microdrip tubing universally delivers 60 gtt/mL. Used when small or very precise volumes are to be infused.
(2) Macrodrip: 10 to 15 gtt/mL (depending on manufacturer). Used to deliver rates greater than 100 mL/h.	There are different commercial parenteral administration sets for macrodrip tubing. Used when large volumes or fast rates are necessary.
f Select one of the following formulas to calculate the minute flow rate (drops per minute) based on drop factor of infusion set:	Once you determine hourly rate, the following formulas compute the correct flow rate.

$mL/h/60\ min = mL/min$

$Drop\ factor \times mL/min = Drops/min$

Or

$mL/h \times Drop\ factor/60\ min = Drops/min$

Example: Calculate minute flow rate for a bag 1000 mL with 20 mEq KCl at 125 mL/h.

Continued

STEP	RATIONALE
Microdrip: 125 mL/h × 60 gtt/mL = 7500 gtt/h 7500 gtt ÷ 60 min = 125 gtt/min	When using microdrip, the milliliters per hour (mL/h) value always equals drops per minute (gtt/min).
Macrodrip: 125 mL/h × 15 gtt/mL = 1875 gtt/h 1875 gtt ÷ 60 min = 31 − 32 gtt/min	Multiply volume by drop factor and divide product by time (in minutes).

Implementation

1 **Regulate gravity infusion with roller clamp:**

   a Perform hand hygiene. Ensure that IV container is at least 76.2 cm (30 inches) above IV site for adults (increase height for more viscous fluids). — Reduces transmission of microorganisms. Pressure caused by gravity is necessary to overcome venous pressure and resistance from tubing and catheter.

   b Slowly open roller clamp on tubing until drops in drip chamber are visualized. Hold a watch with second hand at same level as drip chamber and count drip rate for 1 minute. Adjust roller clamp to increase or decrease rate of infusion. — Regulates flow to prescribed rate.

   c Monitor drip rate at least hourly. — Many factors influence drip rate; frequent monitoring ensures IV fluid administration as prescribed.

2 **Regulated EID (infusion pump or smart pump):** Follow manufacturer guidelines for setup. Use infusion tubing compatible with EID: — Smart pumps with medication safety software are designed for administration of IV fluids that contain medications.

   a Close roller clamp on primed IV infusion tubing. — Prevents fluid leakage.

STEP	RATIONALE
b Insert infusion tubing into chamber of control mechanism (see manufacturer directions) (Fig. 53.1). Roller clamp on IV tubing goes between EID and patient.	Most EIDs use positive pressure to infuse. Infusion pumps propel fluid through tubing by compressing and milking IV tubing.

Continued

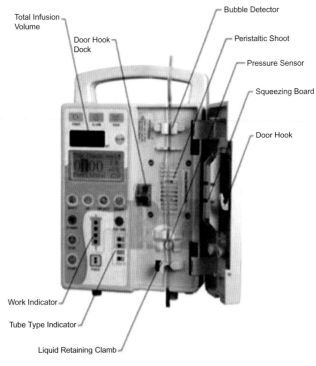

Total Infusion Volume

Door Hook Dock

Bubble Detector

Peristaltic Shoot

Pressure Sensor

Squeezing Board

Door Hook

Work Indicator

Tube Type Indicator

Liquid Retaining Clamb

Fig. 53.1 Electronic infusion device components. Courtesy Medical Shopping Center, Guangzhou, China.

STEP	RATIONALE
c Secure part of IV tubing through "air in line" alarm system. Close door and turn on power button, select required drops per minute or volume per hour, close door to control chamber, and press start button. If infusing medication, access the EID library of medications and set appropriate rate and dose limits. If smart pump alarms immediately and shuts down, settings were outside unit parameters and need to be adjusted.	Ensures safe administration of ordered flow rate or medication dose. Smart pumps require information input (such as medication). Computer will match the pump setting against a drug database (Wolf and Hughes, 2019).

CLINICAL JUDGMENT *An anti-free flow safeguard (preventing bolus infusion in the event of machine malfunction or when tubing is removed from machine) is an important, required element of an EID. Follow manufacturer recommendations for specific device features.*

STEP	RATIONALE
d Open infusion tubing drip regulator completely while EID is in use.	Ensures that pump freely regulates infusion rate.
e Monitor infusion rate and IV site for complications according to agency policy. Use watch to verify rate of infusion, even when using EID.	Flow controllers and pumps do not replace frequent, accurate nursing evaluation. EIDs can continue to infuse IV solutions after a complication has developed (Gorski et al., 2021).
f Assess IV system from container to VAD insertion site when alarm signals.	Alarm indicates situation that requires attention. EID alarms can be triggered by: a solution container that is empty, tubing kinks, closed clamp, infiltration, clotted catheter, air in tubing, and/or low battery.

STEP	RATIONALE
3 Attach label to IV solution container with date and time container changed (check agency policy).	Provides reference to determine appropriate time for container change.
4 Perform postprocedure protocol.	
5 **Changing IV solutions.**	Reduces transmission of infection and contamination of equipment (Gorski et al., 2021). Proper handling of solutions prevents IV site–related complications, such as occlusion. Checking that solution is correct prevents medication error.
a Have next solution prepared at least 1 h before needed. Allow solutions that have been refrigerated to warm to room temperature. Check that solution is correct and properly labeled. Check solution expiration date. Ensure that appropriate precautions are followed for fluids that are light sensitive.	
b Identify patient using at least two identifiers (e.g., name and birthday or name and medical record number) according to agency policy. Compare identifiers with information on patient's medication administration record (MAR) or EHR.	Ensures patient safety. Complies with The Joint Commission standards and improves patient safety (TJC, 2023).

Continued

STEP	RATIONALE
c Perform hand hygiene. Change solution when only the neck of the IV container contains fluid (about 50 mL), when new type of solution has been ordered, or when existing solution hang time has expired.	Reduces transmission of microorganisms. Prevents waste of solution. Prevents exposure to contaminated solution.
d If using plastic solution container, hang on IV pole and remove protective cover from IV tubing port. If using glass bottle, remove metal cap and metal and rubber disks.	Permits quick, smooth, organized change from old to new container.
e Close roller clamp on existing solution to stop flow rate. Remove IV tubing from EID (if used). Then remove old IV solution container from IV pole. Discard in appropriate container or hold old container with tubing port pointing upward.	Prevents solution remaining in drip chamber from emptying while changing solutions. Prevents solution in bag from spilling.
f Quickly remove spike from old solution container and, without touching tip, insert spike into new container (Fig. 53.2).	Reduces risk for solution in drip chamber becoming empty; maintains sterility.

CLINICAL JUDGMENT *If spike becomes contaminated by touching an unsterile object, a new IV tubing set will be needed.*

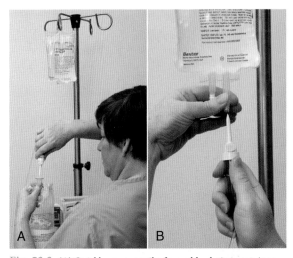

Fig. 53.2 (A) Quickly remove spike from old solution container. (B) Without touching tip, insert spike into new container.

STEP	RATIONALE
g Check for air in IV tubing. If air bubbles have formed, remove by closing roller clamp, stretching tubing downward, and tapping tubing with finger (bubbles rise in fluid to drip chamber).	Reduces risk of air entering tubing. Use of an air-eliminating filter also reduces risk.
h Ensure that drip chamber is one-third to one-half full. If drip chamber is too full, level can be decreased by removing bag from IV pole, pinching off IV tubing below drip chamber, inverting container, squeezing drip chamber (Fig. 53.3), releasing and turning solution container upright, and releasing pinch on tubing.	Reduces risk for air entering IV tubing. If chamber is completely filled, you cannot observe or regulate drip rate.

Continued

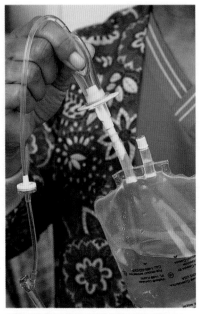

Fig. 53.3 Squeeze drip chamber to empty excess fluid. Be sure chamber is one-third to one-half full.

STEP	RATIONALE
i Regulate flow to ordered rate (Step 1 or 2).	Maintains a rate which restores fluid balance and delivers IV solution as ordered.
j Apply label to bag with time hung, time scheduled for completion, and initials. Option: Add a time tape vertically along bag if regulating using flow clamp.	Time tape provides visual comparison of volume infused compared with prescribed rate of infusion.
k Perform postprocedure protocol.	
6 Changing IV tubing:	
a Coordinate IV tubing changes with solution changes when possible.	Decreases number of times system is open.

STEP	RATIONALE
b Perform hand hygiene. Open new infusion set and connect add-on pieces (e.g., filters, extension tubing) using ANTT aseptic technique. Keep protective coverings over infusion spike and distal adapter. Place roller clamp about 2–2.5 cm (1–2 inches) below drip chamber and move roller clamp to "off" position. Secure all connections.	Reduces transmission of microorganisms. Close proximity of roller clamp to drip chamber allows more accurate regulation of flow rate. Securing connections reduces later risk of air emboli and infection. Protective covers reduce entrance of microorganisms. All connections should be of Luer-Lok type (Gorski et al., 2021).
c Apply clean gloves. If patient's IV cannula hub is not visible, remove IV dressing. Do not remove tape securing cannula to skin.	Cannula hub must be visible to provide smooth transition when removing old and inserting new tubing.
d Prepare IV tubing with new IV container (see Step 3, above).	
e Prepare IV tubing with existing continuous IV infusion bag.	
(1) Be sure roller clamp on new IV tubing is still in the "off" position.	Prevents fluid spillage.
(2) Slow rate of infusion through old tubing to KVO rate using EID or roller clamp.	Prevents occlusion of VAD.
(3) Compress and fill drip chamber of old tubing.	Ensures that drip chamber remains full until new tubing is changed.
(4) Invert container and remove old tubing. Old tubing may be hung on IV pole until end of change is over. Keep spike of tubing sterile and upright.	Solution in drip chamber will continue to run and maintain catheter patency.

Continued

STEP	RATIONALE
(5) Insert spike of new infusion tubing into existing solution container. Hang solution bag on IV pole, compress drip chamber on new tubing, and release, allowing to fill one-third to one-half full.	Permits drip chamber to fill and promotes rapid, smooth flow of solution through tubing.
(6) Prime air out of IV tubing by filling with IV solution: Remove protective cover on end of tubing and slowly open roller clamp to allow solution to flow from drip chamber to distal end of IV tubing. If tubing has Y connector, invert Y connector when solution reaches it to displace air. Return roller clamp to "off" position after priming tubing (filled with IV solution). Replace protective cover on end of IV tubing. Place end of adapter near patient's IV site.	Priming ensures that IV tubing is clear of air before connection with VAD and filling with IV solution. Slow fill of tubing decreases turbulence and chance of bubble formation. Closing clamp prevents accidental loss of fluid.

Maintains sterility. Equipment is positioned for quick connection of new tubing. |
| f Stop EID or turn roller clamp on old tubing to "off" position. | Prevents fluid spillage. |
| g Prepare tubing with extension set or saline lock. | |

STEP	RATIONALE
(1) If short extension tubing is needed, use sterile technique to connect new injection cap to new extension set or IV tubing.	Prepares extension set for connection with IV.
(2) Scrub injection cap with antiseptic swab for at least 15 seconds and allow to dry completely. Attach syringe with 3 to 5 mL of normal saline flush solution and inject through injection cap into extension set.	Ensures effective disinfection (Gorski, 2023). Maintains patency of catheter.
h Reestablish infusion.	
(1) Gently disconnect old tubing from extension tubing (or from IV catheter hub). Quickly insert Luer-Lok end of new tubing or saline lock into extension tubing connection (or IV catheter hub).	Allows smooth transition from old to new tubing, minimizing time system is open.
(2) For continuous infusion, open roller clamp on new tubing and regulate drip rate using roller clamp or insert tubing into EID, program to desired rate, and push "on."	Ensures catheter patency and prevents occlusion.
i Attach label with date and time of IV tubing change onto tubing below drip chamber.	Provides reference to determine next time for tubing change.
j Form loop of tubing and secure to patient's arm with strip of tape.	Avoids accidental pulling against site and stabilizes catheter.

Continued

STEP	RATIONALE
k Remove and discard old IV tubing, if necessary, then apply new dressing (see Skill 52).	Reduces transmission of microorganisms.
l Perform postprocedure protocol.	
7 Whenever regulating IV rates or changing solutions/tubing, instruct or reinforce to patient the purpose of IV, what to report, and how to move and position properly without occluding or pulling on IV tubing.	Prevents accidental occlusion or disconnection and contamination of IV tubing.
8 Evaluate patient response:	
a Observe patient every 1 to 2 h (see agency policy), noting volume of IV fluid infused and rate of infusion; function, patency, and intactness of IV system; and type/amount solution infused.	Ensures delivery of prescribed volume over prescribed time and decreases risk for fluid and electrolyte imbalance.
b Evaluate patient response to IV therapy (e.g., laboratory values, input and output, weights, vital signs). Monitor for signs of fluid volume excess or fluid volume deficit.	Provides ongoing evaluation of patient's fluid status.
c Using ANTT Evaluate condition of IV site at established intervals per agency policy and procedure for signs and symptoms of IV site–related complications.	Prevents complications that compromise integrity of VAD or cause inaccurate IV solution flow rate.

Recording and Reporting

- Record IV solution (and additives), if solution changed, record volume of container, rate of infusion in drops per minute (gtt/min) or milliliters per hour (mL/h), and integrity and patency of system. Use an infusion therapy flow sheet for parenteral solutions per agency policy.
- If using an EID, document type and rate of infusion and device identification number.
- Record tubing change or catheter flushes to include solution, volume, and concentration; rate of newly established infusion.
- Record patient response to therapy and unexpected outcomes.
- Record patient's and family caregiver's understanding following instructions.
- Report to oncoming nursing staff type and rate of infusion and remaining volume; reason for IV solution change (if applicable).
- Report to health care provider any infusion-related complications, IV site complications, interventions, and response to treatment.

UNEXPECTED OUTCOMES	RELATED INTERVENTIONS
1 Sudden infusion of large volume of solution occurs; patient develops dyspnea, crackles in lung, dependent edema (edema in legs), and increased urine output, indicating fluid volume excess.	• Slow infusion rate: KVO rates must have specific rate ordered by health care provider. • Notify health care provider immediately. • Place patient in high-Fowler position. • Anticipate new IV orders. • Anticipate administration of oxygen per order. • Administer diuretics if ordered.
2 IV solution runs slower than ordered.	• Check for patient positional change affecting rate, height of IV container, kinking of tubing, or obstruction. • Check VAD site for complications. • Consult health care provider for new order to provide necessary fluid volume.

Continued

UNEXPECTED OUTCOMES	RELATED INTERVENTIONS
3 Laboratory values and assessment findings suggest fluid and/or electrolyte imbalances.	• Notify health care provider. • Anticipate orders for changes in IV solution or additives.
4 IV patency is lost subsequent to IV solution container running empty.	• Discontinue present IV infusion and restart new short peripheral catheter in new site (see Skill 54).

Peripheral Intravenous Care: Short-Catheter Insertion

A peripheral intravenous (IV) device provides access to the venous system to deliver solutions, medications, whole blood, and/or blood products. Reliable venous access for IV therapy administration is essential. Peripheral venous access is categorized by three types of IV catheters (Gorski et al, 2021): short peripheral (in superficial veins), long peripheral (superficial or deep peripheral veins) and midline (peripheral vein of the upper arm via the basilic, cephalic, or brachial vein with the terminal tip located at the level of the axilla). The short over-the-needle (ONC) catheter is most common. An ONC catheter includes (1) a catheter made of silicone, polyurethane, polyvinyl chloride, or polytetrafluoroethylene (Teflon) that threads into a vein and remains there for the infusion of fluid, and (2) a needle device to pierce the skin, allowing insertion of the catheter. A catheter gauge is selected based on the clinical therapy a patient is ordered to receive. Table 54.1 indicates appropriate uses for the more common short peripheral catheter sizes.

Safety Guidelines

- Clinician competence is required for the placement and management of VADs; the ability to recognize signs and symptoms of VAD-related complications; the use of infusion equipment; and knowledge of all aspects of infusion therapy administration (Gorski et al., 2021).
- Reduce risk for administration set misconnections by tracing the path between an IV fluid container and a patient, labeling administration sets near patient connection and solution container, and routing tubing required for different purposes in different directions. Disconnections to reroute tubing are not recommended for any type of therapy or care activity.
- Maintain sterility of a patent IV system using INS standards for ANTT (Box 54.1).

Delegation

The skill of inserting a short peripheral IV access device cannot be delegated to assistive personnel (AP). Delegation to licensed practical nurses varies by state Nurse Practice Act. Instruct the AP to:

- Report if the patient verbalizes any IV site–related complications such as redness, pain, tenderness, swelling, bleeding, drainage, or leaking from under dressing.

623

TABLE 54.1 Recommendations for Short Peripheral Catheter Selection

Catheter Size (Gauge)	Clinical Indication
16, 18	Trauma, surgery, rapid blood transfusions, rapid fluid replacement
20	Continuous or intermittent infusions in adults, administration of blood transfusions in adults
22	Continuous or intermittent infusions in adults, pediatric patients, neonates, and older adults; administration of blood or blood product in adults, pediatric patients, neonates, and older adults
24–26	Continuous or intermittent infusions in adults, pediatric patients, neonates, and older adults; administration of blood or blood product in adults, pediatric patients, neonates, and older adults

Modified from Gorski L. et al: *Infusion therapy standards of practice*, ed 8. Norwood: Mass, 2021, Infusion Nurses Society (INS).

BOX 54.1 INS Standards to Decrease Intravascular Infection Related to Intravenous Therapy

Aseptic Non Touch Technique (ANTT) is designed for use in the placement, management, and infusion administration of vascular access devices (VAD). ANTT is achieved by integrating standard precautions including hand hygiene, use of personal protective equipment (PPE) with appropriate aseptic field management, non-touch technique, and sterilized supplies.

- Perform hand hygiene following ANTT before inserting and providing any IV-associated interventions.
- Assess the IV catheter--skin junction site and surrounding area for redness, tenderness, swelling, and drainage by visual inspection and palpation and through patient report of symptoms of a complication.
  1. Assess short peripheral IV catheters minimally at least every 4 h or more if clinically indicated.
  2. Assess CVADs and midline catheters at least daily. Assess VADs daily for outpatient or home care patients. For a continuous infusion via a short peripheral catheter in the home, assess every 4 h while patient is awake.
- Change a dressing on any VAD or a peripheral IV site immediately to assess, clean, and disinfect the site in the event of drainage, tenderness, or other signs of infection, or if dressing becomes loose or visibly soiled, or dislodged.
- Change gauze dressing every 2 days.

BOX 54.1 INS Standards to Decrease Intravascular Infection Related to Intravenous Therapy—cont'd

- Change transparent semipermeable membrane dressing every 5 to 7 days.
- Use approved antiseptic agents before venipuncture and when performing skin antisepsis. Preferred solution is greater than 0.5% CHG in alcohol solution. Tincture of iodine, an iodophor (povidone-iodine), or 70% alcohol may be used if CHG solution is contraindicated.
- Allow skin antiseptic to dry fully before dressing placement; alcoholic CHG for at least 30 seconds; iodophors for at least 1.5 to 2 minutes.
- Use catheter stabilization device that allows visual inspection of access site.

CHG, chlorhexidine gluconate. Modified from Gorski L. et al: *Infusion therapy standards of practice*, ed 8. Norwood: Mass, 2021, Infusion Nurses Society (INS).

- Report if the patient's IV dressing becomes wet.
- Report if the level of fluid in the IV bag is low or the electronic infusion device (EID) is alarming.

Collaboration

- Health care provider, certified registered nurse infusion (CRNI), and pharmacist can assist with managing IV therapy.

Equipment

- Short peripheral IV start kit supplies (available in some agencies): single-use tourniquet, plastic tape for short-term wear (Fumarola et al., 2020), transparent semipermeable membrane (TSM) dressing or sterile gauze and sterile tape, antiseptic wipes (chlorhexidine gluconate [CHG] solution preferred, povidone-iodine, or 70% alcohol), 2 × 2 inch gauze pads, and label. *Note:* Plastic tape preferred to prevent medical adhesive--related skin injury (MARSI).
- If kit is not available, gather all items separately use ANTT for setup.
- Appropriate short peripheral IV catheter with safety mechanism for venipuncture
- Clean gloves (latex-free for patients with latex allergy); sterile gloves are needed if palpating the site after skin antisepsis (Gorski et al., 2021)
- Single-use hair clippers or scissors for hair removal if indicated
- Short extension tubing with fused needleless connector or separate needleless connector (also called *injection cap, saline lock, heparin lock, IV plug,* or *PRN adapter*)
- 5-mL prefilled syringe with preservative-free 0.9% sodium chloride (normal saline)
- Antiseptic swabs
- Skin barrier: film, cream, or wipe

- Manufactured catheter stabilization device (if available)
- Prescribed IV solution or medication
- IV infusion set (IV tubing), either macrodrip or microdrip, depending on prescribed rate; if using EID, appropriate administration set for device
- 0.2-micron filter for nonlipid (fat emulsions) solutions (may be incorporated into the infusion set)
- Personal protective equipment: goggles, face shield, and mask (based on agency policy)
- EID and IV pole
- Vein visualization device (*optional,* based on agency policy and availability)
- Stethoscope
- Watch with second hand to calculate drip rate
- Special patient gown with snaps at shoulder seams if available (makes removal with IV tubing easier)
- Needle disposal container (sharps container or biohazard container)

STEP	RATIONALE
1 Perform preprocedure protocol.	

Assessment

• Review electronic health record (EHR) for accuracy of health care provider's order: date and time, IV solution, route of administration, volume, rate, duration, and signature of ordering health care practitioner (Gorski, 2023). Follow the seven rights of medication administration.	Before IV therapy, an order from a health care provider is needed (Gorski et al., 2021). Verification that order is complete prevents medication errors.
• Check drug reference regarding IV solution composition, purpose, potential incompatibilities, adverse reactions, and side effects.	Ensures safe and correct administration of IV therapy and appropriate selection of catheter.
• Review EHR for clinical factors/conditions that will respond to or be affected by administration of IV solutions. Perform hand hygiene and conduct physical examination of following:	Provides baseline to determine effectiveness of prescribed therapy.

STEP	RATIONALE
a Body weight	Changes in body weight can indicate fluid loss or gain (Gorski, 2018).
b Clinical markers of vascular volume:	
(1) Urine output (decreased, dark yellow)	Kidneys respond to extracellular volume (ECV) deficit by reducing urine production and concentrating urine. Kidney disease can also cause oliguria.
(2) Vital signs: blood pressure (BP), respirations, pulse, temperature	Changes in BP may be associated with fluid volume deficit (FVD) seen in postural hypotension. Respiration changes may indicate presence of acid--base imbalances. Elevated body temperature of 38.3 °C (101 °F) to 39.4 °C (103 °F) increases need for fluid replacement (Gorski, 2023).
(3) Distended neck veins (Normally, veins are full when person is supine and flat when person is upright.)	Indicator of fluid volume status: flat or collapsing with inhalation when supine with ECV deficit; full when upright or semi-upright with ECV excess.
(4) Auscultation of lungs	Crackles or rhonchi in dependent parts of lung may signal fluid buildup caused by ECV excess.
(5) Capillary refill	Indirect measure of tissue perfusion (sluggish with ECV deficit).
c Clinical markers of interstitial volume	
(1) Skin turgor. (Pinch skin over sternum or inside of forearm.) Assess skin temperature, color, moisture level, fragility, and overall integrity, including presence of irritation around potential IV site.	Failure of skin to return to normal position after several seconds indicates FVD (Gorski, 2023). Skin characteristics can indicate risk for MARSI (Fumarola et al., 2020).

Continued

STEP	RATIONALE
(2) Dependent edema (pitting or nonpitting)	Edema is not usually apparent until 2 to 4 kg (4.4 to 8.8 lb) of fluid are retained. A weight gain of 1 kg (2.2 lb) is equivalent to the retention of 1 L of body water (Gorski, 2023).
(3) Oral mucous membrane between cheek and gum	More reliable indicator than dry lips or skin. Dry between cheek and gums indicates ECV deficit.
d Thirst	Occurs with hypernatremia and severe ECV deficit. Not a reliable indicator for older adults (Gorski, 2023).
e Behavior and level of consciousness:	
(1) Restlessness and mild confusion	Occurs with FVD or acid-base imbalance.
f Perform hand hygiene after examination.	Reduces transmission of microorganisms.
• Review EHR to determine patient's risk for developing MARSI with use of adhesive devices or tape: Age, dehydration, malnutrition, exposure to radiation therapy, underlying chronic conditions (e.g., diabetes, immunosuppression, edema).	Common risk factors for MARSI (Fumarola et al., 2020).
• Review EHR and ask patient about history of allergy e.g., adhesive, latex, or CHG.	Medications, solutions used during catheter insertion, and use of gloves and tape can cause serious allergic reactions.
• Determine whether patient is to undergo any planned surgeries or procedures.	Allows for selection of appropriate gauge catheter for infusion and avoids placement in an area that will interfere with medical procedures (Gorski et al., 2021).

STEP	RATIONALE
• Assess available laboratory data (e.g., hematocrit, serum electrolytes, arterial blood gases, and kidney functions [blood urea nitrogen, urine specific gravity, and urine osmolality]).	Establishes baseline for determining whether therapy is effective. Laboratory values are an assessment of hydration status (Gorski, 2023).

Implementation

STEP	RATIONALE
1 While collecting equipment select the correct infusion set for the EID being used. Obtain proper adhesive tape to reduce risk of MARSI.	Ensures patient safety. To reduce risk of MARSI consider plastic tape for short-term wear (Fumarola et al., 2020).
2 With patient sitting or lying supine, change patient's gown (if needed) to one more easily removed with snaps at shoulder, if available. Provide adequate lighting.	Use of this gown decreases risk of inadvertently dislodging VAD or administration set when changing gown. Aids in successful vein location.
3 Identify patient using at least two identifiers (e.g., name and birthday or name and medical record number) according to agency policy. Compare identifiers with information on patient's medication administration record or EHR.	Ensures patient safety. Complies with The Joint Commission standards and improves patient safety (The Joint Commission, 2023).
4 Perform hand hygiene. Select appropriate-size catheter based on assessment. Open and prepare sterile packages using sterile ANTT technique.	Reduces transmission of microorganisms. Use smallest-gauge peripheral catheter for prescribed therapy and patient need (Gorski et al, 2021).

Continued

STEP	RATIONALE
5 Prepare a short extension tubing with fused needleless connector or separate needleless connector (injection cap) to be used to attach to catheter hub.	Needleless connectors protect against needlestick injuries. Use of ANTT reduces infection risk (Gorski et al., 2021)
a Remove protective cap from needleless connector and attach syringe with 1 to 3 mL 0.9% sodium chloride (normal saline), maintaining sterility. Slowly inject enough saline to prime (fill) short extension tubing and connector, removing all air. Leave syringe attached to tubing.	Replaces air with normal saline, preventing air from entering patient's vein later during IV catheter insertion.
b Maintain sterility of connector end by reapplying end caps and set aside for attaching to catheter hub after successful venipuncture.	Prevents touch contamination, preventing microorganisms from entering infusion equipment and bloodstream.

CLINICAL JUDGMENT *Short extension sets may be used on short peripheral catheters. Reduces catheter manipulation. For patient safety, all connections should be of Luer-Lok type (Gorski et al., 2021). Many agencies use short extension tubing for continuous infusions and stand-alone saline locks (capped catheters).*

6 Prepare IV tubing and solution for continuous infusion:

STEP	RATIONALE
a Check IV solution using seven rights of medication administration. Review label for name and concentration of solution, type and concentration of any additives, volume, beyond-use and expiration dates, and sterility state. Check bag for leaks or discoloration.	Reviewing label for accuracy reduces risk for medication errors (Gorski et al., 2021). Risk for medication errors can be reduced with safe medication practices, including (Gorski et al., 2021): Do not use IV solutions that are discolored, contain precipitates, or are expired. Risk for infection transmission can be reduced by not using leaking bags because integrity has been compromised. Do not add medications to infusing containers of IV solutions
If using bar code, scan code on patient's wristband and then on IV fluid container. Be sure that prescribed additives such as potassium and vitamins have been added. Check solution for color and clarity. Check bag for leaks.	Barcode system reduces human error (Gorski et al., 2021).
b Open IV infusion set, maintaining sterility. *Note:* EIDs sometimes have a dedicated administration set; follow manufacturer instructions.	Prevents touch contamination, which can allow microorganisms to enter infusion equipment and bloodstream.
c Place roller clamp 2 to 5 cm (1 to 2 inches) below drip chamber and move roller clamp to "off" position.	Close proximity of roller clamp to drip chamber allows more accurate regulation of flow rate. Moving clamp to "off" prevents accidental spillage of IV solution.

Continued

STEP	RATIONALE
d Remove protective sheath over IV tubing port, on plastic IV solution bag (Fig. 54.1) or top of IV solution bottle while maintaining sterility.	Provides access for insertion of IV tubing spike into solution using sterile technique.
e Remove protective sheath from IV tubing spike while maintaining sterility of spike. Insert spike into port of IV bag using a twisting motion.	Flat surface on top of bottled solution may contain contaminants, whereas opening to plastic bag is recessed.

CLINICAL JUDGMENT *If solution container is a glass bottle, clean rubber stopper on glass-bottled solution with antiseptic swab and insert spike into rubber stopper of IV bottle. Bottles require vented tubing. Prevents contamination of bottled solution during spike insertion. If sterility is compromised, discard IV tubing and obtain new one.*

STEP	RATIONALE
f Compress drip chamber and release, allowing it to fill one-third to one-half full (Fig. 54.2).	Creates suction, allowing fluid to enter drip chamber and preventing air from entering tubing.

Fig. 54.1 Remove protective sheath from intravenous tubing port.

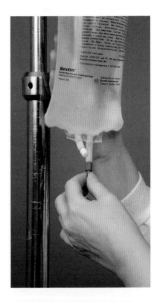

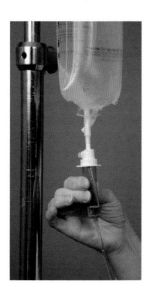

Fig. 54.2 Squeeze drip chamber to fill with fluid.

STEP	RATIONALE
g Prime air out of IV tubing by filling with IV solution: Remove protective cover on end of IV tubing (some tubing can be primed without removing protective cover) and slowly open roller clamp to allow fluid to flow from drip chamber to distal end of IV tubing. If tubing has a Y connector, invert Y connector when fluid reaches it to displace air. Return roller clamp to "off" position after priming tubing (filled with IV fluid).	Priming ensures that IV tubing is clear of air and filled with IV solution before connecting to VAD. Slowly filling tubing decreases turbulence and chance of bubble formation. Closing clamp prevents accidental loss of fluid.
Replace protective cover on distal end of tubing. Label IV tubing with date according to agency policy and procedure.	Maintains sterility. Labeling IV tubing allows for recognition of length of time tubing has been in use and when to change it.

Continued

STEP	RATIONALE
h Be certain that IV tubing is clear of air and air bubbles. Remove small air bubbles by firmly tapping tubing where bubbles are located. Check entire length of tubing.	Large air bubbles may act as emboli (Gorski, 2023).
i If using optional long extension tubing (not short tubing mentioned in Step 5), remove protective cover and attach to distal end of IV tubing, maintaining sterility. Then prime long extension tubing. Insert tubing into EID with power off.	Priming removes air so it does not enter patient's vascular system. Facilitates starting infusion as soon as IV site is ready.
7 Perform hand hygiene.	Decreases transmission of microorganisms.

CLINICAL JUDGMENT *Gloves are not necessary to locate vein but must be applied for VAD insertion using a no-touch technique in which the site is not palpated after skin antisepsis (Gorski et al, 2021).*

8 Apply tourniquet around upper arm about 10 to 15 cm (4 to 6 inches) above proposed insertion site. Do not apply tourniquet too tightly. Check for presence of pulse distal to tourniquet.	Tourniquet should be tight enough to impede venous flow while maintaining arterial circulation. If patient has fragile veins or bruises easily, tourniquet should be applied loosely or not at all to prevent damage to veins and bruising (Gorski et al., 2021).
(*Option A:* Apply tourniquet on top of thin layer of clothing such as gown sleeve to protect fragile or hairy skin.)	Reduces trauma to skin.

STEP	RATIONALE
(*Option B:* BP cuff may be used in place of tourniquet: activate cuff and hold at approximately 50 mm Hg. Avoid inserting catheter tip too close to the BP cuff.)	Excessive back pressure may be seen if venipuncture is performed too close to the BP cuff (Gorski, 2023).
9 Select vein for VAD insertion (Fig. 54.3). Veins on dorsal and ventral surfaces of arms (e.g., metacarpal, cephalic, basilic, or median) are preferred in adults.	Ensures adequate vein that is easy to puncture and less likely to rupture. Better hemodilution is obtained in the larger veins of the forearms (Gorski, 2023).
a Use most distal site in nondominant arm if possible.	Allows patient to perform self-care.

Continued

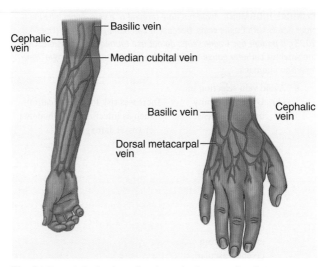

Fig. 54.3 Cephalic, basilic, and median cubital veins are best for intravenous line placement in adults.

STEP	RATIONALE
b With your fingertip, palpate vein at intended insertion site by pressing downward. Note resilient, soft, bouncy feeling while releasing pressure.	Fingertip is more sensitive and better for assessing vein location and condition.
c Select well-dilated vein.	Increased volume of blood in vein at venipuncture site makes vein more visible.
d Methods to improve vascular distention:	
(1) Position extremity lower than heart, have patient open and close fist slowly, and lightly stroke vein downward.	Use of gravity promotes vascular distention (Gorski et al., 2021).
(2) Apply dry heat to extremity for several minutes.	Dry heat has been found to increase successful peripheral catheter insertion (Gorski et al., 2021).

CLINICAL JUDGMENT *Avoid multiple tapping of a vein, especially in older adults with fragile veins, because it can damage the vein (Gorski, 2023). If patient has fragile veins: do not use tourniquet if possible. Use the smallest catheter gauge available. Use a "bevel-up," "low angle" slow insertion approach.*

e Avoid vein selection in:	
(1) Upper extremity on side of breast surgery with axillary node dissection or lymphedema or after radiation, arteriovenous fistulas/grafts; or affected extremity from cerebrovascular accident (Gorski et al., 2021).	Increases risk for complications, such as infection, lymphedema, or vessel damage.

STEP	RATIONALE
(2) Areas with pain on palpation, compromised areas, sites distal to compromised areas (e.g., open wounds, bruising, infection, infiltration, or extravasation) (Gorski et al., 2021).	Assessment of signs or symptoms of complications is more difficult if an IV device is inserted in an area already compromised. Phlebitis is associated with bruised insertion sites (Marsh et al., 2018).
(3) Site distal to previous venipuncture site, sclerosed or hardened veins, areas of venous valves, or phlebitic vessels.	Such sites cause infiltration around newly placed VAD site and vessel damage.
(4) Veins of lower extremities should not be used for routine IV therapy in adults because of risk of tissue damage and thrombophlebitis (Gorski et al., 2021).	Leg Veins have increased risk for infiltration.
(5) Areas of flexion such as wrist or antecubital area and ventral surface of wrist (10 to 12.5 cm [4 to 5 inches]).	Veins have increased risk for infiltration, phlebitis, or dislodgement. Ventral surface of wrist is painful, potential nerve damage.
10 Release tourniquet temporarily.	Restores blood flow and prevents venospasm when preparing for venipuncture.

Continued

STEP	RATIONALE

CLINICAL JUDGMENT *If hair removal is needed, do not shave area with a razor. Shaving increases risk of infection (Gorski et al., 2021). Clip hair with scissors or hair clippers to prepare area for application of TSM dressing, if necessary (explain to patient).*

CLINICAL JUDGMENT *Both topical and injectable local anesthetics can be used to reduce pain, and require a health care provider's order. Apply topical local anesthetic to intended IV site 30 minutes before procedure. Follow manufacturer recommendations and monitor for allergic reaction (Gorski, 2023; Gorski et al., 2021).*

STEP	RATIONALE
11 Perform hand hygiene and apply clean gloves. Wear eye protection and mask (see agency policy) if splash or spray of blood is possible.	Use of ANTT decreases potential risk of microbial contamination and cross-contamination (Gorski et al., 2021).
12 Place adapter end of short extension set (see Step 5) or needleless connector (injection cap) for saline lock nearby in the sterile package.	Permits smooth, quick connection of infusion to short peripheral catheter once vein is accessed. Keeps equipment sterile.
13 If area of insertion is visibly soiled, clean site with antiseptic soap and water first and dry. Then apply alcoholic CHG prep in back-and-forth motion for 30 seconds and allow to dry completely. If using alcohol or povidone-iodine, clean in concentric circle, moving from insertion site outward with swab. Allow drying time between agents if agents are used in combination. Do not touch insertion site after disinfecting.	Drying allows for complete antisepsis; alcoholic CHG solutions for at least 30 seconds; iodophors for at least 1.5 to 2 minutes (Gorski et al., 2021).

CLINICAL JUDGMENT *If vein palpation is necessary after performing skin antisepsis, use sterile gloves for palpation or perform skin antisepsis again. Touching cleaned area introduces microorganisms from your finger to site (Gorski et al., 2021).*

STEP	RATIONALE
14 Reapply tourniquet 10 to 15 cm (4 to 6 inches) above anticipated insertion site. Check for presence of pulse distal to tourniquet.	Pressure of tourniquet promotes vein distention. Diminished arterial flow prevents venous filling.
15 Perform venipuncture: Anchor vein below anticipated insertion site by placing thumb over vein 4 to 5 cm (½ to 2 inches) distal to selected insertion site. Gently stretch skin against direction of insertion. Instruct patient to relax hand.	Stabilizes vein for needle insertion; prevents vein from rolling; and stretches skin taut, decreasing drag during insertion. Some devices require loosening needle (stylet) from catheter before venipuncture. Follow manufacturer directions for use.
a Warn patient of a sharp stick. Hold catheter with needle bevel up. Align catheter on top of vein at 10- to 30-degree angle. Puncture skin and anterior vein wall (See Fig. 54.4).	Accessing vein at an angle reduces risk of puncturing posterior vein wall. Superficial veins require smaller angle. Deeper veins require greater angle.

Continued

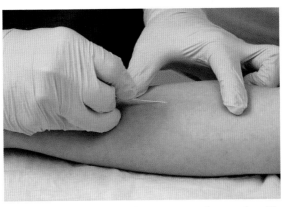

Fig. 54.4 Puncture skin with catheter at 10- to 15-degree angle to skin.

STEP	RATIONALE

CLINICAL JUDGMENT *Use each catheter only once for each insertion attempt.*

---

16 Observe for blood return in catheter or flashback chamber of catheter, indicating that bevel of needle has entered vein (Fig. 54.5). Advance catheter approximately ¼ inch (0.6 cm) into vein and loosen stylet (needle). Continue to hold skin taut while stabilizing catheter and, with index finger on push-off tab, advance catheter off needle into vein until hub rests at venipuncture site. *Do not reinsert stylet into catheter once catheter has been advanced into vein.* Advance catheter while safety device automatically retracts stylet (techniques for retracting stylet vary with different VADs). Place stylet directly into sharps container.

Increased venous pressure from tourniquet causes backflow of blood into catheter and/ or flashback chamber. Some devices have a notch in the stylet, allowing flash of blood into catheter. Stabilizing allows for placement of catheter into vein and advancement of catheter off stylet.

Advancing entire stylet into vein may penetrate wall of vein, resulting in hematoma. Advancing catheter with finger on open hub causes contamination (Gorski et al., 2021).

Reinsertion of stylet can cause catheter to shear off and embolize into vein. Proper sharps disposal prevents needlestick injury (OSHA, n.d.).

CLINICAL JUDGMENT *A single clinician should not make more than two attempts at initiating IV access, and total attempts should be limited to no more than four (Gorski et al., 2021).*

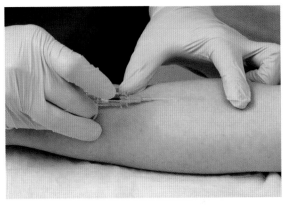

Fig. 54.5 Observe for blood return in catheter or flashback chamber.

STEP	RATIONALE
17 Stabilize catheter hub with nondominant hand and release tourniquet or BP cuff with other. Apply gentle but firm pressure with middle finger of nondominant hand 3 cm (1¼ inches) above insertion site. Keep catheter stable with index finger.	Permits venous flow and reduces backflow of blood. Digital pressure minimizes blood loss and allows attachment of extension set or needleless connector (Gorski et al., 2021).
18 Quickly connect Luer-Lok end of short extension tubing with needleless connector to end of catheter hub. Secure connection. Avoid touching sterile connection ends following ANTT.	Prompt connection maintains patency of vein, minimizes blood loss, and prevents risk of exposure to blood. Maintains sterility.

Continued

STEP	RATIONALE
Option: IV tubing can be attached directly to catheter hub in place of short extension tubing or needleless connector.	
19 Attach prefilled syringe of 0.9% sodium chloride to short extension set and aspirate to remove air and assess blood return. (Do not reinject any air; remove from syringe before flush.) After blood return, slowly inject normal saline from prefilled syringe into catheter (Fig. 54.6). Look for swelling at insertion site. Remove syringe and discard.	Aspirating air prevents air embolism. Blood return that is color and consistency of whole blood confirms placement of catheter in vein (Gorski et al., 2021). Flushing prevents reflux of blood into catheter and occlusion (Gorski et al., 2021). Swelling indicates infiltration, and catheter would need to be removed and restarted.

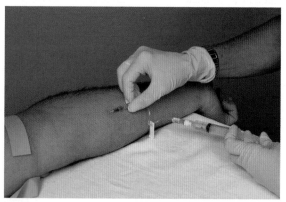

Fig. 54.6 Flush short extension set after aspirating air and assessing blood return.

STEP	RATIONALE
Option: To begin primary infusion, swab needleless connector with antiseptic swab and attach Luer-Lok end of IV tubing to needleless connector. Open roller clamp of IV tubing, turn on EID, and program it. Begin infusion at correct rate. If using gravity flow instead of EID, begin infusion by slowly opening roller clamp to regulate rate.	Initiates flow of fluid through IV catheter, preventing clotting of VAD.

CLINICAL JUDGMENT *Needleless connectors have different internal mechanisms for fluid displacement and vary in the flush-clamp-disconnect sequence to prevent reflux of blood into catheter on disconnection (Gorski et al. 2021). Sequence depends on the type of internal mechanism (Gorski, 2023):*
Neutral displacement devices do not have a specified flush/clamp/ disconnect sequence.
FOR NEGATIVE-PRESSURE displacement devices, flush, clamp catheter while maintaining pressure on flush syringe, and then disconnect syringe.
FOR POSITIVE-PRESSURE displacement, flush, disconnect syringe, and then clamp catheter.

20 Apply protective skin barrier: film, cream, or wipe over area around IV site insertion. Allow to dry completely.	Skin should be protected with a barrier product before an adhesive medical device (including tape) is applied. This should be a standard part of the skin-care protocol to prevent MARSI (Fumarola et al., 2020). Forms a mechanical barrier over the skin; thin and nonmessy if dries thoroughly. Dressings can still adhere to the skin (Fumarola et al., (2020).

Continued

STEP	RATIONALE
21 Apply sterile dressing over site.	
a TSM dressing:	
(1) Continue to hold hub of catheter with nondominant hand. Remove adherent backing of dressing. Apply one edge of dressing and gently smooth over IV insertion site). Do not apply with tension or stretching.	Protects catheter insertion site and minimizes risk for infection (Gorski, 2023). Allows visualization of insertion site and surrounding area for complications (Gorski et al., 2021).
Leave the Luer-Lok connection between tubing and catheter hub uncovered. Apply in the correct orientation to allow for stretching of body part if movement or swelling is anticipated. Smooth into place without gaps or wrinkles. Remove outer covering and smooth dressing gently over site (see Fig. 54.7).	Access to Luer-Lok connection between tubing and catheter hub facilitates changing tubing if necessary. Steps of application follow evidence based guidelines (Fumarola et al., 2020).
(2) Place 2.5 cm (2-inch) piece of tape over Luer-Lok connector. Do not cover connection between connector and catheter hub. Do not apply tape on top of TSM dressing.	Removal of tape from TSM dressing can tear dressing and cause catheter dislodgement. Tape on top of TSM dressing prevents moisture from being carried away from skin.

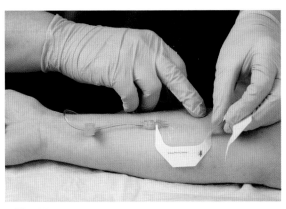

Fig. 54.7 Apply transparent semipermeable membrane dressing.

STEP	RATIONALE

b Sterile gauze dressing:

(1) Be sure skin is dry, then place 5-cm (2-inch) piece of sterile plastic tape over catheter hub. NOTE: plastic tape is preferred over other tapes for short-term wear to prevent MARSI (Fumarola et al., 2020).

Moisture reduces effectiveness of adhesion (Fumarola et al., 2020). Stabilizes catheter under gauze dressing.

(2) Place 2 × 2–inch gauze pad over insertion site and edge of catheter hub. Secure all edges with tape. Do not place tape over insertion site. Do not cover connection between IV tubing and catheter hub.

Use gauze dressings for site drainage, excessive perspiration, or sensitivity/allergic reactions to TSM dressings (Gorski, 2023).

Continued

STEP	RATIONALE
(3) Fold 2 × 2–inch gauze in half and cover with 1-inch-wide (2.5 cm) tape so that about 1 inch will extend on each side of dressing. Place under Luer-Lok connector. Secure Luer-Lok connector and tubing to tape on folded gauze with 2.5-cm (1-inch) piece of tape. Avoid applying tape or gauze around arm.	Tape on top of gauze makes it easier to access hub/tubing junction. Gauze pad elevates hub off skin to prevent pressure area. Prevents back-and-forth motion of catheter.
Do not use rolled bandages with or without elastic to secure catheter. Taping Luer-Lok connection can be eliminated if engineered stabilization device is to be used.	Rolled bandages do not secure VAD adequately, and can impair circulation or flow of infusion, and obscure visualization for complications (Gorski et al., 2021).
22 *Option:* Secure IV catheter using engineered stabilization device (follow manufacturer directions and agency policy).	Devices allow visual inspection of insertion site and can reduce risk of VAD complications (i.e., phlebitis, occlusion/infiltration, dislodgment, and infection) and unintentional loss of IV access (Gorski et al., 2021; Marsh et al., 2018).
a Apply skin protectant to area of skin where stabilization device is to be placed. Allow to dry completely.	Minimizes risk for MARSI, which increases with age, joint movement, and edema (Fumarola et al., 2020).

STEP	RATIONALE
(1) Align anchoring pads with directional arrow pointing to insertion site. Press device retainer over top of Luer-Lok connection while supporting underneath connection.	
(2) Stabilize catheter and peel off one side of liner and press to adhere to skin. Repeat on other side.	
23 *Option:* Apply site protection device.	Reduces risk of VAD dislodgement (Gorski et al., 2021).
24 Loop extension or IV tubing alongside dressing on arm and secure with second piece of tape directly over tubing.	Reduces risk for dislodging catheter if IV tubing is pulled (i.e., loop comes apart before catheter dislodges).
25 For continuous infusion, verify ordered rate of infusion and be sure EID is programmed correctly. If infusing by gravity drip, adjust flow rate to correct drops per minute.	Prevents fluid overload.
26 Label dressing per agency policy. Include date and time of IV insertion, VAD gauge size and length, and initials of person inserting device.	Allows for recognition of type of device and length of time that device has been in place.

Continued

STEP	RATIONALE
27 When disposing of supplies use the appropriate receptacle if patient is receiving hazardous drugs (Oncology Nursing Society, 2018).	Contact with blood can expose nurse to chemotherapeutic agent.
28 Perform postprocedure protocol.	
29 Evaluate patient response:	
a Observe patient every 1 to 2 h or at established intervals per agency policy and procedure for function, intactness, and patency of IV system; correct infusion rate; and accurate type/amount of IV solution infused (by observing level in IV container).	Ensures delivery of prescribed volume over prescribed time and decreases risk for fluid and electrolyte imbalance.
b Review laboratory values, intake and output, weights, vital signs, other physical findings, condition of IV site.	Early recognition of complications leads to prompt treatment.
c Observe for signs and symptoms of phlebitis and infiltration: inspect and gently palpate skin around and above IV site over the dressing.	Identifies complications that compromise integrity of VAD or cause inaccurate IV solution flow rate.
d Monitor IV dressing site for MARSI: mechanical trauma (skin stripping, blistering, skin tears), dermatitis (irritation in response to adhesive), and maceration and folliculitis.	MARSI refers to any skin damage related to the use of medical adhesive products or devices (such as tape).

Recording and Reporting

- Record number of insertion attempts (successful and unsuccessful), precise description of insertion site by location, catheter brand, length, and gauge; IV solution and additives infusing; rate and method of infusion (e.g., gravity or EID); appearance of IV site; patient response to insertion (e.g., what they report).
- Record patient's status and when infusion was started. Record amount of fluid infused on intake and output flow sheet.
- Record tubing or catheter flushes to include solution, volume, and concentration.
- Record patient and family caregiver's level of understanding after instruction.
- Report to oncoming nursing staff placement of catheter, reason for insertion, signs or symptoms of observed or patient-reported IV-related complications, type of fluid, flow rate, status of catheter, amount of fluid remaining in present solution, expected time to hang subsequent IV container, and current patient condition.
- Report to health care provider any adverse events during/after insertion (e.g., persistent pain or suspected nerve damage, hematoma formation, arterial puncture, phlebitis).

UNEXPECTED OUTCOMES	RELATED INTERVENTIONS
1 FVD: decreased urine output, dry mucous membranes, decreased capillary refill, tachycardia, hypotension, shock.	• Notify health care provider. • May require readjustment of infusion rate.
2 Fluid volume excess: dyspnea, crackles in lung, edema, and/or increased urine output.	• Reduce IV flow rate. • Notify health care provider.
3 Electrolyte imbalances: abnormal serum electrolyte levels, changes in mental status, alterations in neuromuscular function, cardiac arrhythmias, and changes in vital signs.	• Notify health care provider. • Adjust additives or IV solution per order.

Continued

UNEXPECTED OUTCOMES	RELATED INTERVENTIONS
4 Infiltration: pain, swelling, coolness to touch, or presence of blanching (white, shiny appearance at or above IV site), or redness (Gorski et al., 2021).	• Notify health care provider or CRNI. • Stop infusion and remove IV catheter at first sign of infiltration. • Elevate affected extremity. • Avoid applying pressure, which can force solution into contact with more tissue, causing tissue damage.
5 Catheter occlusion due to bent catheter, positional catheter (catheter resting against vein wall), kink or knot in infusion tubing, clot formation, or precipitate formation from incompatible medications or solutions.	• Determine cause and consider catheter removal. • Positional catheters can be repositioned to improve IV flow. • Remove occluded IV catheter. Occluded catheters should not be flushed (Gorski, 2023).
6 Phlebitis (i.e., vein inflammation): pain, redness, warmth, swelling, induration, or presence of palpable cord along course of vein. Rate of infusion may be altered.	• Notify health care provider and CRNI. • Determine cause: *Chemical phlebitis:* Apply heat, elevate limb, and consider slowing infusion rate (Gorski et al., 2021). *Mechanical phlebitis:* Apply heat, elevate limb, monitor for 24 to 48 h, consider catheter removal if signs and symptoms persist (Gorski et al., 2021). *Bacterial phlebitis:* Remove IV catheter (Gorski et al., 2021). Evidence does not recommend use of topical agents/interventions in the prevention or treatment of IV-related phlebitis (Goulart et al., 2020).

UNEXPECTED OUTCOMES	RELATED INTERVENTIONS
7 MARSI develops under adhesive covering IV site dressing.	• If IV site is to remain or if decision is made to remove IV and insert new one, protect skin with a skin barrier product. If skin is broken, an alcohol-free product will not irritate skin (Fumarola et al., 2020). • Treat affected skin with appropriate emollient.

Preoperative Teaching

With shortened hospital lengths of stay and growth in ambulatory surgery, there is a greater demand for early patient preparation. Patient education must go beyond providing information. Patients and families must be prepared to understand the expected course of recovery, anticipate possible complications, and participate in recovery activities (e.g., exercise and diet). Comprehensive preoperative patient education has traditionally been provided to patients with the intent of improving patient knowledge, health behaviors, and health outcomes. However the evidence is mixed regarding the efficacy of preoperative education (McDonald et al., 2014). The content of preoperative education varies across settings but frequently includes discussion of presurgical procedures, the actual steps in a surgical procedure, postoperative care (e.g., monitoring, positioning, exercises), scenarios that contribute to potential stress associated with surgery, potential surgical and nonsurgical complications, postoperative pain management, physical movements to avoid after surgery, and how to eliminate high-risk behaviors that can slow recovery (Association of periOperative Registered Nurses, 2019; McDonald et al., 2014; Smetana, 2020).

In the case of orthopedic surgery, patients often undergo rehabilitation that involves formal exercise programs. In patients undergoing total knee and hip arthroplasty, research shows significant improvements in function, postoperative pain, and length of hospital stay in patients who participated in these exercise programs (Moyer et al., 2017). These programs are becoming more of a standard, but research is not conclusive as the quality of the interventions in different studies has varied.

This skill summarizes basic preoperative teaching for patients who undergo general anesthesia or monitored sedation. Much of the education will occur before a patient enters the hospital or surgical center, and is completed through pamphlets and brochures or preoperative classes. Some surgeons have nursing staff contact patients by phone before surgery to provide basic preoperative education.

Safety Guidelines

- Assess a patient's home environment and whether a caregiver is present so that any teaching of skills can be adapted to the patient's setting.

Delegation

The skills of preoperative teaching cannot be delegated to assistive personnel (AP). AP can reinforce and help patients perform postoperative exercises. Instruct the AP about:

- Any precautions or safety issues unique to the patient (e.g., fall precautions, mobility limitations, bleeding precautions, weight-bearing issues, dietary concerns).
- Informing the nurse of any identified concerns (e.g., patient is unable to perform the exercises correctly).

Collaboration

- Physical therapy and/or respiratory therapy can offer support of postoperative exercise education.

Equipment

- Stretcher or bed
- Pillow
- Incentive spirometer
- Preoperative education flow sheet
- Positive expiratory pressure (PEP) device
- Stethoscope
- Equipment for patient self-care skills to be performed after discharge

STEP	RATIONALE
1 Perform preprocedure protocol.	

Assessment

• Ask about patient's previous experiences with surgery and anesthesia.	This allows for individualized teaching and addresses specific patient concerns.
• Identify patient's cognitive level, language, and culture. If patient does not speak English, have a professional interpreter assist with communication. Have family caregiver present if appropriate.	These factors may alter patient's ability to understand meaning of surgery and can affect postoperative healing if there are mixed messages or misunderstandings.

Continued

STEP	RATIONALE
• Assess patient's risk for postoperative respiratory complications. Check electronic health record (EHR) for patient's height and age.	General anesthesia predisposes patient to respiratory problems e.g., atelectasis and pneumonia. Presence of underlying respiratory conditions or patient's inability to perform postoperative respiratory exercises increases patient's risk for pulmonary complications. Height and age are used to set incentive spirometer parameters.
• Assess patient's level of anxiety related to surgery and recovery.	Directs you to provide additional emotional support and indicates patient's readiness to learn.
• Assess family caregiver's willingness to learn and support patient after surgery.	Family caregiver's presence after surgery can be a potential motivating factor for patient recovery. A caregiver can coach patient through postoperative exercise and observe for any postoperative problems.
• Assess patient's understanding of the intended surgery and anesthesia. Ask patient to offer a description rather than asking a simple yes-or-no question (e.g., "Tell me what your surgery will involve."). Ask about patient's and family caregiver's expectations of surgery and care. Include questions concerning time frame for surgery and recovery, fears, cultural practices, and religious or spiritual beliefs.	Patients may have misconceptions and incomplete knowledge. Asking about fears, cultural practices, and religious or spiritual beliefs allows for anticipation of priorities of care and subsequent adaptation of teaching and support.

STEP	RATIONALE
• Assess patient's EHR for type of surgery and approach.	The surgical procedure itself may require patient to limit activities postoperatively. Anticipating limitations that might affect how patient can perform postoperative exercises allows for adaptation of preoperative instruction.

Implementation

STEP	RATIONALE
1 Explain surgery to patient, including the procedure, expected postoperative experiences, and exercises that improve recovery. Inform patient and family caregiver of date, time, and location of surgery; anticipated length of surgery; additional time in postanesthesia recovery area; and where family caregivers can wait during procedure.	Accurate information helps reduce anticipatory stress associated with surgery.

CLINICAL JUDGMENT *Preoperative education is provided by nurses in health care provider offices, surgical centers, and hospitals. Patients usually receive printed information preoperatively. Education is individualized to the type of surgical procedure. Whenever patient interaction is involved, encourage and answer questions to clarify misconceptions and encourage patient participation. Elective surgery allows for more time to prepare patients. Urgent surgery reduces time available for detailed educational instruction.*

2 Preparation before patient comes to a surgical center or hospital:

Continued

STEP	RATIONALE
a Instruct about preoperative skin preparations. Check medical orders and agency policy regarding number of preoperative showers and agent to be used for each shower (2% or 4% chlorhexidine gluconate is most common). After each preoperative shower, instruct patient to rinse the skin thoroughly and dry with a fresh, clean, dry towel. Patient should don clean clothing.	Proper skin preparation is a critical element in preventing surgical site infections. Rinsing skin removes residual antiseptic preparation that may cause skin irritation (Mann, 2020). After use, towels contain microorganisms that can grow in presence of moisture. Using fresh towel after each shower and donning clean clothing minimizes risk of reintroducing microorganisms to clean skin (Berrios-Torres et al., 2017).
b Instruct about bowel preparation for those undergoing major abdominal surgery (guidelines will vary). Explain to patient when to take ordered bowel preparation (e.g., NuLytely) and clear liquids to stay hydrated.	Hyperosmotic laxatives are sometimes used to clear bowel of fecal material, reducing risk of contamination of surgical field when incision is made.
c Instruct patient about extent and purpose of food and fluid restrictions for period specified before surgery (e.g., no clear liquids at least 2 h before surgery, no light meal [e.g., toast and a clear liquid] 6 h or more before surgery, no meat or fried foods 8 h before surgery, unless otherwise specified by surgeon or anesthesiologist) (Crowley, 2019).	During general anesthesia and monitored sedation muscles relax and gastric contents can reflux into esophagus, leading to pulmonary aspiration. Anesthetic eliminates patient's ability to gag.

STEP	RATIONALE
d Review which routine medications patient needs to discontinue before surgery. Some surgeons may allow patients to take medication as prescribed, but with only a sip of water. In many cases patients cannot take any anticoagulant or other medication containing aspirin 5 to 7 days before surgery; however, the health care provider must assess whether this is a risk (Wanderer and Rathmell, 2017). No herbal supplements or preparations should be taken 1 week before surgery.	Some medications are discontinued before surgery to minimize effects that can cause surgical risks. For example, anticoagulants may increase bleeding and are usually discontinued several days before surgery. Insulin dosages are usually adjusted because of reduced intake of food before surgery.
3 Preparation morning of surgery:	
a Describe perioperative routines (e.g., time-out, site marking, intravenous therapy, urinary catheterization, enema, hair clipping or removal, laboratory tests, and transport to operating room).	Allows patient to anticipate and recognize routine procedures, reducing anxiety.
b Describe planned effect of preoperative medications.	Provides information about what to expect, decreasing anxiety.
c Describe perioperative sensations (e.g., blood pressure cuff tightening, electrocardiogram leads, cool room, beep of monitor).	Misconceptions and concerns about anesthesia have been ranked high among preoperative patients.

Continued

STEP	RATIONALE
d Describe pain-control methods to be used after surgery. Many patients have a patient-controlled analgesia pump (see Skill 50).	Explaining pain-management techniques reduces patient fear. Manages expectations surrounding pain (knowing that they will not be pain free), but that their pain will be managed.
e Describe what patient will experience after surgery (e.g., where patient will be on awakening, frequent vital signs, catheters, drains, tubes, alternating pressure from sequential compression device, postoperative exercises).	Provides concrete description of what patient can expect after surgery so that patient is prepared.
4 Postoperative exercises.	
a *Turning.* Instruct patient on turning onto side and sitting up (especially suited for abdominal and thoracic surgery):	Promotes circulation and ventilation.
(1) Turn onto right side: Have patient assume supine position and move to side of bed (in this case left side) if permitted by surgery. Instruct patient to move by bending knees and pressing heels against mattress to raise and move buttocks (Fig. 55.1). Top side rails on both sides of bed should be in up position.	Positioning begins on side of bed so that turning to other side does not cause patient to roll toward edge of bed. Lifting the buttocks prevents shearing force against sheets. If patient's bed has a turn-assist feature, use it to help with positioning.

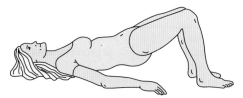

Fig. 55.1 Buttocks lifts for moving to side of bed.

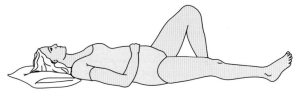

Fig. 55.2 Leg position before turning to right.

STEP	RATIONALE
(2) Have patient splint incision with right hand or with right hand with pillow over incisional area; keep right leg straight and flex left knee up (Fig. 55.2); grab right side rail with left hand, pull toward right, and roll onto right side. Reverse process to turn to left side.	Supports incision and decreases discomfort while turning.
(3) Instruct patient to turn every 2 h from side to side while awake. Patient may require assistance with turning after surgery.	Reduces risk of vascular, pulmonary, and pressure injury complications.

CLINICAL JUDGMENT *Some patients, such as those who have had back surgery or vascular repair, are restricted from flexing their legs after surgery. Some patients are restricted from turning or may need help for positioning.*

Continued

STEP	RATIONALE
b *Sit up on right side of bed.* Elevate head of bed and have patient turn onto right side. While lying on right side, patient pushes on mattress with left arm and swings feet over edge of bed to sit upright with nurse's help. To sit up on left side of bed, reverse this process.	Sitting position lowers diaphragm to permit fuller lung expansion.

CLINICAL JUDGMENT *Caution patient to always ask for assistance, particularly with first time sitting up on side of bed. Orthostatic hypotension will increase risk for a fall.*

c Deep breathing:	Patient may be unable or reluctant to deep breathe because of weakness or pain, resulting in secretions remaining in base of lungs. Collection of secretions increases risk of pulmonary atelectasis and pneumonia.
(1) Assist patient to high-Fowler position in bed with knees flexed, or have patient sit on side of bed or chair in upright position.	Sitting position facilitates diaphragmatic expansion.
(2) Instruct patient to place palms of hands across from one another lightly along lower border of rib cage or upper abdomen (Fig. 55.3).	This allows patient to feel rise and fall of abdomen during deep breathing.

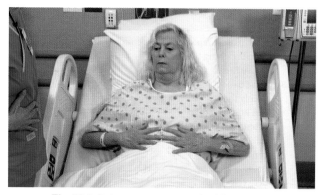

Fig. 55.3 Patient assuming position for deep breathing.

STEP	RATIONALE
(3) Have patient take slow, deep breaths, inhaling through nose. Explain that patient will feel normal downward movement of diaphragm during inspiration. Demonstrate as needed. Encourage patient to relax.	Helps to prevent hyperventilation or panting. Slow, deep breath allows for more complete lung expansion.
(5) Have patient avoid using chest and shoulder muscles while inhaling.	Increases unnecessary energy expenditure and does not promote full lung expansion.
(6) Once breathing pattern established, have patient take slow, deep breath, inhaling through nose; hold for count of 3 seconds; and slowly exhale through pursed lips as if blowing out candle.	Resistance during exhalation helps to prevent alveolar collapse. Deep breaths expand lungs fully so that air moves behind mucus to facilitate coughing.

Continued

STEP	RATIONALE
(7) Have patient repeat deep breathing three to five times.	Repetition reinforces learning.
(8) Have patient inhale deeply the last time and hold breath to count of 3. Cough fully for two to three consecutive coughs without inhaling between coughs.	Deep breathing moves up secretions in respiratory tract to stimulate cough reflex without voluntary effort on part of patient and reduces atelectasis (Conde and Adams, 2020; Lewis et al., 2019).
d Controlled coughing:	
(1) Explain importance of maintaining upright position.	Position facilitates diaphragm excursion and enhances thorax and abdominal expansion.
(2) Demonstrate coughing. Take two slow, deep breaths, inhaling through nose and exhaling through mouth (pursed lips).	Consecutive coughs help remove mucus more effectively and completely than one forceful cough.
(3) To exhale, have patient lean forward, pressing arms against their abdomen. Cough two to three times without inhaling between coughs. Cough through a slightly open mouth. Coughs should be short and sharp. Tell patient to push all air out of lungs.	Clearing throat does not remove mucus from deeper airways. Full, forceful cough is most effective in removing mucus.
(4) Caution patient against just clearing throat instead of coughing deeply.	Clearing throat does not remove mucus from deeper airways.

STEP	RATIONALE
(5) If surgical incision is either thoracic or abdominal, teach patient to place either hands or pillow over incisional area and place hands over pillow to splint incision (Fig. 55.4). During breathing and coughing exercises, press gently against incisional area for splinting and support.	Surgical incision cuts through muscles, tissues, and nerve endings. Deep-breathing and coughing exercises place additional stress on suture line and cause discomfort. Splinting incision with hands or pillow provides firm support and reduces incisional pulling and pain.

Continued

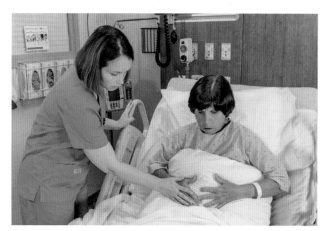

Fig. 55.4 Patient splinting abdomen with pillow.

STEP	RATIONALE
(6) Instruct patient to practice deep breathing and coughing exercises, splinting imaginary incision. Instruct patient to cough two to three times every 2 h while awake after surgery. Have family caregiver coach patient.	Deep coughing with splinting effectively expectorates mucus with minimal discomfort. Frequent pulmonary exercises and movement decrease risk of postoperative pneumonia (Lewis et al., 2019; Smetana, 2020).
(7) Instruct patient to examine sputum for consistency, odor, amount, and color changes and notify a nurse if any changes are noted.	Sputum consistency, odor, amount, and color changes indicate presence of pulmonary complication such as pneumonia.
e Use of an incentive spirometer (see Skill 31)	Provides visual aid of respiratory effort. Encourages deep breathing to loosen secretions in lung bases.
f PEP therapy and "huff" coughing:	PEP therapy creates expiratory flow resistance to increase airway diameter and enhance mucus clearance (Demchuk and Chatburn, 2021).
(1) Set PEP device for setting ordered.	Higher settings require more effort.
(2) Instruct patient to assume semi-Fowler or high-Fowler position in bed or to sit in a chair and place nose clip on patient's nose (Fig.55.5).	Promotes optimum lung expansion and mucus expectoration.

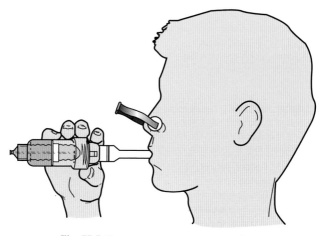

Fig. 55.5 Using positive expiratory pressure device.

STEP	RATIONALE
(3) Have patient place lips around mouthpiece. Instruct patient to take full breath and exhale two or three times longer than inhalation. Repeat pattern for 10 to 20 breaths.	Ensures that patient does all breathing through mouth. Ensures that patient uses device properly. Monitor patient for hyperventilation.
(4) Remove device from mouth and have patient take slow, deep breath and hold for 3 seconds.	Promotes lung expansion before coughing.
(5) Instruct patient to exhale in quick, short, forced "huffs." Repeat exercise every 2 h while awake.	"Huff" coughing, or forced expiratory technique, promotes bronchial hygiene by increasing expectoration of secretions.

Continued

STEP	RATIONALE
g Leg exercises (confirm with health care provider which exercises are allowed):	Nature of patient's surgery may contraindicate certain exercises.

CLINICAL JUDGMENT *Leg exercises are recommended for patients restricted to bed or during times when patients are ambulatory but resting in bed or in a chair. The ideal exercise to promote venous return and improve lung vital capacity is early mobility.*

(1) Position patient supine.	
(2) Instruct patient to rotate each ankle in complete circle and draw imaginary circles with big toe five times	Promotes joint mobility.
(3) Alternate dorsiflexion and plantar flexion while instructing patient to feel calf muscles tighten and relax. Repeat five times	Helps maintain joint mobility and promote venous return to prevent thrombus formation.
(4) Perform quadriceps-setting exercise by tightening thigh and bringing knee down toward mattress and relaxing. Repeat five times.	Quadriceps-setting exercises contract muscles of upper legs, maintain knee mobility, and improve venous return to heart.
(5) Instruct patient to alternate raising one leg straight up from bed surface. Leg should be kept straight. Repeat five times.	Causes quadriceps muscle contraction and relaxation, which help promote venous return.

STEP	RATIONALE
5 Have patient continue to practice all exercises before surgery at least every 2 h while awake. Teach patient to coordinate turning and leg exercises with diaphragmatic breathing and coughing and using incentive spirometer.	Leg exercises stimulate circulation, which prevents venous stasis to help prevent formation of deep vein thrombosis (Lip and Hull, 2020).
6 Verify that patient's expectations of surgery are realistic. Correct expectations as needed.	Can prevent postoperative anxiety or anger.
7 Reinforce therapeutic coping strategies. If ineffective, encourage alternatives.	Therapeutic coping strategies promote postoperative adherence and recovery.
8 Perform postprocedure protocol.	
9 Evaluate patient response:	
a Observe patient demonstrating splinting, turning and sitting, deep breathing, using incentive spirometer, PEP therapy, and leg exercises.	Validates patient's ability to perform postoperative exercises and use devices.
b Ask family to identify location of waiting room and validate or correct as needed.	Establishes family's knowledge of where they can wait for patient information.
c Ask family caregiver to explain how to help prepare patient at home before surgery.	Establishes that postoperative home care is in place for patient on discharge.
d Observe level of emotional support family caregiver provides patient.	Identifies preoperative emotional support for patient.

Recording and Reporting

- Document all preoperative patient and family caregiver teaching and response to teaching.
- Report patient's inability to identify procedure and site of surgery to health care provider.
- Report to charge nurse patient understanding of postoperative exercise(s).

UNEXPECTED OUTCOMES	RELATED INTERVENTIONS
1 Patient identifies incorrect procedure, site, date, or time of surgery.	• Provide correct information verbally and in writing for patient and family caregiver. • Notify health care provider about procedure knowledge.
2 Patient incorrectly performs one of the postoperative exercises.	• Explain and demonstrate correct exercise technique. • Explain importance of the postoperative exercise as it pertains to patient recovery. • Instruct patient to repeat demonstration.

Pressure Bandage

The first step in controlling a hemorrhaging wound or injury is the application of direct pressure. A pressure bandage is a temporary treatment to control excessive, sudden, unanticipated bleeding (Picard, 2017). Applied with elastic bandages, a pressure dressing exerts localized downward pressure over an actual or potential bleeding site. Hemorrhage may occur during or after diagnostic interventions (e.g., cardiac catheterization, arterial puncture, organ biopsy), surgery, or a life-threatening traumatic injury (stabbing, gunshot). Pressure dressings are essential for stopping the flow of blood and promoting clotting at the site (hemostasis) until definitive action can be taken.

Safety Guidelines

- Given the emergent nature of an acute bleeding episode, the aseptic techniques considered essential in most dressing applications are secondary to the goal of halting the bleeding.
- Overly excessive pressure on an affected arm or leg can compromise circulation to an extremity.

Delegation

The skill of applying a pressure dressing in an emergency situation cannot be delegated to assistive personnel (AP). If application requires more than one person, the AP can assist. Direct the AP to:

- Be sure patient does not try to disrupt dressing, and observe the pressure dressing during care activities to make sure that it remains in place and that there is no visible bleeding from the site.
- Observe underneath patient for bleeding after dressing has been applied (and report to health care team as needed).

Collaboration

- Collaborate with health care providers when excessive bleeding occurs to properly prepare patient for future surgery or treatment, such as a chest tube.

Equipment

- Clean gloves
- Necessary dressings: fine-mesh gauze, abdominal gauze pads, hemostatic dressings, elastic roller gauze
- Adhesive tape; hypoallergenic if possible

- Adhesive remover (optional)
- Personal protective equipment (PPE) (e.g., gown, goggles/face mask, mask) as needed
- Equipment for vital signs

STEP	RATIONALE
1 If situation permits, identify patient using two identifiers (e.g., name and birthday or name and medical record number) according to agency policy.	Ensures correct patient. Complies with The Joint Commission standards and improves patient safety (The Joint Commission, 2023). Not always possible in emergent situations.

Assessment

• Perform hand hygiene and apply clean gloves and additional necessary PPE. Anticipate patients at risk for unexpected bleeding: traumatic injury, arterial puncture, donor graft site, postoperative incision, wounds after surgical debridement, and surgical patient with history of bleeding disorder.	Familiarity with conditions associated with unexpected bleeding allows for rapid response to bleeding.
• Look for visible presence of blood, i.e., blood pulsating from arterial site.	These are signs of hemorrhage.

CLINICAL JUDGMENT *If patient is bleeding profusely move immediately to Implementation Phase I, Steps 2 and 3.*

CLINICAL JUDGMENT *If a patient is bleeding from a thoracic or abdominal surgical or traumatic wound, turn patient over to fully assess the amount of hemorrhage.*

STEP	RATIONALE
• If situation permits, assess patient for allergies to antiseptics, tape, or latex. If patient is nonresponsive and no history is available, use nonlatex or nonallergenic supplies where possible.	Prevents localized or systemic allergic reaction.
• Quickly assess patient's anxiety level.	Determines need for education and positive reinforcement during procedure.
• Obtain patient's current vital signs. If bleeding from an extremity, obtain peripheral pulse.	Baseline vital signs indicate status of circulatory function.

Implementation

Phase I: Immediate Action—First Nurse

1 Perform hand hygiene and apply clean gloves. Identify external bleeding site. Turn patient as needed to observe underneath (especially one with a larger abdominal circumference). *Note:* Wounds to groin area (e.g., femoral artery source) also can result in large amounts of blood loss, which is not always visible.	Quick identification increases response time to stop bleeding. Maintaining asepsis and privacy are considered only if time and severity of blood loss permit.
2 Use both hands and press as hard as possible to apply immediate manual pressure to bleeding site.	External pressure over the wound helps control bleeding (Picard, 2017).
3 Remain with the patient and seek help.	Situation potentially life-threatening. Patient should not be left alone.

CLINICAL JUDGMENT *Seek assistance from additional member of the health care team to insert intravenous catheters, prepare dressings, and prepare for emergency transport to the operating room.*

Continued

STEP	RATIONALE

Phase II: Applying Pressure Bandage—Second Nurse

4 If the situation permits, perform hand hygiene and apply clean gloves. Quickly identify source of bleeding:

- *Arterial bleeding* is bright red and gushes forth in waves, related to patient's heart rate; if vessel is very deep, flow is steady.
- *Venous bleeding is* dark red and flows smoothly.
- *Capillary bleeding* is oozing of dark-red blood; self-sealing controls this bleeding.

Determines method of application and supplies to use. First nurse continues to apply pressure.

5 Elevate affected body part (e.g., extremity) if possible.

Helps slow rate of bleeding.

6 First nurse continues to apply direct pressure as second nurse unwraps elastic roller bandage and places within easy reach. Second nurse quickly cuts three to five lengths of adhesive tape and places them within reach; *do not clean wound.*

Pressure dressing controls bleeding temporarily. Preparation allows for securing pressure bandage quickly.

7 In simultaneous coordinated actions:

a Rapidly cover bleeding area with multiple thicknesses of gauze compresses. The first nurse slips fingers out as other nurse exerts adequate pressure to continue controlling bleeding.

Gauze is absorbent. Layers provide bulk against which local pressure can be applied to bleeding site.

STEP	RATIONALE
b Place adhesive strips 7 to 10 cm (3 to 4 inches) beyond width of gauze dressing with even pressure on both sides of fingers as close as possible to central bleeding source. Secure tape on distal end, pull tape across dressing, and keep firm pressure as proximate end of tape is secured.	Tape exerts downward pressure, promoting hemostasis. To ensure blood flow to distal tissues and prevent tourniquet effect, adhesive tape must not be continued around entire extremity.
c Temporarily remove fingers holding pressure against wound and quickly cover center of area with third strip of tape.	Provides pressure to source of bleeding.
d Continue reinforcing area with tape as each successive strip is overlapped on alternating sides of center strip. **Keep applying pressure**.	Prevents tape from loosening.
e When pressure bandage is on extremity, apply gauze directly over bleeding site. Then apply elastic roller bandage over gauze: Apply two circular turns tautly on both sides of fingers that are pressing gauze. Compress over bleeding site. Simultaneously remove finger pressure and apply roller bandage over center. Continue with figure-eight turns. Secure end with two circular turns and strip of adhesive.	Elastic roller bandage acts as pressure bandage, exerting more even pressure over extremity. (**Note**: Gauze roller bandage can be used if elastic not available.)
f Assess whether bleeding has stopped.	

Continued

STEP	RATIONALE

CLINICAL JUDGMENT *Start wrapping a pressure bandage from distal to proximal, working toward the heart. If bleeding continues, contact health care provider.*

8 Perform postprocedure protocol.

9 Evaluate patient response:

a Observe dressing for control of bleeding.	Effective pressure bandage controls bleeding without blocking distal circulation.
b Evaluate adequacy of circulation (distal pulse, skin temperature, and color).	Determines level of perfusion to distal body parts.
c Estimate volume of blood loss (e.g., count number of dressings used, weigh saturated dressing).	Helps to accurately determine blood and fluid replacement needs.
d Monitor vital signs.	Identifies patient's response to blood loss and whether early stages of hypovolemic shock develop.

Recording and Reporting

- Record location of bleeding, vital signs, assessment findings, application and type of pressure dressing, and patient response.
- Report immediately to health care provider present status of patient's bleeding control, time bleeding was discovered, estimated blood loss, nursing interventions (including effectiveness of applied pressure bandage), apical and distal pulses, blood pressure, mental status, signs of restlessness, and any need for prompt attention from health care provider.

UNEXPECTED OUTCOMES	RELATED INTERVENTIONS
1 Bleeding continues. Fluid and electrolyte imbalance, tissue hypoxia, confusion, hypovolemic shock, and cardiac arrest develop.	• Notify health care provider. • Reinforce or adjust pressure dressing. • Initiate intravenous therapy per order. • Monitor vital signs every 5 to 15 minutes (apical pulse, distal pulses, and blood pressure).
2 Pressure dressing is too tight and occludes circulation.	• Inspect areas distal to pressure dressing to ensure that circulation has not been occluded. • Adjust dressing as needed.

Pressure Injury Risk Assessment and Prevention

The goal in preventing the development of pressure injuries (PIs) is early identification of an at-risk patient and the implementation of prevention strategies. The *Prevention and Treatment of Pressure Ulcers/Injuries: Quick Reference Guide 2019* (European Pressure Ulcer Advisory Panel and National Pressure injury Advisory Panel, and Pan-Pacific Pressure Injury Alliance [EPUAP, NPIAP, PPPIA], 2019a) represents findings from an extensive literature review and identifies the best available evidence in the prevention and management of PIs. Overall management goals include the following items:

- Identify individuals at risk for developing PI and initiate an early prevention program.
- Implement appropriate strategies/plans to:
  - Attain/maintain intact skin.
  - Prevent complications.
  - Promptly identify or manage complications.
  - Involve patient and family caregiver in self-management.
  - Implement cost-effective strategies/plans that prevent and treat PIs.

The Braden scale is a reliable clinical assessment tool for prediction of PIs (Borchert, 2022). It has six parameters: sensory perception (ability to respond meaningfully to pressure-related discomfort), moisture (degree to which skin is exposed to moisture), activity (degree of physical activity), mobility (ability to change and control body position), nutrition (usual food intake pattern), and friction and shear (Ayello and Braden, 2002). A modified Norton Scale, optimized Norton Scale (oNS) had high PI injury prediction in critically ill patients. The scale was easier and more critical-care specific and focused on the vulnerabilities of patients with critical illness (Sullivan et al, 2020). The Jackson/Cubbin scale is another option for PI injury risk prediction in critically ill trauma-surgical patients (Delawder et al., 2021; Higgins et al., 2020). It is important to understand how to interpret the meaning of a patient's total score based on the scale utilized.

When performing a skin assessment, inspect all bony prominences when patient is lying and sitting (Fig. 57.1). Palpate any reddened or discolored areas with a gloved finger to determine whether the erythema (redness of the skin caused by dilation and congestion of the capillaries) blanches (lightens in color). *Blanching is normal.* If you palpate an area that

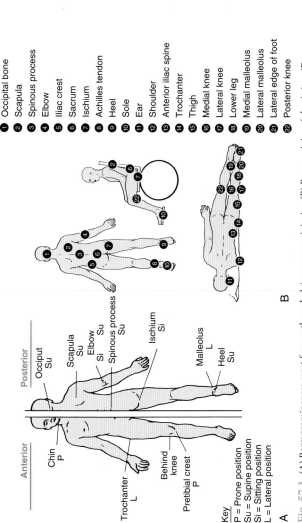

Pressure ulcer sites

1. Occipital bone
2. Scapula
3. Spinous process
4. Elbow
5. Iliac crest
6. Sacrum
7. Ischium
8. Achilles tendon
9. Heel
10. Sole
11. Ear
12. Shoulder
13. Anterior iliac spine
14. Trochanter
15. Thigh
16. Medial knee
17. Lateral knee
18. Lower leg
19. Medial malleolus
20. Lateral malleolus
21. Lateral edge of foot
22. Posterior knee

B

Anterior | Posterior

Chin
P

Occiput
Su

Scapula
Su

Elbow
Si   Su

Spinous process
Su

Ischium
Si

Trochanter
L

Behind
knee

Pretibial crest
P

Malleolus
L

Heel
Su

Key
P = Prone position
Su = Supine position
Si = Sitting position
L = Lateral position

A

Fig. 57.1 (A) Bony prominences most frequently underlying pressure injuries. (B) Pressure injury (ulcer) sites. (From Trelease CC: Developing standards for wound care, *Ostomy Wound Manage* 26:50, 1988.)

does not blanch (abnormal reactive hyperemia), this area is a site for potential skin breakdown and is considered a stage 1 pressure injury. If a patient has a medical device, inspect carefully in areas where the device may cause friction to the skin. Medical device—related PIs (MDRPIs) are PIs that can cause pain, loss of function, increased length of stay, and increased health care costs. Timely assessment of risk for or actual MDPRI provides for prompt prevention or treatment (The Joint Commission [TJC], 2018).

Safety Guidelines

- Pressure injuries pose serious risks to a patient's health. A break in the skin, seen in categories/stages 2 to 4 PIs, eliminates the first line of defense of the body against infection.
- Assess and inspect skin on a schedule based on patient acuity and where there are changes in patient condition.
- Position patients to redistribute the amount and duration of pressure to prevent ischemic tissue injury. The development of PIs, especially stages 3 and 4 and unstageable ulcers, in a care setting is a serious reportable event (Centers for Medicare and Medicaid Services, 2018a).

Delegation

The skill of PI risk assessment cannot be delegated to assistive personnel (AP). Direct the AP to:

- Frequently change a patient's position (recommend specific positions for patient's need).
- Keep a patient's skin dry and provide hygiene after fecal or urinary incontinence and skin exposure from wound drainage.
- Report any changes in a patient's skin, such as redness or a break in the skin.
- Report any redness and/or abrasion from medical devices.

Collaboration

- A wound ostomy care nurse (WOCN) or skin care specialist can assist in identifying skin abnormalities or injuries and recommend preventive approaches.

Equipment

- Risk assessment tool (Use agency-approved tool, see agency policy.)
- Documentation record
- Pressure-redistribution mattress, bed, and/or chair cushion
- Positioning aids
- Clean gloves
- Protective dressing (e.g., silicone, hydrocolloid)

STEP	RATIONALE
1 Perform preprocedure protocol.	

Assessment

• Review patient's electronic health record (EHR), including health care provider's orders, and nurses' notes to assess patient's risk for PI formation:	Determines need to administer preventive care and identifies specific factors that place patient at risk (EPUAP, NPIAP, PPPIA, 2019a, 2019b).
a Paralysis or immobilization caused by restrictive devices	Patient is unable to turn or reposition independently to relieve pressure.
b Presence of medical device such as nasogastric (NG) tube, oxygen equipment, artificial airways, drainage tubing, or mechanical devices (Doughty and McNichols, 2022; TJC, 2018)	Medical devices have potential to exert pressure on patient's skin near or adjacent to devices such as artificial airways and drainage tubes.
(1) If not medically contraindicated, remove medical device to observe and palpate skin and tissues under and around each medical device.	Pressure area assumes same configuration or shape as medical device (Schallom et al., 2015; Wound Ostomy and Continence Nurses Society [WOCN], 2016a).
c Sensory loss (e.g., hemiplegia, spinal cord injury)	Patient is unable to feel discomfort from pressure and does not independently change position.
d Circulatory disorders (e.g., peripheral vascular diseases, vascular changes from diabetes mellitus, neuropathy)	Reduce perfusion of tissue layers of skin.

Continued

STEP	RATIONALE
e Fever	Increases metabolic demands of tissues.
	Accompanying diaphoresis leaves skin moist.
f Anemia	Decreased hemoglobin level reduces oxygen-carrying capacity of blood and amount of oxygen available to tissues.
g Malnutrition	Inadequate nutrition leads to weight loss, muscle atrophy, and reduced tissue mass.
	Nutrient deficiencies result in impaired or delayed healing.
h Fecal or urinary incontinence	Skin becomes exposed to moist environment, which alters skin flora. Excessive moisture macerates skin, which can lead to PI (Bryant and Nix, 2016).
i Heavy sedation and anesthesia	Patient is not mentally alert and does not turn or change position independently. Sedation alters sensory perception (Hotaling and Black, 2021).
j Age	Neonates and very young children are at high risk, with the head being the most common site of PI occurrence (WOCN, 2016a).
	There is loss of dermal thickness in older adults, impairing ability to distribute pressure (Pieper, 2016).
k Dehydration	Results in decreased skin elasticity and turgor.
l Edema	Edematous tissues are less tolerant of pressure, friction, and shear.

STEP	RATIONALE
m Existing pressure injuries	Limit surfaces available for position changes, placing available tissues at increased risk.
n History of pressure injury	Tensile strength of skin from previously healed pressure injury is 80% or less; therefore this area cannot tolerate pressure as much as undamaged skin (Bryant and Nix, 2016).
• Select agency-approved risk assessment tool. Perform risk assessment when patient enters health care setting and repeat at regularly scheduled intervals (at least daily) or when there is significant change in patient's condition (WOCN, 2016a).	Valid and reliable risk assessment tools evaluate patient's risk for developing a pressure injury. Identifying risk factors that contribute to the potential for skin breakdown allows targeting of specific interventions for decreasing risk for skin breakdown.

CLINICAL JUDGMENT *In acute care settings, perform initial assessment within 8 h of admission and reassess every 24 h or as patient condition changes; in critical care areas perform assessment on admission and reassess every 24 h or as patient condition changes; and in long-term and home care settings perform assessment on admission. In long-term care settings reassess weekly and then according to agency standards or when patient condition changes. In home care setting reassess with each registered nurse visit.*

• Obtain risk score and interpret based on patient's unique characteristics and score guidelines. When using the Braden scale there are risk scores identified for specific patient populations: intensive care patients ≤18 (Huang et al., 2020); older adults ≤14 (Alderden et al., 2017).	Risk cutoff score depends on instrument used. Score involves identifying risk factors that contributed to PI and minimizing these specific deficits (Ayello, 2002; EPUAP, NPIAP, PPPIA, 2019a).

Continued

STEP	RATIONALE
• Perform hand hygiene. Assess condition of patient's skin over regions of pressure (Fig. 57.1). Remove medical devices or tape securing these devices, shoes, socks, antiembolic stockings, and heel and elbow protectors to inspect the skin under all medical devices (EPUAP, NPIAP, PPPIA, 2019a; WOCN, 2016a, 2016b). Apply gloves as needed with open and/or draining wounds.	Body weight against bony prominences places underlying skin at risk for breakdown.
a Inspect for skin discoloration (Box 57.1) and tissue consistency (firm or boggy feel) and/or palpate for abnormal sensations.	Indicates that tissue was under pressure; hyperemia is a normal physiologic response to hypoxemia in tissues.
b Palpate discolored area on skin and under and around medical devices, release your fingertip, and look for blanching. If on palpation an area of redness blanches (lightens in color), this indicates normal reactive hyperemia; tissue is not at risk to develop an injury.	Tissue that does not blanch when palpated indicates abnormal reactive hyperemia; indicates possible ischemic injury.
c Inspect for pallor and mottling.	Persistent hypoxia in tissues that were under pressure; an abnormal physiologic response.
d Inspect for absence of superficial skin layers.	Represents early pressure injury formation; usually a partial-thickness wound that may have resulted from shear.

BOX 57.1 Patient-Centered Care for Skin Assessment of Pressure Injuries: Patients With Darkly Pigmented Skin

There is evidence that stage 1 pressure injuries are under-detected in patients with darkly pigmented skin. Areas of redness are more difficult to assess on darker skin tones (EPUAP, NPIAP, PPPIA, 2019a). Patients with darkly pigmented skin cannot be assessed for pressure injury risk by examining only skin color (WOCN, 2016a).

1. Use natural lighting but note that visual inspection techniques to identify pressure injuries are ineffective in darkly pigmented skin.
2. Carefully inspect any discoloration over pressure areas and surrounding skin for temperature changes, edema, change in tissue consistency, and pain (EPUAP, NPIAP, PPPIA, 2019a). Assess localized skin color changes. Any of the following may occur:
   - Color remains unchanged when pressure is applied.
   - Color changes occur at site of pressure and differ from patient's usual skin color.
   - If patient previously had a pressure injury, that area of skin may be lighter than original color.
   - Localized area of skin may be purple/blue or violet instead of red. Purple or maroon discoloration may indicate deep tissue injury (WOCN, 2016a).
3. Assessment of skin temperature changes: Circumscribed area of intact skin may be warm to touch. As tissue changes color, intact skin will feel cool to touch. NOTE: Gloves may decrease sensitivity to changes in skin temperature (EPUAP, NPIAP, PPPIA, 2019a; WOCN, 2016a).
   - Localized heat (inflammation) is detected by making comparisons to surrounding skin. Localized area of warmth eventually will be replaced by area of coolness, which is a sign of tissue devitalization.
4. Edema may occur with induration of more than 15 mm in diameter and may appear taut and shiny.
5. Palpate tissue consistency in surrounding tissues to identify any changes in tissue consistency between area of injury and normal tissue (EPUAP, NPIAP, PPPIA, 2019a).
6. Patient reports discomfort at a site that is predisposed to pressure injury development (e.g., bony prominence, under medical devices).

STEP	RATIONALE
e Inspect for changes in skin temperature, edema, and tissue consistency, especially in patients with darkly pigmented skin.	Localized heat, edema, and induration have been identified as warning signs for pressure injury development. Because it is not always possible to observe changes in skin color on darkly pigmented skin, these additional signs should be considered in assessment (EPUAP, NPIAP, PPPIA, 2019a).
f Inspect for wound drainage.	Wound drainage is caustic to skin, increasing risk for skin breakdown. Tubing from drainage devices causes pressure under device and on adjacent skin (EPUAP, NPIAP, PPPIA, 2019a).
• Assess skin and tissue around and beneath medical devices at least twice daily (EPUAP, NPIAP, PPPIA, 2019a).	Patients at high risk need more frequent assessments and have multiple sites for pressure necrosis in areas other than bony prominences (Chaboyer et al., 2017). These are patients who require mechanical ventilation or who are vulnerable to fluid shifts and/or edema (EPUAP, NPIAP, PPPIA, 2019a). Pressure points around medical devices cause PI in underlying tissue and can become full-thickness PIs (EPUAP, NPIAP, PPPIA, 2019a). Typically the MDRPI conforms to the same size and shape as the medical device that caused the injury (EPUAP, NPIAP, PPPIA, 2019a).
a Nares: NG tube, oxygen cannula	Pressure to nares occurs from tape and other materials used to secure NG tube.

STEP	RATIONALE
b Ears: oxygen cannula, pillow	Oxygen equipment is a significant risk for PIs (Padula et al., 2017). Patients' ears and tips of nares are at risk for pressure from nasal cannula (Schallom et al., 2015; TJC, 2018).
c Tongue and lips: oral airway, endotracheal tube	Mucosal tissues of the mouth are at risk for MDRPI because the devices placed to secure an artificial airway cause pressure on the mucosa, which causes the skin to become ischemic and leads to ulceration (EPUAP, NPIAP, PPPIA, 2019a).
d Forehead: pulse oximetry device	May cause PI to forehead or ears due to the securement device.
e Drainage or other tubing	Stress and pressure against tissue at exit site or from tubing lying under any part of patient's body.
f Indwelling urethral (Foley) catheter	For female patients, catheter can put pressure on labia. For male patients, pressure from catheter not properly anchored can put pressure on tip of penis and urethra (Black et al., 2015).
g Orthopedic and positioning devices: casts, neck collars, splints	Devices have potential to cause pressure to underlying and adjacent skin and tissue (Black et al., 2015).
h Compression stockings	Have potential to cause pressure, especially if they fit poorly or are rolled down (Black et al., 2015).

CLINICAL JUDGMENT *Compression stockings must be completely removed to adequately assess the feet, heels, and legs.*

i Immobilization device and restraints	If device is too tight or poorly placed or if patient strains, pressure points occur under it.
• Remove and dispose of gloves and perform hand hygiene.	Reduces transmission of microorganisms.

Continued

STEP	RATIONALE
• Observe patient for preferred positions when in bed or chair.	Preferred positions result in weight of body being placed on certain bony prominences. Presence of contractures may result in pressure exerted in unexpected places.
• Observe ability of patient to initiate and help with position changes.	Potential for friction and shear increases when patient is completely dependent on others for position changes.

Implementation

1 Implement the following prevention guidelines (WOCN, 2016a, 2016b).	Reduces patient's risk for developing PI.
2 Perform hand hygiene and apply clean gloves.	Reduces transmission of microorganisms.
3 After initial assessment, continue to inspect skin at least once a day.	
a Observe patient's skin; pay particular attention to bony prominences and areas around and under medical devices and tubes (see Assessment). If an area does not blanch, suspect tissue injury and recheck in 1 h. Any discoloration may vary from pink to deep red.	Persistent redness when lightly pigmented skin is pressed can indicate tissue injury. If area of redness blanches (lightens in color), it indicates that skin is not at risk for breakdown.

CLINICAL JUDGMENT *Do not massage reddened areas because doing so may cause additional tissue trauma. Reddened or discolored areas indicate blood vessel damage, and massaging has the potential to damage underlying tissues (Bryant and Nix, 2016; EPUAP, NPIAP, PPPIA, 2019a).*

STEP	RATIONALE
b If patient has darkly pigmented skin, look for color changes that differ from their normal skin color. Also assess temperature, edema, and tissue consistency.	Darkly pigmented skin may not blanch. (see Box 57.1).
4 At each shift, check all treatment and assistive devices (catheters, feeding tubes, casts, braces) for potential pressure points.	Pressure from these devices increases risk for PI on bony prominences and other areas.
a Verify that device is correctly sized, positioned, and secured.	Incorrect size, placement, and securement of medical device can cause excessive pressure and rubbing by device on underlying skin (EPUAP, NPIAP, PPPIA, 2019a; WOCN, 2016a).
b Consider shielding underlying at-risk skin with protective dressing (e.g., silicone, hydrocolloid).	These dressings absorb moisture from body and reduce pressure to underlying skin (EPUAP, NPIAP, PPPIA, 2019a; WOCN, 2016a).

CLINICAL JUDGMENT *Inspect skin around and beneath orthopedic devices. Note any abrasions or warmth in areas where devices can rub against the skin. In addition, a medical device can result in an altered microclimate at the skin–device interface, thus increasing the risks for injury. (EPUAP, NPIAP, PPPIA, 2019a; WOCN, 2016a).*

STEP	RATIONALE
5 Remove and dispose of gloves; perform hand hygiene. Reapply gloves if risk of contact with drainage or other body fluids is anticipated.	Reduces transmission of microorganisms.
6 Review patient's pressure injury risk assessment score.	Risk scores aid in identifying preventive interventions.

Continued

STEP	RATIONALE
7 If immobility, inactivity, or poor sensory perception is a risk factor(s) for patient, consider one of the following interventions (WOCN, 2016a):	Immobility and inactivity reduce patient's ability or desire to independently change position. Poor sensory perception decreases patient's ability to feel sensation of pressure or discomfort.
a Reposition patient on scheduled basis and frequently assess individual's skin condition to identify early signs of pressure damage. If skin changes occur, reevaluate the care plan.	Reduces duration and intensity of pressure. Some patients may require more frequent repositioning.
b When patient is in side-lying position in bed, use 30-degree lateral position (Fig. 57.2). Avoid 90-degree lateral position.	Reduces direct contact of trochanter with support surface.
c Place patient (when lying in bed) on pressure-redistribution surface.	Reduces amount of pressure exerted on tissues.

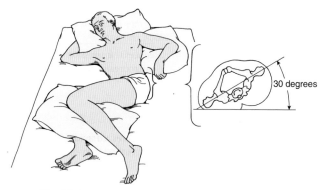

Fig. 57.2 Thirty-degree lateral position with pillow placement.

STEP	RATIONALE
d Place patient (when in chair) on pressure-redistribution device and shift points under pressure at least every hour (WOCN, 2016a).	Reduces amount of pressure on sacral and ischial areas.
8 If friction and shear are identified as risk factors, consider the following interventions:	Friction and shear damage underlying skin.
a Use safe patient-handling guidelines to reposition patient. For example, use slide board or air-assisted transfer device to move patient from bed to stretcher.	Proper repositioning of patient prevents creating shear from dragging patient along sheets. Slide board provides slippery surface to reduce friction. Use of lift team, when appropriate, raises patient's skin off sheets.
b Ensure that heels are free from bed surface by using a pillow under calves to elevate heels or use a heel-suspension device; knees should be in 5- to 10-degree flexion.	"Floating" heels from bed surface offload the heel completely and redistribute the weight of the leg along the calf without applying pressure on the Achilles tendon (Baath et al., 2015).
c Maintain head of the bed at 30 degrees or lower or at the lowest degree of elevation consistent with patient's condition (**do not lower head of bed if patient is at risk for aspiration**) (WOCN, 2016a).	Decreases potential for patient to slide toward foot of bed and incur shear injury.
9 If patient receives low score on moisture subscale, consider one of the following interventions:	Continual exposure of body fluids on patient's skin increases risk for skin breakdown and pressure injury development.

Continued

STEP	RATIONALE
a Apply clean gloves. Clean and dry the skin as soon as possible after each incontinent episode (WOCN, 2016a). Apply moisture barrier ointment to perineum and surrounding skin after each incontinence episode.	Friction and shear are enhanced in the presence of moisture. Protects skin from fecal or urinary incontinence.
b If skin is denuded, use protective barrier paste after each incontinence episode.	Provides barrier between skin and stool/urine, allowing for healing.
c If moisture source is from wound drainage, consider frequent dressing changes, skin protection with protective barriers, or collection devices.	Removes frequent exposure of wound drainage from skin.
10 If friction and shear are risk factors and patient is chair-bound:	Relief of pressure by changing from lying to sitting position is insufficient if sitting lasts a prolonged time. The maximum amount of time a patient can sit before there is a need to reposition is unknown (WOCN, 2016a).
a Tilt patient's chair seat slightly backward to prevent sliding forward, and support arms, legs, and feet to maintain proper posture (EPUAP, NPIAP, PPPIA, 2019a).	
b Limit amount of time patient spends in a chair without pressure relief (EPUAP, NPIAP, PPPIA, 2019a).	
c For patients who can reposition themselves while sitting, encourage pressure relief every 15 minutes using chair push-ups, forward lean, or shifting side to side (WOCN, 2016a).	

STEP	RATIONALE
11 Educate patient and family regarding specific pressure injury risk factors and prevention.	Helps patients and family understand and adhere to interventions (Berlowitz et al., 2022).
12 Perform postprocedure protocol.	
13 Evaluate patient response:	
a Observe patient's skin for areas at risk for tissue damage, noting change in color, appearance, or texture.	Enables evaluation of success of prevention techniques.
b Observe tolerance of patient for position change by measuring level of comfort on pain scale.	Position changes sometimes interfere with patient's sleep and rest pattern.
c Compare subsequent risk assessment scores and skin assessments.	Provides ongoing comparison of patient's risk level to facilitate appropriateness of plan of care.

Recording and Reporting

- Record any skin changes, patient's risk score, and skin assessment. Describe positions, turning intervals, pressure-redistribution devices, and other prevention measures. Note patient's response to the interventions.
- Record evaluation of patient's and family caregiver's understanding of the need for frequent skin and pressure injury assessment education.
- Report need for additional consultations for a high-risk patient to health care provider.

UNEXPECTED OUTCOMES	RELATED INTERVENTIONS
1 Skin becomes mottled, reddened, purplish, or bluish.	• Refer patient to wound, ostomy, and continence nurse (WOCN); dietitian; clinical nurse specialist (CNS); nurse practitioner (NP); and/or physical therapist as needed. • Reevaluate position changes and bed surface.
2 Areas under pressure develop persistent discoloration, induration, or temperature changes.	• Refer patient to WOCN, dietitian, CNS, NP, and/or physical therapist as needed. • Modify patient's positioning and turning schedule.

Pressure Injury Treatment

The principles of managing patients with pressure injuries (PIs) include reducing or eliminating the cause of skin breakdown, and management that promotes healing. Know a patient's risks for developing a PI. Wound assessment tools such as the Bates-Jensen Wound Assessment Tool (BWAT) (Bryant and Nix, 2016) and the Pressure Ulcer Scale for Healing (PUSH) tool can help to determine the individual treatment goals for different PIs.

The best environment for wound healing is moist and free of necrotic tissue and infection. When a wound is contaminated with debris, necrotic tissue, or heavy drainage, use a cleaner e.g. normal saline that is noncytotoxic to healthy tissue. If the tissue in the wound is devitalized, consult with a patient's health care provider to consider debridement, which is the removal of devitalized tissue. The choice of the type of debridement depends on a patient's overall condition, the condition of the wound, and the type of devitalized tissue (Wound, Ostomy and Continence Nurses Society [WOCN], 2016a).

Choose wound dressings based on the characteristics of the wound bed (Bryant and Nix, 2016). The type of dressings needed will change as the pressure injury characteristics change; frequent wound assessment is key. Categories of wound dressings to use in treating PIs include transparent films, hydrocolloids, hydrogels, foams, calcium alginates, gauze, and antimicrobial dressings (see Skills 17 and 18).

For more extensive PIs, negative-pressure wound therapy may be most effective to facilitate healing and collect wound fluid (Netsch, 2016) (see Skill 43).

Safety Guidelines

- Position patients to redistribute the amount and duration of pressure to prevent ischemic tissue injury. The development of pressure injuries—especially stages 3 and 4 and any unstageable ulcers—in a care setting is a serious reportable event.
- Clean patients who are incontinent of stool or urine as soon as possible.
- Use approaches to minimize shear: lift sheets when repositioning patients, raise the head of the bed no more than 30 degrees (unless medically contraindicated) (WOCN, 2016a).

Delegation

The skill of treating PIs and dressing changes cannot be delegated to assistive personnel (AP). Instruct the AP to:

- Report immediately any change in skin integrity, pain, fever, or any wound drainage.

- Report any potential contamination to existing dressing such as patient incontinence or dislodgement of the dressing.

Collaboration

- Plan a dressing change with the wound care team to assess the status of the wound together to determine effectiveness of the treatment plan.

Equipment

- Personal Protective equipment: clean gloves. Option: goggles, face shield, cover gown
- Sterile gloves (optional)
- Plastic bag for dressing disposal
- Wound-measuring device
- Sterile cotton-tipped applicators (check agency policy for use of sterile applicators)
- Normal saline or cleansing agent (as ordered)
- Topical agent or solution (as ordered) such as enzyme debriding agent, antibiotic
- Dressing of choice based on patient wound characteristics
- Skin barrier, e.g., liquid barrier or Stomahesive
- Hypoallergenic tape (if needed)
- Irrigation syringe (optional)
- Scale for assessing wound healing

STEP	RATIONALE
1 Perform preprocedure protocol.	
Assessment	
• Review patient's electronic health record (EHR), including health care provider order/ nurse's notes for type of dressing, previous dressing change and wound assessment, types of topical medications, types of analgesia if needed, and wound care supplies.	Identifies purpose of treatment of pressure injury. Ensures consistent administration of proper medications and treatments for specific wound care needs.

CLINICAL JUDGMENT *Determine whether the medical order is consistent with established wound care guidelines and outcomes for a patient. If the order is not consistent with guidelines or varies from the identified outcome for a patient, review with the health care team.*

STEP	RATIONALE
• Assess character of patient's pain and severity on a pain scale of 0 to 10. If patient is in pain, determine if pain medication as needed has been ordered and administer medication before dressing change.	Dressing change should not be traumatic for patient; evaluate wound pain before, during, and after wound care management (Bryant and Nix, 2016).
• Ask patient to describe history of allergies: known type(s) of allergies and normal allergic reaction(s). Focus on latex and topical agents.	Allows for prevention of exposure to allergic agent and anticipation of possible reactions. Topical agents could contain elements that cause localized skin reactions.
• Position patient to allow dressing removal and position plastic bag for dressing disposal.	Provides an accessible area for dressing change. Proper disposal of old dressing promotes proper handling of contaminated waste.
• Perform hand hygiene and apply clean gloves. Remove and discard old dressing.	Reduces transmission of microorganisms and prevents accidental exposure to body fluids.
• Assess wound using wound parameters. *Note:* This may be done during wound care procedure. a *Wound location:* Describe body site where wound is located.	Determines effectiveness of wound care and guides treatment plan of care (WOCN, 2016a).
b *Stage of wound:* Describe extent of tissue destruction.	Staging assesses a pressure injury based on depth of tissue destruction. Wounds are documented as unstageable if wound base is not visible (European Pressure Ulcer Advisory Panel and National Pressure injury Advisory Panel, and Pan Pacific Pressure Injury Alliance [EPUAP, NPIAP, PPPIA], 2019b).

Continued

STEP	RATIONALE
c *Wound size:* Length, width, and depth of wound are measured per agency protocol. Use disposable measuring guide for length and width. Use cotton-tipped applicator to assess depth (Fig. 58.1).	Injury size changes as healing progresses; therefore, longest and widest areas of wound change over time. Measuring width and length by measuring consistent areas provides consistent measurement (Bryant and Nix, 2016).
d *Presence of undermining, sinus tracts, or tunnels:* Use sterile cotton-tipped applicator to measure depth, undermining, or sinus tracts.	Wound depth determines amount of tissue loss.

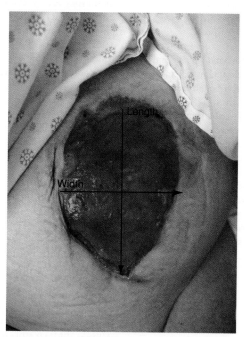

Fig. 58.1 Measuring wound width, length, and undermining of skin. (From Bryant RA, Nix DP: Acute and Chronic Wounds Current Management Concepts, ed 5, 2016, St Louis, Elsevier.)

STEP	RATIONALE
e *Condition of wound bed:* Describe type and percentage of tissue in wound bed.	Approximate percentage of each type of tissue in wound provides critical information on progress of wound healing and choice of dressing. Wound with black tissue may require debridement; yellow tissue or slough tissue may indicate presence of infection; granulation tissue indicates that wound is moving toward healing (EPUAP, NPIAP, PPPIA, 2019a).
f *Volume of exudate:* Describe amount, characteristics, odor, and color.	Amount and type of exudate may indicate type and frequency of dressing changes required (Bates-Jensen, 2022).
g *Condition of periwound skin:* Examine skin for breaks, dryness, and presence of rash, swelling, maceration, redness, or warmth. Modify assessment based on patient's skin color (see Skill 57).	Impaired periwound skin indicates progressive tissue damage (EPUAP, NPIAP, PPPIA, 2019b). Maceration on periwound skin shows need to alter choice of wound dressing. Condition determines whether skin barrier needed.

CLINICAL JUDGMENT *Any signs of skin stripping, blister, tears, skin maceration or contact dermatitis on the periwound skin may indicate medical adhesive--related skin injury (MARSI) and not an extension of a PI (Fumarola et al., 2020).*

STEP	RATIONALE
h *Wound edges:* With a gloved finger, examine wound edges for condition of tissue.	Gives information regarding epithelialization, chronicity, and etiology.
• Remove gloves and discard in appropriate receptacle. Perform hand hygiene.	Reduces transmission of microorganisms. Repeated hand hygiene is needed to assess other pressure areas. Different organisms contaminate different wounds.

Continued

STEP	RATIONALE
• Identify whether patient is at risk for MARSI from adhesives: age, dehydration, malnutrition, exposure to radiation therapy, underlying chronic conditions (e.g., diabetes, immunosuppression) and edema of skin. Factors raise your level of observation as long as patient has a dressing with adhesive closure.	Common risk factors for MARSI (Fumarola et al., 2020). May indicate need to use skin barrier and different type of tape.
• Assess for factors affecting wound healing: poor perfusion and nutrition, immunosuppression, or preexisting infection.	Factors affect treatment choice.

CLINICAL JUDGMENT *When malnutrition is suspected, consider a nutrition consultation to modify patient's diet to promote wound healing.*

• Select appropriate dressing based on pressure injury characteristics:	
(1) Gauze—Apply as moist dressing, a dry cover dressing when using enzymes or topical antibiotics, or a means to deliver solution to wound.	Dressing will either promote moisture or have absorptive properties for drainage. Saline-moistened gauze enables granulation tissue to grow and the wound to heal (Al Aboud and Manna, 2022).
(2) Transparent film dressing—Apply over superficial injuries with minimal or no exudate and skin subjected to friction (see skill 18).	Maintains moist environment and offers intact skin protection.

STEP	RATIONALE
(3) Hydrocolloid dressing (See skill 17)	Maintains moist environment for wound healing and protects wound base.
(4) Hydrogel – sheet or tube	Maintains moist environment for wound healing.
(5) Calcium alginate (See skill 17)	Highly absorbent of wound exudate in heavily draining wounds.
(6) Foam dressings (see skill 17)	Protective and prevents wound dehydration; also absorbs moderate to large amounts of drainage.
(7) Silver-impregnated dressings/gels	Controls bacterial burden in wound.
(8) Wound fillers	Fills shallow wounds, hydrates, and absorbs.

Implementation

1 Many PIs are chronic. Ensure that patient and family caregivers understand likely causes of patient's PI and how to prevent development and/or worsening.	Ongoing care is needed for existing chronic wounds and prevention of new ones.
2 Perform hand hygiene and apply clean gloves. Open sterile packages and topical solution containers. Keep dressings sterile. Wear goggles, mask, and moisture-proof cover gown if potential for contamination from spray exists when cleaning wound.	Reduces transmission of microorganisms.
3 Remove bed linen and arrange patient's gown to expose injury and surrounding skin. Keep remaining body parts draped.	Prevents unnecessary exposure of body parts.

Continued

STEP	RATIONALE
4 Clean wound thoroughly with normal saline or prescribed wound-cleaning agent from least contaminated to most contaminated area. For deep injuries, clean with saline delivered with irrigating syringe as ordered (see skill 83). Remove gloves and discard.	Cleaning wound removes wound exudate, unwanted substances from the skin's surface, and/or dressing residue, which reduces surface bacteria (EPUAP, NPIAP, PPPIA, 2019b).
5 Perform hand hygiene and apply clean or sterile gloves. (Refer to agency policy.)	Maintains aseptic technique during cleaning, measuring, and application of dressings.
6 Protect periwound by applying a skin barrier, e.g., liquid barrier or Stomahesive	Skin barriers form a protective interface between the skin and adhesive, thus reducing the risk of adhesive trauma (Fumarola et al., 2020).
7 Apply topical agents to wound using cotton-tipped applicators or gauze as ordered:	
a Enzymes	Follow manufacturer directions for method and frequency of application.
(1) Apply small amount of enzyme debridement ointment directly to necrotic areas in pressure injury. *Do not apply enzyme to surrounding skin because it may macerate the surrounding skin.*	Thin layer absorbs and acts more effectively than thick layer. Excess medication irritates surrounding skin (Al Aboud and Manna, 2022). Proper distribution of ointment ensures effective action.

CLINICAL JUDGMENT *If using an enzymatic debriding agent, do not use wound-cleaning agents with metals.*

STEP	RATIONALE
(2) Place moist gauze dressing directly over injury and tape in place. When using enzymes, follow specific manufacturer recommendation for type of dressing material to use to cover a pressure injury. Tape dressing in place.	Protects wound and prevents removal of ointment during turning or repositioning.
b Antibacterial (e.g., bacitracin, metronidazole)	Reduces bacterial growth.
8 Apply prescribed wound dressing:	
a Hydrogel	Hydrogel dressings hydrate wound (Al Aboud and Manna, 2022).
(1) Cover surface of injury with thick layer of amorphous hydrogel or cut sheet to fit wound base.	Provides moist environment to facilitate wound healing.
(2) Apply secondary dressing such as dry gauze; tape in place using nonallergenic tape.	Holds hydrogel against wound surface because amorphous hydrogel (in tube) or sheet form does not adhere to wound and requires secondary dressing to hold it in place.
(3) If using impregnated gauze, pack loosely into wound; cover with secondary gauze dressing and tape.	A loosely packed dressing delivers gel to wound base and allows any wound debris to be trapped in gauze.

Continued

STEP	RATIONALE
b Calcium alginate	Absorbs serous fluid or exudate, forming a nonadhesive hydrophilic gel, which conforms to shape of wound (Al Aboud and Manna, 2022). Use in heavily draining wounds.
(1) Lightly pack wound with alginate using sterile cotton-tipped applicator or gloved finger.	The dressing swells and increases in size; tight packing can compromise blood flow to the tissues.
(2) Apply secondary dressing and tape in place.	
(3) Obtain hypoallergenic tape or adhesive dressing sheet	Used to secure nonadherent dressing. Prevents skin irritation and tearing.
c Transparent film dressing, hydrocolloid, and foam dressings (Skills 17 and 18)	

CLINICAL JUDGMENT *Use transparent dressings for autolytic debridement of noninfected superficial PIs. Use a hydrocolloid dressing to protect skin from friction. Some brands have custom shapes available for specific anatomical parts.*

---

9 Perform postprocedure protocol.	
10 Evaluate patient response:	
a Observe periwound skin and PI for inflammation, blisters, edema, and tenderness, and drainage.	Determines progress of wound healing and whether MARSI is developing.
b Inspect dressings and exposed injuries, observing for drainage, foul odor, and tissue necrosis. Monitor patient for signs and symptoms of infection: fever and elevated white blood cell count.	PIs can become infected.

STEP	RATIONALE
c Compare subsequent injury measurements, using one of the scales designed to measure wound healing such as PUSH tool or BWAT.	Allows comparison of serial measurements to evaluate wound healing. Provides standard method of data collection that demonstrates wound progress or lack thereof.

Recording and Reporting

- Record type of wound tissue present in PI, stage of PI, injury measurements, periwound skin condition, character of drainage or exudate, type of topical agent used, dressing applied, and patient's response.
- Document evaluation of patient's and family caregiver's understanding of preventive measures and need to frequently observe and measure wound..
- Report any deterioration in injury appearance to nurse in charge or health care provider.

UNEXPECTED OUTCOMES	RELATED INTERVENTIONS
1 Skin surrounding injury becomes macerated and inflamed.	• Reduce exposure of surrounding skin to topical agents and moisture. • Select dressing that has increased moisture-absorbing capacity. • Avoid washing the skin too much and use a pH-balanced soap substitute to avoid drying the skin (Fumarola et al., 2020).
2 Injury becomes deeper with increased drainage and/or development of necrotic tissue.	• Review current wound care management. • Consult with interdisciplinary team regarding changes in wound care. • Obtain wound cultures.

Continued

UNEXPECTED OUTCOMES	RELATED INTERVENTIONS
3 PI extends beyond original margins.	• Monitor for systemic signs and symptoms of poor wound healing such as abnormal laboratory results (white blood cell count, hemoglobin/hematocrit levels, serum albumin, serum prealbumin, total proteins), weight loss, and fluid imbalances. • Assess and revise current turning schedule. • Consider pressure-redistribution devices.

Pulse: Apical

The apical pulse is the most reliable, noninvasive way to assess cardiac function. The apical pulse rate is the assessment of the number and quality of apical heart sounds that occur in 1 minute. A single apical pulse is the combination of two heart sounds, S_1 and S_2. As you listen for sound waves with a stethoscope, you will hear the characteristic "lub-dub" (S_1 and S_2) as a single pulsation.

Safety Guidelines

- Use an organized, systematic approach when taking an apical pulse to ensure accurate findings.
- When you have difficulty measuring a radial pulse, make the clinical judgment to assess the apical pulse instead.

Delegation

The skill of apical pulse measurement cannot be delegated to assistive personnel (AP). You will measure an apical pulse when there is an irregular radial pulse or when a patient's condition requires a more accurate assessment.

Collaboration

- When an apical pulse deficit is identified, collaborate with cardiac health care providers (e.g., advanced practice nurse or cardiologist) to determine whether interventions such as medications are needed.

Equipment

- Stethoscope
- Wristwatch with second hand or digital display
- Pen and vital sign flow sheet in chart, or electronic health record (EHR)
- Antiseptic swab

STEP	RATIONALE
1 Perform preprocedure protocol.	
Assessment	
• Review patient's EHR to determine need to assess apical pulse: a History of heart disease b Cardiac dysrhythmia	Certain conditions place patients at risk for heart rate (HR) alterations.

Continued

STEP	RATIONALE
c Onset of sudden chest pain or acute pain from any body site	
d Invasive cardiovascular diagnostic tests	
e Surgery	
f Large volume of intravenous (IV) fluid	
g Internal or external hemorrhage	
h Administration of medications that alter cardiac function	
• Determine previous pulse rate and measurement site (if available) from patient's record.	Allows assessment for change in condition. Provides comparison with current and future pulse measurements.
• Assess for factors in patient's history that normally influence apical pulse rate and rhythm:	Allows you to anticipate factors that alter apical pulse.
a Age	Infant's HR at birth ranges from 100 to 159 beats/min at rest; by age 2 pulse rate slows to 70 to 120 beats/min; by adolescence, rate varies between 59 and 90 beats/min, where it remains throughout adulthood (Hockenberry et al., 2019).
b Exercise	Physical activity increases HR. A well-conditioned patient may have a slower-than-usual resting HR that also quickly returns to resting rate after exercise.
c Position changes	HR increases temporarily when changing from lying to sitting or standing position.
d Medications	Antidysrhythmics, sympathomimetics, and cardiotonics affect rate and rhythm of pulse; large doses of opioid analgesics can slow HR; general anesthetics slow HR; central nervous system stimulants (such as caffeine) can increase HR.

STEP	RATIONALE
e Temperature	Fever or exposure to warm environments increases HR; HR declines with hypothermia.
f Sympathetic stimulation	Emotional stress, anxiety, or fear stimulates sympathetic nervous system, which increases HR.
• Perform hand hygiene.	Reduces transmission of microorganisms.
• Assess for signs and symptoms of altered cardiac function such as dyspnea, fatigue, chest pain, orthopnea, syncope, palpitations, edema of dependent body parts, cyanosis, or pallor of skin.	Physical signs and symptoms often indicate alteration in cardiac function, which affects HR and rhythm.
• Ask patient about allergies, with focus on latex allergy. If patient has latex allergy, ensure that stethoscope is latex free. Check patient's wristband.	Reduces risk of allergic reaction to stethoscope.
• Determine whether patient measures apical HR at home. Assess patient's knowledge and skill level.	Determines level and type of instruction required by patient or family caregiver.
Implementation	
1 Help patient to supine or sitting position. Move aside bed linen and gown to expose sternum and left side of chest.	Exposes part of chest wall for selection of auscultatory site. To hear heart sounds more clearly, place the stethoscope diaphragm directly on skin. Placing the stethoscope over a gown or clothing creates extraneous sounds and produces an inaccurate count.

Continued

STEP	RATIONALE
2 Explain to patient that you will listen to their heart for a pulse rate. Encourage patient to relax and not speak. If patient has been active, wait 5 to 10 minutes before assessing pulse. If patient has been smoking or ingesting caffeine, wait 15 minutes before assessing pulse.	Anxiety, activity, caffeine, and smoking elevate HR. Patient's voice interferes with the ability to hear sound when measuring apical pulse. Assessing apical pulse rate at rest allows for objective comparison of values.
3 Locate anatomical landmarks to identify point of maximal impulse (PMI), also called apical *impulse*. The heart is located behind and to left of sternum with base at top and apex at bottom. Find angle of Louis just below suprasternal notch between sternal body and manubrium; it feels like a bony prominence (Fig. 59.1A). Slip fingers down each side of angle to find second intercostal space (ICS) (Fig. 59.1B). Carefully move fingers down left side of sternum to fifth ICS and laterally to left midclavicular line (MCL) (Fig. 59.1C). A light tap felt within area 1 to 2.5 cm (½ to 1 inch) of PMI is reflected from apex of heart (Fig. 59.1D).	Use of anatomical landmarks allows correct placement of stethoscope over apex of heart. This position enhances ability to hear heart sounds clearly. If unable to palpate PMI, reposition patient on left side. In presence of serious heart disease, you may locate PMI to left of MCL or at sixth ICS. PMI may be difficult to palpate in obese adults or patients with severe pulmonary disease that has changed shape of thorax.
4 Place diaphragm of stethoscope in palm of hand for 5 to 10 seconds.	Warming a metal or plastic diaphragm prevents patient from being startled and promotes comfort.

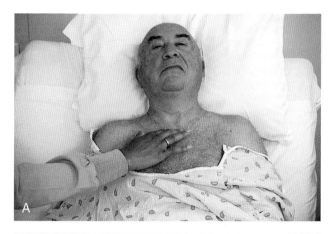

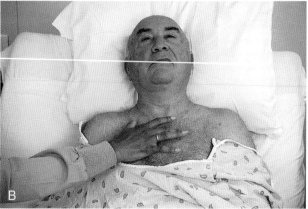

Fig. 59.1   (A) Nurse locates sternal notch. (B) Nurse locates second intercostal space.

Continued

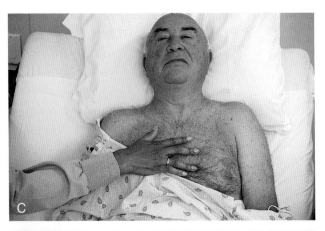

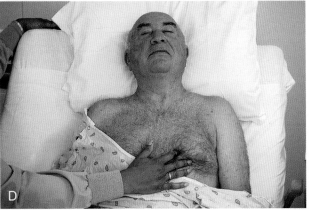

Fig. 59.1, cont'd (C) Nurse locates fifth intercostal space. (D) Nurse locates point of maximal impulse at fifth intercostal space at left midclavicular line.

STEP	RATIONALE
5 Place diaphragm of stethoscope over PMI at fifth ICS, at left MCL, and auscultate for normal S_1 and S_2 heart sounds (heard as lub-dub) (Fig. 59.2).	Allow stethoscope tubing to extend straight without kinks that would distort sound transmission. Normal sounds S_1 and S_2 are high pitched and best heard with diaphragm.
6 When you hear S_1 and S_2 with regularity, use second hand of watch or digital display and begin to count rate: when sweep hand hits starting number on dial, start counting with zero, then one, two, and so on. Count for 1 minute.	Apical rate can only be determined accurately after sounds have been auscultated clearly. Timing begins with zero. Count of one is first sound auscultated after timing begins.
7 If apical rate is regular, count for 30 seconds and multiply by 2.	A regular apical rate can be assessed within 30 seconds.

CLINICAL JUDGMENT *When HR is irregular or patient is receiving cardiovascular medication, count for a full 1 minute (59 seconds). An irregular rate is more accurately assessed when measured over a longer interval.*

8 Note consistent occurrence of any dysrhythmia (S_1 and S_2 occurring early or late after previous sequence of sounds) (e.g., every third or every fourth beat is skipped).	Consistent occurrence of a dysrhythmia within 1 minute indicates inefficient contraction of heart and potential alteration in cardiac output.

CLINICAL JUDGMENT *If apical rate is abnormal or irregular, repeat measurement or have another nurse conduct measurement. Original measurement may be incorrect. Second measurement confirms initial findings of an abnormal HR.*

9 Replace patient's gown and bed linen. Help patient to a comfortable position.	Restores comfort and sense of well-being.

Continued

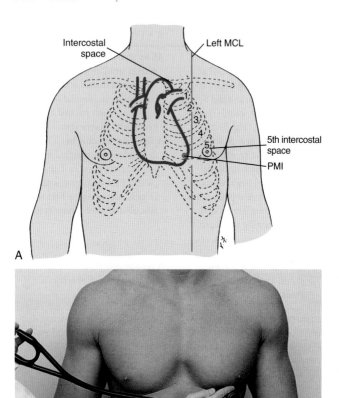

Fig. 59.2 (A) Location of PMI in adult. (B) Listening to PMI in adult. (*MCL*, midclavicular line; *PMI*, point of maximal impulse.)

STEP	RATIONALE
10 Inform patient of pulse rate and record per agency policy.	Promotes participation in care and understanding of health status.
11 Perform postprocedure protocol.	
12 Clean earpieces and diaphragm of stethoscope with alcohol swab routinely after each use.	Stethoscopes are frequently contaminated with microorganisms. Regular disinfection can control nosocomial infections.
13 Evaluate patient response:	
a If assessing pulse for first time, establish apical rate as baseline, if it is within an acceptable range.	Used to compare future pulse assessments.
b Compare apical rate and character with patient's previous baseline and acceptable range of HR for patient's age.	Allows assessment of change in patient's condition and presence of cardiac alteration.

Recording and Reporting

- Record apical pulse rate and rhythm on vital sign flow sheet or in EHR. If apical pulse not found at fifth ICS and left MCL, document location of PMI.
- Document measurement of apical pulse rate after administration of specific therapies per agency policy.
- Document evaluation of patient and family caregiver learning.
- Report abnormal findings including pulse deficit to nurse in charge or health care provider.

UNEXPECTED OUTCOMES	RELATED INTERVENTIONS
1 Adult patient's apical pulse is greater than 100 beats/min (tachycardia).	• Assess for factors that increase apical pulse such as fever, acute pain, fear or anxiety, recent exercise, low blood pressure, blood loss, or inadequate oxygenation. • Observe for signs and symptoms associated with abnormal cardiac function, including dyspnea, fatigue, chest pain, orthopnea, syncope, palpitations, edema of body parts, cyanosis, or dizziness.
2 Patient's apical pulse is less than 59 beats/min (bradycardia).	• Assess for factors that decrease HR such as beta blockers and antiarrhythmic drugs. • Observe for signs and symptoms associated with abnormal cardiac function, including dyspnea, fatigue, chest pain, orthopnea, syncope, palpitations, edema of body parts, cyanosis, or dizziness. • Have another nurse assess apical pulse. • Report findings to nurse in charge and/or health care provider. It may be necessary to withhold prescribed medications that alter HR until health care provider can evaluate need to alter dosage.

UNEXPECTED OUTCOMES	RELATED INTERVENTIONS
3 Patient's apical rate and rhythm differ from radial pulse. (A pulse deficit is the difference between the apical HR and radial pulse rate when obtained simultaneously over 1 minute.)	• Assess for pulse deficit: (1) nurse auscultates apical pulse while second provider palpates radial pulse. (2) Nurse begins 59-second pulse count by calling out loud when to begin counting pulses; (3) if pulse count differs, assess for other signs and symptoms of decreased cardiac output. • Report findings to nurse in charge and/or health care provider, who may order an electrocardiogram to detect cardiac conduction alteration.

Pulse Oximetry

Pulse oximetry is the noninvasive measurement of arterial blood oxygen saturation, the percent to which hemoglobin is filled with oxygen. A pulse oximeter is a probe with a light-emitting diode (LED) connected by cable to an oximeter. The LED emits light wavelengths that are absorbed differently by the oxygenated and deoxygenated hemoglobin molecules. The more hemoglobin saturated by oxygen, the higher the oxygen saturation.

- Normal oxygen saturation (SpO_2) is greater than 95%.
- A saturation less than 90% is a clinical emergency in a patient without a chronic respiratory condition.

There are portable oximeters (Fig. 60.1), pulse oximeters that sit on tabletops, and devices that are integrated into electronic monitoring systems. Pulse oximetry is indicated in patients who have an unstable oxygen status or are at risk for impaired gas exchange. A vascular, pulsatile area such as a nail bed is needed to detect the change in the transmitted light when making measurements with a finger probe. Conditions that decrease arterial blood flow such as peripheral vascular disease, hypothermia, pharmacologic vasoconstrictors, hypotension, or peripheral edema affect accurate determination of SpO_2 in these areas. For patients with decreased peripheral perfusion, use an earlobe or forehead sensor (Seifi et al., 2018). Factors that influence light transmission such as outside light sources or patient motion also affect SpO_2 measurement. Carbon monoxide in the blood, jaundice, and intravascular dyes influence the light reflected from hemoglobin molecules. In adults, reusable and disposable oximeter probes can be applied to the earlobe, finger, toe, bridge of the nose, or forehead.

Safety Guidelines

- Skin under disposable probe adhesive may become moist and harbor pathogens. Risk also increases for medical adhesive-related skin injury (MARSI).
- Disposable probes contain latex.

Delegation

The skill of SpO_2 measurement can be delegated to assistive personnel (AP). Direct AP by:

- Explaining specific factors related to the patient that can falsely lower SpO_2.
- Informing AP about appropriate sensor site and probe and to report any skin irritation from probe.

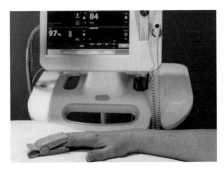

Fig. 60.1 Pulse oximeter.

- Clarifying frequency of SpO2 measurements.
- Instructing to report any reading lower than SpO$_2$ of 95% or value for specific patient.
- To not use pulse oximetry to obtain heart rate (will not detect accurate pulse).

Collaboration

- Respiratory therapy and pulmonary health care providers are resources for airway clearance measures, inhaled medications, or oxygen therapy for patients with persistently decreased SpO$_2$.

Equipment

- Oximeter and probe appropriate for patient
- Acetone or nail polish remover
- Pen and vital sign flow sheet or electronic health record (EHR)

STEP	RATIONALE
1 Perform preprocedure protocol.	
Assessment	
• Review EHR for history of acute or chronic compromised respiratory problems, change in oxygen therapy, chest wall injury, recovery from anesthesia, hypotension.	Risk factors for reduced SpO$_2$.

Continued

STEP	RATIONALE
• Determine whether patient is receiving oxygen therapy, respiratory therapy (e.g., postural drainage and percussion), and medications such as bronchodilators.	Factors can increase SpO_2.
• Review EHR to determine patient's risk for developing MARSI: age, dehydration, malnutrition, exposure to radiation therapy, underlying chronic conditions (e.g., diabetes, immunosuppression), and edema of skin.	Common risk factors for MARSI (Fumarola et al., 2020).
• Review relevant laboratory findings (i.e., hemoglobin).	Level of hemoglobin is correlated with SpO_2.
• Perform hand hygiene. Assess respiratory rate, depth, and rhythm; lung sounds; color of nail beds, lips, mucous membranes, or skin; presence of restlessness, difficulty breathing. If nail polish is present, remove using acetone.	Alterations in findings can reflect symptoms of alterations in SpO_2. Assessing nail color and measuring SpO_2 requires removing nail polish.
• Ask patient to describe history of allergies (especially latex and adhesive), known type(s) of allergies, and type(s) of reaction. Check patient's allergy wristband.	Confirms presence of allergies. Disposable probes contain latex and adhesive.
• Refer to medical order sheet or agency policy for frequency of SPO_2 measurement.	

Implementation

1 Perform hand hygiene.

Reduces transmission of microorganisms.

STEP	RATIONALE
2 Determine most appropriate patient-specific site (e.g., finger, earlobe, bridge of nose, forehead) for sensor probe placement by measuring capillary refill. If capillary refill time is greater than 2 seconds, select alternative site: a A finger free of black or brown nail polish is preferred. b If patient has tremors or is likely to move, use earlobe or forehead. Motion artifact is the most common cause of inaccurate readings. c If patient's finger is too large for the clip-on probe (can occur with obesity or edema), the clip-on probe may not fit properly; obtain a disposable (tape-on) probe.	Ensures accurate reading. Site must have adequate local circulation and be free of moisture.
3 Explain to patient the way that oxygen saturation will be measured and the importance of breathing normally until reading is complete.	Hyper- or hypoventilation can affect SpO_2 level.
4 Attach sensor to monitoring site (Fig. 60.2). If using finger, remove fingernail polish from digit with acetone or polish remover. Instruct patient that clip-on probe will feel like a clothespin on the finger but will not hurt.	Finger must be polish free.

Continued

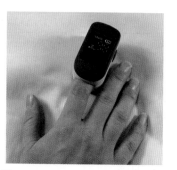

Fig. 60.2 Clip-on pulse oximetry sensor.

STEP	RATIONALE

CLINICAL JUDGMENT *Do not attach probe to finger, ear, or bridge of nose if area is edematous or skin integrity is compromised. Do not use earlobe and bridge of nose sensors for infants and toddlers because of skin fragility. Do not attach sensor to fingers that are hypothermic. Select ear or bridge of nose if adult patient has a history of peripheral vascular disease. Do not place sensor on same extremity as electronic blood pressure cuff. Blood flow to finger will be interrupted temporarily when cuff inflates, which can cause inaccurate reading, triggering oximeter alarms.*

STEP	RATIONALE
5 Once sensor is in place, turn on oximeter by activating power button. Observe pulse waveform/intensity display an audible beep. Assess whether oximeter pulse rate correlates with patient's radial pulse.	
6 Leave sensor in place 10 to 30 seconds or until oximeter readout reaches consistent value and pulse display reaches full strength during each cardiac cycle. Inform patient that oximeter alarm will sound if sensor falls off or patient moves it. Read SpO$_2$ on digital display.	Ensures an accurate reading.

STEP	RATIONALE
7 If continuous SpO_2 is ordered, verify SpO_2 alarm limits preset by manufacturer e.g. a low of 85% and a high of 100%. Determine limits for SpO_2 and pulse rate as indicated by patient's condition. Verify that alarms are on.	Alarm setting must be able to detect SpO_2 levels that indicate abnormalities in patient condition.
a Assess skin integrity under sensor probe every 2 h; relocate sensor at least every 4 h and more frequently if skin integrity is altered or tissue perfusion compromised.	Continued application of device can cause pressure injury.
8 If intermittent or spot-checking of SpO_2 is ordered, remove probe and turn oximeter power off.	Reduces ongoing risk of pressure injury.
9 Discuss findings with patient.	Includes patient as a partner in care.
10 Perform postprocedure protocol.	
11 Clean sensor and device per agency policy and store sensor in appropriate location. Perform hand hygiene.	
12 Evaluate patient response:	
a Compare SpO_2 with patient's previous baseline or normally, acceptable SpO_2. Correlate reading with data obtained from respiratory rate, depth, and rhythm assessment.	Determines patient's oxygenation status.

Recording and Reporting

- Record SpO$_2$ on vital sign flow sheet in chart or EHR, indicate type and amount of oxygen therapy used by patient during assessment, record any signs or symptoms of alterations in oxygen saturation in narrative form.
- Report abnormal findings to nurse in charge or health care provider.

UNEXPECTED OUTCOMES	RELATED INTERVENTIONS
1 SpO$_2$ is less than 90%.	• Verify that oximeter probe is correctly in place. Reposition probe if needed. • Assess for signs and symptoms of decreased oxygenation, including anxiety, restlessness, tachycardia, and cyanosis. • Verify that supplemental oxygen is delivered as ordered and is functioning properly. • Minimize factors that decrease SpO$_2$ value, such as lung secretions, increased activity, and hyperthermia. • Implement measures to reduce energy consumption. • Assist patient to a position that maximizes ventilatory effort; for example, place an obese patient in a high-Fowler position. • If value is outside ordered limits, notify health care provider.
2 Pulse waveform/intensity display is dampened or irregular.	• Locate different site and reposition pulse oximeter probe. • Use another sensor if available.

Rectal Suppositories

A rectal suppository is a form of medication that acts when it melts and is absorbed into the rectal mucosa. Rectal medications exert either local effects on gastrointestinal (GI) mucosa (e.g., promoting defecation) or systemic efwfects (e.g., relieving nausea or providing analgesia).

Rectal suppositories are thinner and more bullet-shaped than vaginal suppositories (Fig. 61.1). The rounded end prevents anal trauma during insertion. When administering a rectal suppository, place it past the internal anal sphincter and against the rectal mucosa. Improper placement can result in expulsion of the suppository before the medication dissolves and is absorbed into the mucosa. The rectal route is not as reliable as oral or parenteral routes in terms of drug absorption and distribution. However, medications that are administered rectally are relatively safe because they rarely cause local irritation or side effects.

Safety Guidelines

- Rectal medications are contraindicated in patients with recent surgery on the rectum, bowel, or prostate gland; rectal bleeding or prolapse; and low platelet counts (Burchum and Rosenthal, 2022).

Delegation

The skill of rectal medication administration cannot be delegated to assistive personnel (AP). Instruct the AP about:

- Reporting common, expected effects on fecal discharge or bowel movement.
- Reporting the occurrence of potential side effects of medications.
- Informing nurse if patient reports any rectal pain or bleeding.

Equipment

- Rectal suppository
- Water-soluble lubricating jelly
- Clean gloves
- Tissue
- Drape
- Medication administration record (MAR) (electronic or printed)

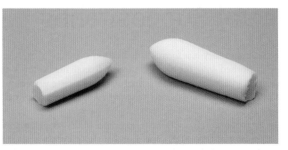

Fig. 61.1 Vaginal suppositories (*right*) are larger and more oval than rectal suppositories (*left*).

STEPS	RATIONALE

1 Perform preprocedure protocol.

Assessment

- Check accuracy and completeness of each MAR or computer printout with health care provider's written medication order. Verify patient's name, medication name and dosage, route of administration, and time of administration.

The order sheet is the most reliable source and only legal record of medications that patient is to receive. Ensures that patient receives the correct medications (Palese et al., 2019). Transcription errors are a source of medication errors (Palese et al., 2019).

- Review electronic health record (EHR): assess patient's medical and medication history.

Determines need for medication or possible contraindications for medication administration.

- Review drug reference information for medication action, purpose, normal dose, side effects, time of peak onset, and nursing implications.

Allows safe administration of medication and monitoring of patient's response to therapy.

STEPS	RATIONALE
• Ask patient to describe history of allergies: known type(s) of allergies and normal allergic reaction(s). List drug allergies on each page of MAR. Check patient's allergy wristband. Do not prepare medication if there is a known patient allergy.	Communication of patient allergies is essential part of safe medication administration.
• Perform hand hygiene.	Reduces transmission of microorganisms.
• Review any presenting signs and symptoms of GI alterations (e.g., constipation or diarrhea). Palpate abdomen for distention.	Provides a baseline to determine patient response to therapy.
• Assess patient's ability to hold suppository and position self to insert medication.	Determines whether instruction needed to prepare patient for safe self-administration.

Implementation

1	Discuss purpose of each medication, action, indication, and possible adverse effects. Allow patient to ask any questions.	Allows patient participation in care, which minimizes anxiety. Prepares patient to self-administer medication, which increases feelings of independence.
2	Prepare medication without interruptions/distractions. Create a quiet environment. Keep all pages of MARs or computer printouts for one patient together or look at only one patient's electronic MAR at a time.	Interruptions contribute to medication errors (Palese et al., 2019).

Continued

STEPS	RATIONALE
3 Perform hand hygiene. Prepare medications for one patient at a time using aseptic technique. Suppositories are usually stored in refrigerator. Check label of medication carefully with MAR or computer printout twice when preparing medication.	Ensures that medication is sterile. *These are the first and second checks for accuracy* and ensure that correct medication is administered.
4 Take medication(s) to patient at correct time (see agency policy). Medications that require exact timing include stat, first-time or loading doses, and one-time doses. Give non–time-critical scheduled medications within a range of 1 or 2 h of scheduled dose (Institute for Safe Medication Practices [ISMP], 2011). During administration apply seven rights of medication administration.	Clinical agencies must adopt medication administration policy and procedure for timing of medication administration that considers nature of the prescribed medication, specific clinical application, and patient needs (ISMP, 2011; US Department of Health and Human Services, 2020).
5 Identify patient using at least two identifiers (e.g., name and birthday or name and medical record number) according to agency policy. Compare identifiers with information on patient's MAR or medical record.	Ensures correct patient. Complies with The Joint Commission (TJC) standards and improves patient safety (TJC, 2023).
6 At patient's bedside, again compare MAR or computer printout with names of medications on medication labels and patient name. Ask patient about history of any allergies.	*This is the third check for accuracy* and ensures that patient receives correct medication. Confirms patient's allergy history.

STEPS	RATIONALE
7 Perform hand hygiene and apply clean gloves. Help patient assume left side-lying Sims position with upper leg flexed upward.	Reduces transmission of microorganisms. Position facilitates suppository insertion.
8 If patient has mobility impairment, obtain help to turn patient and use pillows under upper arm and leg.	
9 Keep patient draped with only anal area exposed.	Promotes patient comfort and privacy.
10 Visually examine condition of anus externally.	
Option: Apply pair of clean gloves and palpate rectal walls if impaction is suspected. After palpation dispose of gloves by turning them inside out and placing them in proper receptacle.	Reduces transmission of microorganisms. Data provides baseline to determine patient progress.

CLINICAL JUDGMENT *Do not palpate patient's rectum if there is a recent history of rectal surgery. A suppository is contraindicated in the presence of active bleeding and diarrhea (Burchum and Rosenthal, 2022).*

STEPS	RATIONALE
11 Perform hand hygiene and apply pair of clean gloves.	Reduces transmission of microorganisms.
12 Remove suppository from foil wrapper and lubricate rounded end with water-soluble lubricant (Fig. 61.2). Lubricate gloved index finger of dominant hand. If patient has hemorrhoids, use liberal amount of lubricant and touch area gently.	Lubrication reduces friction against rectal mucosa.
13 Ask patient to take slow, deep breaths through mouth and relax anal sphincter.	Eases suppository insertion.

Continued

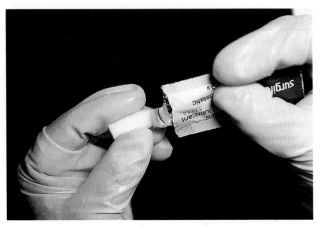

Fig. 61.2 Lubricate tip of suppository.

STEPS	RATIONALE
14 Retract patient's buttocks with nondominant hand. With gloved index finger of dominant hand, insert suppository gently through anus, past internal sphincter, and against rectal wall, 10 cm (4 inches) in adults or 5 cm (2 inches) in infants and children. You should feel rectal sphincter close around your finger.	Correct placement of suppository ensures drug absorption.

CLINICAL JUDGMENT *Do not insert suppository into a mass of fecal material; this will reduce effectiveness of medication.*

15 *Option:* A suppository may be given through a colostomy (not ileostomy) if ordered. Patient should lie supine. Use small amount of water-soluble lubricant for insertion.

STEPS	RATIONALE
16 Withdraw finger and wipe patient's anal area. Ask patient to remain flat or on side for 5 minutes.	Patient position reduces likelihood of suppository expulsion.
17 If suppository contains laxative or fecal softener, place call light within reach of patient.	Ensures that patient can obtain help to reach bedpan or toilet.
18 Perform postprocedure protocol.	
19 If suppository was given for constipation, remind patient not to flush commode after bowel movement.	Allows assessment of characteristics of patient stool.
20 Evaluate patient response:	
a Return to bedside within 5 minutes to determine whether suppository was expelled.	Determines medication efficacy.
b Evaluate patient for any continuing GI symptoms, palpate abdomen for distention.	Determines patient response to medication.

Recording and Reporting

- Record the drug, dosage, route, and actual time and date of administration on MAR immediately after administration. Record patient response to medication.
- Document evaluation of patient learning.
- Report adverse effects/patient response and/or withheld drugs to nurse in charge or health care provider.

UNEXPECTED OUTCOMES	RELATED INTERVENTIONS
1 Patient unable to have bowel movement or there is no relief of symptoms, e.g., pain.	• Consult with health care provider; consider repeating suppository or administering different medication.

Respiration Assessment

Respiration is the exchange of respiratory gases, oxygen (O_2) and carbon dioxide (CO_2), between cells of the body and the atmosphere. Three processes of respiration are ventilation (mechanical movement of gases into and out of the lungs), diffusion (movement of oxygen and carbon dioxide between the alveoli and the red blood cells), and perfusion (distribution of red blood cells to and from the pulmonary capillaries).

You assess ventilation by observing the rate, depth, and rhythm of respiratory movements. Accurate assessment of respirations incorporates the recognition of normal thoracic and abdominal movements. Normal breathing is both active and passive. On inspiration the diaphragm contracts, and the abdominal organs move down to increase the size of the chest cavity. At the same time the ribs and sternum lift outward to promote lung expansion. On expiration the diaphragm relaxes upward, and the ribs and sternum return to their relaxed position (Fig. 62.1). During quiet breathing, the chest wall gently rises and falls. Expiration is an active process only during exercise or voluntary hyperventilation, and in certain disease states.

Safety Guidelines

- Altered breathing tends to be the first sign of clinical deterioration and is a better predictor than blood pressure or pulse of patient deterioration (Takayama et al., 2019).
- Avoid counting respirations for 15 seconds and multiplying by 4 or counting for 30 seconds and multiplying by 2; these methods contribute to errors (Daw et al., 2017; Rolfe, 2019).

Delegation

The skill of counting respirations can be delegated to assistive personnel (AP) unless the patient is considered unstable (i.e., complaints of dyspnea). Instruct the AP by:

- Communicating the frequency of measurement and factors related to patient history or risk for increased or decreased respiratory rate or irregular respirations.
- Reviewing any unusual respiratory values and significant changes to report.

Collaboration

- If patient has severe shortness of breath or persistent tachypnea, refer to a pulmonary health care provider, e.g., advanced practice nurse or a respiratory therapist, for additional interventions such as medications or pulmonary chest physiotherapy.

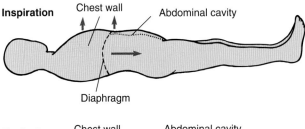

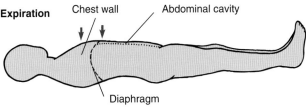

Fig. 62.1 Diaphragmatic and chest wall movement during inspiration and expiration.

Equipment

- Wristwatch with second hand or digital display
- Pen and vital sign flow sheet in chart or electronic health record (EHR)

STEP	RATIONALE
1 Perform preprocedure protocol.	
Assessment	
• Review patient's EHR to assess for factors that influence the patient's respirations.	Allows for anticipation of factors that influence respirations, ensuring a more accurate interpretation.
a Fever	Elevated body temperature increases oxygen demand, respiration rate, and depth.
b Exercise	Respirations increase in rate and depth to meet need for additional oxygen and rid body of carbon dioxide.

Continued

STEP	RATIONALE
c Diseases or trauma of chest wall or muscles (e.g., fractured ribs, thoracic surgery, asthma, chronic lung disease)	Certain conditions affect inspiration and/or expiration.
d Smoking	Chronic smoking changes pulmonary airways, resulting in increased respiratory rate at rest when not smoking.
e Medications	Opioid analgesics, general anesthetics, and sedative hypnotics depress rate and depth; amphetamines and cocaine increase rate and depth; bronchodilators dilate the airways, which ultimately slows respiratory rate.
f Neurologic injury	Damage to brainstem impairs respiratory center and inhibits rate and rhythm.
• Assess pertinent laboratory/ clinical values:	
a *Arterial blood gases (ABGs):* Normal ranges (values vary slightly among agencies): pH, 7.35 to 7.45 $PaCO_2$, 35 to 45 mm Hg HCO_3, 22 to 28 mEq/L PaO_2, 80 to 100 mm Hg SaO_2, 95% to 100%	ABG values measure arterial blood pH, partial pressure of oxygen and carbon dioxide, and arterial oxygen saturation, which reflect patient's ventilation and oxygenation status.
b *Pulse oximetry (SpO₂):* Normal SpO_2 ≥95% to 100%; less than 90% is a clinical emergency (see Skill 60).	SpO_2 <90% is often accompanied by changes in respiratory rate, depth, and rhythm. Exceptions: patients with chronic obstructive pulmonary disease have lower SpO_2 (88% to 92%). Older adults commonly have SpO_2 at 95% (Pagana et al., 2021).

STEP	RATIONALE
c *Hemoglobin (Hgb), or complete blood count (CBC):* Normal CBC for adults (values vary within agencies): Hemoglobin: 14 to 18 g/100 mL, males; 12 to 16 g/100 mL, females Hematocrit: 42% to 52%, males; 37% to 47%, females	CBC measures concentration of hemoglobin. Decreased hemoglobin levels lower amount of oxygen carried in blood, which results in increased respiratory rate to increase oxygen delivery.
• Determine previous baseline respiratory rate (if available) from patient's record.	Assesses for change in condition. Provides comparison with future respiratory measurements.
• Perform hand hygiene.	Reduces transmission of microorganisms.
• Assess for signs and symptoms that influence the patient's respirations:	
a Acute pain	Increases oxygen demand and alters rate and rhythm of respirations; breathing becomes shallow. Patient inhibits or splints chest wall movement when pain is in area of chest or abdomen.
b Constrictive chest or abdominal dressings	Dressings can restrict ease with which a patient is able to breathe deeply.
c Anxiety	Increases oxygen demand and causes increase in respiration rate and depth because of sympathetic nervous system stimulation.
d Body position	Standing or sitting erect promotes full ventilatory movement and lung expansion; stooped or slumped posture impairs ventilatory movement; lying flat prevents full chest expansion.

Continued

STEP	RATIONALE
• Assess for signs and symptoms of respiratory alterations:	Physical signs and symptoms indicate alterations in respiratory status.
a Bluish or cyanotic appearance of nail beds, lips, mucous membranes, and skin	
b Restlessness, irritability, confusion, reduced level of consciousness	
c Pain during inspiration	
d Labored or difficult breathing	
e Orthopnea	
f Use of accessory muscles	
g Inability to breathe spontaneously	
h Thick, frothy, blood-tinged, or copious sputum production	

Implementation

STEP	RATIONALE
1 If patient has been active, wait 5 to 10 minutes before assessing respirations.	Exercise increases respiratory rate and depth. Assessing respirations while patient is at rest allows for objective comparison of values.
2 Ensure that patient is in sitting or lying position with head of bed elevated 45 to 60 degrees.	Sitting erect promotes full ventilatory movement. Position of discomfort causes patient to breathe more rapidly.

CLINICAL JUDGMENT *Patients with difficulty breathing (dyspnea), such as those with heart failure or abdominal ascites or in late stages of pregnancy should be assessed in the position of greatest comfort. Repositioning may increase the work of breathing, which increases respiratory rate.*

STEP	RATIONALE
3 Ensure that patient's chest is visible. If necessary, move bed linen or gown.	Ensures clear view of chest wall and abdominal movements.

STEP	RATIONALE
4 Assess respirations after pulse measurement in an adult, thus doing so when patient is not aware.	Count respirations in such a manner that patient is not aware of the assessment. Patient awareness of breathing can alter the respiratory rate, which prevents a true assessment (Hill et al., 2018; Rolfe, 2019).
5 Perform hand hygiene and place patient's arm in relaxed position across abdomen or lower chest, leaving fingertips on the wrist, or place your hand directly over patient's upper abdomen. Patient's arm or your hand rises and falls during respiratory cycle.	A similar position used during pulse assessment allows respiratory rate assessment to be inconspicuous. Patient awareness of monitoring reduces respiratory rate by 2 breaths/min (Hill et al., 2018).
6 Observe complete respiratory cycle (one inspiration and one expiration).	Rate is accurately determined only after viewing a complete respiratory cycle. An inspiratory breath is half as long as an expiratory breath (Rolfe, 2019).
7 After observing a cycle, look at second hand of watch and begin to count rate: when sweep hand hits determined number on dial, begin time frame, counting one with first full respiratory cycle.	Timing begins with count of one. Respirations occur more slowly than pulse; therefore, timing does not begin with zero.
8 If rhythm is regular, count number of respirations in 30 seconds and multiply by 2. However, if rhythm is irregular, less than 12, or greater than 20, count for 1 full minute. Respiratory rate is equivalent to number of respirations per minute.	Using a consistent counting method when obtaining the respiratory rate increases accuracy (Brabrand et al., 2018). Suspected irregularities require assessment for at least 1 minute. Shorter count durations overestimate respiratory rate by 2 to 4 breaths (Takayama et al., 2019).

Continued

STEP	RATIONALE
9 Note depth of respirations by observing degree of chest wall movement while counting rate. In addition, assess depth by palpating chest wall excursion or auscultating posterior thorax after you have counted rate. Describe depth as shallow, normal, or deep.	Character of ventilatory movement reveals specific disease states restricting volume of air from moving into and out of lungs.
10 Note rhythm of ventilatory cycle. Normal breathing is regular and uninterrupted. Sighing should not be confused with abnormal rhythm.	Character of ventilations reveals specific types of alterations. Periodically people unconsciously take single deep breaths or sighs to expand small airways prone to collapse.

CLINICAL JUDGMENT *Any irregular respiratory pattern or periods of apnea (cessation of respiration for several seconds) are symptoms of underlying disease in the adult and need to be reported to the health care provider or nurse in charge. Further assessment and immediate intervention are often necessary.*

11 Replace bed linen and patient's gown.	Promotes sense of well-being.
12 Inform patient of respiratory rate	Promotes participation in care and understanding of health status.
13 Perform postprocedure protocol.	
14 Evaluate patient response:	
a If assessing respirations for first time, establish rate, rhythm, and depth as baseline if within acceptable range.	Used to compare future respiratory assessment.

STEP	RATIONALE
b Compare respirations with patient's previous baseline and usual rate, rhythm, and depth.	Allows you to assess for changes in patient's condition and presence of respiratory alterations.
c Correlate respiratory rate, depth, and rhythm with data obtained from pulse oximetry and ABG measurements, if available.	Evaluations of ventilation, perfusion, and diffusion are interrelated.

Recording and Reporting

- Record respiratory rate, depth, and rhythm on vital sign flow sheet or EHR.
- Document respiratory rate after administration of specific therapies (e.g., nebulizer) per agency policy.
- Document evaluation of patient and family caregiver learning.
- Record type and amount of oxygen therapy, if used.
- Report abnormal findings to nurse in charge or health care provider.

UNEXPECTED OUTCOMES	RELATED INTERVENTIONS
1 Adult patient's respiratory rate is below 12 breaths/min (bradypnea) or above 20 breaths/min (tachypnea). Breathing pattern is sometimes irregular. Depth of respirations is increased or decreased; observe dyspnea. Patient reports shortness of breath.	• Assess for related factors, including obstructed airway, abnormal breath sounds, productive cough, restlessness, anxiety, and confusion. • Help patient to supported sitting position (semi- or high-Fowler) unless contraindicated. • Provide oxygen as ordered. • Assess for environmental factors that influence patient's respiratory rate such as secondhand smoke, poor ventilation, or gas fumes. • Notify health care provider or nurse in charge if alteration continues. Even small deviations from normal (3 to 5 breaths/min) can indicate a change in the patient's condition and are often the first sign of deterioration (Wheatley, 2019).
2 Patient demonstrates Kussmaul, Cheyne-Stokes, or Biot respirations.	• Notify health care provider for additional evaluation and possible medical intervention.

Restraint Application (Physical)

A restraint is a chemical or physical method of restricting an individual's freedom of movement, including physical activity or normal access to their body that (1) is not a usual part of a medical diagnostic or treatment procedure, (2) is not indicated to treat the individual's medical condition, or (3) does not promote the individual's independent functioning (The Joint Commission [TJC], 2020a). Three forms of restraints are used in health care settings: physical, chemical, and seclusion. Physical restraints are any manual method, physical or mechanical device, material, or equipment that immobilizes or prevents a patient from moving any part of the body freely, or restricts normal access to the patient's own body (Centers for Medicare and Medicaid Services [CMS], 2020). Physical restraint may involve:

- Applying a wrist, elbow, ankle, or waist restraint
- Tucking in a sheet tightly enough that a patient cannot move
- Keeping all side rails up to prevent a patient from getting out of bed
- Preventing a patient in a recliner, wheelchair or enclosed bed from freely exiting on their own

Physical restraints are most commonly used in health care agencies to protect the integrity of medically necessary devices (e.g., drainage tubes, catheters, intravenous [IV] catheters), to prevent ambulation when it is unsafe to do so, or when patients are physically aggressive towards caregivers or others (Springer, 2015). The use of restraints is most common in the critical care setting, where patients who are acutely ill often unknowingly try to remove their endotracheal tubes or other life sustaining medical devices (Perez et al, 2019).

Safety Guidelines

- Restraint application requires continuous assessment by all health care providers to determine appropriateness of use, type of restraint or safety device to use, and patient's tolerance of the device.
- The CMS standards emphasize that restraint or seclusion may be used only to ensure the immediate physical safety of a patient, a staff member, or others and must be discontinued at the earliest possible time (CMS, 2020).
- When the use of a restraint is necessary, the least restrictive method must be used to ensure a patient's safety (CMS, 2020).

- The CMS standards note that there is no evidence that the use of physical restraint (including, but not limited to, raised side rails) will prevent or reduce falls (CMS, 2020).
- The use of restraints is associated with serious complications, including pressure injuries, hypostatic pneumonia, constipation, incontinence, and death.

Delegation

The skill of assessing a patient's behavior, orientation to the environment, need for restraints, and appropriate use of restraints cannot be delegated to assistive personnel (AP). The application and routine checking of a restraint can be delegated to trained AP. CMS (2020) requires training of all direct care staff who apply restraints. Instruct the AP about:

- Appropriate restraint to use and correct placement of restraint.
- When and how to change patient's position and provide range-of-motion exercises, hydration, toileting, skin care, and time for socialization.
- When to report signs and symptoms of patient not tolerating restraint and what actions to take.

Collaboration

- Inform physical or occupational therapists and IV nurses regarding the patient behavior leading to use of restraints and how the patient reacts when restraint is removed for therapy.

Equipment

- Proper-size restraint
- Padding (if needed)

STEP	RATIONALE
1 Perform preprocedure protocol.	

Assessment

• Review electronic health record (EHR) to assess for underlying cause(s) of agitation and cognitive impairment or presence of depression or dementia that may lead to patient-initiated medical device removal (Bradas et al., 2020).	Physiologic and cognitive alterations can lead to accidental patient-initiated medical device removal (Bradas et al., 2020). Knowing causes allows for use of preventive measures that can make restraints unnecessary.

STEP	RATIONALE
• Perform hand hygiene (as needed) if assessment is required related to abrupt change in perception, attention, or level of consciousness. Assess for respiratory and neurologic alterations, fever and sepsis, hypoglycemia and hyperglycemia, alcohol or substance withdrawal, and fluid and electrolyte imbalance.	Reduces transmission of microorganisms. Factors can develop quickly that affect patient cognition.

CLINICAL JUDGMENT *Notify health care provider of change in mental status and compromised physiologic status so a restraint order (if appropriate) can be made.*

• Refer to agency policy for the use of restraints.	A licensed health care provider's order based on a face-to-face, thorough assessment is needed to implement use of restraints. A patient's or family caregiver's informed consent is necessary in the long-term care setting.
• Obtain baseline or previous cognitive function from family caregivers.	Excellent sources of information for patient's behavior patterns and history.
• Review medications that can cause risk for falling (American Geriatrics Society, 2019; Bradas et al., 2020) and changes in mental status: a Benzodiazepines b Antipsychotics, antidepressants c Opiates, barbiturates, sedatives d Antihistamines e Anticonvulsants f Antihypertensives g Diuretics	Medications can alter cognition, cause drowsiness and postural hypotension, and create other risks.

Continued

STEP	RATIONALE
• Review current laboratory values (e.g., electrolytes, blood glucose, blood culture, urinalysis).	May reveal a fluid and electrolyte imbalance or other problems, all of which can cause sudden confusion in the elderly (National Health Service, 2018).
• Assess patient's current behavior (e.g., confusion, disorientation, restlessness, combativeness, inability to follow directions, wandering or repeated removal of therapeutic devices). Assess whether patient creates a risk to other patients.	If patient's behavior continues despite treatment or restraint alternatives, use of least restrictive restraint might be indicated. Cognitively impaired are at risk for exiting bed without asking for assistance.

CLINICAL JUDGMENT *In the case of alcohol withdrawal, resistance against restraints can increase temperature, produce rhabdomyolysis, and cause physical injury (Hoffman and Weinhouse, 2021).*

• If earlier restraint alternatives have failed, confer with health care provider. Review agency policies and state laws regarding restraints. **Obtain current health care provider's order for restraint,** including purpose, type, location, and time or duration of restraint. Determine whether signed consent for use of restraint is necessary (long-term care). For nonviolent/ non–self-destructive patients, orders are renewed per hospital policy.	A restraint order that is being used for violent or self-destructive behavior has a definite time limit (e.g., every 4 h for adults, every 2 h for children and adolescents ages 9 to 17); these orders may be renewed according to the prescribed time limits for a maximum of 24 consecutive hours (CMS, 2020). A health care provider's order for least restrictive type of restraint is required (CMS, 2020).

CLINICAL JUDGMENT *A licensed independent health care provider responsible for the care of the patient evaluates the patient in person within 1 h of the initiation of restraint used for the management of violent or self-destructive behavior that jeopardizes the physical safety of the patient, staff, or others. A registered nurse, an advanced practice nurse, or a physician assistant may conduct the in-person evaluation if trained in accordance with the requirements and consults with the aforementioned health care provider after the evaluation as determined by hospital policy (CMS, 2020).*

STEP	RATIONALE
• Review manufacturer instructions for restraint application. Determine most appropriate size restraint. Be familiar with all devices	Incorrect sizing and application of restraint device can result in patient injury or death.

Implementation

STEP	RATIONALE
1 Perform hand hygiene. Prepare restraint, ensuring it is intact.	Reduces transmission of microorganisms. Ensures restraint is in condition for correct use.
2 Explain to patient and family caregiver the choice of restraint, how it will be applied, length of time to be used, and procedure and rationale for ongoing assessment.	Promotes patient/family cooperation and helps to minimize any anxiety.
3 Adjust bed to proper height and lower side rail on side of patient contact. Be sure that patient is comfortable and in proper body alignment.	Allows repositioning of patient during restraint application without injuring self or patient. Proper alignment prevents contracture formation with restraint in place.
4 Inspect area where restraint is to be placed. Note whether there is any nearby tubing or device. Assess condition of skin, sensation, adequacy of circulation, and range of joint motion.	Restraints sometimes compress and interfere with functioning of devices or tubes. Assessment provides baseline to monitor patient's response to restraint, condition of patient's skin, and presence of pressure injuries.
5 Pad skin and bony prominences (as necessary) that will be under restraint.	Reduces friction and pressure from restraint to skin and underlying tissue.
6 Apply proper-size restraint. *Note:* Refer to manufacturer directions.	

Continued

STEP	RATIONALE
a *Mitten restraint:* Thumbless mitten device restricts patient's use of hands for dislodging or removing medical device, removing dressings, or scratching. Place hand in mitten, ensuring that Velcro strap is around wrist and not forearm (Fig. 63.1).	Hand mitt is considered a restraint if (TJC, 2020b): (1) The mitts are pinned or otherwise attached to the bed/bedding, or wrist restraints are used in conjunction, and/or (2) The mitts are applied so tightly that the patient's hands or finger are immobilized, and/or (3) The mitts are so bulky that the patient's ability to use their hands is significantly reduced, and/or (4) The mitts cannot be easily removed intentionally by the patient in the same manner it was applied by staff considering the patient's physical condition and ability to accomplish the objective.

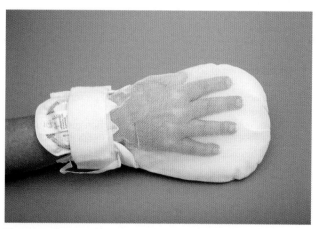

Fig. 63.1 Mitten restraint. (From Sorrentino SA, Remmert LN: *Mosby's textbook for nursing assistants*, ed 10, St Louis, 2021, Elsevier.)

STEP	RATIONALE

CLINICAL JUDGMENT *Mittens are considered a restraint alternative if untethered and patient is physically and cognitively able to remove the mitten.*

b *Elbow restraint (freedom splint):* Restraint consists of rigidly padded device that wraps around arm and is closed with Velcro. The upper end has a clamp that hooks to sleeve of patient's gown or shirt. Center splint over elbow with opening facing away from patient. Secure splint by threading hook and loop strap through buckle and back onto itself. (Fig. 63.2).

The restraint makes it difficult to remove or disrupt a medical device near the face or neck. It does not impede removing abdominal or urinary medical devices. With freedom splints, patients have difficulty bending their arms. The splints may not prevent a patient from removing IV lines.

Continued

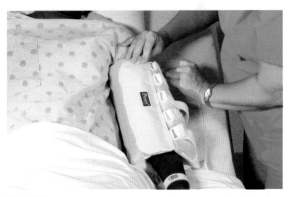

Fig. 63.2 Freedom elbow restraint. (Copyright © Mosby's *Clinical skills: essentials collection.*)

STEP	RATIONALE

c *Self-Releasing Roll Belt Restraint* (Fig. 63.3).

(1) While patient is out of bed, center belt on bed at patient waist level with belt label facing head of bed.

(2) Position the long straps so they hang off each side of the mattress. Attach straps to bed frame by releasing the quick release (QR) buckle and looping strap around a moveable part of the bed frame.

(3) Reconnect the QR buckle, pull on the strap end to tighten strap to bed; repeat on other side of bed.

(4) To attach belt to patient, open the QR buckle and the belt, place patient on the bed with belt at waist level. Bring belt around patient waist and secure hook and loop fastener and QR buckle.

(5) Ensure belt is snug but does not restrict breathing. Ensure bed frame straps are snug to the mattress and won't slide or move if bed is adjusted.

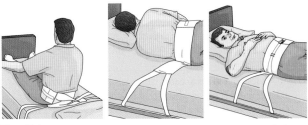

Fig. 63.3 Properly applied roll belt restraint allows patient to turn in bed. (From Sorrentino SA, Remmert LN: *Mosby's textbook for nursing assistants*, ed 10, St Louis, 2021, Elsevier.)

STEP	RATIONALE
d *Soft extremity (ankle or wrist) restraint:* Restraint made of soft quilted material or sheepskin with foam padding. Wrap limb restraint around wrist or ankle with soft part toward skin and secure snugly (not tightly) in place with Velcro strap (Fig. 63.4A). Insert two fingers under secured restraint (see Fig. 63.4B).	Appropriate for patients who are becoming increasingly agitated, cannot be redirected with distraction, and keep trying to remove needed medical devices. Restraint designed to immobilize one or all extremities. Tight application interferes with circulation and potentially causes neurovascular injury.

Continued

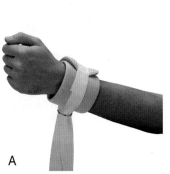
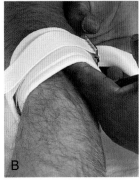

Fig. 63.4 (A) Extremity restraint. (B) Check restraint for constriction by inserting two fingers under restraint.

STEP	RATIONALE

CLINICAL JUDGMENT *Patient with wrist and ankle restraints is at risk for aspiration if positioned supine. Place patient in lateral position or with head of bed elevated rather than supine.*

7 Attach restraint straps to part of bedframe that moves when raising or lowering head of bed. Be sure that straps are secure. *Do not attach to side rails.* Attach restraint to chair frame for patient in chair or wheelchair, being sure that buckle is out of patient's reach.	Properly positioned strap does not tighten and restrict circulation when bed is raised or lowered.
8 Secure restraints on bedframe with quick-release buckle (Fig. 63.5). *Do not tie strap in a knot.* Be sure that buckle is out of patient reach.	Allows for quick release in emergency.

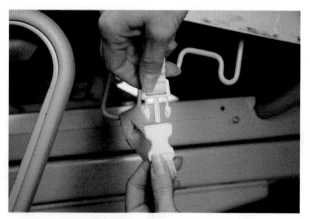

Fig. 63.5 Quick-release buckle.

STEP	RATIONALE
9 Double-check by inserting two fingers under secured restraint one more time. Assess proper placement of restraint, including skin integrity, pulses, skin temperature and color, and sensation of restrained body part. Place bed in lowest position after restraint(s) applied.	Provides baseline to later evaluate if injury develops from restraint. Provides safest environment in which to leave a patient who is restrained.
10 Perform hand hygiene. Remove restraint at least every 2 h (TJC, 2020a) or more frequently as determined by agency policy. Reposition patient, provide comfort and toileting measures, and evaluate patient condition each time. If patient is agitated, violent, or nonadherent, remove one restraint at a time and/or have staff assistance while removing restraints.	Provides opportunity to attend to patient's basic needs and determine need for continuation of restraints. A temporary, directly supervised release of a restraint that occurs for the purpose of caring for a patient's needs (e.g., toileting, feeding, or range of motion exercises) is **not** considered a discontinuation of the restraint.

CLINICAL JUDGMENT *Restraints cannot be ordered on an as-needed basis. If a patient was recently released from restraint and exhibits behavior that can be handled only through the reapplication of restraint or seclusion, a new order is required (CMS, 2020).*

CLINICAL JUDGMENT *Do not leave a patient who is violent or aggressive unattended while restraints are off. Monitoring violent/self-destructive patients placed in restraints is continuous (by way of video or audio) versus every 2 h for nonviolent patients.*

11 Perform postprocedure protocol.

Continued

STEP	RATIONALE
12 Evaluate patient response:	
a *Nonviolent patients:* Conduct evaluation for signs of injury (e.g., circulation, range of motion, vital signs, skin condition), behavior and psychological status, and readiness for discontinuation (frequency based on agency policy) (TJC, 2020a).	Frequent evaluation prevents injury to patient and ensures removal of restraint at earliest possible time. Frequency of monitoring guides staff in determining appropriate intervals for evaluation based on patient's needs and condition, type of restraint used, risk associated with use of chosen intervention, and other relevant factors.
(1) *Violent/self-destructive patients:* Conduct same evaluation every 15 minutes. Perform visual checks if patient is too agitated to approach (TJC, 2020a).	
b Evaluate patient's need for toileting, nutrition and fluids, and hygiene, and release restraint at least every 2 h.	Prevents injury to patient and attends to basic needs.
c Evaluate patient for any complications of immobility.	Early detection of skin irritation, restricted breathing, or reduction in mobility prevents serious adverse events.

STEP	RATIONALE
d Observe IV catheters, urinary catheters, and drainage tubes to determine that they are positioned correctly and that therapy remains uninterrupted.	Reinsertion is uncomfortable and increases risk for infection or interrupts therapy.
13 Renewal of restraints (CMS, 2020):	Ensures that restraint application continues to be medically appropriate.
a Nonviolent patients may have renewal of restraints based on hospital policy. However, the restraint must be discontinued at the earliest possible time, regardless of the scheduled expiration of the order.	
b Violent/self-destructive patients may have restraints renewed within the following limits:	
• 4 h for adults 18 years of age or older	
• 2 h for children and adolescents 9 to 17 years of age	
• 1 h for children under 9 years of age	
Orders may be renewed according to the time limits for a maximum of 24 consecutive hours.	

Recording and Reporting

- Record restraint alternatives used and patient's response, patient's current behavior and medical condition, level of orientation, and patient or family member's statement of understanding of the purpose of restraint and consent for application (if required by agency).
- Record placement and purpose for restraint, type and location of restraint, time applied, and patient's behavior after restraint application. Record times patient was assessed, attempts to use alternatives to restraint and patient's response, times restraint was released (temporarily and permanently), and patient's response when restraint was ended.
- Report any injury resulting from a restraint to registered nurse in charge and health care provider immediately.
- During hand-off report, note the location and type of restraint, last time assessment was conducted, and findings.

UNEXPECTED OUTCOMES	RELATED INTERVENTIONS
1 Patient experiences impaired skin integrity.	• Evaluate need for continued use of restraint and determine whether alternatives can be used. • If restraint is still needed, be sure that it is applied correctly and provide adequate padding. • Check skin under restraint for abrasions and remove restraints more often. Provide appropriate skin care and change wet or soiled restraints.
2 Patient becomes more confused or agitated.	• Reassess cause of behavior and eliminate if possible; consult with health care provider. • Determine need for more or less sensory stimulation, and ensure that stimulation provided is meaningful. • Reorient as needed and try restraint-free options.

UNEXPECTED OUTCOMES	RELATED INTERVENTIONS
3 Patient has neurovascular injury (e.g., cyanosis, pallor, and coldness of skin, or patient complains of tingling, pain, or numbness).	• Remove restraint immediately, stay with patient, and notify health care provider, or delegate someone to do so. • Protect extremity from further injury.

Restraint-Free Environment

A restraint-free environment is the first goal of care for all patients in hospitals or long-term care settings. A restraint is any method (chemical or physical) of restricting an individual's freedom of movement, including physical activity or normal access to their body that (1) is not a usual part of a medical diagnostic or treatment procedure, (2) is not indicated to treat the individual's medical condition, or (3) does not promote the individual's independent functioning (The Joint Commission, 2022). Serious and often fatal complications can result from the use of restraints, such as bruises, pressure injuries, musculoskeletal injury, suffocation and respiratory complications, and urinary incontinence. Because of the risks associated with the use of restraints, current legislation emphasizes reducing this use. Federal and state laws prohibit Medicare and Medicaid-certified nursing homes from using restraints unless medically needed.

In trying to create a restraint-free environment, patients at risk for falling or wandering present special safety challenges and require additional precautions. Wandering is aimless pacing, attempts at elopement, or getting lost on one's own that exposes a patient to harm and is frequently in conflict with boundaries, limits, or obstacles (Butcher, 2018). Many hospitals and long-term care facilities use electronic alarms to notify staff when patients begin ambulating (or when leaving bedside chairs). E-sitting is a technology involving use of in-room cameras, either hard-mounted to the wall or placed on a portable cart, that provides real-time, continuous visibility to trained staff who can observe patient rooms on multiple monitors at a workstation (Deibert, 2021). These staff members are not registered nurses, and are typically called E-sitters.

Safety Guidelines

- The Centers for Medicare and Medicaid Services (CMS) set the original standard that restraint or seclusion may be imposed only to ensure the immediate physical safety of a patient, and must be discontinued at the earliest possible time (CMS, 2018b).

Delegation

The skills of assessing patient behaviors and orientation to the environment and determining the type of restraint-free interventions to use cannot be delegated to assistive personnel (AP). Actions that provide a safe environment can be delegated to AP. Direct the AP about:

- Using specific diversional or activity based measures for creating a safe environment.
- Applying appropriate monitoring or alarm devices.
- Reporting patient behaviors and actions (e.g., confusion, getting out of bed unassisted).

Collaboration

- In the long-term care setting, collaborate with AP and case managers who may observe patient behavior and recognize signs of wandering.
- Physical, speech, and occupational therapists offer exercise options and activities that provide meaningful stimulation.

Equipment

- Visual or auditory stimuli meaningful to patient (e.g., photos, music, streaming devices, calendar, piece of art)
- Diversional activities (e.g., puzzle, game, audiobook, DVD)
- Wraparound belt
- Options: Electronic bracelet continuous video monitoring system, or pressure pad alarm sensor

STEP	RATIONALE
1 Perform preprocedure protocol.	
Assessment	
• Assess patient's medical history for memory impairment and underlying causes of agitation and cognitive impairment (e.g., delirium, dementia, depression). Also assess for the following:	Causes of agitation and wandering are commonly associated with these conditions (Berry and Kiel, 2022).
a Considered dangerous to self or others	
b Disability as result of mental disorder	
c Lacks cognitive ability (either permanently or temporarily) for decision-making	
d Alcohol or substance withdrawal	
e Fluid and electrolyte imbalance	

Continued

STEP	RATIONALE
• In patients with known dementia, assess for signs of restlessness: pacing, fidgeting, repetitive motor movements and repetitive questioning (Regier and Gitlin, 2017).	Being able to distinguish restlessness from other behaviors may assist in recognition and appropriate treatment (Regier and Gitlin, 2017).

CLINICAL JUDGMENT *In a patient with dementia restlessness is not: (1) the disordered locomotion that is the hallmark of wandering behavior, (2) associated with attempts to elope or leave without permission of caregivers from an institution (3) the physiologic effects of a substance (e.g., neuroleptic medication, withdrawal from benzodiazepines) or another medical condition (e.g., hypoglycemia) and (4) a mental disorder, except in cases when associated with dementia. It is a generalized anxiety disorder or movement disorder (e.g., restless legs syndrome, essential tremor, Parkinson disease) (Regier and Gitlin, 2017).*

STEP	RATIONALE
• Review patient's medications for over-the-counter and prescribed medications (see Box 64.1) that pose risk for falling (compare with medications on Beers criteria lists [AGS, 2019]). Assess for interactions and untoward effects.	Medication interactions or side effects often contribute to falling or altered mental status.
• Perform hand hygiene. Assess patient's orientation, level of consciousness, ability to understand and follow directions, combative behaviors, balance, gait, vision, hearing, bowel/bladder routine, level of pain, electrolyte and blood count values, and presence of orthostatic hypotension.	Reduces transfer of microorganisms. Accurate assessment identifies patients with safety risks and the physiological causes for patient behaviors that prompt caregivers to use restraints. Ensures proper selection of nonrestraint interventions.

BOX 64.1 Medications That Create or Increase Risk for Falls

- Benzodiazepines
- Antipsychotics
- Antidepressants
- Opiates
- Barbiturates
- Antihistamines
- Anticonvulsants
- Sedatives
- Antihypertensives
- Diuretics

STEP	RATIONALE
• For patients who wander or have known dementia. Assess patient during time of day when cognition normally decreases (e.g., end of the day or at night screen for cognitive decline using a validated patient assessment tool, such as the General Practitioner Assessment of Cognition (GPCOG), the Memory Impairment Screen (MIS), or the Mini-Cog™ (Alzheimer's Association, 2023)).	Findings assist in determining patient's mental status, predisposition to wandering, and potential interventions. Tools are easily administered by medical staff members who are not physicians and are relatively free from educational, language, and/or cultural bias (Alzheimer's Association, n.d.).
• Assess degree of wandering behavior using Algase Wandering Scale (Version 2) (AWS-V2) (Martin et al., 2015; Nelson and Algase, 2007).	The AWS-V2 is a valid and reliable measure for persistent walking, spatial disorientation, and eloping behavior.
• For patients with dementia, ask family about their usual communication style and cues to indicate pain, fatigue, hunger, and need to urinate or defecate.	Enables utilization of best method to determine patient needs. Wandering or agitation often prompted when needs are unmet.

Continued

STEP	RATIONALE
• Inspect condition of any therapeutic medical devices.	Patients who become restless, agitated, or confused will attempt to remove medical devices and then become candidates for physical restraint.
• Assess whether a medical device is necessary or can be discontinued. Consider alternative therapy (e.g., oral medications instead of intravenous) when possible.	Patients who are agitated often try to remove medical devices.

Implementation

1 Orient patient and family caregiver to surroundings, introduce to staff, and explain all treatments and procedures. Be sure that patient is able to read your name badge.	Promotes patient understanding and cooperation.
2 Assign same staff to care for patient as often as possible. Encourage family and friends to stay with patient. In some agencies volunteers are effective companions.	Increases familiarity with individuals in patient's environment, decreasing anxiety and restlessness. Companions are helpful and prevent patient from being alone.
3 Place patient in room that is easily accessible to care providers.	Allows for frequent observation to reduce falls in high-risk patients.
4 Follow all Universal Fall Precautions (see Skill 28) to create a safe environment (AHRQ, 2013, Dykes and Hurley, 2021).	Reduces environmental risks for falls/injuries.
5 Ensure that patient is wearing glasses, hearing aid, or other sensory-aid devices and that all are functioning.	Improves patient's level of orientation to environment.

STEP	RATIONALE
6 Provide visual and auditory stimuli meaningful to patient (e.g., clock, calendar, streaming devices [with patient's choice of music], television, and family pictures).	Orients patient to day, time, and physical surroundings. Stimuli must be individualized for this to be effective.
7 Anticipate patient's basic needs (e.g., toileting, relief of pain, relief of hunger) as quickly as possible; conduct hourly rounds (Nuckols et al., 2017).	Providing basic needs in timely fashion decreases patient discomfort, anxiety, restlessness, and incidence of falls.
8 Provide scheduled ambulation, chair activity, and toileting (e.g., ask patient every hour during rounds about toileting needs). Organize treatments so patient has uninterrupted periods throughout the day. Consider using a bedside commode for toileting (but insist that patient be assisted out of bed).	Early mobility is essential for all patients. Regular opportunity to void lowers risk of patient trying to reach bathroom alone. Constant activity overstimulates patients. Commode makes toileting more accessible.

CLINICAL JUDGMENT *Caution: A bedside commode can sometimes encourage patients to get up unassisted. Reinforce to patient and family caregiver that assistance is required.*

STEP	RATIONALE
9 Position intravenous (IV) catheters, urinary catheters, and tubes/drains out of patient view. Use commercial tube holders, camouflage by wrapping IV site with bandage or stockinette, use long-sleeved robes and commercial sleeves over arms. Place undergarments on patient with urinary catheter or cover abdominal feeding tubes/drains with loose abdominal binder.	Maintains medical treatment while reducing patient access to tubes/lines needed for treatment delivery.

Continued

STEP	RATIONALE
10 Implement strategies to decrease wandering: a Eliminate environmental stressors such as cold at night, changes in daily routines, and extra visitors.	Reduced stress allows patient's energy to be channeled more appropriately.
b Use stress-reduction techniques such as back rub, massage, and guided imagery.	Reduces anxiety and restlessness.
c Use activity based measures: puzzles, games, music therapy, art therapy, doll therapy, pet therapy, mirrors in front of exit doors, activity apron, and the integration of purposeful activities such as chores (folding towels) and crafts (Neubauer et al., 2018). Ensure that it is an activity in which patient has interest. Involve family caregiver (if appropriate).	Activity based interventions individualized to the patient with dementia have shown improvement in patient engagement, mood, and agitating behaviors (Lourida, et al., 2020).
11 Position patient comfortably in chair or wheelchair with a wraparound safety belt.	Wraparound belt offers security but allows patient independence.

STEP	RATIONALE
12 Use motion or bed occupancy alarm system for unsteady patients who forget or do not call for assistance when getting out of bed or chair (Dykes and Hurley, 2021). See manufacturer's directions and agency policy.	Alarms alert staff to patient who is standing or rising from bed or chair without help.

CLINICAL JUDGMENT *In any situation in which an alarm is used, timeliness of response is a key factor in preventing falls. Staff response times using video surveillance have been shown to be faster than traditional call lights (Quigley et al., 2019).* ***Always respond quickly to any alarm.***

---

a Explain use of device to patient and family caregiver.	Promotes patient and family cooperation.
b When patient is in chair, position a chair pad alarm so it is correctly positioned under patient's buttocks.	System responds to a change in pressure, requiring accurate placement.
c Test bedside alarm by applying and releasing pressure.	Ensures that alarm is audible through call-light system.
d Be sure video and audio systems are operational.	Ensures observer can interact with patient.
13 Use available locating technology (i.e., global positioning system [GPS], radio frequency, Bluetooth, and Wi-Fi) for patients who wander. Follow manufacturer's directions.	Tag in bracelet or wearable device contains radio frequency circuit that communicates with detection sensor usually installed at an exit door or elevator. Distance between tag and monitor is constantly measured with an alarm, which sounds when predetermined distance is exceeded.

Continued

STEP	RATIONALE
14 Minimize invasive treatments (e.g., tube feedings, blood sampling) as much as possible.	Stimuli increase patients' restlessness.
15 Perform postprocedure protocol.	
16 Evaluate patient response:	
a Monitor patient's behavior routinely and check condition of medical devices.	Will determine whether agitation, wandering, or attempt to remove medical devices has been prevented.
b Observe patient and inspect condition of skin for any injuries.	Patient should be injury free.
c Observe patient's behavior toward staff, visitors, and other patients.	Ensures that patient's behavior does not cause injury to others.

Recording and Reporting

- Record all behaviors that relate to cognitive status and ability to maintain safety: orientation to time, place, and person; ability to follow directions; mood and emotional status; understanding of condition and treatment plan; medication effects related to behaviors; restraint alternatives used; and patient response to interventions.
- Document evaluation of patient/family caregiver learning.
- Report to other health care providers all interventions being used to prevent agitation or wandering, and any occurrences of wandering or other behavior that places the patient at risk for injury.
- Report any patient injury from a fall to health care provider immediately and complete an occurrence/incident report.

UNEXPECTED OUTCOMES	RELATED INTERVENTIONS
1 Patient displays behaviors that increase risk for injury to self or others.	• Review episodes for pattern (e.g., activity, time of day) that indicates alternatives that would eliminate behavior. • Discuss alternative interventions with all health care providers and family caregivers.
2 Patient sustains injury, or is agitated and places others at risk for injury.	• Notify health care provider. Complete occurrence report according to agency policy. • Identify alternative measures for safety or behavioral control. • Apply physical restraint (see Skill 63) only after all other interventions have been unsuccessful.
3 Patient wanders away from health care agency.	• Be prepared to follow agency policy, which should include whom to notify; who will search for patient; which areas will be searched and their priority; who will notify authorities, if necessary; who will notify family members; and who will coordinate search efforts.

Seizure Precautions

A seizure is a sudden, abnormal, electrical discharge in the brain causing alterations in behavior, sensation, or consciousness. Any condition that causes an interruption to the normal connections between neurons in the brain can cause a seizure, including a high fever, abnormal blood sugar, alcohol or drug withdrawal, or a brain injury (Johns Hopkins Medicine, 2021). Anyone can have one or more seizures; however, a person who has two or more seizures is considered to have epilepsy.

The two broad categories of epileptic seizures are generalized seizures, which involve both sides of the brain, and partial seizures, which involve one or more areas of one side of the brain. Status epilepticus is a neurologic and medical emergency defined as 5 or more minutes of either continuous seizure activity or repetitive seizures with no intervening recovery of consciousness (Lesser et al., 2018). A seizure can be convulsive (shown by rhythmic jerking of the extremities) or nonconvulsive (seizure activity shown on an electroencephalogram). The Neurocritical Care Society released practice guidelines for patients with status epilepticus (Brophy et al., 2012):

- Priority within the first 2 minutes: establish and protect the airway when a patient loses consciousness.
- Noninvasive airway protection and gas exchange with head positioning should be done immediately, keeping the airway patent and administering oxygen.

Safety Guidelines

- Seizure precautions are guidelines that health care providers follow to minimize injury to a patient during any type of seizure. Observation during a seizure is critical.
- Patients who have undergone seizures, especially grand mal seizures, may suffer bumps, bruises, or cuts. More serious injuries are related to falling and losing awareness or consciousness during or after a seizure, e.g., head trauma, fractures.

Delegation

The skill of assessing a patient's risk for seizures cannot be delegated to assistive personnel (AP). However, AP can assist in creating a safe patient environment and provide ongoing care of patients. Direct the AP about:

- A patient's prior seizure history and factors that may trigger a seizure.
- Taking immediate action in the event of a seizure by protecting the patient from falling or injury.

- Avoiding restraining the patient or placing anything into patient's mouth.
- Reporting immediately when a seizure activity develops and observing the patient's behaviors during the seizure.

Collaboration

- All health care providers should be aware of patients being placed on seizure precautions.

Equipment

- Seizure pads for side rails and headboard
- Suction machine, oral Yankauer suction catheter, oral airway
- Oxygen via nasal cannula or face mask
- Equipment for vital signs, pulse oximetry, and blood glucose testing
- Equipment for intravenous (IV) line insertion; bag of 0.9% normal saline solution
- Emergency antiepileptic medications (National Institute for Health Care Excellence, 2020):
  First-line treatment (tried first and usually used on its own):
  - Focal seizure: carbamazepine, lamotrigine
  - Generalized seizures: sodium valproate, lamotrigine

  Alternative first-line treatment (added to a first-line treatment [used in combination])
  - Focal seizure: levetiracetam, oxcarbazepine, sodium valproate
  - Generalized seizures: carbamazepine, oxcarbazepine
- Clean gloves
- *Option:* Protective head gear

STEP	RATIONALE
1 Perform preprocedure protocol.	
Assessment	
• Review electronic health record (EHR) for medical and surgical conditions that may contribute to or be a cause of a seizure (e.g., brain trauma or tumor, stroke, hypo- or hyperglycemia, infectious disease) and for any bleeding tendencies.	Common conditions that lead to seizures or worsen existing seizure condition. Bleeding conditions predispose patient to injury during a seizure.

Continued

STEP	RATIONALE
• Assess EHR for patient's seizure history (e.g., new diagnosis, seizure within last year), previous precipitating factors (e.g., emotional stress, sleep deprivation), frequency of seizures, presence and type of aura (e.g., reduced vision, visual illusions, noises, metallic taste, noxious odor) (Wolf, 2016), symptoms during a seizure (confusion, staring, loss of consciousness, muscle jerking), and known sequence of seizure events. Family caregiver can be a resource, if needed.	Allows you to eliminate triggers that can cause seizure, anticipate onset of seizure activity, and take appropriate safety precautions.
• Assess medication history (e.g., antidepressants and antipsychotics). Ask patient about adherence to anticonvulsants and review therapeutic drug levels if laboratory test results available.	Certain medications lower seizure threshold. Seizure medications must be taken as prescribed and not discontinued suddenly; cessation of medication may precipitate seizure activity.
• Inspect patient's environment for potential safety hazards (e.g., extra furniture or equipment). Keep bed in low position, with side rails up at head of bed.	Protects patient from injury sustained by striking head or body on furniture or equipment.

Implementation

1	Ensure patient is in a comfortable position. Reduce lighting in room and reduce opportunities for any sudden, loud, unexpected noise.	Startle seizures are most often precipitated by sudden, loud, unexpected noises (Wolf, 2016).

STEP	RATIONALE
2 Inform patient and family caregiver that patient is on seizure precautions and what these precautions entail. Discuss the possible triggers that result in patient's seizure activity. Include discussion of approaches to adopt seizure precautions in the patient's home environment.	May help to relieve patient and family caregiver anxiety and aid in their participation in patient care.
3 For patients with history of seizures, keep bed in lowest position with side rails up (see agency policy). Pad rails if patient is at risk for head injury, and as an option offer protective head gear. Have oral suction and oxygen equipment ready for use.	Modifications to environment minimize risk of injury from seizure activity or related fall. Use padded side rails and head gear only when patient is at risk for head injury.

CLINICAL JUDGMENT *When a patient is placed on* **seizure precautions** *and all side rails are raised, the use of side rails would not be considered restraint. The use of padded side rails in this situation should protect the patient from harm, including falling out of bed should the patient have a seizure (CMS, 2020).*

4 Place patient with history of seizures in room close to nurse's station or room with video monitor (if available).	Improves likelihood of quick identification of seizure and response with emergency equipment.
5 **Partial or general seizure response:** a Position patient safely.	

Continued

STEP	RATIONALE
(1) Guide a patient who is standing or sitting to the floor and protect head by cradling in your lap or place pillow under head. Position patient so as to keep head tilted to maximize breathing (if able). If possible, position patient on side, *but do not force.* Do not lift patient from floor to bed during seizure.	Position protects patient from aspiration and traumatic injury, especially head injury.
(2) If patient is in bed, turn them onto side, if possible *(do not force)* and raise side rails.	
b Note time the seizure began and call for help immediately. Have staff member bring emergency cart to bedside and clear surrounding area of furniture. Provide airway protection and gas exchange by positioning head. Have someone notify health care provider and Rapid Response Team immediately.	Timing and description of seizure may help in ultimate identification of type of seizure. Initial management requires immediate supportive care to maintain ABCs (airway, breathing, circulation) and prompt administration of anti-seizure medications (Drislane, 2022).

STEP	RATIONALE

CLINICAL JUDGMENT *Activate your agency's Rapid Response Team. When a patient demonstrates signs of imminent clinical deterioration, a team of providers is summoned to the bedside to immediately assess and treat the patient with the goal of preventing intensive care unit transfer, cardiac arrest, or death (Agency for Healthcare Research and Quality, 2019).*

c Keep patient in side-lying position (if possible), supporting head and keeping it flexed slightly forward.	Position prevents tongue from blocking airway and promotes drainage of secretions, reducing risk of aspiration.
d **Do not restrain patient**; if patient is flailing limbs, hold them loosely. Loosen restrictive clothing/gown to aid breathing.	Prevents musculoskeletal injury. Promotes free ventilatory movement of chest and abdomen.
e *Never force any object into patient's mouth,* such as fingers, medicine, tongue depressor, or airway when teeth are clenched.	Prevents injury to mouth and possible aspiration.

CLINICAL JUDGMENT *Injury can result from forcible insertion of a hard object into the mouth. Soft objects break and become aspirated. Insert a bite block or oral airway in advance if there is a possibility of a generalized seizure.*

f If possible, provide privacy. Have staff control flow of visitors in area.	Embarrassment is common after a seizure, especially if others witnessed it.

Continued

STEP	RATIONALE
g Observe sequence and timing of seizure activity. Note type of seizure activity (tonic-clonic movements, staring, blinking); whether more than one type of seizure occurs; sequence of seizure progression; level of consciousness; character of breathing; presence of incontinence; presence of autonomic signs of lip smacking, mastication, or grimacing; eye rolling.	Continued observation helps to document, diagnose, and treat seizure disorder.
h As patient regains consciousness, assess vital signs and reorient and reassure. Explain what happened and answer patient's questions. Stay with patient until fully conscious.	Informing patients of type of seizure activity experienced helps them to participate knowledgeably in their care. Some patients remain confused for period of time after seizure or become violent. Confusion predisposes them to falling if they exit a bed too quickly.
6 Status epilepticus is a medical emergency.	
a Follow Steps 5a to 5e to protect patient, and call Rapid Response Team.	Ensures rapid management of airway and breathing.

STEP	RATIONALE
b Assist health care provider with oropharyngeal or nasopharyngeal airway insertion if oxygen saturation is compromised or if seizure lasts ≥ 30 minutes. (*Note:* Apply clean gloves if timing allows.) Physician on team will intubate patient with endotracheal tube when jaw is relaxed (between seizure activity).	Airway promotes oxygenation.
c Access and administer oxygen, turn on suction equipment, keep airway patent with oral suctioning (if possible).	Maintains oxygenation.

CLINICAL JUDGMENT *Never place hands in patient's mouth during a seizure. The patient may accidentally bite your fingers. Do not force any type of airway into mouth.*

d Have another nurse on team measure blood pressure, heart rate, respirations, and oxygen saturation immediately and then every 2 minutes and have team member perform fingerstick to check blood glucose (Sawaf et al., 2021).	Necessary to monitor and support baseline vital signs and determine whether patient is hypoglycemic (common cause of seizure).

Continued

STEP	RATIONALE
e Member of team will prepare for and insert IV catheter (if one is not in place) with infusion of 0.9% sodium chloride, and administer IV antiseizure medications (see Skill 54).	Provides route for IV medication to stop seizure, for fluid resuscitation, and to collect electrolytes, hematology, toxicology screen and anticonvulsant levels (Sawaf et al., 2021).
f As seizure subsides, suction patient's airway if secretions have accumulated. If oral airway was inserted, be sure that it remains in correct position. Continue oxygen administration.	Maintains open airway, decreases chance of aspiration, and promotes oxygenation.
g Keep patient in a side-lying position of comfort in bed with side rails up and bed in lowest position.	Provides for continued safety to reduce risk of aspiration of secretions as patient regains consciousness; lessens risk of fall with injury if patient tries to exit bed.
7 As patient regains consciousness, reorient and reassure. Explain what happened and provide quiet, nonstimulating environment (e.g., lights low, minimal care interruptions).	Provides for continued safety. Patients are often confused and lethargic after seizure (postictal). Patient at risk for falls if they attempt to get out of bed.
8 Instruct patient not to get out of bed without help.	Ensures patient safety.
9 Perform postprocedure protocol.	

STEP	RATIONALE

10 Evaluate patient response:

   a Check vital signs and oxygen saturation every 15 minutes during postictal phase and maintain patent airway. — Determines patient's cardiopulmonary status and response to seizure episode.

   b Recheck blood glucose per health care provider order or agency protocol. — Determines whether normal blood glucose level has been reached.

   c Examine patient for injury, including oral cavity (broken teeth, laceration of tongue or mucosa), skin, and extremities. — Determines presence of any traumatic injuries resulting from seizure activity.

CLINICAL JUDGMENT *If onset of seizure was not witnessed and it is suspected that patient fell and struck head, treat as a closed head injury or spinal injury. Place a cervical collar on patient before attempting to turn or reposition. If patient is taking anticoagulants there is a high risk of intracranial bleeding if head injury occurred.*

   d Evaluate patient's mental status after seizure (level of consciousness, confusion, hallucinations). Ask whether the patient is aware of seizure triggers. — Temporary mental status changes are common after seizure.

   e Assist health care provider in conducting neurologic examination of patient and collect any ordered blood specimens (see Skill 81). — Evaluates for any head trauma and life-threatening metabolic conditions (Sawaf et al., 2021).

Recording and Reporting

- Record in nurses' notes observations before, during, and after seizure. Provide detailed description of the type of seizure activity and sequence of events (e.g., presence of aura [if any], level of consciousness, vital signs and oxygen saturation, color, movement of extremities, incontinence, patient's status immediately after seizure, and time frame of events).
- Record treatments administered for the seizure: establishing IV line, fluid infusion, airway stabilization.
- When a patient has had a seizure, report to oncoming staff a detailed description of seizure and patient's response.
- Alert health care provider immediately as seizure begins. Status epilepticus is an emergency situation requiring immediate medical therapy.

UNEXPECTED OUTCOMES	RELATED INTERVENTIONS
1 Patient sustains traumatic injury.	• Continue to protect patient from further injury. • Notify health care provider immediately. • Administer prescribed treatments. • Reassess patient's environment and eliminate any safety hazards. • Complete agency occurrence/incident report.
2 Patient aspirates oral secretions.	• Turn onto side, insert oral or nasal airway, and apply suction to remove material in oral pharynx, and maintain patent airway. • Administer oxygen as needed per order.

Sequential Compression Devices and Elastic Stockings

Venous thromboembolism (VTE) is a blood clot in a vein. There are two types: deep vein thrombosis (DVT), which is a clot in a deep vein, usually involving the leg or pelvis, but which can also occur in the arms, and pulmonary embolus, a deep vein clot that breaks free from a vein wall, travels to the lungs, and blocks some or all of the blood supply (American Heart Association, 2017). VTE is a result of immobility.

What follows are clinical standards for the prevention of VTE, published by the American Society of Hematology (Schünemann et al., 2018):

- Provision of pharmacologic VTE prophylaxis (anticoagulant therapy) in acutely or critically ill inpatients at acceptable bleeding risk.
- Use of mechanical prophylaxis (compression stockings, intermittent compression) when bleeding risk is unacceptable.
- Conditional recommendation: Do **not** use VTE prophylaxis routinely in long-term care patients or outpatients with minor VTE risk factors.
- Conditional recommendation: Use graduated compression stockings or low-molecular-weight heparin in long-distance travelers only if they are at high risk for VTE.

Nurses play a critical role in promoting mechanical prophylaxis in at-risk patients, including early ambulation and application of intermittent sequential compression devices (SCDs) or compression stockings. SCDs limit patient's ability to ambulate while device is in place, while mechanical compression devices (MCDs) allow for ambulation. Mechanical compression of veins reduces venous stasis by displacing blood from the leg veins into the more proximal vein system segments, thereby increasing the speed and volume flow of the blood in the lower limb deep venous system (Tamowicz et al., 2019). When compression is applied (uniformly or sequentially) the increase in the arterial-venous pressure gradient enables an increase in arterial blood flow and decreases peripheral vascular resistance. An additional benefit of circumferential compression is the increase in hydrostatic pressure on the extracellular interstitial spaces, which may augment blood flow and decrease edema (Weinberger and Cipolle, 2016). An SCD exerts a calculated compression on the lower limbs in the following sequence: from the ankles, through the calves, to the thighs (Tamowicz et al., 2019). The device delivers a preset rate of compression cycle repetitions;

the compression lasts about 10 to 20 seconds, after which the cuffs relax, letting out the air and allowing the veins to be filled again with blood. By increasing blood flow, the SCDs also prevent blood accumulation in the lower limbs and blood clot formation (Tamowicz et al., 2019).

Using an additional device, such as an intermittent SCD plus graduated compression stockings, offers no additive benefit regarding VTE outcomes (Weinberger and Cipolle, 2016).

Safety Guidelines

- Select the appropriate-size SCD or MCD stocking and ensure that the patient follows all recommendations for keeping the device on correctly (Tamowicz et al., 2019). The wrong size or constriction around an extremity can impair circulation.
- Contraindications for SCDs, MCDs, or compression stockings include advanced leg ischemia, skin or tissue necrosis or local skin infections, massive edema of the lower limbs or pulmonary edema due to congestive heart failure, extreme cases of lower limb distortions, acute DVT, and the presence of malignant neoplasms within the limbs (Tamowicz et al., 2019).

Delegation

The skill of applying and maintaining graduated stockings and SCDs or MCDs may be delegated to assistive personnel (AP). The nurse determines the size of the device and assesses the patient's lower extremities for any signs and symptoms of a DVT or impaired circulation. Direct the AP to:

- Remove the SCD sleeves (exception: MCDs may remain on) before allowing a patient to get out of bed. Do not allow a patient with MCD to ambulate without assistance.
- Report if a patient's calf appears larger than the other or is red or hot, and/or if the patient reports calf pain.
- Report if there is redness, itching, or irritation on the legs (signs of allergic reactions to elastic).
- Report if the patient is routinely removing the device from the legs.

Equipment

- Tape measure
- Graduated compression stockings or Velcro compression device sleeves; SCD/MCD insufflator with air hoses attached
- Compression device pump
- *Option:* cotton stockinette with MCD
- Hygiene supplies and clean gloves (optional)

STEP	RATIONALE
1 Perform preprocedure protocol.	

Assessment

• Review electronic health record (EHR) for order for SCDs/MCDs or graduated compression stocking. Order should include whether single or bilateral, whether knee or thigh length, duration, and criteria for discontinuing.	Order typically required, may not include all elements. Order may be part of an evidence-based protocol in some cases (see agency policy).
• Review EHR for risk factors for developing DVT.	Common risk factors for DVT include conditions that influence the Virchow triad: hypercoagulability (e.g., inherited clotting disorders, fever, dehydration, pregnancy), venous wall abnormalities (e.g., orthopedic surgery, varicose veins), and blood flow stasis (e.g., immobility after serious injury, illness, or long-term travel; obesity).
• An option is to use the Wells score to determine patient's risk for a DVT (Box 66.1)	Wells score is an objective and widely used measure for determining a patient's risk for a DVT (Wells et al., 1998; Modi et al., 2016) .
• Perform hand hygiene. Apply clean gloves if lesions or wounds on extremities. Assess for contraindications for use of elastic stockings or compression devices:	
a Dermatitis or open skin lesions on area to be covered by stockings/sleeves	Device can increase irritation.

Continued

BOX 66.1 Wells Score

Parameter	Score[a]
Active cancer (patient receiving treatment for cancer within previous 6 months or currently receiving palliative treatment)	1
Paralysis, paresis, or recent plaster immobilization of lower extremities	1
Recently bedridden for 3 days or more, or major surgery within previous 12 weeks requiring general or regional anesthesia	1
Localized tenderness along distribution of the deep vein system	1
Entire leg swollen	1
Calf swelling at least 3 cm (1.2 inches) more when compared with asymptomatic leg	1
Pitting edema localized to symptomatic leg	1
Collateral superficial veins	1
Previously documented DVT	1
Alternative diagnosis as likely or greater than that of DVT	-2

[a] Wells scoring system for DVT: -2 to 0, low probability; 1 to 2, moderate probability; 3 to 8, high probability.

DVT, deep vein thrombosis.

From Modi S et al: Wells criteria for DVT is a reliable clinical tool to assess the risk of deep venous thrombosis in trauma patients. *World J Emerg Surg.* 11: 24, 2016. Published online 2016 Jun 8. https://doi.org/10.1186/s13017-016-0078-1.

STEP	RATIONALE
b Recent skin graft to lower leg	Compression could cause graft to fail.
c Decreased arterial circulation in lower extremities as evidenced by cyanotic, cool extremities, and/or gangrenous conditions affecting the lower limb(s)	Further compression from a device will more seriously impair circulation.
d Presence of signs or symptoms of a DVT	(Manipulation could cause a clot in vein within the leg to dislodge.)

STEP	RATIONALE
• Assess condition of patient's skin and circulation to the legs. Measure circumference of extremity. Palpate pedal pulses, note any palpable veins, and inspect skin over lower extremities for edema, skin discoloration, warmth, presence of lesions. *If a DVT is suspected, keep patient calm and quiet in bed and notify the health care provider*	Signs of a DVT usually occur on one side of the body at a time, including swelling in the affected leg or arm; warm, cyanotic skin; and pain or tenderness in the affected extremity. A patient may report cramping or soreness. Increased activity/stimulation could dislodge clot in extremity.
• Ask patient to describe history of allergies: known type(s) of allergies and normal allergic reaction(s).	Prevents exposure to allergic agent and allows anticipation of possible reactions. Elastic may cause localized skin reactions.
• Remove and discard gloves (if worn). Perform hand hygiene.	

Implementation

STEP	RATIONALE
1 Perform hand hygiene. Assist patient to supine position in bed. Bathe patient's legs as needed. Dry thoroughly. Perform hand hygiene.	Clean, dry extremity makes it easier to apply stockings. Reduces transmission of microorganisms.
2 Apply graduated compression stocking:	
a Use tape measure to measure patient's leg to determine proper elastic stocking size (follow package directions).	Necessary for proper and safe compression.
b Turn elastic stocking inside out: Place one hand into stocking, holding heel of stocking. Take other hand and pull stocking inside out until reaching the heel (Fig. 66.1).	Allows for easier stocking application.

Continued

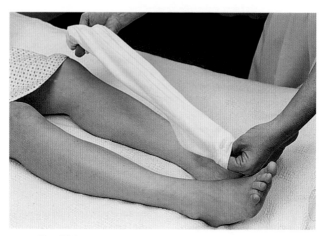

Fig. 66.1 Turn stocking inside out, hold heel, and pull through.

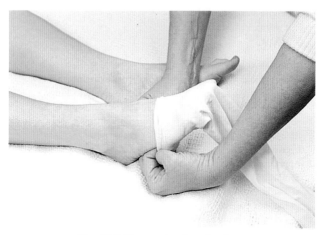

Fig. 66.2 Place toes into foot of stocking.

STEP	RATIONALE
c Place patient's toes into foot of elastic stocking up to the heel, making sure that stocking is smooth (Fig. 66.2).	Wrinkles can constrict circulation.

STEP	RATIONALE
d Slide remaining portion of stocking over patient's foot, making sure that toes are covered. Make sure that foot fits into toe and heel position of stocking. Stocking will now be right side out (Fig. 66.3).	Proper fit ensures proper compression.
e Slide stocking up over patient's calf until sock is completely extended. Ensure that stocking is smooth and that no ridges or wrinkles are present (Fig. 66.4).	
f Instruct patient to refrain from rolling stockings partially down, to avoid wrinkles, to avoid crossing legs, and to elevate legs while sitting.	

Continued

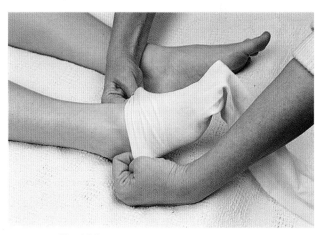

Fig. 66.3 Slide remaining part of stocking over foot.

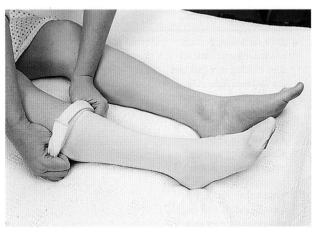

Fig. 66.4 Slide sock up leg until completely extended.

STEP	RATIONALE
3 Apply SCD sleeve(s):	
a Select appropriate-size SCD (see package directions). Remove SCD sleeves from plastic cover; unfold and flatten onto bed.	Necessary for proper and safe compression.
b Arrange SCD sleeve under patient's leg according to leg position indicated on inner lining of sleeve.	
c Place patient's leg on SCD sleeve. Back of ankle should line up with ankle marking on inner lining of sleeve.	Proper placement ensures proper compression.
d For thigh length, position back of knee with popliteal opening on inner sleeve.	A full length sleeve must be properly positioned to cover upper and lower extremity.

STEP	RATIONALE
e Wrap SCD sleeve securely around patient's leg. Check fit of SCD sleeve by placing two fingers between patient's leg and sleeve (Fig. 66.5).	If sleeve is too tight, inflation may compromise circulation.
f Attach SCD sleeve connector to plug on mechanical unit. Arrows on connector line up with arrows on plug from mechanical unit.	
g Turn mechanical unit on. Green light indicates that unit is functioning. Monitor functioning SCD through one full cycle of inflation and deflation.	Ensures proper function of device.

Continued

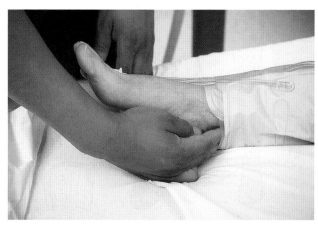

Fig. 66.5 Check fit of sequential compression device sleeve.

STEP	RATIONALE
4 Apply MCD sleeve:	
a Select appropriate-size MCD (see package directions). Example shown is knee-high length. A cotton stockinette is provided along with the calf sleeves. Apply over patient's calves.	Reduces skin irritation
b Wrap the sleeve smoothly around the patient's calf and fasten it beginning at the top, moving toward the bottom.	Avoids wrinkles that are constricting.
c Place two fingers between patient's calf and sleeve to be sure it is snug but not too tight (Fig. 66.6)	If sleeve is too tight, inflation may compromise circulation.

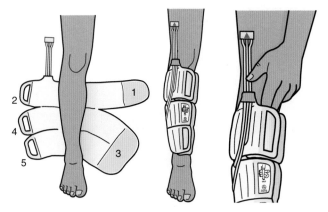

Fig. 66.6 Applying mechanical compression device sleeve to patient calf.

STEP	RATIONALE
d In example shown the device has two identical extension tubes. Use either end of the extension tube to connect to the sleeve or device pump.	
(1) Connect one end of the extension tube to the sleeve connector. The white arrows should be pointed toward each other.	
(2) Connect the other end of the extension tube to the device pump. The white arrow should be facing up.	
e Press the power switch located at the back of the device to ON position. After turning the device on, a configuration setup screen is shown on the liquid crystal display (LCD) screen and the sleeves should immediately start to inflate, from the bottom to the top.	Inflation sequence Is initiated.
f Wait 60 seconds for the automatic operation of the device. The device automatically identifies which sleeves are connected, selects the suitable treatment mode, and displays information on the main LCD screen.	Ensures proper functioning of device.

Continued

STEP	RATIONALE
5 Position patient comfortably. When wearing MCD sleeves a patient may walk with device in place (Fig. 66.7).	Advantage of MCD is patient can initiate early mobility and the design of the device limits risk of falling.

CLINICAL JUDGMENT *Caution patient not to exit bed and walk with SCDs in place. Have patient call for assistance. However, the patient may walk with an MCD in place. Continue any fall prevention measures based on patient risk (Skill 28).*

6 Perform postprocedure protocol.
7 Evaluate patient response:

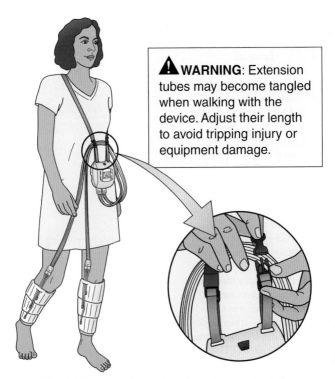

WARNING: Extension tubes may become tangled when walking with the device. Adjust their length to avoid tripping injury or equipment damage.

Fig. 66.7 Patient walking with mechanical compression device.

STEP	RATIONALE
a Remove compression stockings or SCD/MCD sleeves every 8 h or when patient reports discomfort. During this time inspect skin for irritation or breakdown; evaluate patient's comfort level; assess for tingling feeling in extremities; and measure pulses in extremities and circumference of extremity.	Evaluates patient tolerance and determines skin condition and status of circulation.

Recording and Reporting

- Record the condition of lower extremities before application and during routine removal of device, application and size of stockings/SCDs/MCDs.
- Document evaluation of patient learning.
- Report to health care provider or nurse in charge any signs that may indicate formation of DVT.

UNEXPECTED OUTCOMES	RELATED INTERVENTIONS
1 Patient reports discomfort from sleeve and develops edema of extremity.	• Resize stocking or compression device • Keep edematous extremity elevated when possible
2 Patient removes sleeve without informing nurse.	• Determine source of discomfort (e.g., pain, sweating under sleeve). • Explain implications of device not remaining in place.

Sterile Gloving

Sterile gloves help prevent the transmission of pathogens by direct and indirect contact with contaminated surfaces or substances. Nurses apply sterile gloves before performing sterile procedures such as inserting urinary catheters, assisting with surgical procedures, or applying sterile dressings. Sterile gloves do not replace hand hygiene.

It is important to verify whether the patient or health care providers have a latex allergy. When allergies are present, select latex-free gloves. Box 67.1 lists risk factors for a latex allergy. Latex proteins enter the body through skin or mucous membranes, intravascularly, or via inhalation. Reactions to latex range from mild to severe (Box 67.2).

Gloves must be the proper size. The gloves should not stretch so tightly over the fingers that they can tear easily, but need to be tight enough that objects can be picked up easily. Sterile gloves are available in various sizes (e.g., 6, 6½, 7). They are also available in "one size fits all" or "small," "medium," and "large."

Safety Guidelines

- Repeated exposure to latex can lead to a latex allergy, in which case latex-free gloves would need to be used.

Delegation

Assisting with skills that include the application and removal of sterile gloves may be delegated to assistive personnel (AP). However, most procedures that require the use of sterile gloves cannot be delegated to AP. Instruct the AP about:

- The reason for using sterile gloves for a specific procedure.

Equipment

- Package of proper-size sterile gloves, latex or synthetic nonlatex. If patient has a latex allergy, ensure that gloves are latex free and powder free.

BOX 67.1 Conditions That Contribute to Risk for Latex Allergy

- Spina bifida
- Multiple surgeries or medical procedures
- High latex exposure: health care workers, housekeepers, food handlers, tire manufacturers, workers in industries that use gloves routinely
- Rubber industry workers
- Personal or family history of allergies
- Allergy to avocados, bananas, chestnuts, kiwis, and passion fruit. There is a connection between an allergy to latex and allergy to these foods. . These foods have some of the identical allergens that are found in latex.

From Mayo Clinic: *Diseases and conditions: latex allergy*: 2020, http://www.mayoclinic.org/diseases-conditions/latex-allergy/basics/risk-factors/con-20024233. Accessed September 2022.

BOX 67.2 Levels of Latex Reactions (in Order of Severity)

1. *Irritant dermatitis*: Skin reaction isolated to the area of contact
   a. Acute reaction: Red, dry, itchy, and irritated
   b. Chronic reaction: Dry, thick skin; crusting and possibly cracking or peeling, resulting in open sores
2. *Type IV delayed hypersensitivity*: Allergic reaction to chemicals used in latex processing
   a. Acute reaction: Dry, red, rash, itchy, hives, small blisters
   b. Chronic reaction Dry, thickened skin; crusting; scabbing sores; vesicles; peeling (appears 4 to 96 h after exposure)
3. *Type I immediate hypersensitivity*: Could be life-threatening; reactions can start as soon as 2 to 3 minutes after contact up to several hours
   a. Acute reaction: Hives, swelling, runny nose, nausea, abdominal cramps, dizziness, low blood pressure, bronchospasm, anaphylaxis (shock)

From Centers for Disease Control and Prevention. *Frequently asked questions. Contact dermatitis & latex allergy*, 2016, https://www.cdc.gov/oralhealth/infectioncontrol/faqs/latex.html. Acessed September 2022.

STEP	RATIONALE
1 Perform preprocedure protocol.	

Assessment

- Consider the type of procedure to be performed and consult agency policy on use of sterile gloves. In some institutions double gloving is recommended for the operating room (AlJehani, 2018). | Ensures proper use of sterile gloves when needed. Evidence supports the use of double gloving and double gloving with an indicator glove system to decrease the risk of percutaneous injury; this provides an effective barrier to bloodborne pathogen exposure (Association of periOperative Registered Nurses [AORN], 2020).

- Assess patient's risk for infection (e.g., preexisting condition and size or extent of area being treated). | Knowledge of risk directs you to follow added precautions (e.g., use of additional protective barriers) if necessary.

- Select correct size and type of gloves and examine glove package to determine if it is dry and intact with no water stains. | Torn or wet package is considered contaminated. Signs of water stains on package indicate previous contamination by water.

- Inspect condition of your hands for cuts, hangnails, open lesions, or abrasions. In some settings covering any open lesion with a sterile, impervious transparent dressing is permitted (check agency policy). In some cases presence of such lesions may prevent you from participating in a procedure. | Cuts, abrasions, and hangnails tend to ooze serum, which possibly contains pathogens. Breaks in skin integrity permit microorganisms to enter, increasing the risk for infection for both patient and nurse (AORN, 2020).

STEP	RATIONALE
• Assess patient for the following risk factors before applying latex gloves:	Risk factors determine level of patient's risk for latex allergy.
a Previous reaction to the following items within hours of exposure: adhesive tape, dental or face mask, golf club grip, ostomy bag, rubber band, balloon, bandage, elastic underwear, intravenous (IV) tubing, rubber gloves, condom	Items are known to lead to latex allergy.
b Personal history of asthma, contact dermatitis, eczema, urticaria, rhinitis	Patients with a history of these conditions are at higher risk of having a reaction to latex.
c History of food allergies, especially avocado, banana, peach, chestnut, raw potato, kiwi, tomato, papaya	Patients with a history of food allergies are at higher risk of developing a latex reaction.
d Previous history of adverse reactions during surgery or dental procedure	Previous history suggests allergic response.
e Previous reaction to latex product	Previous reaction suggests allergic response.

CLINICAL JUDGMENT *Synthetic nonlatex gloves (latex free/powder free) must be used when patients are at risk for, or if nurse has sensitivity or allergy to, latex.*

Implementation

1 Apply sterile gloves.

a Perform thorough hand hygiene. Place glove package near work area.	Hand hygiene reduces number of bacteria on skin surfaces and transmission of infection. Proximity to work area ensures availability before procedure.
b Remove outer glove package wrapper by carefully separating and peeling apart sides (Fig. 67.1).	Proper removal prevents inner glove package from accidentally opening and touching contaminated objects.

Continued

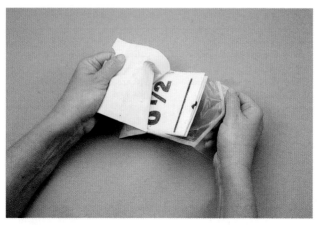

Fig. 67.1 Open outer glove package wrapper.

STEP	RATIONALE
c Grasp inner package and lay on clean, dry, flat surface at waist level. Open package, keeping gloves on inside surface of wrapper (Fig. 67.2).	Sterile object held below waist is contaminated. Inner surface of glove package is sterile.
d Identify right and left glove. Each glove has a cuff approximately 5 cm (2 inches) wide. Glove dominant hand first.	Proper identification of gloves prevents contamination by improper fit. Gloving of dominant hand first improves dexterity.
e With thumb and first two fingers of nondominant hand, grasp glove for dominant hand by touching only inside surface of cuff.	Inner edge of cuff will lie against skin and thus is not sterile.
f Carefully pull glove over dominant hand, leaving a cuff and being sure that cuff does not roll up wrist. Be sure that thumb and fingers are in proper spaces (Fig. 67.3).	If outer surface of glove touches hand or wrist, it is contaminated.

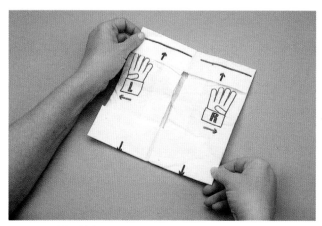

Fig. 67.2 Open inner glove package on work surface.

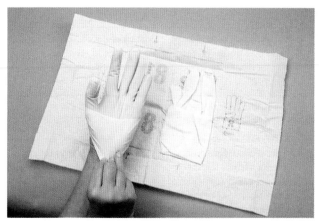

Fig. 67.3 Pick up glove for dominant hand, insert fingers, and pull glove completely over dominant hand (example is for left-handed person).

STEP	RATIONALE
g With gloved dominant hand, slip fingers underneath cuff of second glove (Fig. 67.4).	Cuff protects gloved fingers. Sterile touching sterile prevents glove contamination.

Continued

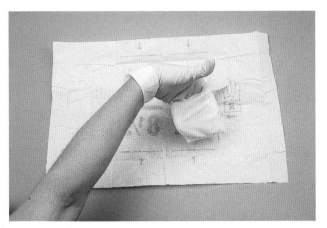

Fig. 67.4 Pick up glove for nondominant hand.

STEP	RATIONALE
h Carefully pull second glove over fingers of nondominant hand (Fig. 67.5).	Contact of gloved hand with exposed hand results in contamination.

CLINICAL JUDGMENT *Do not allow fingers and thumb of gloved dominant hand to touch any part of exposed nondominant hand. Keep thumb of dominant hand abducted back.*

i After second glove is on, interlock hands together and hold away from body above waist level until beginning procedure (Fig. 67.6).	Ensures smooth fit over fingers and prevents contamination.

2 Perform ordered procedure.
3 Remove gloves:

a Grasp outside of one cuff with other gloved hand; avoid touching wrist.	Procedure minimizes contamination of underlying skin.
b Pull glove off, turning it inside out, and place it in gloved hand.	Outside of glove does not touch skin surface.

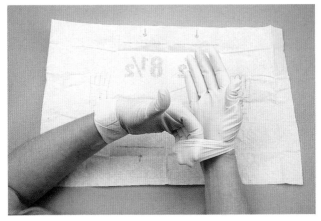

Fig. 67.5 Pull second glove over nondominant hand.

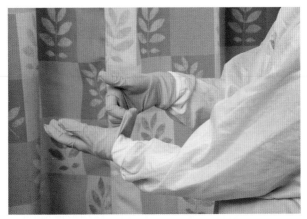

Fig. 67.6 Carefully remove first glove by turning it inside out.

STEP	RATIONALE
c Take fingers of bare hand and tuck inside remaining glove cuff (Fig. 67.7). Peel glove off inside out and over previously removed glove. Discard both gloves in receptacle.	Fingers do not touch contaminated glove surface.

Continued

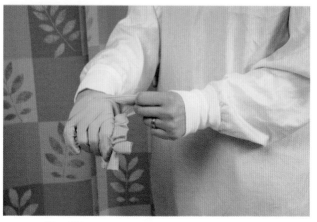

Fig. 67.7 Remove second glove by turning it inside out.

STEP	RATIONALE
d Perform thorough hand hygiene.	Hand hygiene protects health care worker from contamination resulting from any unseen tears or pinholes in gloves; also removes powder from hands to prevent skin irritation.
4 Perform postprocedure protocol.	
5 Evaluate patient response:	
a Assess patient for signs of infection, focusing on area treated.	Improper technique contributes to development of an infection.
b Assess patient for signs of latex allergy.	Assessment establishes baseline for patient's reaction to latex.

Recording and Reporting

- It is not necessary to record glove application. Record specific procedure performed, patient's response, and patient status.
- In the event of a latex allergy reaction, record patient's response on flow sheet or in nurses' notes in electronic health record or chart. Note type of response and patient's reaction to emergency treatment.
- In the event of a patient latex allergy, report the patient response and reaction to healthcare provider.

UNEXPECTED OUTCOMES	RELATED INTERVENTIONS
1 Patient develops localized signs of infection (e.g., urine becomes cloudy or odorous; wound becomes painful, edematous, or reddened with purulent drainage).	• Contact health care provider and implement appropriate treatments as ordered.
2 Patient develops systemic signs of infection (e.g., fever, malaise, increased white blood cell count).	• Contact health care provider and implement appropriate treatments as ordered.
3 Patient develops allergic reaction to latex (see Box 67.2).	• Immediately remove source of latex. • Bring emergency equipment to bedside. Have epinephrine injection ready for administration, and be prepared to initiate IV fluids and oxygen.

Sterile Field Preparation

When performing sterile aseptic procedures, a sterile work area in which objects can be handled with minimal risk for contamination is needed. A sterile field provides a sterile surface for placement of sterile equipment. Sterile drapes establish a sterile field around a treatment site such as a surgical incision, venipuncture site, or site for introduction of an indwelling urinary catheter. Sterile drapes also provide a work surface for placing sterile supplies and manipulating items with sterile gloves. After a sterile disposable kit is opened, the inside surface of the cover or container can be used as a sterile field.

Safety Guidelines

- Once you create a sterile field, you are responsible for performing the procedure and making sure that the field is not contaminated.

Delegation

Surgical technicians may prepare a sterile field (see agency policy); however, assistive personnel (AP) cannot. Direct the AP to:

- Help with patient positioning and obtaining any necessary supplies.

Collaboration

- All members of the surgical team remain mindful to ensure that all maintain a sterile field.

Equipment

- Sterile pack (commercial or institution wrapped)
- Sterile drape or kit that is to be used as a sterile field
- Sterile gloves (optional)
- Sterile solution and equipment specific to a procedure
- Waist-high table/countertop surface
- Appropriate personal protective equipment (PPE): gown, mask, cap, protective eyewear (see agency policy)

STEP	RATIONALE
1 Perform preprocedure protocol for the ordered procedure.	
Assessment	
• Ask patient to describe history of allergies and normal allergic reaction(s). When allergies are present, patient should wear an allergy bracelet. Check patient's allergy wristband. Inquire about latex allergies.	A review may reveal latex allergies and determine the need to use latex-free supplies.
• Verify in agency policy and procedure manual that procedure requires surgical aseptic technique.	Some procedures require medical rather than surgical aseptic technique.
• Assess patient's comfort, positioning, oxygen requirements, and elimination needs before preparing for procedure.	Certain procedures requiring a sterile field may last a long time. Anticipates patient's needs so patient can relax and avoid any unnecessary movement that might disrupt procedure.
• Instruct patient and family caregiver not to touch work surface or equipment during procedure.	Prevents contamination of sterile field.
• Check sterile package integrity for punctures, tears, discoloration, moisture, or any other signs of contamination. Check expiration date if applicable. If using commercially packaged supplies or those prepared by agency, check for sterilization indicator (marker that changes color when exposed to heat or steam).	Inspection of packaging ensures that only sterile items are presented to sterile field (Association of periOperative Registered Nurses [AORN], 2020).

Continued

STEP	RATIONALE
• Anticipate number and variety of supplies needed for procedure.	

Implementation

STEP	RATIONALE
1 Complete all other nursing interventions (e.g., medication administration, suctioning patient) before beginning procedure.	Prepare sterile field as close as possible to time of use to reduce potential for contamination (AORN, 2020).
2 Explain to patient importance of keeping work area sterile. If any health instruction is necessary do it at this time.	Explanation ensures patient's ability to cooperate with procedure. Completing instruction before beginning procedure avoids talking over sterile field.
3 Perform hand hygiene.	Reduces transmission of microorganisms.
4 Apply PPE as needed (see Skill 36).	PPE controls spread of airborne microorganisms.
5 Select a clean, flat, dry work surface above waist level.	A dry work surface is needed for a sterile field. A sterile object placed below a person's waist is considered contaminated.
6 Prepare sterile work surface:	
a Sterile commercial kit or pack containing sterile items.	
(1) Place sterile kit or pack on a dry and clean work surface.	Sterile object placed above waist is considered sterile.
(2) Open outside cover (Fig. 68.1) and remove sterile package from dust cover. Place on work surface.	Inner kit remains sterile.

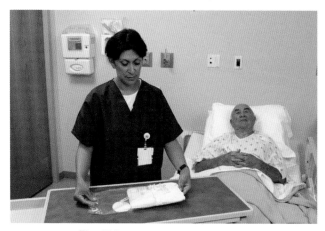

Fig. 68.1 Open outside cover of sterile kit.

STEP	RATIONALE
(3) Grasp outer surface of tip of outermost flap.	Outer surface of package is not sterile. There is a 2.5-cm (1-inch) border around any sterile drape or wrap that is considered contaminated and can be touched with clean fingers.
(4) Open outermost flap away from body, keeping arm outstretched and away from sterile field (Fig. 68.2).	Reaching over sterile field contaminates it.
(5) Grasp outside surface of edge of first side flap.	Outer border is considered unsterile.
(6) Open side flap, pulling to side, allowing it to lie flat on table surface. Keep arm to side and away from sterile surface (Fig. 68.3).	Drape or wrapper should lie flat so it does not accidentally rise up and contaminate inner surface or sterile contents.

Continued

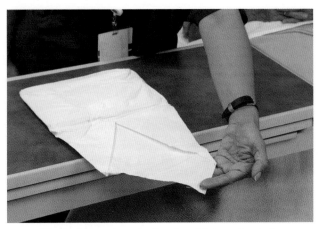

Fig. 68.2 Open outermost flap of sterile kit away from body.

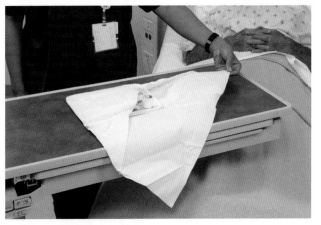

Fig. 68.3 Open first side flap, pulling to side.

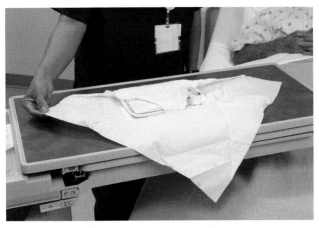

Fig. 68.4 Open second side flap, pulling to side.

STEP	RATIONALE
(7) Repeat Step (6) for second side flap (Fig. 68.4).	
(8) Grasp outside border of last and innermost flap (Fig. 68.5). Stand away from sterile package and pull flap back, allowing it to fall flat on table. Kit is ready to be used.	Outer border is considered unsterile. Never reach over a sterile field.
b Open sterile linen-wrapped package.	
(1) Place package on clean, dry, flat work surface above waist level.	Sterile items placed below waist level are considered contaminated.

Continued

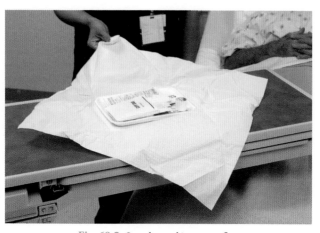

Fig. 68.5 Open last and innermost flap.

STEP	RATIONALE
(2) Remove sterilization tape seal and unwrap both layers following same steps (see Steps 6a[2] through 6a[8]) as for sterile kit.	Linen-wrapped items have two layers. The first is a dust cover. The second layer must be opened to view chemical indicator.
(3) Use opened package wrapper as sterile field.	Inner surface of wrapper is considered sterile.
c Prepare sterile drape.	
(1) Place pack containing sterile drape on flat, dry surface and open as described (see Steps 6a[2] through 6a[8]) for sterile package.	Packaged drape remains sterile.

STEP	RATIONALE
(2) Apply sterile gloves (*optional, see agency policy*). The outer 2.5-cm (1-inch) border of drape can be touched without wearing gloves.	Sterile object remains sterile only when touched by another sterile object. Gloves are not necessary as long as fingers grasp the 2.5-cm (1-inch) unsterile border of the drape.
(3) Using fingertips of one hand, pick up folded top edge of drape along 2.5-cm (1-inch) border. Gently lift drape up from its wrapper without touching any object. Discard wrapper with other hand.	If sterile object touches any nonsterile object, it becomes contaminated.
(4) With other hand, grasp an adjacent corner of drape and hold it straight up and away from body. Allow drape to unfold, keeping it above waist and work surface and away from body (Fig. 68.6). (Carefully discard wrapper with other hand.)	An object held below a person's waist or above chest is contaminated. Drape can now be placed properly with two hands.
(5) Holding drape, position bottom half over top half of intended work surface (Fig. 68.7).	Proper positioning prevents nurse from reaching over sterile field.

Continued

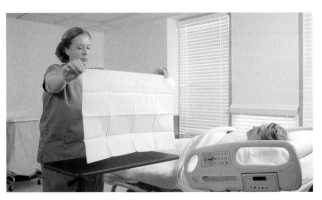

Fig. 68.6 Grasp corners of sterile drape, then hold up and away from body. (From Elsevier: *Clinical skills: essentials collection*, St Louis, 2021, Mosby.)

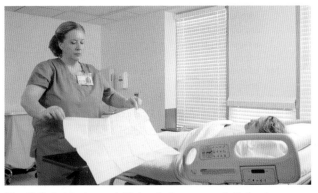

Fig. 68.7 Position bottom half of sterile drape over top half of work space. (From Elsevier: *Clinical skills: essentials collection*, St Louis, 2021, Mosby.)

STEP	RATIONALE
(6) Allow top half of drape to drop over bottom half of work surface (Fig. 68.8).	Proper positioning creates flat, sterile work surface for placement of sterile supplies.
7 Add sterile items to sterile field:	

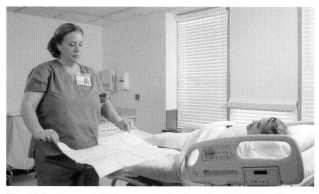

Fig. 68.8 Allow top half of drape to be placed over bottom half of work surface. (From Elsevier: *Clinical skills: essentials collection*, St Louis, 2021, Mosby.)

STEP	RATIONALE
a Open sterile item (following package directions) while holding outside wrapper in nondominant hand.	Use of nondominant hand frees dominant hand for unwrapping outer wrapper
b Carefully peel wrapper over nondominant hand.	Item remains sterile. Inner surface of wrapper covers hand, keeping it sterile.
c Ensure that the wrapper does not fall down onto the sterile field. Place the item onto the field at an angle (Fig. 68.9). **Do not hold arms over sterile field.**	Secured wrapper edges prevent flipping wrapper and contaminating contents of sterile field (AORN, 2020).

CLINICAL JUDGMENT *Do not flip or toss objects onto sterile field.*

d Dispose of outer wrapper.	Disposal prevents accidental contamination of sterile field.

Continued

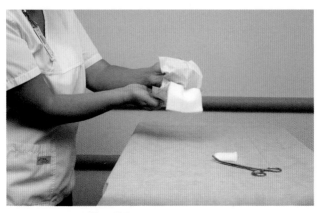

Fig. 68.9 Add items to sterile field.

STEP	RATIONALE
8 Pour sterile solutions:	
a Verify contents and expiration date of solution.	Verification ensures proper solution and sterility of contents.
b Place receptacle for solution near table/work surface edge. Sterile kits have cups or plastic molded sections into which fluids can be poured.	Proper placement prevents reaching over sterile field while pouring solution.
c Remove sterile seal and cap from bottle in upward motion.	Upward movement prevents contamination of bottle lip.
d With solution bottle held away from field and bottle lip 2.5 to 5 cm (1 to 2 inches) above inside of sterile receiving container, slowly pour needed amount of solution into container. Hold bottle with label facing palm of hand.	Edge and outside of bottle are considered contaminated. Slow pouring prevents splashing. Sterility of contents cannot be ensured if cap is replaced. Prevents label from becoming wet and illegible.

STEP	RATIONALE

CLINICAL JUDGMENT *When liquids permeate sterile field or barrier, it is called strikethrough, which results in contamination of the sterile field.*

9 Perform postprocedure protocol.

10 Evaluate patient response:

   a Observe for breaks in sterile field (contaminated object touches field).   A break in sterile field requires setup of new sterile field.

Recording and Reporting

▪ No recording or reporting is required for this set of skills.

UNEXPECTED OUTCOMES	RELATED INTERVENTIONS
1 Sterile field comes in contact with contaminated object, or liquid splatters onto drape, causing strikethrough.	• Discontinue field preparation and start over with new equipment.
2 Sterile item falls off sterile field.	• As long as field does not become contaminated, open another package containing new sterile item and add to field. If field becomes contaminated, a new sterile field should be established.

Subcutaneous Injections

Subcutaneous injections deposit medication into the loose connective tissue underlying the dermis (Fig. 69.1). Because subcutaneous tissue does not contain as many blood vessels as muscles, medications are absorbed more slowly than with intramuscular injections. Physical exercise or application of hot or cold compresses influences the rate of drug absorption by altering local blood flow to tissues. Any condition that impairs blood flow is a contraindication for subcutaneous injections.

Subcutaneous tissue is sensitive to irritating solutions and large volumes of medications. Only administer small volumes (0.5 to 1.5 mL) of water-soluble medications subcutaneously to adults. Children receive smaller volumes, up to 0.5 mL (Hockenberry et al., 2022).

The best subcutaneous injection sites include the outer aspect of the upper arms, the abdomen from below the costal margins to the iliac crests, and the anterior aspects of the thighs (Fig. 69.2). These areas are easily accessible and are large enough to allow rotating multiple injections within each anatomical location.

A patient's body weight indicates the depth of the subcutaneous layer. Choose a needle length and angle of insertion based on a patient's weight and an estimation of the amount of subcutaneous tissue (Larkin et al., 2018b).

- Use a 25-gauge, ⅝ -inch (16-mm) needle inserted at a 45-degree angle or a ½ -inch (12-mm) needle inserted at a 90-degree angle to administer medications to a normal-size adult.
- Some children require only a ½-inch needle.
- Needle length varies for obese or very thin patients. If 2 inches (5 cm) of tissue can be grasped, insert the needle at a 90-degree angle; if 2.5 cm (1 inch) of tissue can be grasped, insert the needle at a 45-degree angle.
- Research shows that insulin needles that are ⁵⁄₁₆ inch (8 mm) or longer enter the muscles of men and people with a body mass index of 25 or less. Shorter (³⁄₁₆-inch or 4- to 5-mm) needles were associated with less pain, adequate control of blood glucose, and risk of bleeding and bruising (Gorska-Ciebiada et al., 2020). When giving insulin, use needles of 3/16 inch (4–5 mm) administered at a 90-degree angle to reduce pain and achieve adequate control of blood sugars with minimal adverse effects for people of all BMIs, including children (Gorska-Ciebiada et al., 2020; Weinstock, 2022).

Injection pens are a technology that patients can use to self-administer subcutaneous medications (e.g., epinephrine, insulin, or interferon). In many health care settings, nurses administer insulin using pens. Pens are

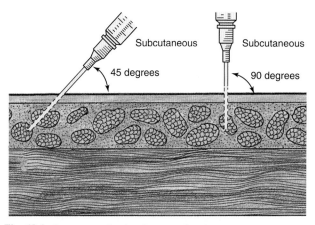

Fig. 69.1 Comparison of angles of insertion for subcutaneous 45- and 90-degree injections.

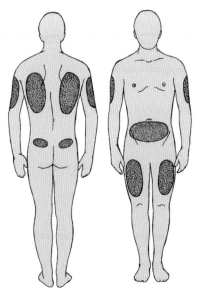

Fig. 69.2 Subcutaneous sites for injections.

convenient and relatively easy for patients to use. The disadvantages of this technology include increased risk for needlestick injury and lack of user knowledge and skill in administration technique (ISMP, 2017).

Safety Guidelines

- Be vigilant during medication administration. Avoid distractions.
- If the patient is receiving a small dose (less than 5 units) of insulin, a pen injector should not be used because there is a 50% chance of dose errors (McCulloch et al.,2020).
  - The timing of insulin injections is critical to correct insulin administration. Health care providers plan insulin injection times based on blood glucose levels and when a patient will eat. Know the peak action and duration of the insulin before you administer.
  - Patients receiving heparin are at risk for bleeding, including bleeding gums, hematemesis, hematuria, or melena.
  Results from coagulation blood tests (e.g., activated partial thromboplastin time and partial thromboplastin time) allow for monitoring of heparin response.

Delegation

The skill of administering subcutaneous injections cannot be delegated to assistive personnel (AP). Direct the AP about:

- Potential medication sides effects and the need to immediately report their occurrence.
- Reporting any change in the patient's condition.

Collaboration

- Diabetes nurse educator and endocrinologist are resources for diabetes management

Equipment

- Proper-size syringe and sharp with engineered sharps injury protection needle
  - Subcutaneous: syringe (1 to 3 mL) or tuberculin syrine
  - Insulin prefilled pen
- Needles
  - Immunizations: 23- to 25-gauge, ⅝-inch needle (Centers for Disease Control and Prevention, 2023)
  - Subcutaneous U-100 insulin: insulin syringe (1 mL) with preattached needle (28 to 31 gauge [⁵⁄₁₆ to ³⁄₁₆ inch])
  - Subcutaneous U-500 insulin: 1 mL tuberculin (TB) syringe with needle (25 to 27 gauge, ½ to ⅝ inch)
- Small gauze pad *(optional)*

- Antiseptic swab
- Medication vial
- Clean gloves
- Medication administration record (MAR) or computer printout
- Puncture-proof container

STEP	RATIONALE
1 Perform preprocedure protocol.	

Assessment

• Check accuracy and completeness of each MAR or computer printout with health care provider's written medication order. Check patient's name, medication name and dosage, route of administration, and time of administration.	The order sheet is the most reliable source and only legal record of medications that patient is to receive. Ensures that patient receives the correct medications (Palese et al., 2019). Transcription errors are a source of medication errors (Zhu and Weingart, 2022).
• Review electronic health record (EHR): assess patient's medical and medication history.	Determines need for medication or possible contraindications for medication administration.
a Conditions contraindicating heparin: cerebral or aortic aneurysm, cerebrovascular hemorrhage, severe hypertension, and blood dyscrasias	Supplements can interact with heparin
b Medications that increase risk of hemorrhage: over-the-counter and herbal supplements (e.g., garlic, ginger, ginkgo, horse chestnut, or feverfew); medications including aspirin, nonsteroidal anti-inflammatory drugs, cephalosporins, antithyroid agents, probenecid, and thrombolytics	Medications combined with heparin increase hemorrhage risk

Continued

STEP	RATIONALE
• Review drug reference information for medication action, purpose, normal dose, side effects, time and peak of onset, and nursing implications.	Allows you to safely administer medication and monitor patient's response to therapy.
• Review EHR for relevant laboratory results (e.g., blood glucose, partial thromboplastin).	Provides baseline for measuring drug response.
• Ask patient to describe history of allergies: known type(s) of allergies and normal allergic reaction(s). Check patient's allergy wristband.	Do not prepare medication if there is known patient allergy.
• Perform hand hygiene. Assess condition of skin for contraindication to subcutaneous injections: circulatory shock or reduced local tissue perfusion. Assess adequacy of adipose tissue.	Reduced tissue perfusion interferes with drug absorption and distribution. Amount of adipose tissue influences needle length selection.
• Assess patient's symptoms before initiating medication therapy.	Provides information to evaluate desired effect of medication.

Implementation

1	Explain to patient signs and symptoms to expect from medications.	Lessens anxiety by helping patient know what to expect, promoting self-care.
2	Prepare medication without interruptions/ distractions. Keep all pages of MARs or computer printouts for one patient together, or look at only one patient's electronic MAR at a time.	Interruptions contribute to medication errors (Palese et al., 2019).

STEP	RATIONALE
3 Perform hand hygiene. Prepare medications for one patient at a time using aseptic technique. See Skill 49. Check label of medication carefully with MAR or computer printout when removing medication from storage and after preparing medication. Check drug expiration date.	Prevents transmission of pathogens. Ensures that medication is sterile. *These are the first and second checks for accuracy* and ensure that correct medication is administered. Dose potency increases or decreases when outdated.
4 Take medication(s) to patient at correct time (see agency policy). Give non–time-critical scheduled medications within a range of 1 to 2 h of scheduled dose (CMS, 2020). During administration, apply seven rights of medication administration.	Hospitals must adopt medication administration policy and procedure for timing of medication administration that considers nature of the prescribed medication, specific clinical application, and patient needs (CMS, 2020; US Department of Health and Human Services, 2020).

CLINICAL JUDGMENT *Timing of insulin injections is critical. A patient must eat immediately after injecting fast-acting insulin. Short-acting insulins begin to work within 30 minutes, so injection needs to be given 30 minutes before eating. Insulin combinations can be taken before a meal to provide a stable level of insulin for some time after the meal (ADA, 2022).*

5 Identify patient using at least two identifiers (e.g., name and birthday or name and medical record number) according to agency policy. Compare identifiers with information on patient's MAR or medical record.	Ensures correct patient. Complies with The Joint Commission standards and improves patient safety (TJC, 2023). Some agencies use a barcode system for patient identification.

Continued

STEP	RATIONALE
6 At patient's bedside again compare MAR or computer printout with names of medications on medication labels and patient name. Confirm whether patient has allergies.	*This is the third check for accuracy* and ensures that patient receives correct medication. Confirms patient's allergy history.
7 Perform hand hygiene and apply clean gloves. Keep sheet or gown draped over body parts not requiring exposure.	Reduces transmission of infection. Respects dignity of patient while exposing injection area.
8 Position patient comfortably for site assessment. Select appropriate injection site (see Fig. 69.2). Inspect skin surface over sites for bruises, inflammation, or edema. Do not use an area that is bruised or has signs associated with infection.	Injection sites are free of abnormalities that interfere with drug absorption. Sites used repeatedly become hardened from lipohypertrophy (increased growth in fatty tissue).

CLINICAL JUDGMENT *Applying ice to an injection site for 1 minute before the injection may decrease a patient's perception of pain (Hockenberry et al., 2019).*

9 Palpate sites. Avoid masses or areas of tenderness. Ensure that needle is correct size by grasping skinfold at site with thumb and forefinger. Measure fold from top to bottom. Make sure that needle is one-half length of fold.	Subcutaneous injections can mistakenly be given in muscle, especially in abdomen and thigh sites. Appropriate size of needle is needed to reach subcutaneous tissue (Drutz, 2020).
a When administering insulin or heparin, use abdominal injection sites first, followed by thigh injection site.	Risk for bruising is not affected by site.

STEP	RATIONALE
b When administering low-molecular-weight heparin, choose site on right or left side of abdomen, at least 5 cm (2 inches) away from umbilicus.	Decreases pain and bruising at injection site.
c Rotate insulin site within an anatomical area (e.g., abdomen) and systematically rotate sites within that area.	Rotating injection sites within same anatomical site maintains consistency in day-to-day insulin absorption.
10 Assist patient into comfortable position. Have patient relax arm, leg, or abdomen, depending on site selection.	Relaxation of site minimizes discomfort.
11 Relocate site using anatomical landmarks.	Injection into correct anatomical site prevents injury to nerves, bone, and blood vessels.
12 Clean site with antiseptic swab. Apply swab at center of site and rotate outward in circular direction for about 5 cm (2 inches) (Fig. 69.3)	Mechanical action of swab removes secretions containing microorganisms.
13 Hold swab or gauze between third and fourth fingers of nondominant hand.	Swab or gauze remains readily accessible for use when withdrawing needle after the injection.
14 Remove needle cap or protective sheath by pulling it straight off.	Preventing needle from touching sides of cap prevents contamination.
15 Hold syringe/injection pen between thumb and forefinger of dominant hand; hold as if holding a dart.	Quick, smooth injection requires proper manipulation of syringe/pen parts.

Continued

Fig. 69.3 Cleansing
injection site using
circular motion with
swab.

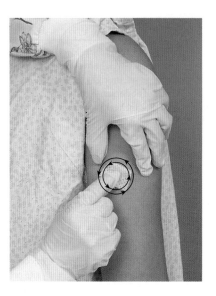

STEP	RATIONALE
16 Administer injection (via syringe):	
a For average-size patient, hold skin across injection site or pinch skin with nondominant hand.	Needle penetrates tight skin more easily than loose skin. Pinching elevates subcutaneous tissue and desensitizes area.
b Inject needle quickly and firmly at 45- to 90-degree angle (Fig. 69.4). Release skin if pinched. *Option:* When giving heparin, continue to pinch skin while injecting medicine	Quick, firm insertion minimizes discomfort. (Injecting medication into compressed tissue irritates nerve fibers.) Correct angle prevents accidental injection into muscle.
c For a patient with obesity, pinch skin at site and inject needle at 90-degree angle below tissue fold.	Obese patients have fatty layer of tissue above subcutaneous layer.

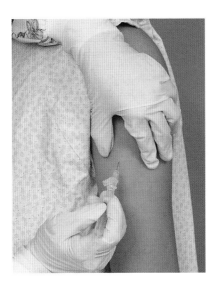

Fig. 69.4 Inserting needle into subcutaneous tissue at 45-degree angle.

STEP	RATIONALE
d After needle enters site, grasp lower end of syringe barrel with nondominant hand to stabilize it. Move dominant hand to end of plunger and slowly inject medication over several seconds. When giving heparin, inject over 30 seconds (Hull et al., 2019). Avoid moving syringe.	Movement of syringe may displace needle and cause discomfort. Slowly injecting medication minimizes discomfort.

CLINICAL JUDGMENT *Aspiration after injecting a subcutaneous medication is not necessary. Piercing a blood vessel in a subcutaneous injection is very rare. Aspiration after injecting heparin and insulin is not recommended (Lilley et al., 2020; CDC, 2022).*

Continued

STEP	RATIONALE
e Withdraw needle quickly while placing antiseptic swab or gauze gently over site.	Supporting tissues around injection site minimizes discomfort during needle withdrawal. Dry gauze may minimize patient discomfort associated with alcohol on nonintact skin.
17 Administer injection (via injection pen):	
a Prime the insulin pen, which removes air bubbles from the needle. The pen must be primed before each injection.	Ensures that the needle is open and working.
b To prime the insulin pen, turn the dosage knob to the 2 units indicator. With the pen pointing up, push the knob all the way. At least one drop of insulin should appear. This step may need to be repeated until a drop appears.	
c Select the dose of insulin that has been prescribed by turning the dosage knob.	A clicking sound is heard when the dial is turned.
d Remove the pen cap. Insert the needle with a quick motion into the skin at a 90-degree angle. The needle should go all the way into the skin.	Safety pen needle has a removable outer cover, but the inner cover is a fixed safety shield that is not removed. The shield will be pushed back, exposing the needle as the injector is pressed against the injection site.
e Slowly push the knob of the pen all the way in to deliver the full dose. Hold the pen at the site for 6 to 10 seconds, and then pull the needle out. Place antiseptic swab or gauze gently over site.	Supporting tissues around injection site minimizes discomfort during needle withdrawal. Dry gauze may minimize patient discomfort associated with alcohol on nonintact skin.

STEP	RATIONALE
f Replace the pen cap and store at room temperature.	Pen can be used again as long as chamber continues to contain medication.
18 Apply gentle pressure to site. *Do not massage site.* (If heparin is given, or if patient is taking an oral anticoagulant, hold alcohol swab or gauze to site for 30 to 60 seconds.)	Aids absorption. Massage can damage underlying tissue. Time interval prevents bleeding at site.
19 Discard uncapped needle or needle enclosed in safety shield and attached syringe in puncture- and leak-proof receptacle.	Prevents injury to patients and health care personnel. Recapping needles increases risk for a needlestick injury (Occupational Safety and Health Administration, nd[a]).
20 In the case of a vaccine, stay/ monitor patient for several minutes and observe for any allergic reactions.	Dyspnea, wheezing, and circulatory collapse are signs of severe anaphylactic reaction.
21 Perform postprocedure protocol.	
22 Evaluate patient response:	
a Return to room in 15 to 30 minutes and ask whether patient feels any acute pain, burning, numbness, or tingling at injection site.	Continued discomfort may indicate injury to underlying bones or nerves.
b Inspect site, noting any bruising or induration. Provide warm compress to site.	Bruising or induration indicates complication associated with injection.
c Observe patient's response to medication at times that correlate with onset, peak, and duration of medication. Review laboratory results as appropriate (e.g., blood glucose, partial thromboplastin).	Adverse effects of parenteral medications develop rapidly. Evaluate effect of medication on basis of onset, peak, and duration of action.

Recording and Reporting

- Immediately after administration, record medication, dose, route, site, time, and date given in EHR or chart. Correctly sign MAR according to agency policy.
- Record any undesirable effects from the injection.
- Record patient teaching, validation of understanding, and patient's response to medication.
- Report any undesirable effects from medication to patient's health care provider.

UNEXPECTED OUTCOMES	RELATED INTERVENTIONS
1 Patient complains of localized pain, numbness, tingling, or burning at injection site.	• Assess injection site; may indicate potential injury to nerve or tissues. • Notify patient's health care provider and do not reuse site.
2 Patient displays adverse reaction with signs of urticaria, eczema, pruritus, wheezing, and dyspnea.	• Monitor patient's heart rate, respirations, blood pressure, and temperature. • Follow agency policy or guidelines for appropriate response to allergic reactions (e.g., administration of antihistamine such as diphenhydramine or epinephrine) and notify patient's health care provider immediately. • Add allergy information to patient's medical record.
3 Hypertrophy of skin develops from repeated subcutaneous injection.	• Do not use same anatomical area for future injections. • Instruct patient not to use site for 6 months.

Suctioning: Open and Closed, for Nasotracheal/ Pharyngeal and Artificial Airways

Suctioning the pharyngeal and tracheal airways is necessary when patients are unable to clear respiratory secretions. When secretions are only in the mouth, oropharyngeal suction (Skill 71) is indicated. Secretions that are not removed from the pharynx are more likely to be aspirated into the lungs, increasing the risk for infection, ventilator-associated pneumonia (VAP), and respiratory failure.

Open vs Closed Suction

Suctioning through the nose into the trachea and pharynx and in established tracheostomies is more commonly performed using open suction. Open suctioning is performed with the suction catheter directly inserted through the nasotrachea or with the disconnection of a patient from a ventilator and the introduction of the suction catheter into the artificial airway. Open suctioning is necessary with ventilated patients who have artificial airways and need to have sputum specimens obtained. Closed suctioning involves use of a suction catheter system that is included in the ventilatory circuit of a patient on a mechanical ventilator. Closed suction used on new artificial airways allows introduction of the suction catheter into the airways without disconnecting a patient from the ventilator. When comparing open versus closed suction, there is a decreased risk of infection for a health care provider from exposure to patient secretions with a closed system (Letchford and Bench, 2018; Urden et al., 2020).

Artificial Airway Suctioning

Endotracheal tubes (ETs) and tracheostomy tubes (TTs) are artificial airways that provide a route for mechanical ventilation, permit easy access for secretion removal, and protect the airway from gross aspiration. Artificial airway suctioning is a sterile procedure, indicated to remove respiratory secretions and maintain optimum ventilation and oxygenation in patients who are unable to remove these secretions independently. The exception is a well-established tracheostomy in which clean, medically aseptic technique can be used.

Endotracheal Tubes

An ET is inserted through the nares (nasotracheal tube) or more commonly through the mouth (oral ET), past the epiglottis and vocal cords and into the trachea (Fig. 70.1). Adult (and some pediatric) sizes of ETs have a cuff molded onto the tube. When the cuff is inflated, it seals the airway around the tube to prevent the aspiration of oral secretions or gastric contents into the lung and/or to obstruct air escaping from mechanical ventilator breaths through the upper airway. Newer ETs also contain a port that can be connected to a syringe or suction for subglottal suctioning (removal of secretions that accumulate above the cuff).

Tracheostomy Tubes

A TT can be temporary or permanent, depending on a patient's condition. It is inserted either surgically or percutaneously directly into the trachea through a small incision made in a patient's neck. Reasons for a TT include the need for prolonged mechanical ventilation, upper airway obstruction secondary to trauma or tumor, or difficulties with airway clearance that can occur in conditions such as spinal cord injury or neuromuscular disease (Urden et al., 2020). Tracheal suctioning has potential complications, including hypoxemia, cardiac dysrhythmias,

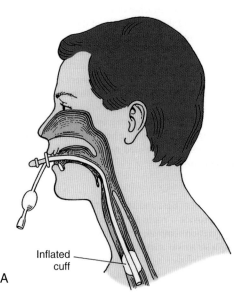

Inflated cuff

A

Fig. 70.1 Endotracheal tube inserted via mouth into trachea with inflated cuff.

changes in blood pressure (either hypertensive or hypotensive), laryngospasm or bronchospasm, pain, infection, or bradycardia. Bradycardia is associated with stimulation of the vagus nerve. Respiratory or cardiac arrest can even occur as a result of tracheal suctioning.

Safety Guidelines

- The length of time that an ET remains in place is controversial. Complications from long-term intubation include laryngeal and tracheal stenosis or a cricoid abscess (Urden et al., 2020). Sources differ on when a patient should be changed from an ET to a TT. The range of recommended length of time to be endotracheally intubated is 7 to 14 days (Urden et al., 2020; Wang et al., 2019).
- VAP is pneumonia that develops more than 48 h after patients have been on mechanical ventilation and is considered a type of ventilator-associated event (Khobodi et al, 2022; Ferrer and Torres, 2018). The use of a care bundle has demonstrated efficacy in reducing VAP (Box 70.1).
- Use caution when suctioning patients with head injuries. The suction procedure causes an elevation in intracranial pressure (ICP) (Harding et al., 2021; Urden et al., 2020). Reduce this risk by providing presuctioning hyperventilation, which results in hypocarbia. This in turn induces vasoconstriction, thereby reducing the risk of elevated ICP.

Delegation

The skill of suctioning directly nasotracheally or newly inserted artificial airways cannot be delegated to assistive personnel (AP). At some agencies, the AP may suction a patient with a well-established tracheostomy that has been determined to be stable. Direct the AP about:

- How to modify suctioning, such as the need for supplemental oxygen or clean versus sterile technique.
- Appropriate suction limits and risks of applying excessive or inadequate suction pressure.
- Reporting any changes in patient's respiratory status, vital signs, unresolved gagging or coughing, level of consciousness, pain, restlessness, and amount and color of secretions.
- Reporting any signs of skin injury around tracheal stoma and peristomal area.

Collaboration

- Respiratory therapist or health care provider may determine any needed alterations to the suctioning procedure, such as no increases in oxygen before suctioning or refraining from changing patient position.

BOX 70.1 Care Bundle to Prevent Ventilator-Associated Pneumonia

- Use proper hand hygiene with universal precautions.
- Elevate the head of the bed to at least 30 degrees, unless contraindicated.
- Perform oral hygiene with chlorhexidine at least twice a day.[a]
- Institute peptic ulcer prophylaxis as ordered.[b]
- Institute venous thromboembolism prophylaxis (anticoagulants, venous sequential compression).
- Provide daily disruption of sedation.
- Encourage early mobilization.
- Initiate enteric feedings earlier rather than later.
- Provide subglottic secretion drainage.
- Maintain artificial airway cuff pressure between 20 and 30 mm Hg.[c]
- Have respiratory therapy change ventilator circuits only when dirty or contaminated and not routinely.[c]

[a] American Association of Critical Care Nurses (AACN): *AACN practice alert: oral care for acutely and critically ill patients*, 2017, https://www.aacn.org/clinical-resources/practice-alerts/oral-care-for-acutely-and-critically-ill-patients. Accessed March, 2021; Alja'afreh M, et al: The effects of oral care protocol on the incidence of ventilator-associated pneumonia in selected intensive care units in Jordan, *Dimensions Critical Care Nurs* 38(1): 5, 2019.
[b] Virk H, Wiersinga J: Current place of probiotics for VAP, *Crit Care* 23:46, 2019.
[c] American Association of Critical Care Nurses (AACN): *AACN practice alert: prevention of ventilator-associated pneumonia in adults*, 2017, https://www.aacn.org/clinical-resources/practice-alerts/ventilator-associated-pneumonia-vap. Accessed April 2020.

- Respiratory therapist is often responsible for suctioning the patient. Communicate frequency of suctioning and patient response to suctioning.
- Collaborate with physical therapy, occupational therapy, or speech therapy. Their interventions may increase the need for you to suction the patient before and during therapies.

Equipment

- Stethoscope
- Pulse oximeter (option for artificial airway suction: end-tidal CO2 monitor)
- Suction machine/wall source with pressure regulator
- Connecting tubing (4-6 feet [1.2 to 1.8 meters])
- Bedside table
- Clean gloves, sterile gloves
- Mask, goggles, or face shield; gown if isolation procedures dictate
- Water-soluble lubricant (nasal approach)

- Open suctioning: Appropriate-size suction catheter. It should be the smallest diameter that will remove secretions effectively, preferably one that is no more than half of the internal diameter of the artificial airway to minimize the decrease in PaO2 (Billington and Luckett, 2019).
  - Sterile basin or solution container
  - Normal sterile saline or solution of sterile water (100 mL)
- Closed suctioning: Closed-system or in-line suction catheter, appropriately sized.
  - 5 to 10 mL normal saline in syringe or vial
- Manual self-inflating resuscitation bag-valve device with appropriate-size mask
- Clean towel or paper drape
- Positive end-expiratory pressure valve for resuscitation bag

STEP	RATIONALE
1 Perform preprocedure protocol.	
Assessment	
• Review patient's electronic health record (EHR): history of abnormal anatomy or head and neck surgery/trauma, tumors involving lower airway, pneumonia, chronic obstructive pulmonary disease, neurologic abnormalities.	Changes in neurologic status and neuromuscular impairment increase likelihood that patient is unable to clear respiratory secretions. Abnormal anatomy or head and neck surgery/trauma and tumors in and around lower airway impair normal secretion clearance. Accumulating pulmonary secretions impede patient's ability to effectively clear airway through cough mechanism (Urden et al., 2020).
• Review EHR for normal pulse oximeter and end-tidal CO_2 values, vital sign trends, previous response and tolerance to suctioning procedure, and color and quantity of sputum.	Knowing the patient condition, medical history, and past response to suctioning helps predict or prevent unexpected outcomes.

Continued

STEP	RATIONALE
• Review sputum microbiology data in laboratory report.	Certain bacteria are easier to transmit or require isolation because of virulence or antibiotic resistance.
• Perform hand hygiene and apply clean gloves or other personal protective equipment (PPE) if risk of exposing self to secretions or if patient condition indicates.	Prevents transmission of microorganisms.
• Assess for signs and symptoms of upper and lower airway obstruction requiring suctioning: abnormal respiratory rate, adventitious lung sounds, secretions in the airway, gurgling, drooling, restlessness, gastric secretions or vomitus in mouth, and coughing without clearing airway secretions and/or improving adventitious lung sounds.	Physical signs and symptoms result from secretions in upper and lower airways and decreased oxygen to the tissues. Presuction assessment provides baseline data to identify need for suctioning and measures the effectiveness of suction procedures (Wiegand, 2017).
• Auscultate lungs and assess vital signs and oximetry for signs and symptoms associated with respiratory distress or hypoxia and hypercapnia: decreased pulse oximetry (SpO_2), increased pulse and blood pressure, bradycardia, tachypnea, decreased breath sounds, apprehension, anxiety, lethargy, pallor, and cyanosis (a late sign of hypoxia). Keep pulse oximeter on patient for continuous assessment of SpO_2.	Physical signs and symptoms resulting from decreased tissue oxygenation. Provides presuction baseline to measure patient tolerance to suctioning and effectiveness of suctioning on SpO_2 levels.

STEP	RATIONALE
• Assess for risk factors for upper and lower airway obstruction, including chronic obstructive pulmonary disease, impaired mobility, decreased level of consciousness, nasal feeding tube, decreased cough or gag reflex, and decreased swallowing ability.	Risk factors can impair patient's ability to clear secretions from airway, increase risk for retaining secretions, and necessitate nasopharyngeal or nasotracheal suctioning (Urden et al., 2020).
• Assess for excessive amounts of secretions visible in the artificial airway, signs of respiratory distress from obstructed airway (increased work of breathing, increased respiratory rate), presence of rhonchi on auscultation, excessive coughing, increased peak inspiratory pressures (if on mechanical ventilator), sawtooth pattern on ventilator monitor, or changes in capnography waveform (if patient on mechanical ventilator) or decrease in patient pulse oximeter (Wiegand, 2017).	All factors indicate need for tracheal suctioning.

CLINICAL JUDGMENT *Suctioning should only be performed as patient assessment and condition indicates and not in a scheduled fashion such as hourly (Harding et al., 2021; Wiegand, 2017).*

STEP	RATIONALE
• Assess patency of ET with capnography/end-tidal carbon dioxide (CO_2) detector.	ET may become displaced or blocked by secretions.
• Assess factors that may affect volume and consistency of secretions: a Fluid balance	Thickened or copious secretions increase risk for airway obstruction. Fluid overload increases amount of secretions. Dehydration can lead to thicker secretions.

Continued

STEP	RATIONALE
b Lack of humidity	Environment influences secretion formation and gas exchange.
c Infection (e.g., pneumonia)	Patients with respiratory infections are prone to increased secretions that are thicker and sometimes more difficult to expectorate.
• For endotracheal suctioning, assess patient's peak inspiratory pressure when on volume-controlled ventilation or check tidal volume during pressure-controlled ventilation.	Increased peak inspiratory pressure or decreased tidal volume may indicate airway obstruction (Urden et al., 2020; Weigand, 2017).

CLINICAL JUDGMENT *Assess a patient's vital signs, pulse oximetry, end-tidal CO_2, ventilator pressures and volumes (if receiving mechanical ventilation), and respiratory status before and continuously throughout suctioning (Wiegand, 2017).*

• Identify contraindications to nasotracheal suctioning: occluded nasal passages; nasal bleeding; croup; acute head, facial, or neck injury or surgery; coagulopathy or bleeding disorder; irritable airway; laryngospasm or bronchospasm; gastric surgery with high anastomosis; myocardial infarction (Hockenberry et al., 2019; Wiegand, 2017).	These conditions contraindicate suctioning because passage of suction catheter through nasal route causes trauma to existing facial trauma/surgery, increases nasal bleeding, or causes severe bleeding in presence of coagulopathy or bleeding disorders. In presence of epiglottitis or croup, laryngospasm, or irritable airway, passage of suction catheter through nose causes intractable coughing, hypoxemia, and severe bronchospasm. Hypoxemia could worsen cardiac damage in myocardial infarction.

STEP	RATIONALE
• Remove and dispose of gloves. Perform hand hygiene. (Other PPE may remain in place for actual suctioning.)	Reduces transmission of microorganisms.
• Assess level of patient's apprehension, anxiety, decreased ability to concentrate, lethargy, decreased level of consciousness (especially acute), increased fatigue, dizziness, and/or behavioral changes (especially irritability).	These are signs and symptoms of hypoxia and/or hypercapnia, which can indicate need for suction. These signs can also help to identify patient's ability to cooperate with procedure.

CLINICAL JUDGMENT *It is important to ensure that the patient's SpO_2 and $EtCO_2$ values return to their own personal normal baseline values after suctioning. Patients with chronic pulmonary disease may have lower than normal SpO_2 or higher than normal $EtCO_2$ values.*

Implementation

1 Perform hand hygiene and apply appropriate PPE, if not already applied during assessment (mask with face shield or goggles; gown).	Reduces transmission of microorganisms.
2 If not already present, place pulse oximeter on patient's finger. Take reading and leave oximeter in place.	Provides continuous SpO_2 value to determine patient's response to suctioning.
3 Assist patient to comfortable Semi-Fowlers or high Fowlers position. Explain that temporary coughing, sneezing, gagging, or shortness of breath is normal during procedure.	Positioning reduces stimulation of gag reflex, promotes patient comfort and secretion drainage, and prevents aspiration. Explanation can reduce anticipatory anxiety.

Continued

STEP	RATIONALE
4 Connect one end of connecting tubing to suction device (usually installed into wall) and place other end in convenient location near patient. Turn suction device on and set pressure to the lowest level possible that still allows for effectively clearing secretions. This value is typically between 80 and 150 mm Hg (Mwakanyanga et al., 2018). Occlude end of suction tubing to check pressure.	Ensures equipment function. Excessive negative pressure damages tracheal mucosa and induces greater hypoxia (Wiegand, 2017).
5 Open suctioning:	
A Using aseptic technique, open suction kit or catheter package. If sterile drape is available, place it across patient's chest or on bedside table. Do not allow suction catheter to touch any nonsterile surfaces.	Prepares catheter, maintains asepsis, and reduces transmission of microorganisms. Provides sterile surface on which to lay catheter between passes.
B Unwrap or open sterile basin and place on bedside table. Be careful not to touch inside of basin. Fill with about 100 mL sterile normal saline solution or water.	Saline or water is used to clean tubing after each suction pass.
C Open packet of water-soluble lubricant and apply small amount to sterile field. Note: Lubricant is not necessary for tracheal airway.	Water-soluble lubricant helps avoid lipid aspiration pneumonia. Excessive amount of lubricant occludes catheter.
D Apply sterile gloves to each hand or clean glove to nondominant hand and sterile glove to dominant hand (see agency policy)	Reduces transmission of microorganisms and maintains sterility of suction catheter.

STEP	RATIONALE
E Pick up suction catheter with dominant hand without touching nonsterile surfaces. Pick up connecting tubing with nondominant hand. Secure catheter to tubing (Fig. 70.2).	Maintains catheter sterility. Connects catheter to suction.
F Place tip of catheter into sterile basin and suction small amount of normal saline solution from basin by occluding suction vent.	Ensures equipment function. Lubricates internal catheter and tubing.
G Suction nasotracheally and nasopharyngeally:	
(1) Ask patient to extend head back. Have patient take deep breaths (if able) or increase oxygen flow rate with delivery device through cannula or mask (if ordered).	Position opens access to airway. May help to decrease risks of hypoxemia.

Continued

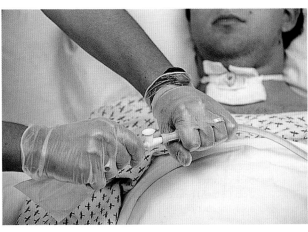

Fig. 70.2 Attaching suction catheter to suction tubing.

STEP	RATIONALE
(2) Lightly coat distal 6 to 8 cm (2 to 3 inches) of catheter with water-soluble lubricant.	Lubricates catheter for easier insertion.
(3) Remove oxygen-delivery device, if applicable, with nondominant hand. Keep device close to patient's mouth/nose.	Allows access to nares and catheter. Provides oxygen source.

CLINICAL JUDGMENT *Be sure to insert catheter during patient inhalation, especially if advancing it into trachea, because epiglottis is open. Do not insert during swallowing or catheter will most likely enter esophagus.* **Never apply suction during insertion.** *Patient should cough. If patient gags or becomes nauseated, catheter is most likely in esophagus and should immediately be removed (Wiegand, 2017).*

STEP	RATIONALE
(4) Nasotracheal: Ask patient to extend head back. As patient takes deep breath, advance catheter (without applying suction) following natural course of naris. Advance catheter slightly slanted and downward to just above larynx (Fig. 70.3). Then as patient takes another deep breath, quickly insert catheter through larynx. Patient will begin to cough; then pull back catheter 1 to 2 cm (½ inch) before applying suction.	Ensures that catheter tip reaches trachea for suctioning.

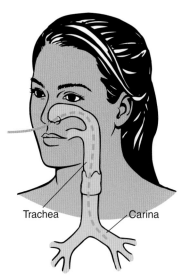

Fig. 70.3 Extent of nasotracheal catheter insertion.

Trachea   Carina

STEP	RATIONALE

CLINICAL JUDGMENT *If resistance is met during insertion, you may need to try the other naris. Do not force the catheter into the nares because this will cause mucosal damage.*

a Apply intermittent suction for no more than 10 to 15 seconds by intermittently placing and releasing nondominant thumb over catheter vent. Slowly withdraw catheter while rotating it back and forth between thumb and forefinger.	Intermittent suction up to 10 to 15 seconds safely removes tracheal secretions. Suction time longer than 15 seconds increases risk for suction-induced hypoxemia (AARC, 2010; Urden et al., 2020; Wiegand, 2017). Intermittent suction and rotation of catheter prevent injury to tracheal mucosa. If catheter "grabs" mucosa, remove thumb to release suction.

CLINICAL JUDGMENT *When there is difficulty passing the catheter, ask patient to cough or say "ahh" or try to advance the catheter during inspiration. Both measures help to open the glottis to permit passage of the catheter into the trachea.*

Continued

STEP	RATIONALE
b Once withdrawn, irrigate the catheter with the sterile water or saline after each suction pass.	Keeps lumen of suction catheter cleared of secretions.
c If it is necessary to suction again, relubricate the catheter. Allow for a 30- to 60-second interval between each suctioning for ventilation and oxygenation (AARC, 2010). Limit to two passes for each suction event. Ask patient to deep breathe and cough.	Prevents oxygen desaturation. Coughing can expectorate secretions, avoiding need to suction a second time.
d If pharyngeal secretions are present, suction just before removing catheter from naris. **Do not suction nasally again after suctioning mouth**.	Catheter is used for sterile airways first, then nonsterile pharyngeal cavity.

CLINICAL JUDGMENT *When using the nasal approach, perform tracheal suctioning before oropharyngeal suctioning whenever possible. The mouth and pharynx contain more bacteria than the trachea. If copious oral secretions are present before beginning the procedure, suction mouth with oral suction device first (see Skill 72).*

STEP	RATIONALE

CLINICAL JUDGMENT *If patient develops respiratory distress, immediately withdraw catheter (without applying suction) and supply additional oxygen and breaths as needed. In an emergency, administer oxygen directly through the catheter. Disconnect suction and attach oxygen at prescribed flow rate through the catheter. If the patient does not tolerate the suctioning procedure, switching to closed (in-line) suctioning (Step 6) or allowing longer recovery times may need to be considered. Notify health care provider if patient develops significant cardiopulmonary compromise during suctioning (Urden et al., 2020; Wiegand, 2017).*

STEP	RATIONALE
(5) Nasopharyngeal: As patient takes deep breath, insert catheter (without applying suction) following natural course of naris; slightly slant catheter downward and advance to back of pharynx. Do not force through naris. In adults insert catheter approximately 16 cm (6.5 inches); in older children, 8 to 12 cm (3 to 5 inches); in infants and young children, 4 to 7.5 cm (1.5 to 3 inches). Rule of thumb is to insert catheter distance from tip of nose (or mouth) to angle of mandible.	Ensure that catheter tip reaches back of pharynx for suctioning.

Continued

STEP	RATIONALE
a Apply intermittent suction for no more than 10 to 15 seconds by placing and releasing nondominant thumb over catheter vent. Slowly withdraw catheter while rotating it back and forth between thumb and forefinger.	Suction time longer than 15 seconds increases risk for suction-induced hypoxemia (AARC, 2010; Urden et al., 2020). Intermittent suction and rotation of catheter prevents injury to mucosa. If catheter "grabs" mucosa, remove thumb to release suction.
b Once withdrawn, irrigate the catheter with the sterile water or saline after each suction pass.	Keeps lumen of suction catheter cleared of secretions.
c If it is necessary to suction again, relubricate the catheter. Allow for a 30- to 60-second interval between each suctioning for ventilation and oxygenation (AARC, 2010). Limit to two passes for each suction event. Ask patient to deep breathe and cough.	Prevents oxygen desaturation. Coughing can expectorate secretions, avoiding need to suction a second time.

STEP	RATIONALE
H Suction established tracheostomy.	
(1) Remove oxygen-delivery device over trachea with nondominant hand. Keep device close to opening of tracheal stoma.	Provides oxygen source during suctioning.
(2) Advise patient that you are about to begin suctioning. Have patient inhale deeply and then insert catheter gently and quickly into tracheostomy without applying suction using dominant thumb and forefinger (it is best to try to time catheter insertion into artificial airway with inspiration). Advance catheter (usually 0.5 to 1 cm below the level of the tube), until patient coughs, then pull back 1 cm (0.4 inch) before applying suction (Billington and Luckett, 2019).	Application of suction pressure while introducing catheter into trachea increases risk for damage to tracheal mucosa and increased hypoxia. Pulling back stimulates cough and removes catheter from mucosal wall so that catheter is not resting against tracheal mucosa during suctioning. (AARC, 2010; Wiegand, 2017).

Continued

STEP	RATIONALE
(3) Apply intermittent suction for 10 to 15 seconds by placing and releasing nondominant thumb over valve of catheter; slowly withdraw catheter while rotating it back and forth between dominant thumb and forefinger. Do not use suction for longer than 15 seconds. Encourage patient to slowly deep breathe and cough. Watch for respiratory distress.	Suction time longer than 15 seconds increases risk for suction-induced hypoxemia (AARC, 2010; Urden et al., 2020; Wiegand, 2017). Intermittent suction and rotation of catheter prevent injury to tracheal mucosa. If catheter "grabs" mucosa, remove thumb to release suction.
(4) Once withdrawn, irrigate the catheter with the sterile water or saline after each suction pass.	Keeps lumen of suction catheter cleared of secretions.
(5) If it is necessary to suction again allow for a 30- to 60-second interval between each suctioning for ventilation and oxygenation (AARC, 2010). Limit to two passes for each suction event.	Prevents oxygen desaturation. Coughing can expectorate secretions, avoiding need to suction a second time.

STEP	RATIONALE
6 Closed suctioning	
a Turn suction device on, set vacuum regulator to appropriate negative pressure (usually 80 to 150 mm Hg), and check pressure. See manufacturer guidelines for recommended pressure to use with the agency's brand of catheter.	Excessive negative pressure damages tracheal mucosa and induces greater hypoxia (Wiegand, 2017).
b Attach suction. In many agencies a respiratory therapist attaches the catheter to the mechanical ventilator circuit. If closed-system catheter is not already in place, apply sterile gloves or sterile glove for dominant hand and clean glove for nondominant hand (see agency policy), Open suction catheter package using aseptic technique and attach closed-system suction catheter to ventilator circuit by removing swivel adapter and placing closed-system suction catheter apparatus on ET or TT. Connect mechanical ventilator circuit to closed-system suction catheter with flex tubing (Fig. 70.4).	Maintains surgical asepsis during suctioning.

Continued

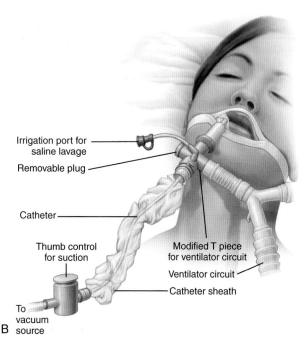

Irrigation port for saline lavage

Removable plug

Catheter

Thumb control for suction

To vacuum source

B

Modified T piece for ventilator circuit

Ventilator circuit

Catheter sheath

Fig. 70.4 Closed suction system attached to an endotracheal tube. (From Blanchard B: Thoracic surgery, In Rothrock JC, McEwen DR, editors, *Alexander's care of the patient in surgery*, ed 14, St Louis 2011, Mosby.)

STEP	RATIONALE
c With assistance from respiratory therapy when patient has an artificial airway and is on a ventilator, hyperoxygenate patient (usually 100% oxygen) for at least 30 seconds by adjusting the fraction of inspired oxygen (FiO_2) setting on the ventilator or by using a temporary oxygen-enrichment program available on microprocessor ventilators according to agency policy or protocol. (Manual ventilation is not recommended.)	Preoxygenation decreases risk of decreased arterial oxygen levels while ventilation or oxygenation is interrupted and volume is lost during suctioning (AARC, 2010; Wiegand, 2017). Some models of resuscitation bags do not deliver 100% oxygen; therefore, this is not the best way to hyperoxygenate patient (Wiegand, 2017).

CLINICAL JUDGMENT *Suctioning can cause elevations in ICP in patients with head injuries. Reduce this risk by performing presuction hyperoxygenation, which results in hypocarbia, which in turn induces vasoconstriction. Vasoconstriction reduces the potential for an increase in ICP (Urden et al., 2020).*

d Unlock suction control mechanism, if required by manufacturer. Open saline port and attach saline syringe or vial.	Saline allows for irrigation of catheter lumen.
e Pick up suction catheter enclosed in plastic sleeve with dominant hand.	Keeps catheter system sterile.

Continued

STEP	RATIONALE
f Apply suction. Wait until patient inhales to insert catheter. Then insert catheter using a repeating maneuver of pushing catheter gently and sliding plastic sleeve back between thumb and forefinger until resistance is felt or patient coughs.	Enhances entrance into tracheal airway, keeping catheter sterile.

CLINICAL JUDGMENT *If unable to insert catheter past the end of the ET, the catheter is probably caught in the Murphy eye (i.e., side hole at the distal end of the ET that allows for collateral airflow in the event of tracheal main-stem intubation). If this happens, rotate the catheter to reposition it away from the Murphy eye or withdraw it slightly and reinsert with the next inhalation. Usually the catheter meets resistance at the carina. One indication that the catheter is at the carina is acute onset of coughing because the carina contains many cough receptors. Pull the catheter back 1 cm (½ inch) (Billington and Luckett, 2019).*

STEP	RATIONALE
g Pull back 1 cm (0.4 inches) before applying suction. Note: If patient has a history of bleeding during previous suction procedures, take care to avoid hitting the carina with the suction catheter.	Avoids damage to tracheal carina.
h Encourage patient to cough and apply suction by squeezing on suction control mechanism while withdrawing catheter. Note: It is difficult to apply intermittent pulses of suction and nearly impossible to rotate the catheter compared with a standard catheter	Enhances suctioning of deeper secretions.

STEP	RATIONALE
i Apply continuous suction for 10 seconds as you remove the suction catheter (AARC, 2010; Wiegand, 2017). Be sure to withdraw the catheter completely into the plastic sheath and past the tip of the airway so that it does not obstruct airflow.	Time for suctioning reduces incidence of oxygen desaturation.
j Reassess cardiopulmonary status, including pulse oximetry (SpO$_2$) and ventilator measures. Repeat Steps 7f to 7i one more time to clear secretions if patient condition indicates. Allow adequate time (at least 1 full minute) between suction passes for ventilation and reoxygenation.	Determines need for additional suctioning and monitors patient response to suctioning. Prevents oxygen desaturation.
k When airway is clear, withdraw catheter completely into sheath. Be sure that colored indicator line on catheter is visible in the sheath. Squeeze the vial or push the syringe attached to saline port while applying suction. Note: Do not let the saline go down the ET or TT. Use at least 5 to 10 mL of saline to rinse the catheter until it is clear of retained secretions, which can cause bacterial growth and increase the risk for infection (AARC, 2010; Wiegand, 2017). Lock suction mechanism if applicable and turn off suction.	Ensures complete removal of catheter from airway. Saline rinses inner lumen of catheter.

Continued

STEP	RATIONALE
l Hyperoxygenate for at least 30 seconds by following the same technique used to preoxygenate (Wiegand, 2017).	Prevents hypoxemia.
m If patient requires oral Skill 71 or nasal suctioning (Step 5G(5)), perform with separate Yankauer or standard suction catheter.	Clears oral and nasal passages of mucous secretions.

CLINICAL JUDGMENT *In the past, the practice of instilling normal saline into an artificial airway was performed to try to thin the secretions, making them easier to suction out of the airway. Evidence indicates that this practice should no longer be performed and actually causes more damage to the lungs (Larrow and Klich-Heartt, 2016; Wiegand, 2017).*

---

7 When suctioning is complete, disconnect catheter from connecting tubing. (Exception: in-line catheter remains in place.) Roll catheter around fingers of dominant hand. Pull glove off inside out so that catheter remains coiled in glove. Pull off other glove over first glove in same way. Discard in appropriate receptacle. Turn off suction device.	Seals contaminants in gloves. Reduces transmission of microorganisms.
8 Remove towel, place in laundry or appropriate receptacle, and reposition patient. (Apply clean gloves to continue personal care.)	Reduces transmission of microorganisms. Promotes comfort.

STEP	RATIONALE
9 If oxygen level was changed during procedure, readjust oxygen to original ordered level because patient's blood oxygen level should have returned to baseline.	Prevents absorption atelectasis (i.e., tendency for airways to collapse if proximally obstructed by secretions). Prevents oxygen toxicity while allowing patient time to reoxygenate blood.
10 Discard remainder of normal saline into appropriate receptacle. If basin is disposable, discard into appropriate receptacle. If basin is reusable, rinse it out and place it in soiled utility room.	Reduces transmission of microorganisms.
13 Help patient to comfortable position and provide oral hygiene as needed.	Work of breathing is decreased when in a comfortable position. Oral hygiene promotes comfort.
14 Perform postprocedure protocol.	
15 Evaluate patient response:	
a Compare patient's vital signs, cardiopulmonary assessments, and EtCO$_2$ and SpO$_2$ values before and after suctioning. If patient is on a ventilator, compare FiO$_2$ and tidal volumes and peak inspiratory pressures.	Identifies physiologic effects of suction procedure to restore airway patency. Auscultation of lungs offers information about change in lung sounds.
b Ask patient if breathing is easier and if congestion is decreased.	Provides subjective confirmation that suctioning procedure has relieved airway.
c Observe character and amount of airway secretions.	Provides data to document presence or absence of respiratory tract infection or thickened secretions.

Recording and Reporting

- Record pre- and postsuctioning vital signs and cardiovascular assessments; amount, consistency, color, and odor of secretions; catheter size; route of suctioning; and patient's response to suctioning.
- Record need for hyperoxygenation, type of hyperoxygenation, and percentage of oxygenation used.
- Document evaluation of patient and family learning.
- Report patient's tolerance of and response to procedure, need for hyperoxygenation, frequency of suctioning, and the quantity and quality of the secretions.
- Report unexpected physiologic changes to health care provider.

UNEXPECTED OUTCOMES	RELATED INTERVENTIONS
1 Patient has decrease in overall cardiopulmonary status: decreased SpO_2, increased $EtCO_2$, continued tachypnea, continued increased work of breathing, and cardiac dysrhythmias.	• Limit length of suctioning. • Determine need for more frequent suctioning, possibly of shorter duration. • Determine need for supplemental or increase in supplemental oxygen. Supply oxygen between suctioning passes. • Notify health care provider.
2 Bloody secretions are returned after suctioning.	• Determine amount of suction pressure used. May need to be decreased. • Ensure that suction is completed correctly using intermittent suction and catheter rotation. Do not apply suction until after catheter has been pulled back 1 cm (0.4 inches) to prevent applying suction while catheter is touching carina. • Evaluate suctioning frequency. • Provide more frequent oral hygiene. • Notify health care provider.

UNEXPECTED OUTCOMES	RELATED INTERVENTIONS
3 Patient has paroxysms of coughing or bronchospasm.	• Administer supplemental oxygen. • Allow patient to rest between passes of suction catheter. • Consult with health care provider regarding need for inhaled bronchodilators or topical anesthetics.
4 Inability to obtain secretions during suction procedure.	• Evaluate patient's fluid status and adequacy of humidification on oxygen-delivery device. • Assess for signs of infection. • Determine need for chest physiotherapy.

Suctioning: Oropharyngeal

A Yankauer suction catheter is used for oropharyngeal suctioning (i.e., the removal of pharyngeal secretions through the mouth) (Fig. 71.1). The catheter is made of rigid, minimally flexible plastic. The tip of this suction catheter usually has one large and several small openings through which the mucus enters when negative pressure is applied. The Yankauer suction catheter is angled to facilitate removal of secretions through a patient's mouth. Oropharyngeal suctioning only removes secretions from the mouth and back of the throat. Perform oral suctioning when a patient is able to cough effectively but is unable to clear secretions, such as for a patient with a neuromuscular injury who cannot manage their own oral secretions or a patient with an artificial airway and impaired swallowing.

Safety Guidelines

- Oropharyngeal suctioning does not replace subglottic suctioning for patients with tracheal or endotracheal tubes. Instead, use the special subglottic suction port on the tracheostomy tube (Tracheostomy Education, 2020).
- Use caution when suctioning patients with head injuries. Suctioning elevates intracranial pressure (Harding et al., 2021; Urden et al., 2020). Reduce this risk by hyperventilating before suction, which results in hypocarbia. This in turn induces vasoconstriction, thereby reducing the risk of elevated intracranial pressure.

Delegation

The skill of performing oropharyngeal suctioning can be delegated to assistive personnel (AP). Do not delegate this skill for patients with oral or neck surgery in the immediate postoperative period. You are responsible for assessing the patient's respiratory status. Direct the AP about:

- Factors (e.g., expected frequency of suctioning, and expected color and volume of secretions) for individualizing approach to suctioning patient.
- The risks of applying excessive or inadequate suction pressure.
- Avoiding mouth sutures, applying suction against sensitive tissues, and dislodging tubes in the patient's nose or mouth.

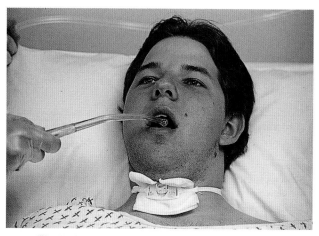

Fig. 71.1 Oropharyngeal suctioning using Yankauer catheter.

- How to avoid stimulating the gag reflex.
- Immediately reporting any change in vital signs, pulse oximetry (SpO2), sputum (i.e., bloody), difficulty breathing, or discomfort during or after the procedure.

Collaboration

- Inform respiratory therapy about the need for oropharyngeal suctioning, and the frequency of suctioning and the amount and characteristics of the secretions.
- Physical therapists, occupational therapists, or speech therapists need to be aware of patient pulmonary status and need for suctioning before implementing their prescribed interventions.

Equipment

- Clean, nonsterile Yankauer or tonsillar tip suction catheter
- Clean gloves
- Other personal protective equipment (PPE): mask, goggles, or face shield; gown if indicated, respiratory protection, if indicated
- Disposable cup or nonsterile basin
- Tap water or normal saline (about 100 mL)
- Suction machine or wall suction device with regulator
- Connecting tubing (6 feet [1.8 meters])
- Oral airway (if indicated)
- Washcloth

- Towel, cloth, or disposable paper drape
- Pulse oximeter
- Stethoscope
- Manual self-inflating resuscitation bag (bag-valve-mask) with oxygen-connecting tubing

STEP	RATIONALE
1 Perform preprocedure protocol.	

Assessment

• Review patient's electronic health record (EHR), including health care provider's order and nurses' notes for patient's normal pulse oximeter values, respiratory rate and effort of breathing, and vital signs. Note medical history for pulmonary or neurologic conditions, frequency of suctioning, and response to suctioning.	Knowing the patient condition and medical history helps to identify cause and need for suctioning, patient's risk for aspiration, and prediction of the patient response to interventions.
• Identify risk factors for airway obstruction: impaired cough or gag reflex, weakened respiratory muscles, impaired swallowing, and decreased level of consciousness.	Risk factors prevent patient from protecting airway from aspiration or clearing secretions safely.

CLINICAL JUDGMENT *If the presence of secretions is noted and/or upper airway obstruction is suspected, immediate suctioning is warranted and should be performed before assessing further.*

• Review EHR for conditions including recent head and neck surgery, mouth trauma.	May contraindicate suctioning or require you to adapt oral suctioning approach
• Perform hand hygiene. Apply gloves and any other PPE equipment as patient condition dictates (e.g., risk of splashing).	Reduces transmission of microorganisms.

STEP	RATIONALE
• Assess patient's level of consciousness and obtain vital signs and pulse oximetry, noting signs and symptoms of hypoxia: anxiety, change in level of consciousness, change in vital signs (see Skill 47). Do not remove oximetry probe until after the oropharynx is suctioned.	Clearing the oropharynx of secretions assists in improving oxygenation. Use of oximetry assesses patient during and after oropharyngeal suctioning.
• Assess for signs and symptoms of upper airway obstruction: gurgling on inspiration or expiration, restlessness, obvious excessive oral secretions, drooling, gastric secretions or vomitus in mouth, or coughing without clearing secretions from upper airway.	Secretions pool in upper airway, which can cause total airway obstruction and hypoxia. The risk for aspiration of gastric contents and airway obstruction is increased in patients with vomiting; delayed gastric emptying; impairment in esophageal sphincter control, cough, swallowing, or gag reflex; or those receiving enteral feedings.
• Auscultate for presence of adventitious sounds.	Determines whether lower airway secretions are present and establishes baseline.
• Assess patient's and/or caregiver's ability to hold or manipulate catheter.	Physical factors such as impaired mobility of upper extremities prevent patient from using catheter to help control oral secretions.

CLINICAL JUDGMENT *In patients with chronic pulmonary disease, the SpO_2 value may remain the same after oropharyngeal suctioning. This baseline value may be lower than the typical normal values of greater than 95%.*

Implementation

1	Assist patient to semi-Fowler or high-Fowler position.	Reduces stimulation of gag reflex, promotes secretion drainage, and prevents aspiration.

Continued

STEP	RATIONALE
2 Explain to patient that coughing, gagging, or (less commonly) sneezing is normal and lasts only a few seconds. Encourage patient to cough out secretions and demonstrate how to splint painful areas during procedure. Practice coughing if able.	Gagging or coughing occurs when posterior pharynx is suctioned or as a result of excess secretions. Coughing secretions out of lower airway or posterior pharynx decreases amount of suctioning required. Splinting reduces abdominal incision discomfort during coughing or gagging.
3 Perform hand hygiene. Apply clean gloves. Apply mask or face shield if splashing is likely. Wear gown and respirator if isolation precautions are indicated.	Reduces transmission of microorganisms.
4 Place towel, cloth, or paper drape across patient's neck and chest. Place pulse oximeter on finger, if not already in place.	Pulse oximetry continuously monitors patient's oxygenation level.
5 Fill cup or basin with approximately 100 mL of water or normal saline.	Helps to clean catheter after suctioning and assesses equipment functioning.
6 Connect one end of connecting tubing to suction machine and other to Yankauer suction catheter. Turn on suction machine; set vacuum regulator to suction, typically between 80 and 120 mm Hg (Wiegand, 2017).	Prepares suction apparatus. Excessive pressures should be avoided because elevated pressure settings increase risk for trauma to oral mucosa (Wiegand, 2017).
7 Check that suction machine is functioning properly by placing tip of catheter in water or normal saline and suctioning small amount from cup or basin.	Ensures that equipment functions and lubricates catheter.

STEP	RATIONALE
8 Remove patient's oxygen mask if present. Nasal cannula may remain in place. Keep oxygen mask near patient's face.	Allows access to mouth. Reduces chance of hypoxia.

CLINICAL JUDGMENT *Be prepared to quickly reapply supplemental oxygen if SpO$_2$ value falls below 90% or respiratory distress develops. Be prepared to use the bag-valve-mask if patient has serious acute respiratory distress or decline in SpO$_2$.*

CLINICAL JUDGMENT *If patients have been tracheally or endotracheally suctioned before oropharyngeal suctioning, they may require some recovery from the suctioning procedure before oropharyngeal suctioning begins. Allow for recovery by reapplying the oxygen mask until just before oropharyngeal suctioning.*

9 Insert catheter into mouth along gum line to pharynx. Move catheter around mouth until secretions have cleared. Encourage patient to cough. Replace oxygen mask.	Movement of catheter prevents suction tip from invaginating (turning inside out) the oral mucosal surfaces and causing trauma. Coughing moves secretions from lower airway into mouth and upper airway.

CLINICAL JUDGMENT *Use caution with a patient who has had recent oral or head/neck surgery. Aggressive suctioning and excessive coughing should not be used or encouraged in patients who have undergone throat surgery such as a tonsillectomy. Irritating the operative site can increase the risk of infection or bleeding (Urden et al., 2020).*

10 Rinse catheter with water or normal saline in cup or basin until connecting tubing is cleared of secretions. Turn off suction. Place catheter in clean, dry area. Remove and dispose of gloves (and any other PPE). Perform hand hygiene.	Rinses catheter and reduces probability of transmission of microorganisms. Clean suction tubing enhances delivery of set suction pressure.

Continued

STEP	RATIONALE
11 Observe respiratory status. Repeat procedure if indicated. May need to use standard suction catheter to reach into trachea if respiratory status not improved (see Skill 70).	Directs you to continue or stop suctioning, or choose another intervention.
12 Remove towel, cloth, or disposable drape. Reposition patient comfortably in Sims or side-lying position, especially if patient has decreased level of consciousness.	Reduces transmission of microorganisms. Facilitates drainage of oral secretions.

CLINICAL JUDGMENT *Keep catheter in nonairtight container such as brown paper or plastic bag attached to bed rail or in suction canister. Do not store the catheter where it will come in contact with secretions or excretions, which promote bacterial growth.*

13 Apply clean gloves to wash the patient's face or perform oral hygiene.	Promotes comfort.
14 Perform postprocedure protocol.	
15 Evaluate patient response:	
a Compare assessment findings before and after procedure.	Identifies physiologic response to suction procedure.
b Auscultate chest and airways for adventitious sounds.	Presence of lower airway adventitious sounds suggests need for lower airway suctioning.
c Inspect mouth for any vomitus, remaining secretions, or oral trauma.	Clear, uninjured oral airway is necessary to prevent aspiration.

Recording and Reporting

- Record the amount, consistency, color, and odor of secretions; number of times suctioned; patient's respiratory assessment findings including patient's oxygen saturation and vital signs before and after suctioning. Document evaluation of patient learning.
- Document evaluation of patient learning.
- Report any unresolved outcomes, such as worsening respiratory distress, to the health care provider.
- During shift change report the frequency of suctioning and patient response to suction.

UNEXPECTED OUTCOMES	RELATED INTERVENTIONS
1 Patient's respiratory distress increases.	• Suction further or implement nasal or tracheal suctioning (Skill 70). • Evaluate need for other means to protect airway (e.g., oral intubation, oral airway, positioning). • Provide supplemental oxygen. • Notify health care provider.
2 Bloody secretions are suctioned.	• Assess oral cavity for trauma or lesions. • Reduce amount of suction pressure. • Observe catheter tip for nicks, which can cause mucosal trauma. • Increase frequency of oral hygiene. • Notify the health care provider.

Suprapubic Catheter Care

A suprapubic catheter is a urinary drainage tube inserted surgically through a small incision in the abdominal wall above the symphysis pubis into the bladder (Fig. 72.1). The catheter may be sutured to the skin, secured with a nonallergenic adhesive material, or retained in the bladder with a fluid-filled balloon (similar to an indwelling catheter). Suprapubic catheters are placed when there is blockage of the urethra (e.g., enlarged prostate, urethral stricture, after urologic surgery) and in situations when a long-term urethral catheter causes irritation or discomfort or interferes with sexual functioning. A review of scientific studies suggests that when placed correctly, there are rarely any complications from the use of suprapubic catheters (Schaeffer et al., 2021a).

Safety Guidelines

- Care requires the use of aseptic technique and the catheter should be connected to a sterile, closed urinary drainage system.

Delegation

The skill of caring for a newly established suprapubic catheter cannot be delegated to assistive personnel (AP); however, care of an established suprapubic catheter may be delegated (refer to agency policy). Direct the AP to:

- Report patient's discomfort (bladder fullness, spasm, abdominal pain) related to the suprapubic catheter.
- Empty drainage bag before it becomes three-quarters full; document urinary output on intake and output (I&O) record.
- Report any change in the amount and character of the urine.
- Report any signs of redness, skin irritation, foul odor, or drainage around catheter insertion site.

Collaboration

- The surgeon and wound ostomy care nurse (WOCN) can assist with problems managing the catheter and any need for bladder training after removal.
- Infection control staff can recommend infection prevention measures.

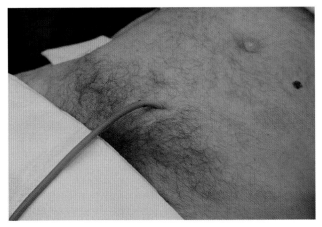

Fig. 72.1 Suprapubic catheter without a dressing.

Equipment

- Clean gloves (sterile may be necessary in some cases, see agency policy)
- Cleaning agent (sterile normal saline solution)
- Sterile cotton-tipped applicators
- Sterile surgical drainage gauze (split gauze)
- Sterile gauze dressing
- Washcloth, towel, soap and water
- Nonallergenic tape: plastic tape recommended for short-term wear; and paper/cloth tape for long-time wear (Fumarola et al., 2020)
- Velcro tube holder or tube stabilizer (optional)
- Option: Skin barrier, e.g., liquid barrier or stoma adhesive

STEP	RATIONALE
1 Perform preprocedure protocol.	

Assessment

• Review electronic health record (EHR) for history of allergies. Ask patient to describe history of allergies (focus on latex): known type(s) of allergies and normal allergic reaction(s). Check patient's allergy wristband.	Determines supplies needed for catheter care. Identifies known patient allergies to avoid patient exposure.

Continued

STEP	RATIONALE
• Inspect urine in drainage bag for amount, clarity, color, odor, and sediment.	Abnormal findings indicate potential complications, such as urinary tract infection (UTI), decreased urinary output, and catheter occlusion.
• Perform hand hygiene and apply clean gloves. Observe dressing around catheter insertion site for drainage and intactness.	Reduces transmission of infection. Drainage indicates potential complication, such as infection. Dressing may become nonocclusive because of tape choice or drainage.
• Assess catheter insertion site (may be deferred until site is cleaned) for signs of inflammation (i.e., pain, erythema, edema, blistering, drainage) and for growth of overgranulation tissue. Assess for pain at suprapubic site; if present, have patient rate on scale of 0 to 10. Remove gloves and perform hand hygiene.	If insertion is new, slight inflammation may be expected as part of normal wound healing but can also indicate infection. Overgranulation tissue can develop at insertion site as reaction to catheter. Irritation and blistering around insertion site could be from medical adhesive--related skin injury (MARSI).
• Assess for elevated temperature and chills.	Increased temperature may indicate UTI or skin site infection.

Implementation

1	Discuss with patient signs and symptoms of UTI. If applicable, teach patient and family caregiver how to perform suprapubic catheter hygiene.	Reduces anxiety and promotes cooperation. Self-care supports patient's sense of autonomy.
2	Perform hand hygiene.	Reduces transmission of infection.
3	Prepare supplies and open gauze packets in same manner as for applying dry dressing (see Skill 16).	Keeps dressing sterile until application.

STEP	RATIONALE
4 Apply clean gloves. Loosen tape and gently remove existing dressing. Note type and presence of drainage and irritation around exit site. Remove gloves and perform hand hygiene.	Provides baseline for condition of suprapubic wound. Reduces transmission of infection from dressing.
5 Clean insertion site using sterile aseptic technique for **newly established catheter:** (*Option:* Review agency policy or consider individual patient need for type of asepsis.)	Catheter site is made surgically and therefore is treated similarly to other incisions as designated by agency policy. Confirm whether use of either medical aseptic or sterile technique is recommended.
a Apply sterile or clean gloves (see agency policy). In some agencies, clean gloves are appropriate.	
b Without creating tension, hold catheter perpendicular with nondominant hand while cleaning. Use sterile gauze moistened in saline and clean skin around insertion site in circular motion, starting near insertion site and continuing in outward, widening circles for approximately 5 cm (2 inches) (Fig. 72.2).	Moves from area of least contamination to area of most contamination. Tension on catheter may create discomfort or damage to bladder wall or cause catheter to slip out of place.
c With fresh, moistened gauze, gently clean base of catheter, moving up and away from insertion site (proximal to distal).	Removes microorganisms that reside on any drainage that adheres to tubing.

Continued

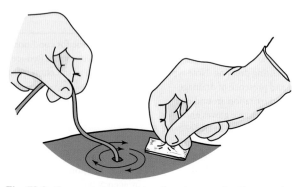

Fig. 72.2 Clean around suprapubic catheter in outward, widening circles.

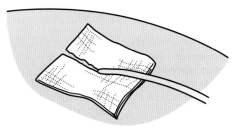

Fig. 72.3 Split drain dressing for suprapubic catheter.

STEP	RATIONALE

CLINICAL JUDGMENT *Reddening, blistering, or maceration around suprapubic site are signs of MARSI. Protect area around site by applying a skin barrier, e.g., liquid barrier or stoma adhesive. Allow skin barrier to dry. Skin barriers form a protective interface between the skin and adhesive, reducing the risk of adhesive trauma (Fumarola et al., 2020).*

STEP	RATIONALE
d Once insertion site is dry, use sterile gloved hand to apply drain dressing (split gauze) around catheter (Fig. 72.3). Tape in place.	Moist skin can cause maceration and breakdown. Dressing collects drainage that develops around catheter insertion site.

STEP	RATIONALE

6 Clean insertion site using medical aseptic technique for **long-term/established catheter**:

   a Apply clean gloves.

   b Without creating tension, hold catheter perpendicular with nondominant hand while cleaning. Clean with soap and water in circular motion, starting near catheter insertion site and continuing outward, widening circles for approximately 5 cm (2 inches).

Cleaning and drying suprapubic insertion site requires general hygienic measures; dressing is optional if drainage is not present.

   c With a fresh washcloth or gauze, gently clean base of catheter, moving up and away from insertion site (proximal to distal).

Removes microorganisms that reside in any drainage that adheres to tubing.

   d *Option:* Apply skin barrier if signs of irritation are seen. Apply drain dressing (split gauze) around catheter and tape in place.

7 Secure catheter to lateral abdomen with nonallergenic plastic or cloth tape or hook-and-loop fastener (Velcro) multipurpose tube holder.

Secures catheter and reduces risk of excessive tension on suture and/or catheter. Nonallergenic tape prevents MARSI.

8 Coil excess tubing on bed. Keep drainage bag below level of bladder at all times.

Maintains free flow of urine, thus decreasing risk for catheter-associated UTI (Fekete, 2021; McNeill, 2017).

Continued

STEP	RATIONALE
9 Perform postprocedure protocol.	Promotes patient comfort and safety.
10 Evaluate patient response:	
a Ask patient to rate pain or discomfort from suprapubic catheter on scale of 0 to 10.	Determines whether bladder is draining and patient is free of infection and bladder spasm.
b Monitor for signs of infection (e.g., fever, elevated white blood cell count) and observe urine for clarity, sediment, unusual color, or odor.	Suprapubic catheters increase risk for UTI.
c Observe catheter insertion site for erythema, edema, blistering discharge, tenderness. Check dressing at minimum of every 8 h.	Indicators of an insertion site infection or MARSI.

Recording and Reporting

- Record condition of insertion site and surrounding skin, character of urine, type of dressing change and tape, and patient's comfort level with the catheter and dressing change.
- Record urine output on I&O flow sheet. In a situation in which there is both a suprapubic and a urethral catheter, record outputs from each catheter separately.
- Document evaluation of patient learning.
- Report condition of insertion site, character of urine, type of dressing change, and patient's comfort level with the catheter and dressing change.
- Report any complications with catheter or skin site to health care provider.

UNEXPECTED OUTCOMES	RELATED INTERVENTIONS
1 Patient develops symptoms of UTI or catheter site infection.	• Increase fluid intake to at least 2200 mL in 24 h (unless contraindicated). • Monitor vital signs, I&O; observe amount, color, consistency of urine; assess site. • Notify health care provider.
2 Suprapubic catheter becomes dislodged.	• Cover site with sterile dressing. • Notify health care provider. If newly established catheter, it will need to be reinserted immediately.
3 Skin surrounding catheter exit site becomes red, irritated, or blistered and/or develops open areas.	• Notify health care provider. • Change dressing (if used) more frequently to keep site dry. • Use skin barrier around suprapubic site. • Change type of securement device. • Consult with WOCN nurse.

Suture and Staple Removal

Sutures are threads made with metal or other materials used to sew body tissues together. Sutures are available in a variety of materials, including silk, steel, cotton, linen, wire, nylon, and Dacron. Sutures made from polydioxanone, Vicryl, and Monocryl can be absorbed; others, such as nylon, silk, and steel, are nonabsorbable and must be removed. The choice of suture technique depends on the type and anatomical location of the wound, skin thickness, degree of tension, and desired cosmetic effect (Fig. 73.1) (Bryant and Nix, 2016). A patient's history of wound healing, wound site, tissues involved, and the purpose of the sutures determine the suture material selected. Removal requires the use of sterile scissors.

Staples are stainless steel wires that are quick to use and provide strength. The location of the incision sometimes restricts their use because there must be adequate distance between the skin and structures that lie below the skin, including bone and vascular structures. Staples are used for skin closure of abdominal incisions and orthopedic surgery when appearance of the incision is not critical. Removal requires a sterile staple extractor and aseptic technique. The health care provider must determine and order removal of all sutures or staples at one time, or removal of every other suture or staple as a first phase, with the remainder removed in the second phase.

Sutures and staples generally are removed within 7 to 14 days after surgery if healing is adequate (Bryant and Nix, 2016). Retention sutures usually remain in place 14 to 21 days. Timing the removal of sutures and staples is important. They must remain in place long enough to ensure initial wound closure with enough strength to support internal tissues and organs. The inflammatory process may cause the skin around staples to appear slightly red and edematous. After sutures or staples have been removed, Steri-Strips are often applied over the incision to provide support. Steri-Strips are not removed and are allowed to fall off gradually.

Safety Guidelines

- If there is any sign of suture line separation during removal, leave the remaining sutures or staples in place, document the finding and report to the health care provider.

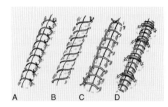

Fig. 73.1 Types of sutures. (A) Intermittent. (B) and (C) Continuous. (D) Blanket.

Delegation

The skill of staple and/or suture removal cannot be delegated to assistive personnel (AP). Agency policy determines whether only a health care provider or nurse may remove sutures and staples. Direct the AP to:

- Report any drainage, bleeding, swelling at the incision site, elevation in patient's temperature, or patient complaint of pain.
- Provide patient proper hygiene after suture removal.

Equipment

- Disposable waterproof biohazard bag
- Sterile suture removal set (forceps and scissors) or sterile staple extractor
- Sterile antiseptic swabs
- Gauze pads
- Steri-Strips or butterfly adhesive strips, as needed
- Clean gloves (sterile gloves optional)

STEP	RATIONALE
1 Perform preprocedure protocol.	
Assessment	
• Review patient's electronic health record (EHR), including health care provider's order and nurses' notes for the following information:	Health care provider's order is required for removal of sutures
a Specific directions related to suture or staple removal.	Indicates specifically which sutures are to be removed (e.g., every other suture).

Continued

STEP	RATIONALE
b History of conditions that pose risk for impaired wound healing: advanced age, cardiovascular disease, diabetes, immunosuppression, radiation, obesity, skin barrier, e.g., liquid barrier or stoma adhesive, smoking, poor nutrition, and infection.	Preexisting health disorders affect speed of healing and sometimes result in dehiscence if sutures removed too early.
• Ask patient to describe history of allergies: known type(s) of allergies and normal allergic reaction(s) (focus on antiseptic and adhesives). Check patient's allergy wristband.	Determines whether patient is sensitive to antiseptic or adhesive if Steri-Strips are to be used. Communication of patient allergies is essential part of safe medication administration.
• Assess character of patient's pain and rate acuity on pain scale of 0 to 10.	Provides baseline of patient's comfort level to determine response to therapy.
• Defer direct assessment of wound to implementation, just before suture removal.	Provides for more efficient procedure. Limits wound exposure when dressing is in place.

CLINICAL JUDGMENT *If wound edges are separated or signs of infection are present, the wound has not healed properly. Notify the health care provider because sutures or staples may need to remain in place and/or other wound care may need to be initiated.*

Implementation

1 Explain to patient how you will remove staples or sutures and that removal is usually not a painful procedure but patient may feel pulling or tugging of skin.	Gains patient cooperation and reduces anxiety.

STEP	RATIONALE
2 Administer prescribed analgesic if needed at least 30 minutes before procedure.	Promotes patient comfort to help minimize movement during suture removal.
3 Perform hand hygiene and position patient comfortably while exposing suture line. Ensure that direct lighting is on suture line.	Reduces transmission of microorganisms. Aids visibility and correct placement of forceps or extractor during removal process, ultimately reducing soft tissue injury.
4 Place cuffed waterproof disposal bag within easy reach.	Provides for easy disposal of contaminated sutures and dressings (if present) and prevents passing items over sterile work area.
5 Open sterile packages of equipment needed for suture/staple removal:	Ensures an organized procedure.
a Open sterile suture removal kit or staple extractor kit.	
b Open sterile antiseptic swabs and place on inside surface of kit.	Avoids contamination of the antiseptic swabs.
c Obtain gloves (sterile gloves if policy indicates).	
6 Perform hand hygiene. Apply clean gloves. Remove any gauze dressing covering wound. Dispose of soiled dressing in proper receptacle. Inspect incision for healing ridge and skin integrity of suture line for uniform closure of wound edges, normal color, and absence of drainage and inflammation (Fig. 73.2). Palpate around suture line gently, looking for expression of drainage, and note any tenderness. Remove and dispose of gloves. Perform hand hygiene.	Indicates adequate wound healing for support of internal structures without continued need for sutures or staples (Whitney, 2016). Reduces transmission of infection.

Continued

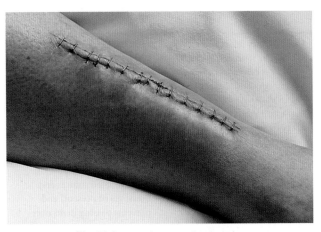

Fig. 73.2 Suture line secured with staples.

STEP	RATIONALE
7 Apply clean or sterile gloves as required by agency policy.	Reduces transmission of infection.
8 Clean sutures or staples and healed incision with antiseptic swabs. Start at sides next to incision and then wipe across suture line using new antiseptic swab for each swipe.	Removes surface bacteria from incision and sutures or staples.
9 Remove staples: a Place lower tips of staple extractor under first staple. As the handles are closed, upper tip of extractor depresses center of staple, causing both ends of staple to be bent upward and simultaneously exit their insertion sites in dermal layer (Fig. 73.3).	Avoids excess pressure on suture line and secures smooth removal of each staple.

STEP	RATIONALE
b Carefully control staple extractor.	Avoids pressure on suture line and patient discomfort.
c As soon as both ends of staple are visible, lift up and move it away from skin surface (Fig. 73.4) and continue until staple is over refuse bag. In some health care facilities, contaminated staples may be disposed of in a sharps container.	Prevents scratching tender skin surface with sharp pointed ends of staple for comfort and infection control.
d Release handles of staple extractor, allowing staple to drop into refuse bag.	Avoids contaminating sterile field with used staples.
e Repeat Steps 9a through 9d until all staples have been removed.	

Continued

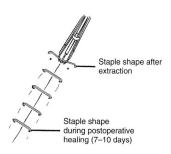

Fig. 73.3 Staple extractor placed under staple.

Staple shape after extraction

Staple shape during postoperative healing (7–10 days)

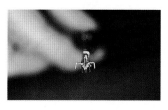

Fig. 73.4 Metal staple removed by extractor.

STEP	RATIONALE
10 Remove interrupted sutures:	
a Place gauze a few inches from suture line. Hold scissors in dominant hand and forceps (clamp) in nondominant hand.	Gauze serves as receptacle for removed sutures. Placement of scissors and forceps allows for efficient suture removal.

CLINICAL JUDGMENT *Placement of scissors and forceps is very important. Avoid pinching the skin around the wound when lifting up the suture. Likewise avoid cutting the skin around the wound by accident when snipping the suture.*

b Grasp knot of suture with forceps and gently pull up knot while slipping tip of scissors under knot of suture near skin (Fig. 73.5).	Releases suture.
c Snip suture as close to skin as possible at end distal to knot.	

CLINICAL JUDGMENT *Never snip both ends of suture; there will be no way to remove the part of the suture situated below the surface.*

Fig. 73.5 Removing an intermittent suture. Cut suture as close to skin as possible, away from knot.

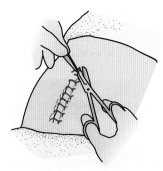

STEP	RATIONALE
d Grasp knotted end with forceps and in one continuous smooth action pull suture through from the other side. Place removed suture on gauze.	Smoothly removes suture without additional tension on suture line.

CLINICAL JUDGMENT *Never pull exposed surface of any suture into tissue below epidermis. The exposed surface of any suture is considered contaminated.*

e Observe healing level. Based on observations of wound response to suture removal and health care provider's original order, determine whether remaining sutures will be removed at this time. If so, repeat Steps 10a through 10d until you have removed all sutures.	Determines status of wound healing and whether suture line will remain closed after all sutures have been removed.
f If there is any doubt about appropriateness of suture removal, stop and notify health care provider.	
11 Remove continuous and blanket stitch sutures:	
a Place sterile gauze a few inches from suture line. Grasp scissors in dominant hand and forceps in nondominant hand.	Gauze serves as receptacle for removed sutures. Placement of scissors and forceps allows for efficient suture removal.
b Snip first suture close to skin surface at end distal to knot.	Releases suture.

Continued

STEP	RATIONALE
c Snip second suture on same side.	Releases interrupted sutures from knot.
d Grasp knotted end and gently pull with continuous smooth action, removing suture from beneath skin. Place suture on gauze.	Smoothly removes sutures without additional tension to suture line. Prevents pulling contaminated part of suture through skin.
e Repeat Steps 11a to 11d in consecutive order until entire all sutures are removed.	
12 Inspect incision to make sure that all sutures have been removed and identify any trouble areas. Gently wipe suture line with antiseptic swab to remove debris and clean incision.	Reduces risk for further incision line separation.
13 Apply Steri-Strips if *any* separation greater than two stitches or two staples in width is apparent, to maintain contact between wound edges. Note condition of skin where Steri-Strips are to be applied.	Steri-Strips support wound by distributing tension across wound and eliminate scarring from closure techniques. Steri-Strips can cause inflammation, burning, blistering if patient develops medical related-- adhesive injury (MARSI); assessment provides a baseline (Fumarola et al., 2020).
a Cut Steri-Strips to allow strips to extend 4 to 5 cm (1½ to 2 inches) on each side of incision.	
b Remove from backing and apply across incision.	

STEP	RATIONALE
c Instruct patient to take showers rather than soak in bathtub according to health care provider's instructions.	Steri-Strips are not removed; strips loosen over time (5 to 7 days) and are allowed to fall off gradually.
14 Remove and discard gloves. Perform hand hygiene and apply new pair of gloves if applying dressing. Apply light gauze dressing or expose to air if clothing will not contact suture line. Instruct patient about applying own dressing if needed at home.	Healing by primary intention eliminates need for dressing.
15 Dispose of sharps (disposable staple extractor and/or scissors) in designated sharps disposal bin.	Prevents exposure to bloodborne organisms. Instruments are sharp and contaminated.
16 Perform postprocedure protocol.	Increases patient safety.
17 Evaluate patient response:	
a Examine site where sutures or staples were removed; inspect condition of soft tissues, including surrounding skin. Look for any pieces of removed suture left behind.	Ensures that sources of infection have been removed.
b Determine whether patient has pain along incision using pain rating scale.	Determines comfort level and can indicate whether suture material remains in skin.

Continued

Recording and Reporting

- Record the time the sutures or staples were removed and the number of sutures or staples removed; document the cleaning of the suture line, appearance of the wound and surrounding skin edges, level of healing of the wound, and type of dressing applied; document patient's response to suture or staple removal.
- Document evaluation of patient learning.
- Immediately report to the health care provider if suture line separation, dehiscence, evisceration, bleeding, or purulent drainage occurs.
- Report during hand-off the removal of the staples or sutures, the integrity of the incision, the use of a dressing (if indicated), and the patient's response to the removal of the staples or sutures.

UNEXPECTED OUTCOMES	RELATED INTERVENTIONS
1 Retained suture is present.	• Notify health care provider. • Instruct patient to notify health care provider if signs of suture line infection develop after discharge from agency.
2 Patient experiences wound separation or drainage secondary to healing problems.	• Leave remaining sutures or staples in place. • Place Steri-Strip closures across suture line. • Notify health care provider.
3 Skin underlying Steri-Strips becomes inflamed, irritated, blistered.	• Early signs of MARSI (Fumarola et al., 2020). • Consider removing Steri-Strips after consulting with health care provider.

Topical Medications to the Skin

Topical administration of medication involves applying drugs locally to the skin, mucous membranes, or tissues. Topical drugs such as lotions, patches, pastes, and ointments primarily produce local effects. Systemic effects can occur if the skin is thin, drug concentration is high, contact with the skin is prolonged, or the drug is applied to skin that is not intact. In addition, skin hydration and environmental humidity affect absorption of a topical medication. An increase in skin hydration increases absorption. Always remove skin encrustations and dead tissue before applying medication because both can harbor microorganisms and block contact of medications with the affected tissue or membrane.

Safety Guidelines

- Apply topical medications using gloves and applicators to protect from accidental exposure.
- Never apply new medication over a previously applied medication because doing so will decrease the therapeutic benefit to a patient.

Delegation

The skill of administering most topical medications, including skin patches, cannot be delegated to assistive personnel (AP). However, some agencies (e.g., long-term care) may allow AP to apply some forms of topical agents. Check agency policies. Instruct the AP to:

- Report immediately any skin irritation, burning, blistering, or increased itching.
- Not apply any dressing over the topical medication unless instructed.

Collaboration

- A wound care nurse specialist can assist with treating continuing skin condition problems.

Equipment

- Clean gloves (for intact skin) or sterile gloves (for nonintact skin)
- Cotton-tipped applicators or tongue blades *(optional)*
- Ordered medication (powder, cream, lotion, ointment, spray, patch)

- Basin of warm water, washcloth, towel, nondrying soap
- Sterile dressing, nonallergenic tape
- Felt-tip pen *(optional)*
- Medication administration record (MAR) (electronic or printed)
- Plastic wrap, transparent dressing (optional, if ordered*)*

STEP	RATIONALE
1 Perform preprocedure protocol.	
Assessment	
• Check accuracy and completeness of MAR or computer printout with health care provider's original medication order. Check patient's name, medication name and dosage, route of administration, and time of administration.	The order sheet is the most reliable source and only legal record of medications that patient is to receive. Ensures that patient receives the correct medications (Palese et al., 2019). Transcription errors are a source of medication errors (Palese et al., 2019).
• Review drug reference information for medication action, purpose, normal dose, side effects, time of peak onset, and nursing implications.	Allows safe medication administration and monitoring of patient's response to therapy.
• Ask patient to describe history of allergies (medications and latex): known type(s) of allergies and normal allergic reaction(s). Check patient's allergy wristband.	Do not prepare medication if there is a known patient allergy. Communication of patient allergies is essential for safe medication administration.

STEP	RATIONALE
• Perform hand hygiene and assess condition of skin or membrane where medication is to be applied (this step can be delayed until ready for application). If there is an open wound, apply clean gloves. First wash site thoroughly with mild, nondrying soap and warm water, rinse clean, and dry. Be sure to remove any previously applied medication or debris. Also remove any blood, body fluids, secretions, or excretions. Assess for symptoms of skin irritation such as pruritus or burning. Remove gloves when finished. Perform hand hygiene.	Cleaning site thoroughly promotes proper assessment of skin surface. Assessment provides baseline to determine change in condition of skin after therapy. Application of certain topical agents can lessen or aggravate these symptoms. Cleaning removes any residual medication from the previous dose, which reduces potential adverse medication reactions or skin irritation (Burchum and Rosenthal, 2022).
• Determine amount of topical agent required for application: review health care provider's order, and read application directions carefully (a thin, even layer is usually adequate).	An excessive amount of topical agent can irritate skin chemically, negate effectiveness of drug, and/or cause adverse systemic effects.
• Determine whether patient or family caregiver is physically able to apply medication by assessing grasp, hand strength, reach, and coordination.	Necessary if patient is to self-administer medication at home.

Continued

STEP	RATIONALE
Implementation	
1 Explain purpose and side effects of each medication to patient. If applicable, teach patient how to report any side effects. Be specific if patient wishes to self-administer medications. Allow sufficient time for patient to ask questions.	Patient has the right to be informed, and patient's understanding of each medication improves adherence to therapy. Promotes feelings of independence.
2 Prepare medication without interruptions/distractions. Create a quiet environment. Keep all pages of MARs or computer printouts for one patient together or look at only one patient's electronic MAR at a time.	Interruptions contribute to medication errors (Palese et al., 2019).
3 Perform hand hygiene. Prepare medications for one patient at a time using aseptic technique. Check label of medication carefully with MAR or computer printout when removing from storage and after preparation. Preparation usually involves taking bottle or tube of lotion, cream, ointment, or patch out of storage and to patient's room. Check expiration date on medication container.	Ensures that medication is sterile. *These are the first and second checks for accuracy* and ensure that correct medication is administered. Dose potency increases or decreases when outdated.

STEP	RATIONALE
4 Take medication(s) to patient at correct time (see agency policy). Give non–time-critical scheduled medications within a range of 1 to 2 h of scheduled dose (Centers for Medicare and Medicaid Services [CMS], 2020). During administration, apply seven rights of medication administration.	Hospitals must adopt medication administration policy and procedure for timing of medication administration that considers nature of the prescribed medication, specific clinical application, and patient needs (CMS, 2020; US Department of Health and Human Services, 2020).
5 Assist patient to comfortable position. Arrange supplies at bedside.	Allows easy access to application site.
6 Identify patient using at least two identifiers (e.g., name and birthday or name and medical record number) according to agency policy. Compare identifiers with information on patient's MAR or medical record.	Ensures correct patient. Complies with The Joint Commission (TJC) standards and improves patient safety (TJC, 2023).
7 At patient's bedside again compare MAR or computer printout with names of medications on medication labels and patient name. Ask patient about history of allergies.	*This is the third check for accuracy* and ensures that patient receives correct medication. Confirms patient's allergy history.
8 Perform hand hygiene. If patient's skin is broken, apply sterile gloves. Otherwise, apply clean gloves.	Reduces transmission of microorganisms.

Continued

STEP	RATIONALE
9 Apply topical creams, ointments, and oil-based lotions:	
a Expose affected area while keeping unaffected areas covered.	Provides visualization for application and protects privacy.
b Wash, rinse, and dry affected area before applying medication if not done earlier (see Assessment).	Cleaning removes microorganisms from remaining debris and any surface medication (Burcham and Rosenthal, 2022).
c If skin is excessively dry and flaking, prepare to apply topical agent while skin is still damp.	Increased skin hydration and surface humidity enhance absorption of topical medication (Goldstein and Goldstein, 2022).
d Remove gloves, perform hand hygiene, and apply new clean or sterile gloves.	Sterile gloves are used when applying agents to open, noninfectious skin lesions. Changing gloves prevents cross contamination of infected or contagious lesions. Gloves also protect you from topical absorption of the medication and subsequent drug effects.
e Place required amount of medication in palm of gloved hand and soften by rubbing briskly between hands.	Softening topical agent makes it easier to spread on skin.
f Tell patient that initial application of agent may feel cold. Once medication is softened, spread it evenly over skin surface, using long, even strokes that follow direction of hair growth. Do not vigorously rub skin. Apply to thickness specified by manufacturer instructions.	Ensures even distribution and sufficient dosage of medication. Technique prevents irritation of hair follicles.

STEP	RATIONALE
g Explain to patient that skin may feel greasy after application.	Ointments often contain oils.
10 Apply antianginal (nitroglycerin) ointment:	
a Remove previous dose paper. Fold used paper containing any residual medication with used sides together and dispose in biohazard trash container. Wipe off residual medication with tissue.	Prevents overdose that can occur with multiple dose papers left in place. Proper disposal protects you and others from accidental exposure to medication.
b Write date, time, and your initials on printed side of new application paper.	Label provides reference to prevent missing doses.
c Antianginal (nitroglycerin) ointments are usually ordered in inches and are measured on small sheets of paper marked off in 1.25 cm (½-inch) markings. Unit-dose packages are available. Apply desired dose (in inches) of ointment on the side of the application paper that is NOT PRINTED to (Fig. 74.1).	Ensures correct dose of medication.
	Rationale: When nitroglycerine contacts print on application paper it will cause the print to leak into medication.

CLINICAL JUDGMENT *Unit-dose packages are available. Note: One package equals 2.5 cm (1 inch); smaller amounts should not be measured from this package.*

Continued

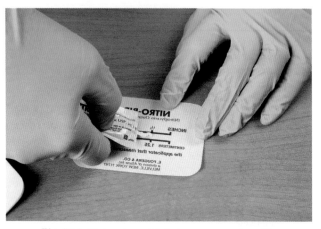

Fig. 74.1 Ointment spread in inches over measuring guide.

STEP	RATIONALE
d Select new application site: Apply nitroglycerin to chest area, back, abdomen, or anterior thigh (Burchum and Rosenthal, 2022). Do not apply on nonintact skin or hairy surfaces or over scar tissue.	Application sites are rotated to reduce skin irritation. Application on nonintact skin may result in increased absorption of medication. Application on hairy surfaces or scar tissue may decrease absorption (Burchum and Rosenthal, 2022).
e Apply ointment to skin surface by holding edge or back of paper measuring guide and placing ointment and wrapper directly on skin (Fig. 74.2). Do not rub or massage ointment into skin.	Minimizes chance of ointment covering gloves and later touching nurse's hands. Medication is designed to absorb slowly over several hours; massaging increases absorption rate.

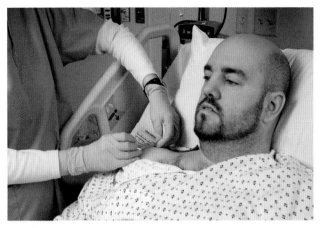

Fig. 74.2 Nurse applies wrapper with medication to patient's skin.

STEP	RATIONALE
f Secure ointment and paper with transparent dressing or strip of nonallergenic tape. Apply transparent dressing or plastic wrap only when instructed by pharmacy (Burchum and Rosenthal, 2022).	Prevents staining of clothing or inadvertent removal of medication. Covering topical medications with dressing or plastic wrap increases heat and skin humidity and rate of absorption of medication (Goldstein and Goldstein, 2022).
11 Apply transdermal patches (e.g., analgesic, nicotine, nitroglycerin, estrogen):	
a If old patch is present, remove it and clean area. Be sure to check between skinfolds for patch.	Failure to remove old patch can result in overdose. Many patches are small, clear, or flesh-colored and can be easily hidden between skinfolds. Cleaning removes residual medication traces of previous patch.

Continued

STEP	RATIONALE
b Dispose of old patch by folding in half with sticky sides together. Some facilities require patch to be cut before disposal (see agency policy). Dispose in biohazard trash bag.	Proper disposal prevents accidental exposure to medication.
c Date and initial outer side of new patch before applying it and note time of administration. Use soft-tip or felt-tip pen.	Visual reminder prevents missing or extra doses. Ballpoint pen damages patch and alters medication delivery.
d Choose a new site that is clean, intact, dry, and free of hair. Some patches have specific instructions for placement locations (e.g.,Testoderm patches are placed on scrotum; a scopolamine patch is placed behind the ear; *never apply* an estrogen patch to breast tissue or waistline). Do not apply patch on skin that is oily, burned, cut, or irritated in any way.	Ensures complete medication absorption. Estrogen patches should never be placed on the breast, genitals, or other reproductive organs. There is a risk for systemic absorption of the hormone, which can increase patient's risk for breast, testicular, or ovarian cancers (Burchum and Rosenthal, 2022).
e Carefully remove patch from protective covering by pulling off liner. Hold patch by edge without touching adhesive edges.	Touching only edges ensures that patch will adhere and that medication dose has not changed. Removing protective covering allows medication to be absorbed through skin.
f Apply patch. Hold palm of one hand firmly over patch for 10 seconds. Make sure that it sticks well, especially around edges. Apply overlay if provided with patch.	Adequate adhesion prevents loss of patch, which results in decreased dose and effectiveness.

STEP	RATIONALE

CLINICAL JUDGMENT *Never apply heat (such as with a heating pad) over a transdermal patch because this results in an increased rate of absorption with potentially serious adverse effects.*

g Do not apply patch to previously used sites for at least 1 week.

Rotating application sites reduces skin irritation from medication and adhesive (Burchum and Rosenthal, 2022).

h Instruct patient that transdermal patches are never to be cut in half; a change in dose would require prescription for new strength of transdermal medication.

Cutting patch in half would alter intended medication delivery of transdermal system, resulting in inadequate or altered drug levels.

CLINICAL JUDGMENT *It is recommended to have a daily "patch-free" interval of 10 to 12 h because tolerance develops if patches are used 24 h a day every day (Burchum and Rosenthal, 2022). Apply a new patch each morning, leave in place for 12 to 14 h, and remove in the evening.*

i Instruct patient to always remove old patch and clean skin before applying new one. Patients should not use alternative forms of same medication when using patches. For example, patients should not apply nitroglycerin ointment in addition to patch unless specifically ordered to do so by their health care provider.

Using a patch with additional or alternative drug preparation can result in toxicity or other side effects.

12 Administer aerosol sprays (e.g., local anesthetic sprays):

a Shake container vigorously. Read container label for recommended distance to hold spray from area, usually 15 to 30 cm (6 to 12 inches).

Mixing ensures delivery of fine, even spray. Proper distance ensures that fine spray hits skin surface. Holding container too close results in thin, watery distribution.

Continued

STEP	RATIONALE
b Ask patient to turn face away from spray or briefly cover face with towel while spraying neck or chest.	Prevents inhalation of spray.
c Spray medication evenly over affected site (in some cases, time spray for a period of seconds).	Ensures that affected area of skin is covered with thin spray.
13 Apply suspension-based lotion:	
a Follow Steps 9a through 9d for skin preparation	
b Shake container vigorously.	Mixes powder throughout liquid to form well-mixed suspension.
c Apply small amount of lotion to small gauze dressing or pad and apply to skin by stroking evenly in direction of hair growth.	Method of application leaves protective film of powder on skin after water base of suspension dries. Technique prevents irritation to hair follicles.
d Explain to patient that area will feel cool and dry.	Water evaporates to leave thin layer of powder.
14 Apply powder:	
a Follow steps 9a through 9d for skin preparation.	
b Ensure that skin surface is thoroughly dry. With your nondominant hand, fully spread apart any skinfolds such as between toes or under axilla and dry with towel.	Minimizes caking and crusting of powder. Fully exposes skin surface for application.
c If application site is near face, ask patient to turn face away from powder or briefly cover face with towel.	Prevents inhalation of powder.

STEP	RATIONALE
d Dust skin site lightly with dispenser so that area is covered with fine, thin layer of powder. *Option:* Cover skin area with dressing if ordered by health care provider.	Thin layer of powder has slight lubricating properties, which reduces friction and promotes drying (Burchum and Rosenthal, 2022).
15 Help patient to comfortable position, reapply gown, and cover with bed linen as desired.	Provides for patient's sense of well-being.
16 Perform postprocedure protocol.	
17 Evaluate patient response:	
a Inspect condition of skin between applications. *Note:* Observe primary area being treated but also note if there is any irritation or blisters under area where adhesive was applied	Determines whether skin condition is improving or verifies that skin is intact and not irritated. Irritation and blisters are signs of medical adhesive—related skin injury (MARSI) (Fumarola et al., 2020)
b Have patient keep diary of doses taken.	Confirms adherence to prescribed therapy.
c Observe patient or family caregiver apply topical medication.	Return demonstration measures learning.

Recording and Reporting

- Record drug, dose or strength, application site, and time administered immediately after administration, not before on MAR.
- Record condition of skin before each topical application of medication.
- Document evaluation of patient learning.
- Report adverse effects or changes in appearance and condition of skin lesions to health care provider.

UNEXPECTED OUTCOMES	RELATED INTERVENTIONS
1 Skin site appears inflamed and edematous with blistering and oozing of fluid from lesions. These signs indicate subacute inflammation or eczema that can develop if skin lesions are getting worse, or signs of MARSI.	• Withhold medication. • Notify health care provider; alternative therapies may be needed.
2 Patient is unable to explain information about drug or does not administer as prescribed.	• Identify possible reasons for nonadherence and explore alternative approaches or options.

Tracheostomy Care

A tracheostomy is a stoma or artificial opening into the trachea, created surgically or by an incision through the neck, that allows for the insertion of an artificial airway, tracheostomy tube (TT). Patients with TTs require long-term airway management because of airway obstruction, airway clearance needs, and/or long-term need for mechanical ventilation (Bolsega and Sole, 2018). A TT offers advantages over long-term endotracheal tube (ETT) placement such as decreased risk of laryngeal and tracheal injury, less sedation, shorter ventilator weaning time (time it takes to transition a patient from ventilator to other oxygen sources), and improved comfort for the patient. Some TTs even allow more patient freedom in performing activities of daily living such as feeding, speaking, and mobility (Wang et al., 2019).

TTs have several components (Fig. 75.1). The shaft is the main component that sits inside the trachea, keeping the airway open. Flanges rest against the patient's neck and prevent the TT from migrating into the trachea. The 15-mm connector is located on the shaft or the inner cannula and is where the ventilator tubing or resuscitation bag attaches to the TT. The obturator is placed inside the TT and used during the TT insertion process. It is replaced with an inner cannula (if necessary) once inserted. The inner cannula is located inside the shaft of the TT and is a safety feature because it can be quickly removed and replaced if obstructed. TTs are curved and are commonly made of a synthetic material such as polyvinyl chloride, silicone, or polyurethane. The curved nature of the TT improves the ability of the tube to fit within the trachea. Metal tubes are rarely used today.

The pressure exerted by a TT against the neck creates the risk for medical device related pressure injuries (MDRPI). The AARC developed a tracheostomy bundle for presenting MDRPI (Mussa et al., 2021). The bundle consists of 4 components: (1) placement of a hydrocolloid dressing underneath the tracheostomy flange in the post procedure (trach creation) period, (2) removal of plate sutures within 7 days of the tracheostomy procedure, (3) placement of a polyurethane foam dressing after suture removal, and (4) neutral positioning of the head.

A TT is cuffed or uncuffed. A cuff on a TT is made of a balloon-like inflatable plastic, typically inflated with air, although there are brands that are inflated with liquid such as water or saline. When the cuff is inflated, it prevents the aspiration of mucous or regurgitated gastric contents into the trachea. Uncuffed tubes allow patients the ability to clear the airway, but they provide no protection from aspiration. It is also more difficult to use positive-pressure ventilation in patients with uncuffed TTs (Wiegand, 2017).

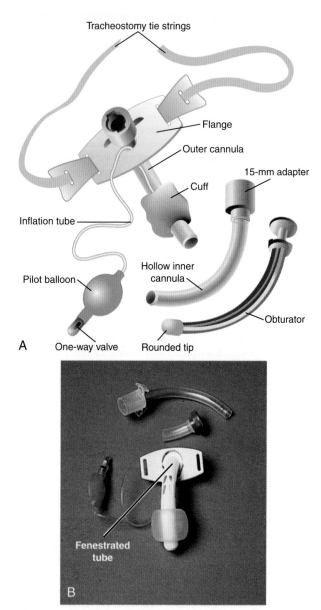

Fig. 75.1 (A) Parts of tracheostomy tube. (B) Fenestrated tracheostomy tube with cuff, inner cannula, decannulation plug, and pilot balloon. (From Harding MM, et al: *Medical-surgical nursing: assessment and management of clinical problems*, ed 11, St Louis, 2021, Mosby.)

There are speaking valves that can be used with TTs. The patient must have a cuffless or fenestrated TT in place or be able to tolerate the cuff being deflated without risk of respiratory distress or aspiration. The openings in fenestrated tubes allow air to flow from the lungs over the vocal cords. This type of TT gives patients the ability to verbalize needs, and such communication often provides psychological benefits to the patient.

Safety Guidelines

- Cuffs with speaking valves must be used with caution, and only in patients who can swallow without aspiration.
- Always monitor patients with tracheostomies for emergency events such as tube obstruction or dislodgement (Table 75.1).
- Stabilize TT at all times during tracheostomy care to prevent injury, unnecessary discomfort, or accidental extubation.

TABLE 75.1 Tracheostomy Emergencies

Emergency Type	Signs and Symptoms	Interventions
Tube dislodgement or decannulation	• Unable to pass suction catheter past the length of the tube • Presence of subcutaneous emphysema near stoma • Signs of respiratory distress • High-pressure alarm on ventilator • Flange of TT not flush with neck • Decreased SpO_2 • Patient able to speak around the TT	• Call for help. • If stoma is less than 1 week old, notify surgeon. • Perform bag-mask ventilation. • Prepare for intubation or surgical reinsertion of new TT. • If stoma is well established (typically greater than 1 week old), replace with a new TT, inserting at a 90-degree angle into the trachea, then angling downward another 90 degrees.

Continued

TABLE 75.1 Tracheostomy Emergencies—cont'd

Emergency Type	Signs and Symptoms	Interventions

Tube obstruction	• Respiratory distress
	• Unable to pass suction catheter
	• Resistance felt when using the self-inflating resuscitation bag
		• Ensure TT is in correct position.
		• Call for help.
		• Remove and inspect the inner cannula (if one present); clean or replace with a new one.
		• Established tracheostomy:
		  a Replace the TT (if changing inner cannula did not work).
		  b Patient may need bronchoscopy.
		• New tracheostomy:
		  a Prepare for oral endotracheal intubation, tracheostomy revision, or placement of a longer TT.

Hemorrhage	• More than minimal bleeding at stoma site	• Notify health care provider. • Provide oxygen, if not already in place.

TT, tracheostomy tube.
Data from Billington J, Luckett A: Care of the critically ill patient with a tracheostomy, *Nursing Standard* 34(2):59, 2019; Urden L, et al: *Priorities in critical care nursing,* ed 8, St Louis, 2020, Elsevier; Wiegand D: *AACN procedure manual for high acuity, progressive, and critical care,* ed 7, St Louis, 2017, Elsevier.

Delegation

The skill of performing tracheostomy care is not routinely delegated to assistive personnel (AP). The exception is in long-term care settings where patients have permanent or well-established TTs. The nurse is responsible for assessing a patient and evaluating for proper artificial airway care, often in collaboration with a respiratory therapist. The nurse is also responsible for educating the patient and caregivers regarding care of an established tracheostomy in the home. Direct the AP to:

- Immediately report any changes in patient's respiratory status, level of consciousness, confusion, restlessness or irritability, or level of comfort.
- Immediately report any dislodgement or excessive movement of the TT.
- Immediately report abnormal color of the tracheal stoma and drainage.

Collaboration

- Respiratory therapists are often responsible for the care of the mechanical ventilator, as well as performing TT care.
- Physical and occupational therapists need to be aware of the signs of TT dislodgment that can occur during their prescribed exercises.
- Speech therapists are often responsible for assessing the patient's ability to swallow and assisting a patient in learning how to speak with a TT in place.

Equipment

- Bedside table
- Person to assist with changing the tracheostomy tie/holder
- Towel
- Artificial airway suction supplies (see Skill 71)
- Oropharyngeal suction supplies (Yankauer catheter, saline)
- Sterile tracheostomy care kit, if available (be sure to collect supplies listed that are not available in kit)
- Three sterile 4 × 4-inch gauze pads
- Sterile cotton-tipped applicators
- Sterile hydrocolloid dressing or polyurethane foam dressing. (if not available can use precut and sewn surgical gauze dressing)
- Sterile basin
- Sterile normal saline or water
- Small sterile brush (or disposable inner cannula)
- Commercial tracheostomy holder or roll of twill tape, tracheostomy ties
- Scissors
- Inner cannula that fits the patient's TT (disposable if patient's is disposable)
- Cuff pressure manometer
- Pulse oximeter, end-tidal CO_2 detector

- Clean gloves (two pairs)
- Personal protective equipment (PPE): goggles, gown, or face shield if concern regarding contact with secretions
- Self-inflating manual resuscitation bag-valve device and appropriate-size mask
- Extra sterile tracheostomy kit
- Stethoscope
- Oxygen source
- 10-mL syringe
- Three-way stopcock
- Padded hemostats
- Tongue depressor
- Reintubation equipment (at the bedside in case of accidental TT dislodgment)
- Extra TTs (one same size as current patient tube, and one a size smaller, in case of accidental dislodgment)

STEP	RATIONALE
1 Perform preprocedure protocol.	
Assessment	
• Review the patient's electronic health record (EHR): time care was last performed; tolerance to procedure; type and size of TT and inner cannula, if present; any specific provider orders regarding the TT care; amount of air or fluid in TT cuff; and trends in patient vital signs and respiratory assessments.	Knowing the patient information guides the care delivery and ensures patient safety. Tracheostomy care is provided at least every 4 to 8 h and more often if indicated (e.g., increased airway or stoma secretions, infection [airway or stoma]) (Wiegand, 2017).
• Perform hand hygiene and apply clean gloves and other PPE as patient condition dictates.	Reduces transmission of microorganisms.

STEP	RATIONALE
• Observe for tube dislodgement/decannulation and tube obstruction; signs and symptoms of gurgling on expiration, decreased exhaled tidal volume (mechanically ventilated patient), signs and symptoms of inadequate ventilation (rising end-tidal carbon dioxide concentration [$EtCO_2$], patient-ventilator dyssynchrony, or dyspnea), or spasmodic coughing.	These findings can indicate an underinflated cuff or tube dislodgment (Wiegand, 2017).
• Observe for excess peristomal secretions, excess intratracheal secretions, soiled or damp tracheostomy ties, soiled or damp tracheostomy dressing, diminished airflow through TT, or signs and symptoms of airway obstruction requiring suctioning (see Skill 70).	Indicate need for tracheostomy care caused by presence of secretions at stoma site or within tracheostomy tube. Irritation of mucosa caused by tube itself can also cause increase in secretions (Wiegand, 2017). Assess every 4 h (Billington and Luckett, 2019).
• Observe skin around tracheal stoma, under TT flange, and under tracheal ties for pressure injury: blistering, erythema, drainage, or other discoloration.	Peristomal skin injuries are medical device related pressure injuries (MDRPIs) due to pressure from the tube, flange, or ties. These MDPRIs are one of the most common problems associated with tracheostomies, so patients should be closely monitored for this complication (Carroll et al., 2020).
• Assess patient's hydration status, humidity delivered to airway, status of any existing infection, patient's nutrition status, and ability to cough.	Determines factors that affect amount and consistency of secretions in tracheostomy and patient's ability to clear airway.

Continued

STEP	RATIONALE
• Assess patient's cardiopulmonary status, including pulse oximetry (SpO_2), $EtCO_2$, vital signs, respiratory effort, lung sounds, and level of consciousness. Keep pulse oximeter in place.	Provides baseline to determine patient response to and tolerance of therapy.
• Remove and dispose of gloves. Perform hand hygiene. Keep remaining PPE in place.	Reduces transmission of microorganisms.

Implementation

1	Have another nurse or respiratory therapist assist with procedure. Ensure they also perform hand hygiene, apply clean gloves, and don PPE as patient condition dictates (Wiegand, 2017). All PPE should remain in place until end of procedure.	Assisting with procedure prevents accidental dislodgment of TT.
2	Raise head of bed at least 30 degrees, unless contraindicated. Ensure patient is comfortable. Adjust bed to appropriate height and lower side rail on side nearest you. Ensure bed is locked.	Provides access to site and facilitates completion of procedure. Prepares patient for any required suctioning. Positioning may decrease risk of aspiration (American Association of Critical Care Nurses, 2017b, 2018).
3	Explain patient's need to participate, including trying not to cough when tape or holder is off TT, keeping hands down, and not pulling on staff or tubing.	Encourages cooperation, minimizes risks or accidental dislodgment, and reduces anxiety.

STEP	RATIONALE

CLINICAL JUDGMENT *Patients who do not have or cannot tolerate speaking valves may not be able to verbalize their wants, fears, anxieties, or needs. This impaired ability to communicate can lead to increased anxiety and apprehension. Communication aids should be offered to patients to allow them to ask questions or communicate their concerns (Billington and Luckett, 2019).*

CLINICAL JUDGMENT *At some agencies it is standard practice to have an extra TT that is the same size as the patient's current TT and a TT one size smaller at the bedside at all times in case there is an emergent need to replace the TT because of obstruction or dislodgement (Billington and Luckett, 2019; Higginson et al., 2016).*

STEP	RATIONALE
4 Perform hand hygiene. Apply clean/sterile gloves for suctioning (see Skill 71) and other PPE, if not already in place.	Reduces transmission of microorganisms.
5 Preoxygenate patient for 30 seconds or ask patient to take 5 to 6 deep breaths. Then suction tracheostomy (see Skill 71). Before removing gloves, remove soiled gauze or polyurethane foam tracheostomy dressing and discard. Hydrocolloid and polyurethane foam dressings may remain in place for a week depending on amount of tracheal secretions and manufacturer's directions,.	Removes secretions to avoid occluding outer cannula while inner cannula is removed. Reduces need for patient to cough.
6 Perform hand hygiene. Set up equipment:	Allows for smooth, organized completion of tracheostomy care. Tracheostomy care should be performed twice a day or every 8 h per agency protocol (Billington and Luckett, 2019; Masood et al., 2018).

Continued

STEP	RATIONALE
a Open sterile tracheostomy kit. Open two 4 × 4-inch gauze packages using aseptic technique and pour normal saline on gauze in one package. Leave gauze in second package dry. Open two cotton-tipped swab packages and pour normal saline on swab tip in one package. Do not recap normal saline.	Saline used for cleansing.
b Open sterile hydrocolloid, polyurethane foam or precut gauze dressing.	
c Open sterile basin and pour about 0.5 to 2 cm (0.2 to 1 inch) of normal saline into it.	
d Open small sterile brush package and place aseptically into sterile basin.	
e Prepare TT fixation device.	
(1) If using twill tape: Prepare length of twill tape long enough to go around patient's neck two times, about 60 to 75 cm (24 to 30 inches) for an adult. Cut ends on diagonal. Lay aside in dry area.	Cutting ends of tie on diagonal aids in inserting tie through eyelet.

STEP	RATIONALE
(2) If using commercially available TT holder, open package according to manufacturer directions.	
f Open inner cannula package (if new one is to be inserted, such as with disposable inner cannulas, or if patient does not tolerate being disconnected from oxygen source while cleaning reusable inner cannula).	
7 Apply sterile gloves. Keep dominant hand sterile throughout procedure.	Reduces transmission of microorganisms.
8 Remove oxygen source if present and if patient tolerates.	

CLINICAL JUDGMENT *Stabilize TT at all times to prevent injury, unnecessary discomfort, or accidental extubation. Instruct assistant to stabilize the TT using gloved hands.*

9 Cleanse tracheostomy with reusable inner cannula:	
a Clean TT either twice a day or every 8 h, depending upon agency policy (Billington and Luckett, 2019; Masood et al., 2018). While touching only outer aspect of tube, unlock and remove inner cannula with nondominant hand following line of tracheostomy. Drop inner cannula into normal saline basin.	Removes inner cannula for cleaning. Normal saline loosens secretions from inner cannula.

Continued

STEP	RATIONALE

CLINICAL JUDGMENT *If patient is on mechanical ventilation, instruct assistant to hold and stabilize TT and to remove the ventilator tube from the connection while you remove the inner cannula. This helps to ensure that the TT itself is not removed accidentally if difficulties removing the ventilator from the TT or removing the inner cannula from the TT occur.*

b	Place tracheostomy collar, T-tube, or ventilator oxygen source over outer cannula. (*Note:* You may not be able to attach T-tube and ventilator oxygen devices to all outer cannulas when inner cannula is removed.)	Maintains continuous supply of oxygen to patient as needed.

CLINICAL JUDGMENT *If patient is unable to tolerate being disconnected from the ventilator, replace the inner cannula with a clean new one and reattach the ventilator to the tracheostomy. Then proceed with cleaning the original inner cannula as described in the next steps and store it in a sterile container until the next inner cannula change (Wiegand, 2017).*

c	To prevent oxygen desaturation, quickly pick up inner cannula and use small brush to remove secretions inside and outside inner cannula.	Tracheostomy brush provides mechanical force to remove thick or dried secretions.
d	Hold inner cannula over basin and rinse with sterile normal saline, using nondominant (clean) hand to pour normal saline.	Removes secretions and normal saline from inner cannula.

STEP	RATIONALE
e Remove oxygen source, replace inner cannula (Fig. 75.2), and secure locking mechanism. Reapply ventilator, tracheostomy collar, or T-tube oxygen source. Hyperoxygenate (administer additional oxygen) patient if needed.	Secures inner cannula and reestablishes oxygen supply.
10 Cleanse tracheostomy with disposable inner cannula:	
a Remove new cannula from manufacturer packaging.	Prepares for change of inner cannula. Should be changed twice a day (Masood et al., 2018).
b While touching only outer aspect of tube, withdraw inner cannula and replace with new cannula. Lock into position.	Maintains a clean, sterile inner cannula for patient.

Continued

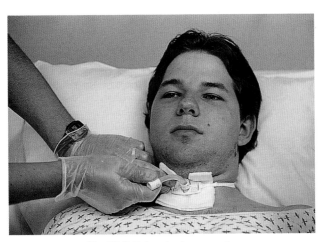

Fig. 75.2 Reinserting inner cannula.

STEP	RATIONALE

CLINICAL JUDGMENT *If patient on mechanical ventilation, instruct assistant to hold and stabilize TT, and remove the ventilator tube from the connection while you remove the inner cannula. This ensures that the TT itself is not removed accidentally if there are difficulties removing the ventilator from the TT or removing the inner cannula from the TT.*

STEP	RATIONALE
c Dispose of contaminated cannula in appropriate receptacle and reconnect TT to ventilator or oxygen supply.	Prevents transmission of infection. Restores oxygen delivery.
11 Using normal saline–saturated cotton-tipped swabs and 4 × 4-inch gauze, clean exposed outer cannula surfaces and around tracheal stoma under faceplate extending 5 to 10 cm (2 to 4 inches) in all directions from stoma. Clean in circular motion from stoma site outward with dominant hand to handle sterile supplies. Do not repeat action over previously cleaned area.	Aseptically removes secretions from stoma site. Moving in outward circle pulls mucus and other contaminants from stoma to periphery (Bolsega and Sole, 2018).
12 Using dry 4 × 4-inch gauze, pat skin lightly and expose outer cannula surfaces. Inspect condition of skin under tracheostomy flange.	Dry surfaces prohibit formation of moist environment for microorganism growth and skin excoriation (Wiegand, 2017). Area under flange common site for MDRPI.
13 Secure tracheostomy.	

CLINICAL JUDGMENT *Some agencies do not recommend changing the securement device for the first 72 h after insertion of the TT because of risk of stoma closure if the tube were to become dislodged accidentally (Wiegand, 2017).*

STEP	RATIONALE
a Tracheostomy tie/twill tape method:	
(1) As assistant continues to hold TT, cut old tracheostomy ties. Do not cut pilot balloon of cuff.	Secures TT to prevent dislodgement. If pilot balloon is cut, there is no ability to inflate cuff (Wiegand, 2017).

CLINICAL JUDGMENT Assistant must not release hold on TT until new ties are firmly tied. If working without an assistant, do not cut old ties until new ties are in place and securely tied (Harding et al., 2020). When working with an assistant and the ties are removed, this is a good time to clean the back of the patient's neck and assess patient's skin under TT flange and under the ties or tube holder, ensuring that skin is intact, free of pressure, and dry before applying securement device.

(2) Take prepared twill tape, insert one end of tie through faceplate eyelet, and pull ends even (Fig. 75.3).	Diagonal cuts ensure ease of threading end of tie through holes of eyelet (Wiegand, 2017).

Continued

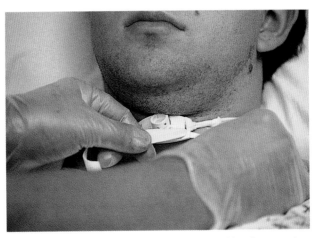

Fig. 75.3 Replacing tracheostomy ties. Do not remove old tracheostomy ties until new ones are secure.

STEP	RATIONALE
(3) Slide both ends of tie behind head and around neck to the other eyelet and insert one tie through second eyelet.	
(4) Pull snugly.	Secures TT.
(5) Tie ends securely in double square knot, allowing space for insertion of only one loose or two snug finger widths between tie and neck.	One finger width of slack prevents ties from being too tight when tracheostomy dressing is in place. Prevents movement of TT into lower airway (Wiegand, 2017).
(6) Insert new hydrocolloid, foam or a 4 × 4–inch gauze precut tracheostomy dressing under clean neck plate. Option: if using gauze dressing apply barrier cream around stoma, if ordered. (see illustration). (Fig. 75.4).	Dressing Absorbs drainage. and protect underlying skin. Dressing prevents pressure on clavicle heads (Bolsega and Sole, 2018; Wiegand, 2017). However, gauze dressings may retain secretions and keep the area moist, leading to increased risk of skin breakdown. Barrier cream helps prevent skin breakdown around the stoma (Carroll et al., 2020).
b TT commercial holder method:	
(1) Instruct assistant to continue holding TT in place. When an assistant is not available, leave old TT holder in place until new device is secure.	Ensures that tracheostomy stays in correct position.

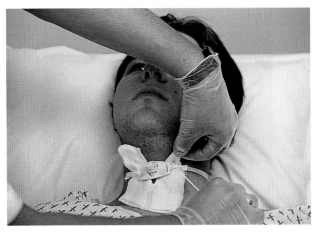

Fig. 75.4 Applying tracheostomy gauze dressing.

STEP	RATIONALE
(2) Align strap under patient's neck. Be sure that Velcro attachments are on either side of TT.	
(3) Place narrow end of ties under and through faceplate eyelets. Pull ends even and secure with Velcro closures (Fig. 75.5).	Ensures proper securement of TT.
(4) Verify that there is space for only one loose or two snug finger widths to be inserted under neck strap.	Ensures proper securement of TT without securement device being too tight.

Continued

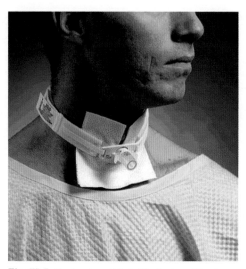

Fig. 75.5 Tracheostomy tube holder in place. (Courtesy Dale Medical Products, Plainesville, MA.)

STEP	RATIONALE
(5) Follow step 13a(6) to apply hydrocolloid, foam or a 4 × 4–inch gauze precut tracheostomy dressing. If using gauze dressing, Apply barrier cream to skin of stoma, if ordered.	Absorbs drainage. Dressing prevents pressure on clavicle heads (Bolsega and Sole, 2018; Wiegand, 2017). However, gauze dressings may retain secretions and keep the area moist, leading to increased risk of skin breakdown. Barrier cream helps prevent skin breakdown around the stoma (Carroll et al., 2020).

CLINICAL JUDGMENT *Never cut a regular gauze pad to fit around TT. The cut fibers from the gauze pad may shed fibers that could be inhaled by patient and lead to pulmonary damage or infection. Use a manufactured pad for this purpose (Wiegand, 2017). Foam dressings have a key hole opening to fit easily around stoma and are ideal be used in patients with excess secretions (Bolsega and Sole, 2018).*

STEP	RATIONALE
14 Ensure the TT is midline and secure and that no excess traction is applied. Assistant may release TT at this time.	Prevents the development of complications such as tracheal erosion or skin ulcerations (Wiegand, 2017).
15 Perform oral care with toothbrush or oral swabs and chlorhexidine rinse. Suction orally if needed. Perform subglottic suctioning if TT equipped with that capability.	Using chlorhexidine may decrease patient risk of developing a ventilator-associated event/ventilator-associated pneumonia and promotes patient comfort (Pozuelo-Carrascosa et al., 2020) Wiegand, 2017).
16 Measure cuff pressure with the manometer; add or remove air/saline/water from cuff to maintain pressure between 20 and 25 mm Hg.	complet at least once per shift or as often as 2 to 4 h (follow agency policy). Prevents aspiration of oral secretions. Prevents tracheal damage (Billington and Luckett, 2019; Wiegand, 2017).

CLINICAL JUDGMENT *If cuff is deflated during use of a speaking valve, then inflate cuff once the use of the valve is finished and measure cuff pressures. Perform oral and/or subglottic suctioning before deflating the cuff (Pozuelo-Carrascosa et al., 2020).*

17 Reposition patient comfortably, with head of bed remaining elevated at least 30 degrees (unless contraindicated) and assess respiratory status.	Promotes comfort. Some patients require posttracheostomy care suctioning. Keeping the head of the bed at 30 degrees helps to decrease risk of ventilator-associated pneumonia (Wiegand, 2017).
18 Be sure that oxygen- or humidification-delivery sources are in place and set at correct levels.	Humidification provides moisture for airway, makes it easier to suction secretions, and decreases risk of mucus plugs.

Continued

STEP	RATIONALE
19 Replace cap on reusable normal saline bottles. Store reusable liquids, date container, and store unused supplies in appropriate place.	Once opened, normal saline is considered free of bacteria for 24 h.
20 Perform postprocedure protocol.	
21 Evaluate patient response:	
a Compare respiratory assessments before and after tracheostomy care.	Determines effectiveness of tracheostomy care and patient's tolerance of procedure.
b Assess fit of newly secured TT and ask patient whether tube feels comfortable. Palpate tube for pulsation for air under the skin.	Tracheostomy ties are uncomfortable and place patient at risk for tissue injury when they are too loose or too tight. A pulsating feeling in the TT can indicate early signs of innominate artery erosion. Air under skin suggests presence of subcutaneous emphysema.
c Inspect inner and outer cannulas for secretions.	Presence of secretions on cannulas indicates need for more frequent tracheostomy care.
d Assess stoma, surrounding skin, and skin under ties/tube holder for pressure injury, inflammation, edema, bleeding, or discolored secretions.	Broken skin places patient at risk for infection. Stoma infection requires change in tracheostomy skin care plan.
e Observe for excessive phonation, presence of gastric secretions in airway secretions, or tracheoesophageal fistula.	Occurs with inadequate or excessive cuff inflation.

Recording and Reporting

- Record respiratory, stoma, and skin assessments before and after care; type and size of TT and inner cannula; frequency and extent of care, including inner cannula, dressing, and securement device changes; type, color, and amount of secretions; patient tolerance and understanding of procedure; and any interventions performed in event of unexpected outcomes.
- Document evaluation of patient/family learning.
- Report any unexpected outcomes to health care provider or nurse in charge.
- During hand-off, report patient status, frequency of care, tolerance and response to care, TT size and type of securement device, and last time care was performed.

UNEXPECTED OUTCOMES	RELATED INTERVENTIONS
1 Cuff leak develops.	• Verify position of tube. • Notify respiratory therapy, and follow agency policy.
2 Inflammation of tracheostomy stoma or pressure area around TT.	• Increase frequency of tracheostomy care. • Apply topical antibacterial solution; apply bacterial barrier if ordered. • Apply hydrocolloid, foam or transparent dressing around stoma to protect skin from breakdown. • Consult with skin care specialist.

Continued

UNEXPECTED OUTCOMES	RELATED INTERVENTIONS
3 Accidental decannulation/ dislodgement.	• Call for help.
	• Notify health care provider and respiratory therapist immediately.
	• Prepare for replacement of old TT with new tube. Some experienced nurses or respiratory therapists may be able to reinsert TT quickly.
	• Same-size endotracheal tube can be inserted in stoma in an emergency.
	• Insert suction catheter to confirm that new tube is in trachea.
	• Be prepared to manually ventilate patients in whom respiratory distress develops with self-inflating resuscitation bag until tracheostomy is replaced.
4 Respiratory distress from mucus plugs in cannula.	• Remove inner cannula if applicable for cleaning or suction cannula.
	• Notify health care provider if TT requires replacement.

Urinary Catheter Insertion: Straight or Indwelling Catheter

Urinary catheterization (straight and indwelling) is the placement of a hollow flexible tube into the bladder to remove urine. Indwelling urinary catheterization may be short term (≤2 weeks) or long term (>14 days) (Fekete, 2021). Intermittent urinary catheterization is the insertion of a flexible single-use straight catheter, indicated for urinary retention and specimen collection. Catheterization is an invasive procedure that requires the order of a health care provider and use of strict sterile technique. The use of an indwelling urinary catheter is associated with numerous complications, particularly catheter-associated urinary tract infection (CAUTI). This results in patient discomfort, increased hospital stays (by as much as 2 to 5 additional days), increased costs, and mortality (from sepsis). Other complications related to indwelling catheterization include prostatitis; cystitis; bladder stones; damage to the kidneys, the bladder, and the urethra; and development of antibiotic resistance (Schaeffer et al., 2021a).

Because of the risk of CAUTI, there are recommendations for the appropriate use of an indwelling catheter (Gould et al., 2019):

- Patient has acute urinary retention or bladder outlet obstruction.
- Need for accurate measurements of urinary output in critically ill patients.
- Perioperative use for selected surgical procedures (e.g., urologic, anticipated prolonged surgery).
- To assist in healing of open sacral or perineal wounds in incontinent patients.
- Patient requires prolonged immobilization.
- End-of-life care.

The steps for inserting an indwelling and an intermittent single-use straight catheter are the same. The difference lies in the inflation of a balloon to keep the indwelling catheter in place and the presence of a closed drainage system. Urinary catheters may have up to three lumens: single-lumen catheters for intermittent catheterization, double for indwelling catheters (one lumen for urinary drainage and a second lumen for balloon inflation), and triple-lumen catheters for continuous bladder irrigation or to instill medications into the bladder. A nurse is responsible for maintaining the sterility of the urinary tract during catheter insertions and in the ongoing care and maintenance of indwelling catheters.

Safety Guidelines

- Insert catheter only for appropriate indications and to reduce incidence of CAUTI; leave in place only as long as needed (Gould et al., 2019).
- Maintain personal safety in handling urine of patients receiving hazardous drugs.
- Inappropriate use of an indwelling catheter includes: as a substitute for nursing care of patient or resident with incontinence; as a means of obtaining urine for culture or other diagnostic tests when patient can voluntarily void; or for prolonged postoperative duration without appropriate indications (Gould et al., 2019).

Delegation

The skill of inserting a straight or indwelling urinary catheter usually cannot be delegated to assistive personnel (AP). The exception is in long-term care facilities where AP have received specialized training. Direct the AP to:

- Assist with patient positioning, focus lighting for the procedure, maintain privacy, empty urine from collection bag, and help with perineal care.
- Report postprocedure patient discomfort or fever.
- Report abnormal color, odor, and amount of urine in drainage bag, and whether the catheter is leaking or causes pain.

Collaboration

- Health care provider and rehabilitation services can assist with management of long-term indwelling catheters.
- Wound ostomy care nurses (WOCN) provide expertise if a catheter is being used for incontinence.

Equipment

- Catheter kit containing sterile items (Note: Contents of catheter kits vary.)
- Straight catheterization kit: single-lumen catheter (12 Fr to 14 Fr), drapes (one fenestrated [has an opening in the center]), sterile gloves, lubricant, cleansing solution incorporated in an applicator or to be added to cotton balls, and specimen container and label
- Indwelling catheterization kit : double-lumen catheter, drapes (one fenestrated [has an opening in the center]), sterile gloves, lubricant, antiseptic cleansing solution incorporated in an applicator or to be added to cotton balls, specimen container and label, and a prefilled

syringe with sterile water (to inflate balloon) (Note: Some kits contain a catheter with attached drainage bag; others contain only a catheter; others have no catheter.)

▪ Sterile drainage tubing and bag (if not included in indwelling catheter insertion kit)
▪ Catheter fixation device (i.e. StatLock® or Stayfix devices).
▪ Extra sterile gloves and catheter (optional, if needed)
▪ Clean gloves
▪ Basin with warm water, washcloth, towel, and soap for perineal care
▪ Flashlight or other additional light source
▪ Bath blanket, waterproof absorbent pad
▪ Measuring container for urine

STEP	RATIONALE
1 Perform preprocedure protocol.	

Assessment

• Review patient's electronic health record (EHR), including health care provider's order and nurses' notes. Note previous catheterization, including catheter size, response of patient, and time of catheterization.	Identifies purpose of inserting catheter (such as for measurement of postvoid residual urine (PVR), preparation for surgery, or specimen collection) and potential difficulty with catheter insertion.
• Review EHR for any pathologic conditions that may impair passage of catheter (e.g., enlarged prostate gland in men, urethral strictures).	Obstruction of urethra may prevent passage of catheter into bladder.
• Assess patient's biological gender and age.	Assists with selection of catheter size.
• Ask patient to describe history of allergies: known type(s) of allergies (including latex and adhesives) and normal allergic reaction(s). Check patient's allergy wristband.	Procedure may involve exposure to latex and adhesive. Use latex-free catheter if patient has a sensitivity.

Continued

STEP	RATIONALE
• Perform hand hygiene. Assess patient's weight, level of consciousness, developmental level, ability to cooperate, and mobility.	Determines positioning to use for catheterization; indicates how much help is needed to properly position patient, ability of patient to cooperate during procedure, and level of explanation needed.
• Assess for pain and bladder fullness. Palpate bladder over symphysis pubis or use bladder scanner (if available) (see Skill 5).	Palpation of full bladder causes pain and/or urge to void, indicating full or overfull bladder.
• Apply clean gloves. Inspect perineal region, observing for perineal anatomical landmarks, erythema, drainage or discharge, and odor. Remove and dispose of gloves and perform hand hygiene.	Assessment of perineum (especially female perineal landmarks) improves accuracy and speed of catheter insertion. Determines whether more frequent perineal care may be required. Reduces transmission of microorganisms.

Implementation

1 Check patient's plan of care for size and type of catheter (if this is a reinsertion). Use smallest-size catheter possible. Size 14 Fr to 16 Fr is most common for adults; for older adults, 12 Fr to 14 Fr; larger sizes (20 Fr to 22 Fr) are needed in special circumstances, such as after urological surgery or in the presence of gross hematuria.	Ensures that patient receives correct size and type of catheter. Larger catheter diameters increase the risk for urethral trauma. Small catheter allows for adequate drainage of periurethral glands.
2 Perform hand hygiene.	Reduces transmission of microorganisms.

STEP	RATIONALE
3 Raise bed to appropriate working height. If side rails are in use, raise side rail on opposite side of bed and lower side rail on working side.	Promotes good body mechanics. Use of side rails in this manner promotes patient safety.
4 Have patient log roll or bend knees and raise hips to place a waterproof pad under patient.	Prevents soiling bed linen.

CLINICAL JUDGMENT *Obtain assistance from additional staff to position and support patients who have mobility restrictions or who are weak, frail, obese, or confused.*

---

5 Position patient:	
a Female patient:	
(1) Assist into dorsal recumbent position (on back with knees flexed). Ask patient to relax thighs so that hips can be gently rotated.	Exposes perineum and allows hip joints to be externally rotated.
(2) Alternative female position: position side-lying (Sims) position with upper leg flexed at knee and hip. Support patient with pillows if necessary to maintain position.	Alternative position is more comfortable if patient cannot abduct leg at hip joint (e.g., patient has arthritic joints or contractures, or recent hip surgery).
b Male patient:	
(1) Position supine with legs extended and thighs slightly abducted.	Comfortable position for patient aids in visualization of penis.

Continued

STEP	RATIONALE
6 Drape patient:	Protects patient dignity and privacy by avoiding unnecessary exposure of body parts.
a Female patient: (1) Drape with bath blanket. Place blanket diamond-fashion over patient, with one corner at patient's midsection, side corners over each thigh and abdomen, and last corner over perineum b Male patient: (1) Drape patient by covering upper part of body with small sheet or towel; drape with separate sheet or bath blanket so that only perineum is exposed.	
7 Position portable light to illuminate genitals or have assistant available to hold light.	Adequate visualization of urinary meatus assists with accuracy of catheter insertion.
8 Apply clean gloves. Clean perineal area with soap and water, rinse, and dry. Use fingers to retract tissues for examining patient and identifying urinary meatus. Remove and discard gloves. Perform hand hygiene.	Hygiene before initiating aseptic catheter insertion removes secretions, urine, and feces that could be incidentally inserted into urethral canal and increase risk for CAUTI. Perform hand hygiene immediately before catheter insertion (Gould et al., 2019).

STEP	RATIONALE
9 Open outer wrapping of catheterization kit. Place inner wrapped catheter kit tray on clean, accessible surface such as bedside table or, if possible, between the patient's open legs. Patient size and positioning dictate exact placement.	Provides easy access to supplies during catheter insertion. Tray provides a sterile field.
10 Remove the cover of the tray by taking the edge of the outer cover, peeling it away to open the tray, and ensuring hand does not extend over the sterile contents (see Skill 68).	Sequence prevents reaching over sterile field.
a Indwelling catheterization open system: *Open separate package containing drainage bag, check to m*ake sure that clamp on drainage port is closed, and place drainage bag and tubing in easily accessible location. Open outer package of sterile catheter, maintaining sterility of inner wrapper.	Open drainage bag systems have separate sterile packaging for sterile catheter, drainage bag and tubing, and insertion kit.
b Indwelling catheterization closed system: All supplies are in sterile tray and arranged in sequence of use.	Closed drainage bag systems have catheter preattached to drainage tubing and bag.

Continued

STEP	RATIONALE
c Straight catheterization: All needed supplies are in sterile tray that contains supplies and can be used for urine collection.	
11 Perform hand hygiene. Apply sterile gloves. *Note:* Special gloves or double gloving needed if patient is receiving hazardous drugs.	Maintains surgical asepsis. If patient is receiving chemotherapy, double gloving is needed (Oncology Nursing Society, 2018).
12 *Option:* Apply sterile drape with ungloved hands when drape is packed as first item. Touch only 2.5 cm (1-inch) edges of drape. Then apply sterile gloves.	Maintains surgical asepsis.
13 Drape perineum, keeping gloves and working surface of drape sterile.	Sterile drapes provide a sterile field for catheterization tasks.
a Drape female patient:	
(1) Pick up square sterile drape touching only edges (2.5 cm [1 inch]).	
(2) Allow drape to unfold without touching unsterile surfaces. Allow top edge of drape (2.5 to 5 cm [1 to 2 inches]) to form cuff over both gloved hands.	When creating cuff over sterile gloved hands, sterility of gloves and workspace is maintained.

STEP	RATIONALE
(3) Place drape with shiny side down on bed between patient's thighs. Slip cuffed edge just under buttocks while asking patient to lift hips. Take care not to touch contaminated surfaces or patient's thighs with sterile gloves. If gloves are contaminated, remove and apply new pair.	
(4) *Option:* Pick up fenestrated sterile drape out of tray. Allow drape to unfold without touching unsterile surfaces. Allow top edge of drape to form cuff over both gloved hands. Apply drape over perineum so that opening is over exposed labia.	Note: Use of fenestrated drape designed to provide additional sterile field, but positioning can create risk of contaminating gloves. Opening in drape creates sterile field around labia.
b Drape male patient:	
(1) Use of square drape is optional; you may apply fenestrated drape instead.	

Continued

STEP	RATIONALE
(2) Pick up edges of square drape and allow to unfold without touching unsterile surfaces. Place over thighs, with shiny side down, just below penis. Take care not to touch contaminated surfaces with sterile gloves.	
(3) Place fenestrated drape with opening centered over penis.	
14 Place sterile tray with cleaning solution (premoistened swab sticks or cotton balls, forceps, and solution), lubricant, catheter, and prefilled syringe for inflating balloon (indwelling catheterization only) on sterile drape close to patient. Arrange any remaining sterile supplies on sterile field, maintaining sterility of gloves.	Provides easy access to supplies during catheter insertion and helps to maintain aseptic technique. Appropriate placement is determined by size of patient and position during catheterization.
a If kit contains sterile cotton balls, open package of sterile antiseptic solution and pour over cotton balls. Some kits contain package of premoistened swab sticks. Open end of package for easy access.	Use of sterile supplies and antiseptic solution reduces risk of CAUTI (Gould et al., 2019).

STEP	RATIONALE
b Open sterile specimen container if specimen is to be obtained.	Makes container accessible to receive urine from catheter if specimen is needed.
c For indwelling catheterization, open sterile inner wrapper of catheter and leave catheter on sterile field or in tray. If part of closed-system kit, remove tray with catheter and preattached drainage bag and place on sterile drape. Make sure that clamp on drainage port of bag is closed. If needed (and if part of sterile tray) attach catheter to drainage tubing.	Indwelling catheterization trays vary. Some have preattached catheters, others need to be attached but are part of the sterile tray, others do not have catheter or drainage system as part of tray.
d Open packet of lubricant and squeeze onto sterile field. Lubricate catheter tip by dipping into water-soluble gel 2.5 to 5 cm (1 to 2 inches) for women and 12.5 to 17.5 cm (5 to 7 inches) for men.	Lubrication minimizes trauma to urethra and discomfort during catheter insertion. Male catheter needs enough lubricant to cover length of catheter inserted.

CLINICAL JUDGMENT Pretesting a balloon on an indwelling catheter by injecting fluid from the prefilled sterile normal saline syringe into the balloon port is **not recommended**. Testing the balloon may distort and stretch it and lead to damage, causing increased trauma on insertion.

Continued

STEP	RATIONALE
15 Clean urethral meatus:	
a Female patient:	
(1) Separate labia with fingers of nondominant hand (now contaminated) to fully expose urethral meatus.	Optimal visualization of urethral meatus is possible.
(2) Maintain position of nondominant hand throughout procedure.	Closure of labia during cleaning means that area is contaminated and requires cleaning procedure to be repeated.
(3) Holding forceps in dominant hand and while maintaining sterility, pick up one moistened cotton ball or pick up one swab stick at a time. Clean labia and urinary meatus from clitoris toward anus. Use new cotton ball or swab for each area that you clean. Clean by wiping far labial fold, near labial fold, and last, directly over center of urethral meatus (Fig. 76.1)	Front-to-back cleaning moves from area of least contamination toward highly contaminated area. Follows principles of medical asepsis. Dominant gloved hand remains sterile, with only cotton balls or swabs touching the labia/meatus during cleaning.

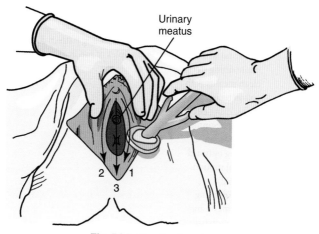

Fig. 76.1 Clean female perineum.

STEP	RATIONALE
b Male patient: (1) With nondominant hand (now contaminated) retract foreskin (if uncircumcised) and gently grasp penis at shaft just below glans. Hold shaft of penis at right angle to body. This hand remains in this position for remainder of procedure.	When grasping shaft of penis, avoid pressure on dorsal surface to prevent compression of urethra. Losing grasp during cleaning means that area is contaminated and requires cleaning procedure to be repeated.

Continued

STEP	RATIONALE
(2) Using dominant hand and while maintaining sterility, clean meatus with cotton balls/swab sticks, using circular strokes, beginning at meatus and working outward in spiral motion (Fig. 76.2).	Circular cleaning pattern follows principles of medical asepsis.
(3) Repeat cleaning three times using clean cotton ball/swab stick each time.	

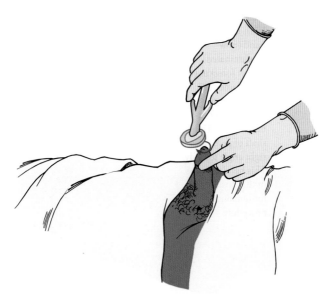

Fig. 76.2 Clean male urinary meatus.

STEP	RATIONALE
16 Pick up and hold catheter 7.5 to 10 cm (3 to 4 inches) from catheter tip with catheter loosely coiled in palm of hand. If catheter is not attached to drainage bag, make sure to position urine tray so that end of catheter can be placed there once insertion begins.	Holding catheter near tip allows for easier manipulation during insertion. Coiling catheter in palm prevents distal end from striking nonsterile surface.
17 Insert catheter. Explain to patient that feeling of discomfort or pressure may be experienced as catheter is inserted into urethra. This sensation is normal and will go away quickly.	Helps to minimize patient anxiety.
a Female patient:	
(1) Ask patient to bear down gently and slowly insert catheter through urethral meatus (Fig. 76.3).	Bearing down may help visualize urinary meatus and promotes relaxation of external urinary sphincter, aiding in catheter insertion.
(2) Advance catheter total of 5 to 7.5 cm (2 to 3 inches) or until urine flows out of catheter. Stop advancing with straight catheter. When urine appears, advance catheter another 2.5 to 5 cm (1 to 2 inches) for indwelling catheter. Do not use force to insert catheter.	Urine flow indicates that catheter tip is in bladder or lower urethra.

Continued

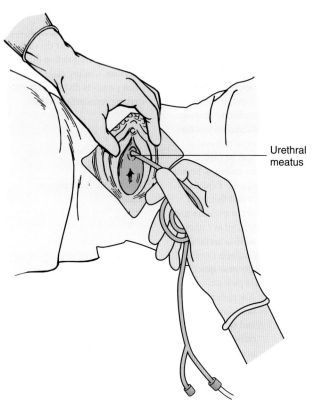

Urethral
meatus

Fig. 76.3 Insert catheter into female urinary meatus.

STEP	RATIONALE
(3) Release labia and hold catheter securely with nondominant hand.	Prevents accidental expulsion of catheter from the patient's bladder.

STEP	RATIONALE
b Male patient:	
(1) Lift penis to position perpendicular (90 degrees) to patient's body and apply gentle upward traction (Fig. 76.4).	Straightens urethra to ease catheter insertion.
(2) Ask patient to bear down as if to void and slowly insert catheter through urethral meatus.	Relaxation of external sphincter aids in insertion of catheter.
(3) Advance catheter 17 to 22.5 cm (7 to 9 inches) or until urine flows out end of catheter. Do not use force to advance catheter.	Length of male urethra varies. Flow of urine indicates that tip of catheter is in bladder or urethra but not necessarily that balloon part of indwelling catheter is in bladder.

Continued

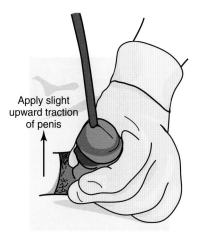

Apply slight upward traction of penis

Fig. 76.4 Insert catheter into male urinary meatus.

STEP	RATIONALE
(4) Stop advancing with straight catheter. When urine appears in indwelling catheter, advance it to bifurcation (inflation and deflation ports exposed) (Fig. 76.5)	Further advancement of indwelling catheter to bifurcation of drainage and balloon inflation port ensures that balloon part of catheter is not still in prostatic urethra.
(5) Lower penis and hold catheter securely in nondominant hand.	Prevents accidental expulsion of catheter from the patient's bladder.
18 Allow bladder to empty fully unless agency policy restricts maximum volume of urine drained (see agency policy).	There is no definitive evidence regarding whether there is benefit in limiting maximal volume drained.

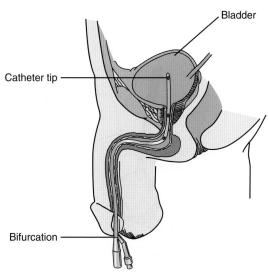

Fig. 76.5 Male anatomy with correct catheter insertion to bifurcation.

STEP	RATIONALE
19 Collect urine specimen as needed. Fill specimen container to 20 to 30 mL by holding end of catheter over the cup. Set container aside. Keep end of catheter sterile.	Sterile specimen for culture analysis can be obtained.
20 Option for straight catheterization: When urine stops flowing, withdraw catheter slowly and smoothly with dominant hand until removed.	Minimizes trauma to urethra.
21 For indwelling catheter: Inflate catheter balloon with amount of fluid designated by manufacturer.	Indwelling catheter balloon should not be underinflated. Underinflation causes balloon distortion and potential bladder damage.
a Continue to hold catheter with nondominant hand.	Holding on to catheter before inflating balloon prevents expulsion of catheter from urethra.
b With free dominant hand, connect prefilled syringe to injection port at end of catheter.	Tight connection needed to instill solution.
c Slowly inject total amount of solution.	Full amount of solution needed to inflate balloon properly.

CLINICAL JUDGMENT *If patient reports sudden pain during inflation of balloon or when resistance is felt during inflation, stop inflation, allow the fluid from the balloon to flow back into the syringe, advance catheter farther, and reinflate balloon. The balloon may have been inflating in the urethra. If pain continues, remove catheter and notify the health care provider.*

Continued

STEP	RATIONALE
d After inflating catheter balloon, release catheter from nondominant hand. *Gently* pull catheter until resistance is felt. Then advance catheter slightly.	By moving catheter slightly back into bladder, pressure on bladder neck is avoided.
e Connect drainage tubing to catheter if it is not already preconnected.	
22 Secure indwelling catheter with catheter fixation device. Leave enough slack to allow leg movement. Attach securement device at tubing just above catheter bifurcation.	Securing catheter reduces risk of movement, urethral erosion, CAUTI, or accidental catheter removal (Gould et al., 2019; McNeill, 2017). Attaching securement device at catheter bifurcation prevents occlusion of catheter.

CLINICAL JUDGMENT *Avoid use of adhesive tape for securing indwelling catheter because doing so creates risk of medical adhesive--related skin injury (Fumarola et al., 2020).*

---

a. Female patient: (1) Secure catheter tubing to inner thigh, allowing enough slack to prevent tension.	
b. Male patient: (1) Secure catheter tubing to upper thigh or lower abdomen (with penis directed toward chest). Allow slack in catheter so that movement does not create tension on catheter.	Anchoring catheter reduces traction on urethra and minimizes urethral injury (Gould et al., 2019; McNeill, 2017).

STEP	RATIONALE
(2) If retracted, replace foreskin over glans penis.	Leaving foreskin retracted can cause discomfort and penial edema, which can harm the patient.
23 Fasten drainage tubing to edge of mattress, using clip provided. Position drainage bag below level of bladder by attaching to bedframe (most have a notch/area for this purpose) (Gould et al., 2019). *Do not attach to side rails of bed and do not rest on floor.*	Keeping the collection bag below the level of the bladder at all times prevents backflow into bladder, which can cause risk for CAUTI (Gould et al., 2019). Bags attached to movable objects such as side rail increase risk for urethral trauma from pulling or accidental dislodgement.
24 Check to ensure that there is no obstruction to urine flow. Coil excess tubing on bed and fasten to bottom sheet with clip or another securement device.	Keeping the catheter and collecting tube free from kinking may reduce risk of CAUTI (Gould et al., 2019).
25 Provide perineal hygiene as needed. Assist patient to comfortable position.	Promotes patient comfort.
26 Label and bag specimen according to agency policy. Label specimen in presence of patient (The Joint Commission, 2021b). Have specimen sent to laboratory as soon as possible.	Fresh urine specimen ensures more accurate findings. Labeling ensures that diagnostic results will be connected to correct patient.
27 Measure urine and record.	Provides baseline for urine output.
28 Perform postprocedure protocol.	
29 Evaluate patient response: a Palpate bladder for distention or use bladder scan (see Skill 5) per agency protocol.	Determines whether distention is relieved.

Continued

STEP	RATIONALE
b During routine perineal hygiene inspect condition of perineal area and note any drainage.	Detects early signs of infection.
c Ask patient to describe level of comfort and whether sensation of bladder fullness was relieved.	Determines whether patient's sensation of discomfort or fullness has been relieved.
d Indwelling catheter: Observe character and amount of urine in drainage system and ensure that there is no urine leaking from catheter or tubing connections.	Determines whether urine is flowing adequately. Prevents injury to patient's skin and ensures closed sterile system.

Recording and Reporting

- Record reason for catheterization, type and size of catheter inserted, amount of fluid used to inflate balloon, specimen collection (if applicable), appearance of periurethral area, characteristics and amount of urine, and patient's response to procedure.
- Record intake and output on flow sheet record.
- Record evaluation of patient learning.
- During hand-offs, report reason for catheterization, type and size of catheter inserted, specimen collection, and verify it was sent to the laboratory (if applicable), characteristics and amount of urine, patient's response to procedure, and any education.
- Report to health care provider persistent catheter-related pain, change in urine appearance and discomfort.

UNEXPECTED OUTCOMES	RELATED INTERVENTIONS
1 Catheter goes into vagina.	• Leave catheter in vagina (allows for visualization of appropriate insertion site). • Clean urinary meatus again. Using another catheter kit, reinsert sterile catheter into meatus (check agency policy). *Note:* If gloves become contaminated, start procedure again. • Remove catheter in vagina after successful insertion of second catheter.
2 Sterility is broken during catheterization.	• Replace gloves if contaminated and start over. • If patient touches sterile field but equipment and supplies remain sterile, avoid touching that part of sterile field. • If equipment and/or supplies become contaminated, replace with sterile items or start over with new sterile kit.
3 Patient reports bladder discomfort, and catheter is patent as evidenced by adequate urine flow.	• Check catheter to ensure that there is no traction on it. • Notify health care provider. Patient may be experiencing bladder spasms or symptoms of urinary tract infection. • Monitor catheter output for color, clarity, odor, and amount.

Urinary Indwelling Catheter Care and Removal

While an indwelling catheter is in place, ongoing monitoring for signs of a urinary tract infection (UTI) along with proper cleansing of the external portion of the catheter and the patient's perineum are necessary to reduce risk of infection. Maintaining a closed drainage system is also essential to reduce entrance of microorganisms into the urinary tract. Timely removal of indwelling catheters has been shown to reduce the risk of catheter-associated UTI (CAUTI)(Schaeffer et al., 2021a). When removing a catheter, always be sure that the catheter balloon is fully deflated to minimize trauma to the urethra.

Evidence is unclear whether the practice of clamping a catheter to achieve bladder fullness for several minutes before removal improves bladder function after removal (Gould et al., 2019). A review of studies showed that catheter clamping before removal was not necessary for short-term patients because clamping carries the risk of complications such as prolonging urinary catheter retention and urinary tract injury (Wang et al., 2016). In a study involving hysterectomy patients bladder reconditioning through indwelling urinary catheter clamping did not restore bladder function in patients after radical hysterectomy (Gong et al., 2017).

All patients should have their voiding monitored after catheter removal for at least 24 to 48 h by using a voiding record or bladder diary to record the time and amount of each voiding, including any incontinence. A bladder scanner can monitor bladder functioning by measuring postvoid residual urine (PVR) (see Skill 5). Abdominal pain and distention, a sensation of incomplete emptying, incontinence, constant dribbling of urine, and voiding in very small amounts can indicate inadequate bladder emptying that requires intervention. Symptoms of infection can develop 2 days or more after catheter removal. Always inform patients about the risk for infection, prevention measures, and signs and symptoms that need to be reported immediately to the health care provider.

Safety Guidelines

- Maintain safe infection control practices in handling urine for patients receiving hazardous drugs (see agency policy). Use eye and/or face protection if liquid could splash (e.g., during emptying of urine drainage bag or obtaining sample) and always in the event of spills (Oncology Nursing Society [ONS], 2018)

Delegation

The skill of performing routine catheter care can be delegated to assistive personnel (AP). The skill of removing an indwelling catheter can be delegated to AP (see agency policy); however, a patient's status must first be assessed and order verified by an RN. Direct the AP to:

- Report characteristics of the urine (color, clarity, odor, and amount) before and after removal.
- Report the condition of the patient's genital area (e.g., color, rashes, open areas, odor, soiling from fecal incontinence, trauma to tissues around urinary meatus).
- Check size of balloon and syringe needed to deflate balloon and report if balloon does not deflate, and/or if there is bleeding after removal.
- Report time and amount of first voiding after catheter is removed and if patient complains of fever, chills, burning, flank pain, back pain, and blood in the urine (signs of kidney infection).
- Report patient complaints of fever, dysuria, hematuria, urgency, frequency, lower abdominal pain, change in mental status, and lethargy (signs of bladder infection).

Collaboration

- Collaborate with wound/ostomy care nurse (WOCN) for specific skin care measures if the patient has perineal skin irritation from catheter, from adhesive of catheter fixation device, or from drainage around catheter insertion.

Equipment

Catheter Care

- Clean gloves, face shield (as needed)
- Waterproof pad
- Bath blanket
- Soap, washcloth, towel, and basin filled with warm water. Option: chlorhexidine gluconate (CHG) 2% cloth

Removing a Catheter

- 10-mL or larger syringe without needle (information on balloon size [in milliliters or cubic centimeters] is printed directly on balloon inflation valve [Fig. 77.1])
- Graduated cylinder to measure urine

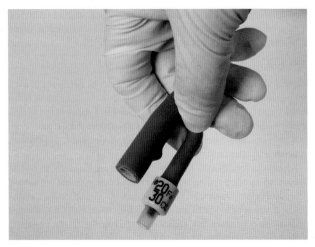

Fig. 77.1 Size of catheter and balloon printed on catheter inflation valve.

- Toilet, bedside commode, urine hat, urinal, or bedpan
- Bladder scanner (if indicated)
- Clean gloves

STEP	RATIONALE
1 Perform preprocedure protocol.	
Assessment	
• Assess need for catheter care:	
a Observe urinary output and urine characteristics.	Sudden decrease in urine output may indicate occlusion of catheter. Cloudy, foul-smelling urine associated with other systemic symptoms may indicate CAUTI.
b Assess for history or presence of bowel incontinence.	Most common bacteria to cause CAUTI is *Escherichia coli,* a major colonizer of the bowel; thus, fecal incontinence increases risk for CAUTI (Fekete, 2021).

STEP	RATIONALE
c Perform hand hygiene. Apply clean gloves. Position patient, then retract labia or foreskin to observe for any discharge, redness, bleeding, or presence of tissue trauma around urethral meatus (this may be deferred until catheter care).	Indicates inflammatory process, possible infection, or erosion of catheter through urethra.
d Remove and dispose of gloves, perform hand hygiene.	Reduces transmission of microorganisms.
• Assess need for catheter removal:	
a Review patient's electronic health record, including health care provider's order and nurses' notes. Note length of time catheter has been in place.	Catheters in place for more than a few days cause higher risk for catheter encrustation and UTI.
b Assess urine color, clarity, odor, and amount. Note any urethral discharge, irritation of genital region, or trauma to urinary meatus (this may be deferred until just before removal).	May be indicator of inflammation or UTI and source of discomfort during catheter removal.
• Determine size of catheter inflation balloon by looking at balloon inflation valve.	Determines size of syringe needed to deflate balloon and amount of fluid expected in syringe after deflation.

Implementation

1 If patient is to be discharged with a catheter, teach patient or family caregiver how to perform catheter hygiene and how to recognize signs/symptoms of UTI.	Reduces anxiety and promotes cooperation. Self-care supports patient's sense of autonomy.

Continued

STEP	RATIONALE
2 Perform hand hygiene.	Reduces transmission of microorganisms.
3 Position patient with waterproof pad under buttocks and cover with bath blanket, exposing only genital area and catheter.	Shows respect for patient dignity by only exposing genital area and catheter.
a If a female patient, place in dorsal recumbent position.	
b If a male patient, place in supine position.	
4 Apply clean gloves.	Reduces transmission of microorganisms.
5 Remove catheter fixation device while maintaining connection with drainage tubing. Inspect skin for redness, blistering, or tears.	Provides ability to easily clean around catheter and to remove it. Skin changes may reflect medical adhesive–related skin injury (Fumarola et al., 2020).
6 Catheter care:	
a *Female:* Use nondominant hand to gently separate labia to fully expose urethral meatus and catheter. Maintain position of hand throughout procedure.	Provides full visualization of urethral meatus. Full separation of labia prevents contamination of meatus during cleaning.
b *Male:* Use nondominant hand to retract foreskin if not circumcised and hold penis at shaft just below glans. Maintain hand position throughout procedure.	Retraction of foreskin provides full visualization of urethral meatus.
c Grasp catheter with two fingers of nondominant hand to stabilize it.	Prevents unnecessary traction on catheter. Pulling on catheter causes discomfort for patient and can damage urethra and bladder neck.

STEP	RATIONALE
d If not performed earlier, assess urethral meatus and surrounding tissues for inflammation, swelling, discharge, or tissue trauma and ask patient whether burning or discomfort is present.	Determines frequency and type of ongoing care required. Indicates possibility of CAUTI or catheter erosion through urethra.
e Provide perineal hygiene using mild soap and warm water. *Option:* Use CHG 2% cloth.	Antiseptic cleaners have not been shown to definitively decrease CAUTI; mild soap and water is appropriate (Schaeffer et al., 2021b). Although CHG 2% cloth can be used, there is no clear scientific evidence for use of antiseptics versus nonantiseptics to reduce rates of CAUTI (Fasugba et al., 2017; Rea et al., 2018).
f Using clean washcloth or CHG cloth, clean along length of catheter.	Removes residue containing microorganisms that can ascend catheter.
(1) Starting on section closest to urinary meatus, clean catheter in circular motion along its length for about 10 cm (4 inches), moving away from body (Fig. 77.2). Remove all traces of soap. *For male patients:* Reduce or reposition foreskin after care.	Moves from an area with potentially more microorganisms to an area of fewer microorganisms.

Continued

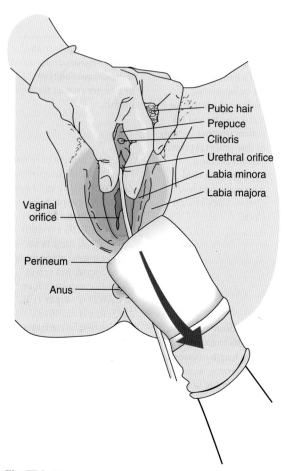

Pubic hair
Prepuce
Clitoris
Urethral orifice
Labia minora
Labia majora
Vaginal orifice
Perineum
Anus

Fig. 77.2 Clean catheter starting at meatus and moving downward while holding it securely.

STEP	RATIONALE
g Reapply catheter fixation device (replace if soiled/damaged). Allow slack in catheter so that movement does not create tension on it. Avoid using adhesive tape.	Securing indwelling catheter reduces risk of urethral trauma, urethral erosion, CAUTI, or accidental removal (Lawrence et al., 2019; Rea et al., 2018). Adhesive can cause medical adhesive–related skin injury.
7 Routinely check drainage tubing and bag that:	Pooling urine can reflux into bladder. Maintaining drainage system in dependent position below bladder prevents CAUTI (Fekete, 2021; Rea et al., 2018).
a Catheter is secured to upper thigh.	Maintains unobstructed flow of urine out of bladder (Gould et al., 2019).
b Tubing is positioned without loops and secured onto bed linen.	
c Tubing is not kinked or clamped.	
d Drainage bag is positioned below level of bladder (attached to the bed frame) with urine flowing freely into bag.	
e Drainage bag is not overfull. Empty drainage bag when one-half full.	Overfull drainage bag creates tension and pulls on catheter, resulting in trauma to urethra and/or urinary meatus. Facilitates unobstructed flow of urine (Gould et al., 2019).

Continued

STEP	RATIONALE
8 Catheter removal: (Perform catheter care [Step 6] before catheter removal.)	
a With clean gloves still on, move syringe plunger up and down to loosen and then pull it back to 0.5 mL. Insert hub of syringe into inflation valve (balloon port). Allow balloon fluid to drain into syringe by gravity. Syringe should fill. Make sure that entire amount of fluid is removed by comparing removed amount with volume needed for inflation.	Partially inflated balloon can traumatize urethral wall during removal. Passive drainage of catheter balloon prevents formation of ridges in balloon. These ridges can cause discomfort or trauma during removal.
b Pull catheter out smoothly and slowly. Examine it to ensure that all surfaces are intact. Catheter should slide out easily. Do not use force. If you note any resistance, repeat Step 8a to remove remaining water.	Nonintact catheter means that pieces of catheter may still be in bladder. Notify health care provider immediately.
c Wrap contaminated catheter in waterproof pad. Unhook collection bag and drainage tubing from bed.	Promotes patient comfort and safety.
d Empty, measure, and record urine present in drainage bag. Ensure proper gloving and use of face shield if patient is taking hazardous drugs.	Documents urinary output. Use of face shield protects against splashing and transmission of chemotherapeutic agent when a patient is taking hazardous drugs (ONS, 2018).

STEP	RATIONALE
e Encourage patient to maintain or increase fluid intake (unless contraindicated).	Maintains normal urine output.
f Initiate voiding record or bladder diary. Instruct patient to tell health care staff when need to empty bladder occurs and that all urine needs to be measured. Make sure that patient understands how to use collection container (hat or other device).	Evaluates bladder function.
g Explain that many patients experience mild burning, discomfort, or small-volume voiding with first voiding, which soon subsides.	Burning results from urethral irritation.
h Measure PVR volume (if ordered) (Skill 5) within 5 to 15 minutes after helping the patient to void.	Bladder scan provides objective PVR reading.
i Inform patient to report any signs of UTI.	
j Ensure easy access to toilet, commode, bedpan, or urinal. Place urine hat on toilet seat if patient is using toilet.	Reduces incidence of falls during toileting. Urine hat collects first voided urine.
9 Provide patient personal hygiene as needed.	Promotes patient comfort and safety.
10 Dispose of all contaminated supplies in appropriate receptacle, remove and dispose of gloves and face shield (if worn), and perform hand hygiene.	Reduces transmission of microorganisms. Use appropriate disposal receptacle and face shield if patient is taking hazardous drugs (ONS, 2018).

Continued

STEP	RATIONALE
11 Perform postprocedure protocol.	
12 Evaluate patient response:	
a Inspect catheter and genital area for soiling, irritation, and skin breakdown. Ask if patient is experiencing any discomfort.	Determines whether area is cleaned properly and/ or whether patient has any irritation.
b Observe time and measure amount of first voiding after catheter removal.	Indicates return of bladder function after catheter removal.
c Evaluate patient for signs and symptoms of UTI.	Any patient who has a catheter or has had a catheter removed recently is at risk for UTI.

Recording and Reporting

- Record time catheter was removed; teaching related to increasing fluid intake and signs and symptoms of UTI; and time, amount, and characteristics of first voiding.
- Record intake and voiding times and amounts on voiding record or bladder diary as indicated.
- Record patient symptoms experienced at time of and after catheter removal.
- Document evaluation of patient learning.
- Report time catheter was removed; teaching related to increasing fluid intake and signs and symptoms of UTI; and time, amount, and characteristics of first voiding.
- Report hematuria, dysuria, inability or difficulty voiding, and any new incontinence after a catheter is removed to health care provider.

UNEXPECTED OUTCOMES	RELATED INTERVENTIONS
1 Normal saline from inflation balloon does not return into syringe.	• Reposition patient; ensure that catheter is not pinched or kinked. • Remove syringe. Attach new syringe and allow enough time for passive emptying. • Attempt to empty balloon by gently pulling back on syringe plunger. • If catheter balloon does not deflate, *do not* cut balloon inflation valve to drain water. Notify health care provider.
2 Patient has cloudy urine, foul urine odor, fever, chills, dysuria, flank pain, back pain, hematuria, urgency, frequency, lower abdominal pain, change in mental status, and lethargy (Fekete, 2021).	• Assess for bladder distention and tenderness. • Monitor vital signs and urine output. • Report findings to health care provider and consult regarding removal of catheter.
3 Patient is unable to void within 6 to 8 h after catheter removal, has sensation of not fully emptying, strains to void, or experiences small voiding amounts with increasing frequency.	• Assess for bladder distention. • Help to normal position for voiding and provide privacy. • Perform bladder scan to assess for excessive urine volume in bladder. • If patient is unable to void within 6 to 8 h of catheter removal and/or experiences abdominal pain, notify health care provider.

Urinary Indwelling Catheter Irrigation

Irrigation of an indwelling urinary catheter is not recommended for preventing a urinary tract infection (UTI) (CDC, 2015). However, after surgery on the bladder and other genitourinary structures, it is common to have hematuria for several days. Intermittent or continuous urinary catheter irrigations are appropriate for maintaining catheter patency by keeping the bladder clear and free of blood clots or sediment. Irrigation must be done maintaining a closed urinary drainage system. Closed catheter irrigations do not disrupt the sterile connection between the catheter and the drainage system (Fig. 78.1). Continuous bladder irrigation (CBI) is an example of a continuous infusion of a sterile solution into the bladder, usually using a three-way irrigation closed system with a triple-lumen catheter.

Safety Considerations

- Bladder irrigation poses a risk for causing a UTI. Use sterile technique.

Delegation

The skill of a closed catheter irrigation cannot be delegated to assistive personnel (AP). Direct the AP to:

- Report if the patient complains of pain, discomfort, or leakage of fluid around the catheter.
- Monitor and record intake and output (I&O); report immediately any decrease in urine output.
- Report any change in the color of the urine, especially the presence of blood clots.

Collaboration

- Collaborate with the urologist or surgeon for support with bladder irrigation needs (e.g., volume to administer, signs and symptoms to report).

Equipment

- Sterile irrigation solution at room temperature (as prescribed)
- Intravenous (IV) pole (closed continuous)

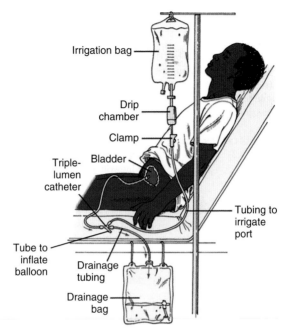

Fig. 78.1 Closed continuous bladder irrigation.

- Antiseptic swabs
- Clean gloves
- Option: Catheter fixation device if changed
- Closed intermittent irrigation
  - Sterile 50-mL syringe to access system: Luer-Lok syringe for needleless access port (per 'manufacturer's instructions)
  - Screw clamp or rubber band (used to occlude catheter temporarily as irrigant is instilled)
- Closed continuous irrigation
  - Irrigation tubing with clamp to regulate irrigation flow rate

STEP	RATIONALE
1 Perform preprocedure protocol.	

Assessment

- Verify in electronic health record (EHR):

Continued

STEP	RATIONALE
a Order for irrigation method (continuous or intermittent), solution type (sterile saline or medicated solution), and amount of irrigant.	Health care provider's order is required to initiate therapy. Frequency and volume of solution used for irrigation may be in the order or standardized as part of agency policy.
b Type of catheter in place (Fig. 78.2).	Triple-lumen catheters are used for continuous closed irrigation. Indwelling urinary catheter is accessed for intermittent irrigation.
• Perform hand hygiene. Palpate bladder for distention and tenderness or use bladder scan (see Skill 5).	Reduces transmission of microorganisms. Bladder distention indicates that flow of urine may be blocked from draining.
• Assess patient for abdominal pain or spasms, sensation of bladder fullness, or urine draining around catheter. Wear clean gloves if risk of contact with urine.	May indicate overdistention of bladder caused by catheter blockage. Offers baseline to determine whether therapy is successful.
• Observe urine for color, amount, clarity, and presence of mucus; clots; or sediment.	Indicates whether patient is bleeding or sloughing tissue, which would require increased irrigation rate or frequency of catheter irrigation.
• Monitor I&O. If CBI is being used, amount of fluid draining from bladder should exceed amount of fluid infused into bladder. Remove and dispose of gloves (if worn) and perform hand hygiene.	If output does not exceed irrigant infused, catheter obstruction (i.e., blood clots, kinked tubing) should be suspected, irrigation stopped, and prescriber notified (Ignatavicius et al., 2021).

Implementation

1 Perform hand hygiene. Raise bed to appropriate working height. If side rails are raised, lower side rail on working side.	Reduces transmission of microorganisms. Promotes use of good body mechanics. Position provides access to catheter.

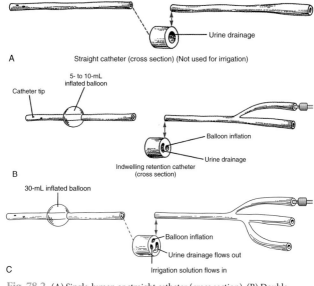

Fig. 78.2 (A) Single-lumen or straight catheter (cross section). (B) Double-lumen or indwelling retention catheter for intermittent closed irrigation (cross section). (C) Triple-lumen catheter for continuous closed irrigation (cross section).

STEP	RATIONALE
2 Position patient supine and expose catheter junctions (catheter and drainage tubing).	Position provides access to catheter and promotes patient dignity/privacy as much as possible.
3 Remove catheter fixation device.	Eases access to catheter parts.
4 Closed continuous irrigation:	
a Close clamp on new irrigation tubing and hang bag of irrigating solution on IV pole. Insert (spike) tip of sterile irrigation tubing into designated port of irrigation solution bag using aseptic technique.	Prevents air from entering tubing. Air can cause bladder spasms. Technique prevents transmission of microorganisms.

Continued

STEP	RATIONALE
b Fill drip chamber half full by squeezing chamber. Remove cap at end of tubing, and then open clamp and allow solution to flow (prime) through tubing, keeping end of tubing sterile. Once fluid has filled tubing, close clamp and recap end of tubing.	Priming tubing with fluid prevents introduction of air into bladder.
c Using aseptic technique, cleanse port on catheter with antiseptic swab, remove cap on tubing, and connect end of tubing securely to port for infusing irrigation fluid into triple-lumen catheter.	Reduces transmission of microorganisms.
d Adjust clamp on irrigation tubing to begin flow of solution into bladder. If set volume rate is ordered, calculate drip rate and adjust rate at roller clamp. If urine is bright red or has clots, increase irrigation rate until drainage appears pink (according to ordered rate or agency protocol).	Continuous drainage is expected. It helps to prevent clotting in presence of active bleeding in bladder and flushes clots from bladder.
e Observe for outflow of fluid into drainage bag. Empty catheter drainage bag as needed.	Discomfort, bladder distention, and possible injury can occur from overdistention of bladder when bladder irrigant cannot adequately flow from bladder. Bag will fill rapidly and may need to be emptied every 1 to 2 h.

STEP	RATIONALE
5 Closed intermittent irrigation:	Fluid is instilled through catheter in a bolus, flushing system. Fluid drains out after irrigation is complete.
a Pour prescribed sterile irrigation solution into sterile container.	
b Draw prescribed volume of irrigant (usually 30 to 50 mL) into sterile syringe using aseptic technique. Place sterile cap on tip of needleless syringe.	Ensures sterility of irrigating fluid.
c Clamp catheter tubing below soft injection port with screw clamp (or fold catheter tubing onto itself and secure with rubber band).	Occluding catheter tubing below point of injection allows irrigating solution to enter catheter and flow into bladder.
d Using circular motion, clean catheter port (specimen port) with antiseptic swab.	Reduces transmission of microorganisms.
e Insert tip of needleless syringe using twisting motion into port.	Ensures that catheter tip enters lumen of catheter.
f Inject solution using slow, even pressure.	Gentle instillation of solution minimizes trauma to bladder mucosa.
g Remove syringe and clamp (or rubber band), allowing solution to drain into urinary drainage bag.	Allows irrigation solution to flow out by gravity. Medications must be instilled long enough to be absorbed by lining of bladder. Clamped drainage tubing and bag should not be left unattended.

CLINICAL JUDGMENT *Some medicated irrigants may need to dwell in the bladder for a prescribed period, requiring the catheter to be clamped temporarily before being allowed to drain.*

Continued

STEP	RATIONALE
6 Anchor catheter with catheter fixation device.	Prevents trauma to urethral tissue caused by pulling catheter.
7 Dispose of all contaminated supplies in appropriate receptacle, remove and dispose of gloves, and perform hand hygiene.	Reduces transmission of microorganisms. Use appropriate disposal receptacle if patient on hazardous drugs (ONS, 2018).
8 Perform postprocedure protocol.	
9 Evaluate patient response:	
a Measure actual urine output by subtracting total amount of irrigation fluid infused from total volume drained into basin.	Determines accurate urinary output.
b Review I&O flow sheet to verify that hourly output into drainage bag is in appropriate proportion to irrigating solution entering bladder. Expect more output than fluid instilled because of urine production.	Determines urinary output in relation to irrigation.
c Inspect urine for blood clots and sediment and be sure that tubing is not kinked or occluded.	Decrease in blood clots means that therapy is successful in maintaining catheter patency. System is patent.
d Evaluate patient's comfort level.	Indicates catheter patency by absence of symptoms of bladder distention.
e Monitor for signs and symptoms of infection.	Patients with indwelling catheters remain at risk for infection.

Recording and Reporting

- Record irrigation method, amount of and type of irrigation solution, amount returned as drainage, characteristics of output, urine output, and patient response.
- Record I&O.
- Document evaluation of patient learning.
- Report status of urine output and occurrence of catheter occlusion, sudden bleeding, infection, or increased pain.

UNEXPECTED OUTCOMES	RELATED INTERVENTIONS
1 Irrigating solution does not return (closed intermittent irrigation) or is not flowing at prescribed rate (CBI).	• Examine tubing for clots, sediment, and kinks. • Notify health care provider if irrigant does not flow freely from bladder, patient complains of pain, or bladder distention occurs.
2 Drainage output is less than amount of irrigation solution infused.	• Examine drainage tubing for clots, sediment, or kinks. • Inspect urine for presence of or increase in blood clots and sediment. • Evaluate patient for pain and distended bladder. • Notify health care provider.
3 Bright-red bleeding with the irrigation (CBI) infusion wide open.	• Assess for hypovolemic shock (vital signs, skin color and moisture, anxiety level). • Leave irrigation infusion wide open, ensuring catheter is draining, and notify health care provider.
4 Patient experiences pain with irrigation.	• Examine drainage tubing for clots, sediment, or kinks. • Evaluate urine for presence of or increase in blood clots and sediment. • Evaluate for distended bladder. • Notify health care provider.

Urostomy Pouching

Patients who have had the bladder removed because of cancer or significant bladder dysfunction require surgical procedures that divert urine to the outside of the body through an opening in the abdominal wall called a stoma. Urinary diversions are created from a section of intestinal ileum to create a storage reservoir or a conduit for urine drainage. Because urine flows more frequently from a urinary diversion, placement of a pouch is more challenging than a fecal diversion (Skill 46). It can be difficult keeping the skin dry as you prepare a pouch application. In the immediate postoperative period, urinary stents extend out from a stoma (Fig. 79.1). The stents prevent stenosis of the ureters at the site where the ureters are attached to the conduit. The stents are removed during the hospital stay or at the first postoperative visit with the surgeon.

The stoma is normally red and moist. A normal stoma protrudes above the skin. An ileal conduit is usually located in the right lower quadrant of a patient's abdomen. While the patient is in bed, the pouch may be connected to a bedside drainage bag to decrease the need for frequent emptying. When the patient goes home, a bedside drainage bag may be used at night to avoid having to get up to empty the pouch. Each type of urostomy pouch comes with a connector for the bedside drainage bag. As in the case of a colostomy or ileostomy pouching (Skill 46), patients are at risk for medical adhesive skin injury (MARSI) unless proper skin barrier and pouch application are performed.

Safety Guidelines

- Know the signs of a healthy stoma and surrounding skin:
  - Color/moisture: Stoma should be red or pink and moist. Report a gray, purple, black, or very dry stoma immediately.
  - Size: In the 4 to 6 weeks after surgery, the stoma will likely decrease in size as postoperative edema and abdominal distention decrease.
  - Peristomal skin: The skin around the stoma is normally intact with some reddening after removal of the adhesive wafer. Presence of blisters, a rash, or excoriated skin is abnormal and could indicate maceration or medical adhesive related–skin injury (MARSI) (Fumarola et al., 2020).
- Use sterile technique when handling stents.

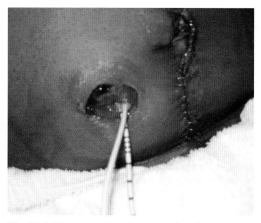

Fig. 79.1 Urostomy stoma with stents in place. (Courtesy Jane Fellows.)

Delegation

The skill of pouching a new incontinent urostomy cannot be delegated to assistive personnel (AP). In some agencies care of an established urostomy (4 o 6 weeks or more after surgery) can be delegated. Direct the AP about:

- Expected appearance of the stoma.
- Expected amount and character of the output and when to report changes.
- Reporting change in appearance of patient's stoma and surrounding skin integrity.
- Special equipment needed to complete procedure.

Collaboration

- A wound, ostomy, continence nurse (WOCN), when available, can assist with postsurgical assessment, pouch selection, and patient education.

Equipment

- Wafer (skin barrier) and clear urinary pouch, one- or two-piece, cut-to-fit or precut size
- Appropriate adapter for connection to bedside drainage bag
- Measuring guide
- Bedside urinary drainage bag

- Clean gloves
- Washcloth
- Towel or disposable waterproof barrier
- Basin with warm tap water
- Scissors
- Adhesive remover
- *Option:* ostomy skin barrier product (e.g., liquid or stoma adhesive)
- Absorbent wick made from gauze rolled tightly (in the shape of a tampon)
- Waterproof bag for disposal of pouch
- Mirror for patient to observe ostomy
- Gown and goggles (optional if there is any risk of splashing when emptying pouch)

STEP	RATIONALE
1 Perform preprocedure protocol.	

Assessment

• Review patient's electronic health record (EHR), including nurses' notes for type of urinary diversion, type of pouching system used, and whether patient has any problems related to stoma or peristomal area.	Allows anticipation of supplies needed and if special skin care is required.
• Ask patient to describe history of allergies: known type(s) of allergies and normal allergic reaction(s). Check patient's allergy wristband. Focus on adhesive and latex.	Reduces risk for exposing patient to allergens that can cause localized or systemic allergic reactions. Any patient sensitivity will affect your choice of a skin barrier and dictate avoiding use of latex.

STEP	RATIONALE
• Identify patient's history for: Age, dehydration, malnutrition, exposure to radiation therapy, underlying chronic conditions (e.g., diabetes, immunosuppression), and edema of skin. Common risk factors for MARSI (Fumarola et al., 2020).	Common risk factors for MARSI (Fumarola et al., 2020). Factors raise level of observation for patient with an adhesive-containing pouching system.
• Have patient assume semi-reclining or supine position. Observe existing skin barrier and pouch for leakage and length of time in place. Pouch should be changed every 3 to 7 days. If urine is leaking under wafer, change pouch.	Assesses effectiveness of pouching system and allows for early detection of potential problems. To minimize skin irritation, avoid changing entire pouching system unnecessarily. Repeated leakage may indicate need for different type of pouch to provide reliable seal.
• Perform hand hygiene and apply clean gloves.	Reduces transmission of infection.
• *Note:* Inspection of pouch and stoma can be deferred until just before pouch change. Observe characteristics of urine in pouch or bedside drainage bag. Empty pouch before it is half full by opening valve and draining it into container for measurement.	There may be blood or large amounts of mucus in urine after surgery, but this should resolve in the first 1 to 2 weeks after surgery. Weight of pouch can disrupt seal. Urine from ileal conduit will contain mucus because of flow through intestinal segment.

CLINICAL JUDGMENT *Repeated leaking may indicate need for different type of pouch or addition of products such as stoma adhesive for pouch application. If the pouch is leaking, change it. Taping or patching it to contain urine leaves the skin exposed to chemical or enzymatic irritation.*

Continued

STEP	RATIONALE
• Remove used pouch and skin barrier gently by pushing skin away from barrier in direction hair grows (Wound, Ostomy, and Continence Nurses Society [WOCN], 2018). Loosen and lift the edge with one hand and press down on the skin near the sticky backing with the other hand. It may be helpful to start at the top and work down to the bottom for better visualization. This will also allow the pouch to catch any urine the stoma produces (WOCN, 2018). Use adhesive remover to facilitate removal of skin barrier. With stoma exposed observe color, location and position, presence of swelling, sutures, or stents.	Method reduces risk of skin stripping or tears. Stoma characteristics influence selection of an appropriate pouching system. Convexity in skin barrier is often necessary with a flush or retracted stoma (WOCN, 2017).
• Assess peristomal skin for temperature, color, moisture level, turgor, fragility, and integrity. Observe for local signs of irritation or skin damage, e.g., stripping or blisters where any adhesive has been or will be applied.	Signs and symptoms of MARSI (Fumarola et al., 2020).
• Remove and dispose of gloves. Perform hand hygiene.	Reduces transmission of microorganisms.
• Explore patient's attitudes, perceptions, knowledge of stoma and ostomy care, and acceptance of stoma and change in function. Discuss interest in learning self-care. Identify others who will be helping patient after leaving hospital.	Determines patient's willingness to learn. Assesses patient's body image. Facilitates teaching plan and timing of care to coincide with availability of family caregivers (WOCN, 2017).

STEP	RATIONALE

Implementation

1 Make patient comfortable, continuing in semireclining or supine position. If possible, provide patient with mirror for observation.

When patient is semireclining versus sitting, there are fewer skin wrinkles, which allows for easier pouch application.

2 Apply clean gloves.

Reduces transmission of microorganisms.

3 Place towel or disposable waterproof barrier under patient and across patient's lower abdomen.

Protects bed linen; maintains patient's dignity/privacy.

4 If not done during assessment, remove used pouch and skin barrier at this time, inspect stoma and peristomal skin, and empty pouch. Dispose of pouch in an appropriate receptacle. Measure output.

Reduces risk for trauma to skin and for dislodging stents. Keeps urine from leaking onto skin. Urine output provides information about renal status and whether volume is within acceptable limits ($\geq$30 mL/h).

5 Place rolled gauze at stoma opening. Maintain gauze at stoma opening continuously during pouch measurement and change.

Using gauze for wick at stoma opening prevents peristomal skin from becoming wet with urine during pouch change.

6 While keeping rolled gauze in contact with stoma, clean peristomal skin gently with warm tap water and washcloth; do not scrub skin. Minor bleeding is normal if stoma is touched. Pat skin dry.

Avoid soap. It leaves residue on skin, which can irritate it. Pouch does not adhere to wet skin.

7 Measure stoma (see Skill 46). Expect size of stoma to change for first 4 to 6 weeks after surgery.

Allows for proper fit of pouch that will protect peristomal skin. Expect normal postoperative swelling.

8 Trace pattern on pouch backing or skin barrier (see Skill 46).

Prepares for cutting opening in pouch.

Continued

STEP	RATIONALE
9 Cut opening in pouch (see Skill 46). If using a moldable or a shape-to-fit barrier, use fingers to mold shape-to-fit stoma.	Customizes pouch to provide appropriate fit over stoma.

CLINICAL JUDGMENT *Instruct patients to remeasure stomas occasionally if they notice that the stoma has changed shape or size (Goldberg, 2018).*

STEP	RATIONALE
10 Remove protective backing from adhesive backing or wafer surface. (see Skill 46). Remove rolled gauze from stoma.	Prepares pouch for application to skin.
11 Apply pouch. Press adhesive barrier firmly into place around stoma and outside edges. Have patient hold hand over pouch 1 to 2 minutes to secure seal.	Pouch adhesives are heat- and pressure-sensitive and will hold more securely at body temperature.
12 Use adapter provided with pouches to connect pouch to bedside urinary bag. Keep tubing below level of bag.	Allows patient to rest without frequent emptying of pouch. Tubing position allows for collection and measurement of urine and prevents backflow of urine into stoma. Risk of reflux is reduced by attaching a urinary pouch to straight drainage when high urinary output is expected.
13 Perform postprocedure protocol.	
14 Evaluate patient response: a Observe appearance of stoma, stents, peristomal skin, and suture line during pouch change.	Determines condition of stoma, stents, and peristomal skin and progress of wound healing.

STEP	RATIONALE
b Evaluate character and volume of urinary drainage.	Determines whether stoma and/or stents are patent. Character of urine reveals degree of concentration and whether there is possible urinary tract infection. (Colwell and Goldberg, 2021).
c Observe patient's and family caregiver's willingness to view stoma and ask questions about procedure.	Determines level of adjustment and understanding of stoma care and pouch application.

Recording and Reporting

- Record type of pouch, time of change, condition and appearance of stoma/stents and peristomal skin, and character of urine.
- Record urinary output on intake and output form.
- Record patient's and family caregiver's reaction to stoma and level of participation. Document evaluation of patient and family caregiver learning.
- Report abnormalities in stoma or peristomal skin and absence of urinary output to nurse in charge or health care provider.

UNEXPECTED OUTCOMES	RELATED INTERVENTIONS
1 Skin around stoma is irritated, blistered, or bleeding; or maceration is noted, signs resulting from chronic exposure to urine or MARSI.	• Check stoma size and opening in skin barrier. • Resize skin barrier opening if necessary. • Remove pouch more carefully. • Consult WOCN.
2 No urine output for several hours, or output is less than 30 mL/h. Urine has foul odor.	• Increase fluid intake (if allowed). • Notify health care provider. • Obtain urine specimen for culture and sensitivity if ordered.

Continued

UNEXPECTED OUTCOMES	RELATED INTERVENTIONS
3 Patient and family caregiver are unable to observe stoma, ask questions, or participate in care.	• Consult WOCN. • Allow patient to express feelings. • Determine source of discomfort or maladjustment to pouch; encourage family support.

Vaginal Medication

Female patients who develop vaginal infections often require the instillation of anti-infective agents. Topical vaginal medications are available in foam, jelly, cream, or suppository form. Medicated irrigations or douches can also be given. However, their excessive use can lead to vaginal irritation.

Vaginal suppositories are oval shaped and come individually packaged in foil wrappers. They are larger and more oval than rectal suppositories (Fig. 80.1). Storage in a refrigerator prevents the solid suppositories from melting. A suppository is inserted into the vagina with an applicator or a gloved hand. After insertion, body temperature causes the suppository to melt for effective medication distribution. Foam, jellies, and creams can be inserted with an inserter or applicator. Patients often prefer administering their own vaginal medications, and should be given privacy to do so.

Safety Precautions

- Vaginal tissue can be traumatized by the forceful use of applicators or fingernails during medication administration, so introduce medications into the vagina gently.
- A female staff member must be present in the room when a male nurse administers a vaginal medication.

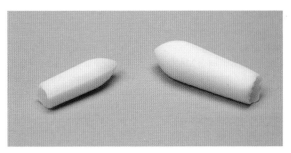

Fig. 80.1 Vaginal suppositories (right) are larger and more oval than rectal suppositories (left).

Delegation

The skill of administering vaginal medications cannot be delegated to assistive personnel (AP). Instruct the AP about:

- Potential side effects of medications and to report their occurrence to the nurse.
- Reporting any change in comfort level or new or increased vaginal discharge or bleeding to the nurse.

Collaboration

- Collaborate with a gynecological specialist if vaginal infection persists or there is a change in color or amount of vaginal discharge.

Equipment

- Vaginal cream, foam, jelly, tablet, suppository
- Applicators (if needed)
- Clean glove
- Tissues, towels, and/or washcloths
- Perineal pad
- Drape or sheet
- Water-soluble lubricant
- Medication administration record (MAR) (electronic or printed)
- *Option:* gooseneck lamp

STEPS	RATIONALE
1 Perform preprocedure protocol.	

Assessment

• Check accuracy and completeness of each MAR or computer printout with health care provider's written medication order. Check patient's name, medication name and dosage, route of administration, and time of administration.	Recopy or reprint any part of MAR that is difficult to read. The order sheet is the most reliable source and only legal record of medications that patient is to receive. Ensures that patient receives the correct medications (Palese et al., 2019).
• Review electronic health record: assess patient's medical and medication history.	Determines need for medication or possible contraindications for medication administration.

STEPS	RATIONALE
• Review drug reference information for medication action, purpose, normal dose, side effects, time of peak onset, and nursing implications.	Allows you to administer medication safely and monitor patient's response to therapy
• Review drug reference information for medication action, purpose, normal dose, side effects, time of peak onset, and nursing implications.	Allows for safe medication administration and monitoring of patient's response to therapy
• Ask patient to describe history of allergies: known type(s) of allergies and normal allergic reaction(s). List drug allergies on each page of MAR. Check patient's allergy wristband. Do not prepare medication if there is a known patient allergy.	Communication of patient allergies is essential part of safe medication administration.
• Perform hand hygiene and apply clean gloves. During perineal care inspect condition of vaginal tissues; note whether drainage is present. Remove gloves and perform hand hygiene.	Reduces transmission of microorganisms. Findings provide baseline to determine patient response to medication.
• Ask whether patient is experiencing any symptoms of pruritus, burning, or discomfort.	Provides baseline to determine patient response to medication.
• Assess patient's ability to manipulate applicator or suppository, and to properly position self to insert medication (may be done just before insertion).	Determines whether instruction is necessary to prepare patient for self-administration.

Continued

STEPS	RATIONALE
• Discuss purpose of each medication, action, and possible adverse effects. Allow patient to ask any questions.	Includes patient as a participant in care, which minimizes anxiety. Prepares patient to self-administer drug, which increases feelings of independence.

Implementation

1 Prepare medication without interruptions/distractions. Create a quiet environment. Keep all pages of MARs or computer printouts for one patient together or look at only one patient's electronic MAR at a time	Interruptions contribute to medication errors (Palese et al., 2019).
2 Perform hand hygiene. Prepare medications for one patient at a time using aseptic technique. Suppositories are usually stored in refrigerator. Check label of medication carefully with MAR or computer printout two times when removing medication from storage and before preparing to take to patient. medication.	Ensures that medication is sterile. *These are the first and second checks for accuracy* and ensure that correct medication is administered.
3 Take medication(s) to patient at correct time (see agency policy). Medications that require exact timing include stat, first-time or loading doses, and one-time doses. Give non–time-critical scheduled medications within a range of 1 or 2 h of scheduled dose (Institute for Safe Medication Practices [ISMP], 2011). During administration apply seven rights of medication administration.	Hospitals must adopt medication administration policy and procedure for timing of medication administration that considers nature of the prescribed medication, specific clinical application, and patient needs (ISMP, 2011; US Department of Health and Human Service, 2020).

STEPS	RATIONALE
4 Identify patient using at least two identifiers (e.g., name and birthday or name and medical record number) according to agency policy. Compare identifiers with information on patient's MAR or medical record.	Ensures correct patient. Complies with The Joint Commission (TJC) standards and improves patient safety (TJC, 2023).
5 At patient's bedside, again compare MAR or computer printout with names of medications on medication labels and patient name. Ask patient about history of allergies.	*This is the third check for accuracy* and ensures that patient receives correct medication. Confirms patient's allergy history.
6 Have patient void (using bathroom facilities or bedpan). Assist to a dorsal recumbent position. Patients with restricted mobility in knees or hips may lie supine with legs abducted.	Suppository insertion can create sensation to void.
7 Keep abdomen and lower extremities draped. Ensure that vaginal orifice is well illuminated by room light. Otherwise, position portable gooseneck lamp.	Maintains patient comfort and privacy. Light improves visibility of vaginal orifice.
8 Perform hand hygiene and apply clean gloves. Provide perineal hygiene if there is vaginal drainage or discharge. (Remove gloves, perform hand hygiene, reapply clean gloves if needed.)	Reduces transmission of microorganisms.

Continued

STEPS	RATIONALE
9 Insert vaginal suppository:	
a Remove suppository from wrapper and apply liberal amount of water-soluble lubricant to smooth or rounded end (Fig. 80.2). Be sure that suppository is at room temperature. Lubricate gloved index finger of dominant hand.	Lubrication eases insertion.
b With nondominant gloved hand, gently separate labial folds in front-to-back direction.	Exposes vaginal orifice.
c With dominant gloved hand, insert rounded end of suppository along posterior wall of vaginal canal, inserting the entire length of finger to ensure placement (7.5 to 10 cm [3 to 4 inches]) (Fig. 80.3)	Placement ensures proper absorption of medication.

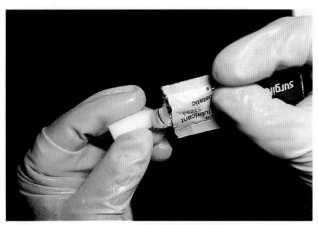

Fig. 80.2 Lubricate tip of suppository.

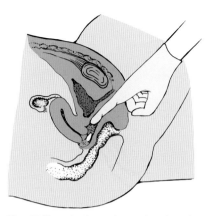

Fig. 80.3 Angle of vaginal suppository insertion.

STEPS	RATIONALE
d Withdraw finger and wipe away remaining lubricant from around orifice and labia with tissue or cloth.	Promotes patient comfort.
10 Apply cream, gel or foam:	
a Fill cream or foam applicator following package directions.	
b With nondominant gloved hand, gently separate labial folds in front-to-back direction.	Exposes vaginal orifice.
c With dominant gloved hand, gently insert applicator approximately 5 to 7.5 cm (2 to 3 inches). Push applicator plunger to deposit medication into vagina (Fig. 80.4).	Ensures proper delivery into vaginal canal.

Continued

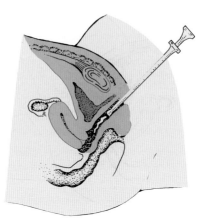

Fig. 80.4 Applicator inserted into vaginal canal. Plunger pushed to instill medication.

STEPS	RATIONALE
d Withdraw applicator and place on paper towel. Wipe off residual cream from labia or vaginal orifice with tissue or cloth.	Promotes patient comfort.
11 Instruct patients who receive cream, gel, or tablet to remain on their backs for at least 10 minutes; 30 minutes after a suppository.	Prevents expulsion of medication.
12 Instruct patient to administer vaginal medicines at bedtime.	Reclined position enhances medication absorption.
13 If using an applicator, wash with soap and warm water, rinse, air dry, and then store for future use.	Reduces transmission of microorganisms.
14 Offer perineal pad when patient resumes ambulation.	Promotes patient comfort.

STEPS	RATIONALE
15 Perform postprocedure protocol.	
16 Evaluate patient response:	
a Thirty minutes after administration, return to patient's room. Perform hand hygiene and apply clean gloves. Inspect condition of vaginal canal and external genitalia between applications. Assess vaginal discharge if present. Remove gloves and perform hand hygiene.	Determines patient response to medication. Reduces transmission of microorganisms.

Recording and Reporting

- Record drug, dose, type of installation, and time administered.
- Document evaluation of patient learning.
- Report to health care provider if symptoms do not improve, or if they worsen.

UNEXPECTED OUTCOMES	RELATED INTERVENTIONS
1 Patient develops tissue irritation, swelling, or redness of vaginal tissues or the patient complains of pain or burning.	• Do not give next scheduled dose of medication. • Confer with health care provider.

Venipuncture: Collecting Blood Specimens and Cultures by Syringe and Vacutainer Methods

Blood tests are one of the most common diagnostic aids in assessing and evaluating patients. Health care providers use blood test results to screen patients for early signs of physical illness, monitor changes in acute or chronic diseases, and evaluate responses to therapies. In some settings nurses are responsible for collecting blood specimens; however, many agencies have specially trained phlebotomists who are responsible for drawing venous blood. Know your agency policies and procedures and your state Nurse Practice Act regarding guidelines for obtaining blood samples.

The two most common methods of obtaining blood specimens are (1) venipuncture and (2) skin puncture. This skill addresses venipuncture. Venipuncture involves inserting a hollow-bore needle into the lumen of a large vein to obtain a specimen using either a needle and syringe or a Vacutainer device that allows the drawing of multiple samples. Because veins are major sources of blood for laboratory testing and routes for intravenous (IV) fluid or blood replacement, maintaining their integrity is essential.

Skin puncture, also called *capillary puncture,* is the least traumatic method of obtaining a blood specimen. A sterile lancet or needle is used to puncture a vascular area on a finger or earlobe in an adult or child. You place a drop of blood on a test slide, wick a drop of blood to a test slide, or collect it within a thin glass capillary tube for laboratory analysis. Point-of-care clinical laboratory tests such as blood glucose monitoring at the bedside typically use skin puncture (Pagana et al., 2021).

Blood cultures are used to detect bacteria in the blood. At least two culture specimens must be drawn from two different venous sites. Because bacteremia may be accompanied by fever and chills, blood culture specimens should be drawn when these symptoms are present (Pagana et al., 2021). Bacteremia exists when both cultures grow the infectious agent. If only one culture grows bacteria, the result is considered a specimen contamination. If antibiotic therapy is ordered, draw all culture specimens before antibiotic therapy begins because the antibiotic may interrupt the growth of an organism in the laboratory. If the patient is already receiving antibiotics, notify the laboratory and inform them of specific antibiotics the patient is receiving (Pagana et al., 2021).

Safety Guidelines

- Observe universal precautions when obtaining a blood specimen.
- Follow the recommended order of draw. Draw specimens into nonadditive tubes before drawing them into tubes without additives (Pagana et al., 2021) (Fig. 81.1).
- Increasing your skill in venipuncture will avoid unnecessary injury to veins.

Delegation

The skill of collecting blood specimens by venipuncture can be delegated to specially trained assistive personnel (AP). In some health care agencies, phlebotomists obtain the samples. Inform the AP to:

- Report any patient discomfort or signs of excessive bleeding from the puncture site.

Equipment

All Procedures

- 70% alcohol or chlorhexidine antiseptic swab (check agency policy)
- Clean gloves
- Small pillow or folded towel
- Sterile 2 × 2-inch gauze pads
- Tourniquet
- Nonallergenic bandage or tape
- Completed identification labels with proper patient identifiers

Blood Draw Order	Tube Color	Description
1	Color Varies	Blood Cultures
2	Light Blue	Sodium Citrate
3	Red	Clot Activator
4	Gold	SST
5	Light Green	Lithium Heparin
6	Dark Green	Sodium Heparin
7	Lavender	EDTA
8	Gray	Sodium Floride
9	Yellow	ACD Solution

Fig. 81.1 Color coding for order of draw in blood specimen collection.

- Completed laboratory requisition (appropriate patient identification, date, time, name of test, and source of culture specimen)
- Small plastic biohazard bag for delivering specimen to laboratory (or container specified by agency)
- Sharps container

Venipuncture with Syringe

- Sterile safety needles (20- to 21-gauge for adults; 23- to 25-gauge for children)
- Sterile 10- to 20-mL Luer-Lok safety syringes
- Needle-free blood transfer device
- Appropriate blood specimen tubes

Venipuncture with Vacutainer

- Vacutainer and safety access device with Luer-Lok adapter
- Sterile double needles (20- to 21-gauge for adults; 23- to 25-gauge for children)
- Appropriate blood specimen tubes

Blood Cultures

- Sterile double needles (20- to 21-gauge for adults; 23- to 25-gauge for children)
- Two 20-mL sterile syringes
- Anaerobic and aerobic culture bottles (check agency policy)

STEP	RATIONALE
1 Perform preprocedure protocol.	
Assessment	
• Review patient's electronic health record (EHR) for health care provider's orders for type of tests. Note if order is stat.	Health care provider's order is required. Stat order requires you to obtain specimen immediately and notify health care provider of results.
• Review EHR for possible risks associated with venipuncture: anticoagulant therapy, low platelet count, bleeding disorders (e.g., hemophilia).	Risks include abnormal clotting abilities caused by low platelet count, hemophilia, or medications that increase risk for bleeding and hematoma formation.

STEP	RATIONALE
• Review policy and procedure for any special conditions needed before and during collection (e.g., patient allowed nothing by mouth, specific time for collection in relation to medication given, and the need to place specimen on ice). Also review type and order of tubes for collection (Fig. 81.1).	Some tests require meeting specific conditions to obtain accurate measurement of blood elements (e.g., fasting blood sugar, drug peak and trough levels, timed endocrine hormone levels). To avoid cross contamination of additives between tubes, blood must be drawn in a specific order (E Phlebotomy Training, nd).

CLINICAL JUDGMENT *Some specimens have special collection requirements before or after specimen collection. Plan ahead; examples follow:*
- *Cryoglobulin levels: Use prewarmed test tubes.*
- *Ammonia and ionized calcium levels: Place tube in ice for delivery to laboratory.*
- *Lactic acid levels: Do not use tourniquet.*
- *Vitamin levels: Avoid exposure of test tube to light.*

• Perform hand hygiene. Assess for contraindicated sites for venipuncture: presence of IV infusion, hematoma at potential site, arm on side of mastectomy, or hemodialysis arteriovenous shunt.	Reduces transmission of microorganisms. Drawing specimens from such sites can result in false test results or may injure patient. Samples taken from vein near IV infusion may be diluted or contain concentrations of IV fluids. Postmastectomy patient may have reduced lymphatic drainage in arm. Never use arteriovenous shunt to obtain specimens because of risks for clotting and bleeding. Hematoma indicates existing injury to vessel wall.

Continued

STEP	RATIONALE
• Ask patient to describe history of allergies: known type(s) of allergies and normal allergic reaction(s). Focus on adhesives, latex, and topicals. Check patient's allergy wristband.	Do not use adhesive or topical agent known to cause patient allergy. Use nonlatex gloves if needed. Adhesive may cause medical adhesive–related skin injury (Fumarola et al., 2020).
• Before drawing blood cultures, assess for systemic signs and symptoms of bacteremia, including fever and chills.	Often two to three blood culture samples are drawn at 30-minute intervals from different sites (Pagana et al., 2021). Also, often drawn when patient has diagnosed fever. Done to detect early signs of sepsis.
• Assess patient's feelings about procedure and possible fear of needlesticks.	Reveals need for patient instruction and/or support. Research shows that needle fear and needle phobia are more prevalent in female patients than in male patients; fear is common when patients undergo venipuncture (McLenon and Rogers, 2019).

Implementation

1 Describe purpose of tests; explain how sensation of tourniquet, alcohol swab, and needlestick will feel.	Anticipatory guidance helps to reduce anxiety.

CLINICAL JUDGMENT *Arrange for extra personnel for confused or pediatric patients who may not be able to remain still during venipuncture.*

STEP	RATIONALE
2 Perform hand hygiene.	Reduces transmission of microorganisms. Correct order prevents additive contamination. Stabilizes extremity because arms are most common sites of venipuncture. Supported position in bed reduces chance of injury to patient if fainting occurs.
3 Organize all necessary blood tubes by order of draw. Help patient to supine or semi-Fowler position with arms extended to form straight line from shoulders to wrists. Place small pillow or towel under upper arm. (*Option:* Lower arm briefly so it fills veins in hand and lower arm with blood.)	
4 Apply tourniquet so it can be removed by pulling an end with single motion.	Tourniquet blocks venous return to heart from extremity, causing veins to dilate for easier visibility.
a Position tourniquet 5 to 10 cm (2 to 4 inches) above selected venipuncture site (antecubital fossa site is commonly used).	
b Cross tourniquet over patient's arm. May place over gown sleeve to protect skin.	Older adults' skin is often very fragile.
c Hold tourniquet between your fingers close to arm. Tuck loop between patient's arm and tourniquet so it can be easily grasped.	Pull free end to release tourniquet after venipuncture.

CLINICAL JUDGMENT *Palpate distal pulse (e.g., radial) below tourniquet. If pulse is not palpable, remove tourniquet, wait 60 seconds, and reapply it more loosely. If tourniquet is too tight, pressure will impede arterial blood flow.*

5 Do not keep tourniquet on patient longer than 1 minute.	Prolonged tourniquet application causes stasis, localized acidemia, and hemoconcentration (American Certification Agency for Healthcare Professionals [ACAHP], 2017).

Continued

STEP	RATIONALE
6 Quickly inspect extremity for best venipuncture site, looking for straight, prominent vein that does not contain swelling or hematoma. Of three veins located in antecubital area, median cubital vein is preferred.	Straight and intact veins are easiest to puncture.
7 Apply clean gloves. Palpate selected vein with finger (Fig. 81.2). Note whether vein is firm and rebounds when palpated or if it feels rigid or cordlike and rolls when palpated. Avoid vigorously slapping vein, which can cause vasospasm.	Patent, healthy vein is elastic and rebounds on palpation. Thrombosed vein is rigid, rolls easily, and is difficult to puncture.
8 Obtain blood specimen.	
a Syringe method:	
(1) Have safety syringe with appropriate needle securely attached.	Needle must not dislodge from syringe during venipuncture.
(2) Clean venipuncture site with antiseptic swab. Use a friction scrub with movement back and forth. Do not use concentric circular motions for cleaning (ACAHP, 2017). Allow to dry.	Antimicrobial agent cleans skin surface of resident bacteria so organisms do not enter puncture site. Friction rub has been found to be superior to concentric circles (ACAHP, 2017). Allowing antiseptic to dry ensures bacteriostasis and reduces "sting" of venipuncture. Alcohol left on skin can cause hemolysis of sample.
(a) If drawing sample for blood alcohol level or blood cultures, use only antiseptic swab rather than alcohol swab.	Ensures accurate test results.

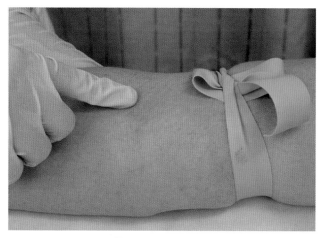

Fig. 81.2 Palpate vein.

STEP	RATIONALE
(3) Remove needle cover and check needle surface for burrs.	Burrs can damage patient's veins.
(4) Place thumb or forefinger of nondominant hand 2.5 cm (1 inch) below site and gently pull skin taut. Stretch skin steadily until vein is stabilized. Inform patient that "stick" will occur, and will last only a few seconds.	Stabilizes vein and prevents rolling during needle insertion. Reduces anticipatory anxiety.
(5) Hold syringe and needle at 15- to 30-degree angle from patient's arm with bevel up.	Reduces chance of penetrating both sides of vein during insertion. Bevel up decreases chance of contamination by not dragging bevel opening over skin and allows point of needle to first puncture skin, reducing trauma.

Continued

STEP	RATIONALE
(6) Slowly insert needle into vein, stopping when "pop" is felt as needle enters vein (Fig. 81.3).	Prevents puncture through vein to opposite side.
(7) Hold syringe securely and pull back gently on plunger.	Prevents needle from advancing. Pulling on plunger creates vacuum needed to draw blood into syringe. If plunger is pulled back too quickly, pressure may collapse vein.
(8) Observe for blood return.	If blood flow fails to appear, needle may not be in vein.
(9) Obtain desired amount of blood, keeping needle stabilized.	Test results are more accurate when required amount of blood is obtained. Movement of needle increases discomfort.
(10) After obtaining specimen, release tourniquet.	Reduces bleeding at site when needle is withdrawn.

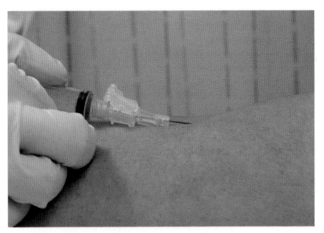

Fig. 81.3 Insert needle into vein.

STEP	RATIONALE
(11) Apply 2 × 2-inch gauze pad or antiseptic pad without applying pressure. Quickly but carefully withdraw needle from vein.	Pressure over needle can cause discomfort. Careful removal of needle minimizes discomfort and vein trauma.
(12) Immediately apply pressure over venipuncture site with 2 × 2-inch gauze or antiseptic pad for 2 to 3 minutes or until bleeding stops. Observe for hematoma. Tape gauze dressing securely.	Hematoma may cause compression injury (ACAHP, 2017).
(13) Activate safety cover and immediately discard needle into appropriate sharps container, and gauze and other supplies in appropriate biohazard container.	Prevents needlestick injury.
(14) Attach blood-filled syringe to needle-free blood transfer device. Attach tube and allow vacuum to fill tube to specified level. Remove and fill other tubes as appropriate (Fig. 81.4). Gently rotate each tube back and forth 8 to 10 times.	Additives prevent clotting. Shaking can cause hemolysis of red blood cells.

Continued

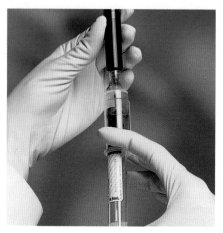

Fig. 81.4 Attach blood-filled syringe to needle-free blood transfer device.

STEP	RATIONALE
b Vacutainer system method:	
(1) Attach double-ended needle to Vacutainer tube.	Long end of needle is used to puncture vein. Short end fits into blood tube.
(2) Have proper blood specimen tube resting inside Vacutainer device but *do not puncture rubber stopper.*	Puncturing causes loss of tube vacuum.
(3) Clean venipuncture site by following Steps 8a(2) and 8a(2a). Allow to dry.	Cleans skin surface of resident bacteria so organisms do not enter puncture site. Drying maximizes effect of antiseptic.
(4) Remove needle cover and inform patient that "stick" will occur, and will last only a few seconds.	Reduces anticipatory anxiety.

STEP	RATIONALE
(5) Place thumb or forefinger of nondominant hand 2.5 cm (1 inch) *below* site and gently pull skin taut. Stretch skin down until vein stabilizes.	Helps to stabilize vein and prevent rolling during needle insertion.
(6) Hold Vacutainer needle at 15- to 30-degree angle from arm with bevel up.	Smallest and sharpest point of needle will puncture skin first. Reduces chance of penetrating sides of vein during insertion. Keeping bevel up causes less trauma to vein.
(7) Slowly insert needle into vein.	Prevents puncture on opposite side.
(8) Grasp Vacutainer securely and advance specimen tube into needle of holder (do not advance needle in vein).	Pushing needle through stopper breaks vacuum and causes flow of blood into tube. If needle in vein advances, vein may become punctured on other side.
(9) Note flow of blood into tube, which should be fairly rapid (Fig. 81.5).	Failure of blood to appear indicates that vacuum in tube is lost or needle is not in vein.
(10) After filling specimen tube, grasp Vacutainer firmly and remove tube. Insert additional specimen tubes as needed. Gently rotate each tube back and forth 8 to 10 times.	Vacuum in tube stops flowing when sufficient amount of blood is collected. Grasping prevents needle from advancing or dislodging. Tube should fill completely because additives in certain tubes are measured in proportion to filled tube. Ensures proper mixing with additive to prevent clotting.

CLINICAL JUDGMENT *Do not shake tubes.*

Continued

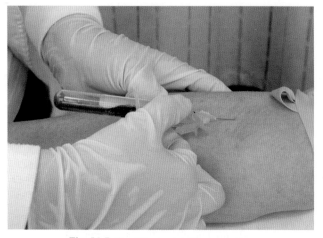

Fig. 81.5 Blood flowing into Vacutainer tube.

STEP	RATIONALE
(11) After last tube is filled and removed from Vacutainer, release tourniquet.	Reduces bleeding at site when needle is withdrawn.
(12) Apply 2 × 2-inch gauze or antiseptic pad over puncture site without applying pressure and quickly but carefully withdraw needle with Vacutainer from vein.	Pressure over needle can cause discomfort. Careful removal of needle minimizes discomfort and vein trauma.

STEP	RATIONALE
(13) Immediately apply pressure over venipuncture site with gauze or pad for 2 to 3 minutes or until bleeding stops (longer time required for patients with coagulopathy). Observe for hematoma. Tape gauze dressing securely.	Direct pressure minimizes bleeding and prevents hematoma formation. Hematoma may cause compression and nerve injury. Pressure dressing controls bleeding.
(14) Dispose of Vacutainer and needle, gauze, and other supplies in appropriate containers.	Safe disposal of supplies exposed to body fluids prevents transfer of microorganisms.
c Blood culture:	
(1) Clean venipuncture site as in Steps 8a(2) and 8a(2)(a) with antiseptic swab. Allow to dry.	Cleans skin surface so organisms do not enter puncture site or contaminate culture. Drying ensures complete bacteriostasis.

CLINICAL JUDGMENT *Culture specimens obtained through an IV catheter are often contaminated, and tests using specimens obtained in this manner are only done when catheter sepsis is suspected (Pagana et al., 2021).*

STEP	RATIONALE
(2) Clean bottle tops of culture bottles for 15 seconds with agency-approved cleaning solution. Allow to dry.	Ensures that bottle top is sterile.
(3) Collect 10 to 15 mL of venous blood using syringe method (see Step 8a) in 20-mL syringe from two different venipuncture sites.	Two to three blood cultures must be collected from different sites to confirm culture growth (Pagana et al., 2021) (see agency policy).

Continued

STEP	RATIONALE
(4) After collecting each specimen, activate safety guard and discard needle in appropriate sharps container, and syringe and gauze in biohazard container. Replace with new sterile needle before injecting each blood sample into culture bottle.	Maintains sterile technique and prevents contamination of specimen.
(5) If both aerobic and anaerobic cultures are needed, fill anaerobic bottle first.	Anaerobic organisms may take longer to grow (Pagana et al., 2021).
(6) Gently mix blood in each culture bottle. Do not shake.	Mixes medium and blood.
9 Check tubes/bottle for any sign of external contamination with blood. Decontaminate with 70% alcohol if necessary.	Prevents cross contamination. Reduces risk for exposure to pathogens present in blood.
10 Remove gloves and perform hand hygiene after specimen is obtained and any spillage is cleaned.	Reduces risk for exposure to bloodborne pathogens.
11 Securely attach label to specimen tube/bottle, with patient's first and last name, patient specific identifier, collection date and time, and the identity of the person that collected the specimen. The labeled tube must be compared with the patient's armband (inpatient). Have the patient verify that the information on the tube is correct. (ACAHP, 2017; The Joint Commission, 2023).	Incorrect identification of specimen could result in diagnostic or therapeutic errors.

STEP	RATIONALE
12 Place specimens in plastic biohazard bag and send to laboratory. Cultures must be sent to laboratory within 30 minutes (Pagana et al., 2021).	Minimizes spread of microorganisms. Prompt analysis ensures accurate results.
13 Perform postprocedure protocol.	
14 Evaluate patient response:	
a Inspect venipuncture site for homeostasis.	Determines whether bleeding has stopped or hematoma has formed.
b Determine whether patient remains anxious or fearful.	Some patients require more blood tests in future. Address concerns and let patient express anxiety.
c Check laboratory report for test results.	Reveals constituents of blood specimen.

Recording and Reporting

- Record method used to obtain blood specimen, date and time collected, type of test ordered, time specimen was sent to the laboratory, and description of venipuncture site.
- Document evaluation of patient and family caregiver learning.
- Report any stat or abnormal test results to health care provider.

UNEXPECTED OUTCOMES	RELATED INTERVENTIONS
1 Hematoma forms at venipuncture site.	• Apply pressure using 2 × 2-inch gauze dressing. • Continue to monitor patient for pain and discomfort.
2 Bleeding at site continues.	• Apply pressure to site; patient may also apply pressure. • Monitor patient. • Notify health care provider if excessive.
3 Signs and symptoms of infection at venipuncture site occur.	• Notify health care provider.

Wound Drainage Evacuation

When drainage accumulates in a wound bed, wound healing is delayed and can lead to infection. Drainage is facilitated when a surgeon inserts either a closed- or an open-drain system, even if the amount of drainage is small. The drain is inserted directly through a small wound/opening created near the suture line into the area of the wound.

An open-drain system (e.g., a Penrose drain [Fig. 82.1]) removes drainage from the wound and deposits it onto the skin surface—that is, passive drainage. A sterile safety pin inserted through this drain, outside the skin, prevents the tubing from moving into the wound.

A closed-drain system such as the Jackson-Pratt (JP) drain (Fig. 82.2) or Hemovac drain is a convenient portable unit that connects to tubular drains lying within a wound bed and exerts a safe, constant low-pressure vacuum to remove and collect drainage. This provides active drainage. A JP drain collects fluid at a rate in the range of 100 to 200 mL/24 h. A Hemovac or ConstaVac drainage system collects larger amounts of drainage (500 mL/24 h). A collection device is connected to a clear plastic drain with multiple perforations. Drainage collects in a closed reservoir or a suction bladder. When the drainage device is half full, you empty the chamber and measure the drainage. After measurement, reestablish the vacuum and ensure that all drainage tubes are patent.

Safety Guidelines

- Unexpected increase in drainage can indicate hemorrhage or infection.
- Empty drainage collection devices routinely to prevent accumulation and possible infection.

Delegation

The skill of emptying a wound drainage system, measuring the amount of drainage, and reporting the amount on the patient's intake and output (I&O) record may be delegated to assistive personnel (AP). A nurse is responsible for wound assessment and management of a drainage system. Direct the AP by:

- Clarifying the need to more frequently empty a drain based on patient condition.
- Instructing to report any change in amount, color, or odor of drainage.
- Reviewing the I&O procedure.

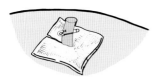

Fig. 82.1 Penrose drain with split drain gauze.

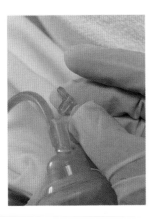

Fig. 82.2 Opening port of Jackson-Pratt wound drainage system.

Collaboration

- Contact wound care team if there are changes in the volume and/or consistency of the drainage, a presence of a strong odor in the drainage, and/or change in wound healing status.

Equipment

- Graduated measuring cylinder or specimen container
- Antiseptic wipes
- Gauze sponges, including split gauze sponges for drain site
- Sterile gauze dressings as needed
- Clean gloves
- Safety pin(s)
- Personal protective equipment: goggles, mask, and gown if risk of spray from drain is present
- Disposable drape or barrier
- *Optional:* Normal saline for cleaning insertion site

STEP	RATIONALE
1 Perform preprocedure protocol.	

Assessment

STEP	RATIONALE
• Review patient's electronic health record (EHR). Note reported presence, location, and purpose of closed wound drain and drainage system as patient returns from surgery (including any notes thereafter).	Identifies type and location of drainage system. Drainage tubing is usually placed near wound through small surgical incision.
• Assess character of patient's pain and rate acuity on a pain scale (0 to 10).	Determines baseline comfort level at wound site.
• Perform hand hygiene. Apply clean gloves. Assess drainage present on patient's surgical dressing. Lift dressing carefully to identify number of wound drain tubes and what each one is draining. Be sure each drain tube is marked with a number or label.	Assigning labeling system to each drain helps with consistent documentation when patient has multiple drainage tubes.
• Inspect system to determine presence of one straight tube or Y-tube arrangement with two tube insertion sites.	Allows for planning of skin care and identifies quantity of sterile dressing supplies needed.
• Inspect system to ensure proper functioning: condition of insertion site, drainage moving through tubing in direction of collection device, patency of drainage tubing, airtight connection sites, and presence of any leaks or kinks in system. Remove and dispose of gloves. Perform hand hygiene.	Properly functioning system maintains suction until reservoir is filled or drainage is no longer being produced or accumulated. Tension on drainage tubing increases injury to skin and underlying muscle.

STEP	RATIONALE
• Determine whether drain tube needs self-suction, wall suction, or no suction by checking health care provider's orders when patient returns from surgery.	Larger drain systems (such as Hemovac) can be used with self-suction or wall suction.
• Identify type of drainage containers that patient has. Remove and dispose of gloves.	Determines frequency for emptying drainage. Reduces transmission of infection.

Implementation

STEP	RATIONALE
1 Perform hand hygiene and apply clean gloves.	Reduces transmission of microorganisms.
2 Place open specimen container or graduate container for measurement on bed between you and patient.	Permits measuring and discarding of wound drainage.
3 Empty Hemovac or ConstaVac:	
a Maintain asepsis while opening plug on port indicated for emptying drainage reservoir.	Avoids entry of pathogens. Vacuum will be broken, and reservoir will pull air in until chamber is fully expanded.
(1) Tilt suction container in direction of plug.	Drains fluid toward plug.
(2) Slowly squeeze two flat surfaces together, tilting toward measuring container.	Prevents splashing of contaminated drainage. Squeezing empties reservoir of drainage.
b Drain all contents into measuring container (Fig. 82.3).	Contents counted as fluid output.
c Hold uncovered antiseptic swab in dominant hand. Place suction device on flat surface with open outlet facing upward; continue pressing downward until bottom and top are in contact.	Cleaning plug reduces transmission of microorganisms into drainage evacuation.

Continued

Fig. 82.3 Hemovac contents drained into measuring container.

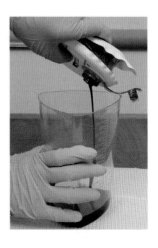

STEP	RATIONALE
d Holding device flat with one hand and using antiseptic swab, quickly clean opening/plug with other hand, and immediately replace plug; secure suction device on patient's bed.	Compressing surface of the Hemovac creates vacuum.
e Check device for reestablishment of vacuum, patency of drainage tubing, and absence of stress on tubing.	Facilitates wound drainage and prevents tension on drainage tubing.
4 Empty Hemovac with wall suction:	Empties drainage and reestablishes suction to wound bed.
a Turn off suction.	
b Disconnect suction tubing from Hemovac port.	Allows port to be opened.
c Empty Hemovac as described in Step 3a-c.	

STEP	RATIONALE
d Holding device flat, use an antiseptic swab to clean port opening and the end of suction tubing. Reconnect tubing to port.	Cleaning plug reduces transmission of microorganisms.
e Set suction level as prescribed or on low if health care provider does not specify suction level.	Reestablishes drain suction.
5 Empty JP suction drain:	
a Open port on top of bulb-shaped reservoir. *Note:* Open device away from you to prevent sprays to face.	Breaks vacuum for drain.
b Tilt bulb in direction of port and drain toward opening. Empty drainage from device into measuring container (Fig. 82.4). Clean end of emptying port and plug with antiseptic wipe.	Reduces transmission of microorganisms.

Continued

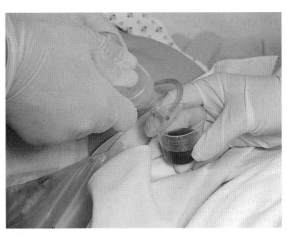

Fig. 82.4 Emptying contents from Jackson-Pratt drainage device.

STEP	RATIONALE
c Compress bulb over drainage container. While compressing bulb, replace plug immediately.	Reestablishes vacuum.
6 Place and secure drainage system below site with safety pin on patient's gown. Be sure that there is slack in tubing from reservoir to wound.	Pinning drainage tubing to patient's gown prevents tension or pulling on tubing and insertion site.
7 Note characteristics of drainage in measuring container; measure volume and discard by flushing in commode.	Contents count as output.
8 Discard soiled supplies and remove and dispose of gloves. Perform hand hygiene.	Reduces transmission of microorganisms.
9 Apply clean gloves. Proceed with dressing change (Skill 16) around drain site and inspection of skin. Split drain gauze dressings are often used around drain tubes and taped in place (Fig. 82.5). Remove gloves and perform hand hygiene after dressing change.	Prevents entrance of bacteria into surgical wound.
10 Perform postprocedure protocol.	
11 Evaluate patient response:	
a Observe for drainage in suction device.	Indicates presence of vacuum, patency of tubing, and functioning of drainage suction device.

CLINICAL JUDGMENT *Inspect for clots or cellular debris. Clots or large collections of debris may block drainage flow. The Y-site in the drainage tubing is especially prone to clogging.*

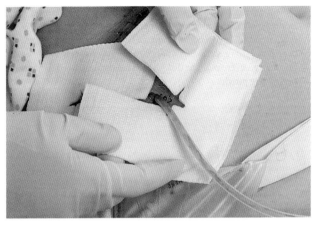

Fig. 82.5 Applying split gauze dressing around Jackson-Pratt drain tube.

STEP	RATIONALE
b Inspect wound for drainage or collection of drainage fluid under skin, which can cause a seroma.	Drainage should not be significant under suture line. May indicate inadequate functioning of drainage suction device.
c Measure drainage from drainage system, and record on I&O form at least every 8 to 12 h and as needed for large drainage volume (check agency policy).	Determines status of wound healing. Collect diagnostic specimen in presence of unexpected findings.

Recording and Reporting

- Record emptying the drainage suction device; reestablishing vacuum in suction device; amount, color, odor of drainage; dressing change to drain site; and appearance of drain insertion site.
- Record amount of drainage on I&O record.

- Document evaluation of patient and family caregiver learning.
- Immediately report a sudden change in amount of drainage (either output or absence of drainage flow) to the health care provider. Also report pungent odor of drainage or new evidence of purulence, severe pain, or dislodgment of the drainage tube to the health care provider.

UNEXPECTED OUTCOMES	RELATED INTERVENTIONS
1 Site where tube exits becomes infected (purulent drainage, odor, reddened site, increased white blood cell count, and temperature elevation).	• Notify health care provider. • Use aseptic technique when changing dressings.
2 Bleeding appears in or around drainage collector.	• Determine amount of bleeding and notify health care provider if excessive. • Assess for tension on patient's drainage tubing. • Secure tubing to prevent pulling and pain.
3 Patient experiences pain.	• Medicate patient as ordered. • Stabilize drainage tubing to reduce tension and pulling against incision. • Notify health care provider if signs of wound infection are present.
4 Drainage suction device is not accumulating drainage.	• Assess drainage tubing for clots. • Assess drainage system for air leaks or kinks. • Notify health care provider.

Performing a Wound Irrigation

Irrigation is a common method for cleansing a wound that contains necrotic tissue. The pressure applied during irrigation removes debris from a wound bed without damaging healthy tissue (Bryant and Nix, 2016). Typically irrigating an open wound involves using clean technique with clean gloves. Review the health care provider's order to determine whether a sterile solution is required. Sterile solutions may be necessary with new traumatic wounds (Bryant and Nix, 2016). Wound irrigation involves the use of a syringe, a combination syringe and catheter, a pulsed lavage device, or a handheld shower. A proper wound-cleaning irrigation does not harm the tissue and uses an adequate force to agitate and wash away surface debris and devitalized tissue that contain bacteria (Jaszarowski and Murphree, 2016).

Safety Guidelines

- Greatest risk of wound irrigation is applying too much pressure, either by occluding a wound with the syringe or catheter tip, or setting pressure too high on a lavage device. Excess pressure can cause further tissue trauma or passage of bacteria and foreign material deeper into a wound (Lewis and Jeffrey, 2023).

Delegation

The skill of wound irrigation cannot be delegated to assistive personnel (AP) unless it is an established chronic wound (see agency policy). The nurse is responsible for assessing and documenting wound characteristics. Direct the AP to:

- Report when the wound is exposed so an assessment can be completed.
- Report the patient's pain, presence of blood, and any drainage.

Collaboration

- Consult with the primary health care provider if there are any questions about wound integrity.
- A wound, ostomy, and continence nurse (WOCN) can offer suggestions if there is a need for a change in dressing covering.

Equipment

- Irrigant/cleaning solution (type per order), volume 1.5 to 2 times the estimated wound volume
- Irrigation delivery system (per order), depending on amount of desired pressure: sterile irrigation 35-mL syringe with sterile soft angiocatheter or 19-gauge needle (Wound, Ostomy and Continence Nurses Society [WOCN], 2016b) or handheld shower
- Personal protective equipment: clean gloves, gown, mask, and goggles/face shield if splash/spray risk exists
- Waterproof underpad if needed
- Dressing supplies as ordered (see Skills 16, 17, and 18)
- Disposable waterproof biohazard bag
- Extra towels and padding (to protect bed)
- Wound assessment supplies: agency wound assessment tool to document assessment: measuring guide; cotton-tipped applicator

STEP	RATIONALE
1 Perform preprocedure protocol.	
Assessment	
• Review patient's electronic health record (EHR), including health care provider's order and nurses' notes. Note status of open wound and type of solution to be used.	Open-wound irrigation requires medical order, including type of solution(s) to use.
• Review EHR for most current signs and symptoms related to patient's open wound:	
a Extent of skin integrity impairment, including size of wound	Provides ongoing data to indicate change in wound status (Bryant and Nix, 2016).
b Number of drains present	Awareness of drain position facilitates safe dressing removal and determines need for special dressings.

STEP	RATIONALE
c Drainage, including amount, color, consistency, and any odor noted	Provides ongoing data; drainage should decrease in healing wound. When drainage increases, it is often related to infection.
d Wound tissue color	Color represents balance between necrotic and new scar tissue. Proper selection of wound care products on basis of wound color facilitates removal of necrotic tissue and promotes new tissue growth (Bryant and Nix, 2016).
e Wound culture reports	Results of culture tests identify type of bacteria and proper treatment. Ongoing wound cultures document resolution of infectious process.
• Assess patient's character of pain and level of acuity on pain scale of 0 to 10.	Provides baseline to determine tolerance to procedure and need to plan for analgesia before irrigation.
• Ask patient to describe history of allergies: known type(s) of allergies and normal allergic reaction(s). Check patient's allergy wristband. Focus on antiseptics, adhesive, and latex.	Reduces risk for exposing patient to allergens that can cause localized or systemic allergic reactions.
• Assess whether patient is taking an anticoagulant or has coagulopathy.	Caution must be used if patient has a bleeding tendency. Irrigation could cause bleeding.
• Perform hand hygiene. Administer analgesic at least 30 minutes before starting wound irrigation procedure.	Promotes pain control, permits patient to move more easily and to be positioned to facilitate wound irrigation (Bryant and Nix, 2016).

Continued

STEP	RATIONALE
Implementation	
1 Position patient comfortably to promote gravitational flow of irrigating solution; wound should be positioned vertical to collection receptacle (Fig. 83.1).	Directing solution from top to bottom of wound and from clean to contaminated area prevents further infection.
2 Ensure that irrigant solution is at room temperature.	Increases comfort and reduces vascular constriction response in tissues.
3 Place padding or extra towel on bed under area where irrigation will take place.	Protects bedding from becoming wet.
4 Perform hand hygiene. Form cuff on waterproof biohazard bag and place near bed.	Reduces transmission of microorganisms. Cuffing maintains large bag opening, permitting placement of contaminated dressings without touching bag itself.
5 Apply gown, mask, and goggles/face shield as indicated; apply clean gloves and remove old dressing. Dispose of dressing in proper biohazard receptacle.	Reduces transmission of microorganisms. Protects you from splashes or sprays of blood and body fluids.

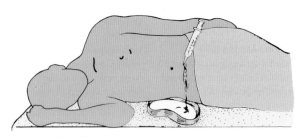

Fig. 83.1 Patient position for wound irrigation.

STEP	RATIONALE
6 Clean wound either with normal saline or cleansing agent recommended by health care provider or WOCN. Dry skin surface. Remove and discard gloves. Perform hand hygiene.	While cleaning wound, use meticulous hand hygiene and proper infection control procedures before and after removing soiled dressings to limit risk for health care–acquired infection (Jaszarowski and Murphree, 2016).
7 Apply clean or sterile gloves (check agency policy). Expose only area near wound and perform wound assessment: condition of wound, depth of wound (using cotton applicator), and length and width. Caution patient against touching wound supplies or wound itself.	Provides privacy and prevents chilling of patient. Provides ongoing wound-healing data. Use sterile precautions when sterile gloves are needed. Patient can contaminate supplies.
8 Irrigate wound with wide opening:	
a Fill 35-mL syringe with irrigation solution.	Irrigating wound uses gentle mechanical force, which helps with separation and removal of necrotic debris and surface bacteria (Jaszarowski and Murphree, 2016). Flushing wound removes debris and facilitates healing by secondary intention.
b Attach 19-gauge angiocatheter.	Catheter lumen delivers ideal pressure for cleaning and removing debris (Lewis and Jeffrey, 2023). Mechanical debridement through use of 35-mL syringe with 19-gauge angiocatheter delivers irrigation pressures between 4 and 15 psi (Gabriel et al., 2021).

Continued

STEP	RATIONALE

CLINICAL JUDGMENT *Pulsatile high-pressure lavage is an alternative to using the 35-mL syringe and the 19-gauge angiocatheter. Studies indicate it is more effective in reducing bacterial populations and removing necrotic tissue and foreign particles versus bulb syringe and other low-pressure systems (Gabriel et al., 2021). However, especially in chronic wounds, high-pressure irrigation systems have been shown to damage granulation and epithelial tissue or cause discomfort to the patient (Gabriel et al., 2021). Follow agency policy if such devices are used.*

STEP	RATIONALE
c Hold syringe tip 2.5 cm (1 inch) above upper end of wound and over area being cleaned.	Prevents syringe contamination. Careful placement of syringe prevents unsafe pressure of flowing solution.
d Using continuous pressure, flush wound; repeat Step 8a and continue flushing until solution draining into basin is clear.	Flushing wound helps to remove debris; clear solution indicates removal of all debris.
9 Irrigate deep wound with very small opening:	
a Attach soft catheter to filled irrigation syringe (see Step 8).	Catheter permits direct flow of irrigant into wound. Expect wound to take longer to empty when opening is small.
b Gently insert tip of catheter into opening about 1.3 cm (0.5 inch).	Prevents tip from touching fragile inner wall of wound.

CLINICAL JUDGMENT *Do not force catheter into the wound because this will cause tissue damage.*

STEP	RATIONALE
c Using slow, continuous pressure, flush wound.	Use of slow mechanical force of stream of solution loosens particulate matter on wound surface and promotes healing.

CLINICAL JUDGMENT *Pulsatile high-pressure lavage pressure settings should be set per provider order, usually between 4 and 15 psi, and should not be used on skin grafts, exposed blood vessels, muscle, tendon, or bone (Gabriel et al., 2021). Use with caution if patient has bleeding tendency.*

STEP	RATIONALE
d While keeping catheter in place, pinch it off just below syringe.	Avoids contamination of sterile solution.
e Remove and refill syringe. Reconnect to catheter and repeat irrigation until solution draining into basin is clear.	
10 Clean wound with handheld shower:	

CLINICAL JUDGMENT *When assisting patient into and out of shower, follow fall precautions (Skill 28).*

a With patient seated comfortably in shower chair or standing (if condition allows), adjust spray to gentle flow; make sure that water is warm.	Useful for patients able to shower with help or independently. May be accomplished at home.
b Shower for 5 to 10 minutes with shower head no closer than 30 cm (12 inches) from wound.	Ensures that wound is cleaned thoroughly.
11 When indicated, obtain wound cultures only after cleaning with nonbacteriostatic saline.	WOCN (2016a) recommends using quantitative bacterial cultures (tissue biopsy or swab cultures). Most common methods for wound cultures are swab technique, aspiration of wound fluid, or tissue biopsy (Stotts, 2016).

CLINICAL JUDGMENT *Obtain a wound culture if indicated by the presence of inflammation around the wound, purulent odor or drainage, new drainage, or a febrile patient.*

12 Dry wound edges with gauze; dry patient after shower.	Prevents maceration of surrounding tissue from excess moisture.

Continued

STEP	RATIONALE
13 Remove and dispose of gloves. Perform hand hygiene. Apply clean or sterile gloves (see agency policy). Apply appropriate dressing and label with time, date, and your initials.	Reduces transmission of microorganisms. Maintains protective barrier and healing environment for wound.
14 Perform postprocedure protocol.	
15 Evaluate patient response:	
a Have patient rate pain acuity on scale of 0 to 10.	Patient's pain should not increase as result of wound irrigation.
b Monitor character and type of tissue in wound bed.	Identifies wound-healing progress.
c Inspect dressing routinely (see agency policy).	Determines patient's response to wound irrigation and need to modify plan of care.
d Inspect periwound skin integrity.	Determines whether extension of wound has occurred or signs of skin maceration or infection are present (warm, red periwound skin).
e Observe for presence of retained irrigant.	Retained irrigant is medium for bacterial growth and subsequent infection.

Recording and Reporting

- Record wound assessment before and after irrigation: size and condition of wound; amount, color, and odor of drainage on dressing removed; amount and type of solution used; irrigation device; patient's tolerance of the procedure; and type of dressing applied after irrigation.
- Record patient's and family caregiver's understanding of wound irrigation.
- Immediately report to the health care provider any evidence of fresh bleeding, increased infection, sharp increase in pain, retention of irrigant, or signs of shock.

UNEXPECTED OUTCOMES	RELATED INTERVENTIONS
1 Bleeding or serosanguineous drainage appears. *Note:* Some bleeding may occur as necrotic tissue is removed and exposes new granulation tissue.	• Flush wound during next irrigation using less pressure. Apply pressure with sterile gauze to wound to stop bleeding. • Notify health care provider.
2 Increased pain or discomfort.	• Decrease force of pressure during wound irrigation. • Assess patient for need for additional analgesia before wound care.
3 Wound opening extends.	• Notify health care provider. • Reevaluate amount of pressure to use for next wound irrigation.

A

AABB (formerly American Association of Blood Banks: Standards for blood banks and transfusion services), ed 32, Bethesda MD, 2020, AABB.

Academy of Nutrition and Dietetics: Nutrition Care Manual, 2022. https://www.nutritioncaremanual.org/auth.cfm.

Agegne M, et al.: Magnitude of Vancomycin-Resistant Enterococci (VRE) Colonization among HIV-Infected Patients Attending ART Clinic in West Amhara Government Hospitals, *International Journal of Microbiology* 1(7), 2018.

Agency for Healthcare Research and Quality (AHRQ): *Preventing Falls in Hospitals: Which fall prevention practices do you want to use?*, Rockville, MD, 2013, AHRQ. https://www.ahrq.gov/patient-safety/settings/hospital/fall-prevention/toolkit/practices.html#3-2. (Accessed 22 February 2021).

Agency for Healthcare Research and Quality (AHRQ): *Preventing Falls in Hospitals: Which fall prevention practices do you want to use?*, Rockville, MD, 2018, AHRQ. https://www.ahrq.gov/professionals/systems/hospital/fallpxtoolkit/fallpxtk3.html#3-2. (Accessed 22 February 2021).

Agency for Healthcare Research and Quality (AHRQ): *Rapid Response Systems*, 2019. https://psnet.ahrq.gov/primers/primer/4/rapid-response-systems. (Accessed 27 August 2020).

Al Aboud AM, Manna B: *Wound Pressure Injury Management*, 2022, National Library of Medicine, StatPearls (Internet). https://www.ncbi.nlm.nih.gov/books/NBK532897/.

Alderden J, et al.: Midrange Braden subscale scores are associated with increased risk for pressure injury development among critical care patients, *J Wound Ostomy Continence Nurs* 44(5):420, 2017.

Alja'afreh M, et al.: The effects of oral care protocol on the incidence of ventilator-associated pneumonia in selected intensive care units in Jordan, *Dimensions of Critical Care Nursing* 38(1):5–12, 2019.

AlJehani R: Factors influencing surgeons' double-gloving practice, *Surgical Infections Society (Larchmont)* Oct 19(7):691–695, 2018.

Allen K, Hoffman L: Enteral nutrition in the mechanically ventilated patient, *Nutrition in Clinical Practice*:1–18, 2019.

Alzheimer's Association: Cognitive assessment toolkit, nd. https://www.alz.org/getmedia/9687d51e-641a-43a1-a96b-b29eb00e72bb/cognitive-assessment-toolkit. Accessed August 27, 2020.

Alzheimer's Association: Cognitive assessment tools, 2023 https://www.alz.org/professionals/health-systems-medical-professionals/clinical-resources/cognitive-assessment-tools.

American Academy of Orthopaedist Surgeons (AAOS): How to use crutches, canes, and walkers, 2015. https://orthoinfo.aaos.org/en/recovery/how-to-use-crutches-canes-and-walkers. Accessed 12/21/20.

American Academy of Otolaryngology-Head and Neck Surgery: Earwax (cerumen impaction), 2021. https://www.enthealth.org/conditions/earwax-cerumen-impaction/. (Accessed 17 February 2021).

American Association Critical Care Nurses (AACN): AACN Practice Alert: Obtaining accurate noninvasive blood pressure measurements in adults, *Crit Care Nurse* 36(3):e12, 2016.

American Association of Critical Care Nurses (AACN): Prevention of ventilator-associated pneumonia in adults, *Crit Care Nurse* 37(3):e22–e25, 2017.

American Association of Critical Care Nurses (AACN): *AACN practice alert: oral care for acutely and critically ill patients*, 2017a. https://www.aacn.org/clinical-resources/practice-alerts/oral-care-for-acutely-and-critically-ill-patients. (Accessed March 2021).

American Association of Critical Care Nurses (AACN): AACN practice alert: prevention of ventilator-associated pneumonia in adults, 2017b. https://www.aacn.org/clinical-resources/practice-alerts/ventilator-associated-pneumonia-vap. Accessed April 2020.

American Association of Critical Care Nurses (AACN): AACN practice alert: Prevention of aspiration, 2018. http://www.aacn.org/wd/practice/content/practicealerts/aspiration-practice-alert.pcms?menu=practice.

American Association of Respiratory Care (AARC): AARC clinical practice guidelines: endotracheal suctioning of mechanically ventilated patients with artificial airways, *Respir Care* 55(6):758, 2010.

American Certification Agency for Healthcare Professionals (ACAHP): New CLSI Venipuncture Guidelines, 2017. http://w.acacert.com/files/ACAreer-Summer_Fall2017.pdf. (Accessed November 2019).

American College of Foot and Ankle Surgeons: Instructions for using crutches, 2020. http://www.acfas.org/footankleinfo/crutches.htm. Accessed 12/21/20.

American Diabetes Association (ADA): The Big Picture: Checking your blood glucose, 2020. http://www.diabetes.org/living-with-diabetes/treatment-and-care/blood-glucose-control/checking-your-blood-glucose.html. Accessed 12/29/2020.

American Diabetes Association (ADA): *Take Care of Your Feet*, 2021. https://www.diabetes.org/diabetes/complications/foot-complications. (Accessed 20 March 2021).

American Geriatrics Society (AGS): For Older People, Medications Are Common; Updated AGS Beers Criteria* Aims to Make Sure They're Appropriate, *Too*, 2019. https://www.americangeriatrics.org/media-center/news/older-people-medications-are-common-updated-ags-beers-criteriar-aims-make-sure. Accessed January 19, 2021.

American Heart Association (AHA): What is Venous thromboembolism: VTE?, 2017. https://www.heart.org/en/health-topics/venous-thromboembolism/what-is-venous-thromboembolism-vte. Accessed April 14, 2021.

American Institute for Ultrasound in Medicine (AIUM): *Practice Parameter for the use of Ultrasound to guide vascular access procedures, J Ultrasound Med* 38(3): E4-E18, 2019. https://www.aium.org/resources/guidelines/usgva.pdf. Accessed 12/31/2020.

American Lung Association (ALA): Measuring your peak flow rate, 2020. https://www.lung.org/lung-health-and-diseases/lung-disease-lookup/asthma/living-with-asthma/managing-asthma/measuring-your-peak-flow-rate.html. (Accessed 20 January 2021).

American Nurses Association (ANA): *Safe patient handling and mobility interprofessional standards*, Silver Spring, MD, 2013, American Nurses Association.

American Nurses' Association (ANA): Position statement: the ethical responsibility to manage pain and the suffering it causes, 2018. https://www.nursingworld.org/~495e9b/globalassets/docs/ana/ethics/theethicalresponsibilitytomanagepainandthesufferingitcauses2018.pdf. (Accessed 16 March 2021).

American Podiatric Medical Association: *What is diabetes?*, 2022. https://www.apma.org/diabetescare. (Accessed 6 July 2022).

American Society for Parenteral and Enteral Nutrition (ASPEN): *Standards*, 2021. https://www.nutritioncare.org/Guidelines_and_Clinical_Resources/Clinical_Practice_Library/Standards/.

American Society of Clinical Oncology (ASCO): ASCO issues new guideline on chronic pain management in adult cancer survivors, 2016. https://ecancer.org/en/news/9846-asco-issues-new-guideline-on-chronic-pain-management-in-adult-cancer-survivors. (Accessed 5 April 2021).

American Society of Pain Management Nursing: Position statement: prescribing and administering opioid doses based solely on pain intensity, 2016. http://www.aspmn.org/Documents/Position%20Statements/Prescribing_and_Administering_Opioid_Doses_Based_Solely_on_Pain_Intensity.pdf. (Accessed 5 March 2021).

American Speech, Language Hearing Association (ASHA): *Adult Dysphagia*, 2020. https://www.asha.org/practice-portal/clinical-topics/adult-. Accessed 12/21/20.

American Thoracic Society (ATS): *Oxygen therapy*, 2020. https://www.thoracic.org/patients/patient-resources/resources/oxygen-therapy.pdf. (Accessed April 2020).

Anderson D, Sexton DJ: Overview of control measures for prevention of surgical site infection in adults, *UpToDate*, 2020. https://www.uptodate.com/contents/overview-of-control-measures-for-prevention-of-surgical-site-infection-in-adults. Accessed February 22, 2021.

Anderson L: Enteral feeding tubes: An overview of nursing care, *British Journal of Nursing* 28(12), 2019, 748754. https://doi.org/10.12968/bjon.2019.28.12.748.

Antoszyk A, et al.: Usability of the ranibizumab 0.5 mg prefilled syringe: Human factors studies to evaluate critical task completion by healthcare professionals, *PDA J Pharm Sci Technol* 72:411, 2018.

Ari A: Patient education and adherence to aerosol therapy, *Respir Care* 60(6):941, 2015.

Armstrong C: *Post-op incentive spirometry: why, when and how, Nursing 2017* 47(6):54–57, 2017.

Armstrong D, et al.: *Basic principles of wound management, UpToDate*, 2022. https://www.uptodate.com/contents/basic-principles-of-wound-management. (Accessed 28 July 2022).

Asai T, et al.: The association between fear of falling and occurrence of falls: A one-year cohort study, *BMC Geriatrics* 22:393, 2022.

Association of periOperative Registered Nurses (AORN): *Perioperative standards and recommended practices*, Denver, CO, 2019, AORN.

Association of periOperative Registered Nurses (AORN): *Guidelines for perioperative practice*, Denver, 2020, AORN.

Ayello EA, Braden B: How and why do pressure ulcer risk assessment, *Adv Wound Care (New Rochelle)* 15(3):125, 2002.

Ayoubi F, et al.: The influence of fear of falling on gait variability: results from a large elderly population-based cross-sectional study, *J Neuroeng Rehabil* 11:128, 2014.

B

Baath C, et al.: Prevention of heel pressure ulcers among older patients from ambulance care to hospital discharge: A multi centre randomized controlled trial, *Appl Nurs Res* 30:170, 2015.

Bagheri N, Wajda B, et al.: *The Wills Eye Manual: Office and Emergency Room Diagnosis and Treatment of Eye Disease*, Philadelphia, PA, 2017, Wolters Kluwer.

Ball J, et al.: *Seidel's guide to physical examination*, ed 9, St Louis, 2019, Mosby.

Barakat-Johnson M, et al.: The incidence and prevalence of medical device-related pressure ulcers in intensive care: a systematic review, *Journal of Wound Care* 28(8):512–521, 2019.

Bard Care: Spirit male external catheters. http://www.bardcare.com/clinicians/products/view-products/incontinence-solutions-male-external-catheters-accessories/spirit-male-external-catheters/, 2019.

Barrett S: Wound-bed preparation: a vital step in the healing process, *Br J Nurs* 26(12):S24, 2017.

Bartlett J: Aspiration pneumonia in adults, *UpToDate*, 2021. https://www.uptodate.com/contents/aspiration-pneumonia-in-adults?search=Bartlett%20J:%20Aspiration%20pneumonia%20in%20adults,%20UpToDate,&source=search_result&selectedTitle=1~150&usage_type=default&display_rank=1. Accessed March 13, 2021.

Bates-Jensen BM: Assessment of the patient with a wound. In *Core curriculum: wound management*, Philadelphia, PA, 2016, Wolters Kluwer.

Bates-Jensen BM: Assessment of the patient with a wound. In *Core curriculum: Wound management*, 2nd ed., Philadelphia, PA, 2022, Wolters Kluwer.

Berlowitz D, et al.: Epidemiology, pathogenesis, and risk assessment of pressure-induced skin and sof tissue injury, *UpToDate*, 2022. https://www.uptodate.com/contents/epidemiology-pathogenesis-and-risk-assessment-of-pressure-induced-skin-and-soft-tissue-injury.

Berrios-Torres, et al.: Centers for Disease Control and Prevention (CDC): Guideline for the Prevention of Surgical Site Infection, *JAMA Surg* 152(8):784–791, 2017.

Berry S, Kiel D: *Falls: prevention in nursing care facilities and the hospital setting, UpToDate*, 2018. https://www.uptodate.com/contents/falls-prevention-in-nursing-care-facilities-and-the-hospital-setting?search=falls-prevention-in-nursing-care-facilities-and-the-hospital-setting.%20Accessed%20July%209&source=search_result&selectedTitle=3~150&usage_type=default&display_rank=3. (Accessed 27 August 2020).

Berry S, Kiel D: *Falls: prevention in nursing care facilities and the hospital setting, UpToDate*, 2020. https://www.uptodate.com/contents/falls-prevention-in-nursing-care-facilities-and-the-hospital-setting/print. (Accessed 13 January 2021).

Berry S, Kiel D: *Falls: Prevention in nursing care facilities and the hospital setting*, 2022, UpToDate. https://www.uptodate.com/contents/falls-prevention-in-nursing-care-facilities-and-the-hospital-setting?search5falls-prevention-in-nursing-care-facilities-and-the-hospital-setting.%20Accessed%20July%209&source5search_result&selectedTitle53~150&usage_type5default&display_rank53.

Billington J, Luckett A: Care of the critically ill patient with a tracheostomy, *Nursing Standard* 34(2):59–65, 2019.

Biswas D, et al.: Role of nurses and nurse practitioners in the recognition, diagnosis, and management of neurogenic orthostatic hypotension: a narrative review, *Int J Gen Med* 12:173–184, 2019. Published online 2019 May 1.

Black J, et al.: Use of wound dressings to enhance prevention of pressure ulcers caused by medical devices, *Int Wound J* 12:322, 2015.

Bochert K: Pressure injury prevention and maintaining a successful plan and program, In McNichol LL, Ratliff CR, Yates S, Ostomy, and Continence Nurses Society, editors: *Wound, Ostomy, and Continence Nurses Society (WOCN) core curriculum*, (2nd ed.)., Philadelphia, PA, 2022, Wolters Kluwer.

Bolsega T, Sole M: Tracheostomy care practices in a simulated setting: an exploratory study, *Clinical Nurs Spec* 32(4):182–188, 2018.

Boltz M, et al.: editors, *Evidence-based geriatric nursing protocols for best practice*, Ed 6, New York, 2020, Springer Publishing Co.

Bonham P: Assessment and management of patients with wounds due to lower extremity arterial disease (LEAD), In McNichol LL, et al., editors: *WOCN core curriculum wound management*, 2nd ed., Philadelphia, PA, 2022, Wolters Kluwer.

Bos EM, et al.: Safety and efficacy of epidural analgesia, *Curr Opin Anesthesiol, Pub Medgov Dec* 30(6):736–742, 2017. https://pubmed.ncbi.nlm.nih.gov/28938298/. (Accessed 23 February 2021).

Boulée D, Kalra S, Haddock A, Johnson T, Peacock W: Contemporary Stethoscope Cleaning Practices: What We Haven't Learned in 150 Years, *Am J Infect Control* 47(3):238–242, 2019 Mar. https://doi.org/10.1016/j.ajic.2018.08.005. Epub 2018 Nov 2.

Boullata J, et al.: ASPEN safe practices for enteral nutrition therapy, *Journal of Parenteral and Enteral Nutrition* 41910:15, 2017.

Bouzat P, et al.: Chest trauma: first 48hours management, *Anaesth Crit Care Pain Med* 36(2):135, 2017.

Boynton T, et al.: Banner Mobility Assessment Tool for nurses instrument validation, *Am J SPHM* 4(3):86, 2014.

Brabrand M, et al.: Measurement of respiratory rate by multiple raters in a clinical setting is unreliable: A cross-sectional simulation study, *J Critic Care* 44:404–406, 2018.

Bradas CM, et al.: Physical restraints and side rails in acute and critical care settings, In Boltz M, et al., editors: *editors, Evidence-based geriatric nursing protocols for best practice*, Ed 6, New York, 2020, Springer Publishing Co.

Braden BJ, Bergstrom N: Clinical utility of the Braden scale for predicting pressure sore risk, *Decubitus* 2(3):44, 1989.

Braden BJ, Bergstrom N: Predictive utility of the Braden scale for predicting pressure sore risk, *Res Nurs Health* 17:459, 1994.

Bravo K, Cochran G: Nursing strategies to increase medication safety in inpatient settings, *J Nurs Care Qual* 31(4):335, 2016.

Brophy GM, et al.: Guidelines for the evaluation and management of status epilepticus, *Neurocrit Care* 17(1):3, 2012. Reference much older than 5 years.

Brudney C, Dunne B: *Epidural management, Epidural Analgesia, Epidural Anesthesia, Thoracic Epidural, Lumbar Epidural, Regional Anesthesia, Critical Care Medicine – Cancer Therapy Advisor*, 2017. https://www.cancertherapyadvisor.com/

home/decision-support-in-medicine/critical-care-medicine/epidural-management-epidural-analgesia-epidural-anesthesia-thoracic-epidural-lumbar-epidural-regionl-anesthesia/. (Accessed 16 March 2021).

Bryant RA, Nix DP: Principles of wound healing and topical management. In Bryant RA, Nix DP, editors: *Acute and chronic wounds: current management concepts*, ed 6, St. Louis, 2024, Mosby.

Burchum J, Rosenthal L: *Lehne's pharmacology for nursing care*, ed 10, St Louis, 2022, Elsevier.

Butcher H: *Nursing Interventions Classification (NIC)*, ed 7, St. Louis, 2018, Elsevier.

C

Caccialanza R, et al.: Subcutaneous infusion of fluids for hydration or nutrition: A review, *Journal of Parenteral and Enteral Nutrition* 42(2):296, 2018.

Caffrey J, Pensa G: Who Gets Constipation? What Are the Causes? What Is an Evidence- Based Approach Management? In Graham A, Carlberg D, editors: *Gastrointestinal Emergencies*, New York, 2019, Springer.

Campbell A: Blood Sugar Chart: What's the Normal Range for Blood Sugar? *Diabetes Self Management*, 2020. https://www.diabetesselfmanagement.com/managing-diabetes/blood-glucose-management/blood-sugar-chart/#:~:text=The%20American%20Diabetes%20Association%20recommends%20a%20fasting%20blood,130%20mg%2Fdl%20for%20most%20nonpregnant%20adults%20with%20diabetes. Accessed 12/29/2020.

Carmel JE, et al., editors: *Wound, Ostomy and Continence Nurses Society (WOCN): Core Curriculum: Ostomy Management*, Philadelphia, PA, 2016, Wolters Kluwer.

Carroll D, et al.: Implementation of an interdisciplinary tracheostomy care protocol to decrease rates of tracheostomy-related pressure ulcers and injuries, *American Journal of Otolaryngology*, 41(4), 2020.

Centers for Disease Control and Prevention (CDC): Summary of Recommendations : Guideline for Prevention of Catheter-Associated Urinary Tract Infections (2009), updated 2015. https://www.cdc.gov/infectioncontrol/guidelines/cauti/recommendations.html. Accessed 3/24/2021.

Centers for Disease Control and Prevention (CDC): *Testing for TB infection*, 2016. https://www.cdc.gov/tb/topic/testing/tbtesttypes.htm.

Centers for Disease Control and Prevention (CDC): *The timed up and go test (TUG)*, 2017. https://www.cdc.gov/steadi/pdf/TUG_Test-print.pdf. (Accessed 21 February 2020).

Centers for Disease Control and Prevention (CDC): FACT SHEET : Risk Factors for Falls, ND. https://www.cdc.gov/steadi/pdf/STEADI-FactSheet-RiskFactors-508.pdf. Accessed 3/9/21.

Centers for Disease Control (CDC): General best practice guidelines for immunization: Best practices guidance of the Advisory Committee on Immunization Practices (ACIP), 2019a. https://www.cdc.gov/vaccines/hcp/acip-recs/general-recs/administration.html#.

Center for Disease Control (CDC): *Healthcare Associated Infections: Pseudomonas aeruginosa in Healthcare Settings*, 2019b. https://www.cdc.gov/hai/organisms/pseudomonas.html. 3/2/2021.

Centers for Disease Control and Prevention (CDC), Siegel JD et al and the Healthcare Infection Control Practices Advisory Committee: 2007 Guideline for isolation precautions: preventing transmission of infectious agents in health care settings, 2007 (last update July 2019), 2019c. https://www.cdc.gov/infectioncontrol/pdf/guidelines/isolation-guidelines-H.pdf. accessed July 2020.

Centers for Disease Control and Prevention (CDC): Tuberculosis (TB), *Guidelines and Recommendations*, 2019d. https://npin.cdc.gov/pages/tuberculosis-tb-guidelines-and-recommendations. Accessed March 9, 2021.

Centers for Disease Control and Prevention (CDC): *Infection control in healthcare Personnel: infrastructure and routine practices for occupational infection prevention and control services*, 2019e. https://www.cdc.gov/infection-control/pdf/guidelines/infection-control-HCP-H.pdf. (Accessed 8 March 2021).

Centers for Disease Control and Prevention (CDC): *Isolation precautions*, 2019f, https://www.cdc.gov/infectioncontrol/guidelines/isolation/index.html. (Accessed 28 April 2022).

Centers for Disease Control and Prevention (CDC): *TB infection control in healthcare settings*, 2019g. https://www.cdc.gov/tb/topic/infectioncontrol/TBhealthCareSettings.htm.

Centers for Disease Control and Prevention: Using Personal Protective Equipment, 2020. https://public4.pagefreezer.com/browse/CDC%20Covid%20Pages/11-05-2022T12:30/https://www.cdc.gov/coronavirus/2019-ncov/hcp/using-ppe.html. Accessed 12/7/2022.

Centers for Disease Control and Prevention (CDC): *Livesaving Naloxone*, 2022, CDC. https://www.cdc.gov/stopoverdose/naloxone/index.html.

Centers for Disease Control and Prevention (CDC): *Vaccine recommendations and guidelines of the ACIP: Vaccine recommendations*, 2023. https://www.cdc.gov/vaccines/hcp/acip-recs/general-recs/administration.html.

Centers for Medicare and Medicaid Services: Interpretive guidelines for hospitals, 482.13(e) Standard: restraint or seclusion, 2008. Available at http://www.cms.gov/Regulations-and-Guidance/Guidance/Transmittals/downloads/R37SOMA.pdf. Accessed January 13, 2021.

Centers for Medicare and Medicaid Services: *Hospital acquired conditions*, 2018. https://www.cms.gov/Medicare/Medicare-Fee-for-Service-Payment/HospitalAcqCond/Hospital-Acquired_Conditions. (Accessed January 2020).

Centers for Medicare and Medicaid Services (CMS): *State Operations Manual Appendix A - Survey Protocol, Regulations and Interpretive Guidelines for Hospitals*, 2018. https://www.cms.gov/Regulations-and-Guidance/Guidance/Manuals/downloads/som107ap_a_hospitals.pdf. (Accessed 10 April 2021).

Centers for Medicare and Medicaid Services (CMS): *State Operations Manual Appendix A - Survey Protocol, Regulations and Interpretive Guidelines for Hospitals*, 2020. https://www.cms.gov/Regulations-and-Guidance/Guidance/Manuals/downloads/som107ap_a_hospitals.pdf. (Accessed 19 January 2021).

Chaboyer W, et al.: Adherence to evidence-based pressure injury prevention guidelines in routine clinical practice: a longitudinal study, *Int Wound J* 14(6):1290, 2017.

Chapman S: Foot care for people with diabetes: prevention of complications and treatment, *Br J Comm Nurs* 22(5):226, 2017.

Chatterjee R: Elbow pain: the 10-minute assessment, *Co-Kinetic Journal* 73:18, 2017.

Chen W: In Cifu DX, editor: *Physical Agent Modalities, in Braddom's Rehabilitation Care: A Clinical Handbook*, 6th edition, 2021, Elsevier.

Chotai P: Tube thoracostomy management, *Medscape*, 2020. https://emedicine.medscape.com/article/1503275-overview. (Accessed 9 January 2021).

Chotai P. Tube thoracostomy management technique. Medscape. 2022 Updated: Feb 09, 2022. https://emedicine.medscape.com/article/1503275-technique?reg=1#c2.

Chou R, et al.: Management of postoperative pain: a clinical practice guideline from the American Pain Society, the American Society of Regional Anesthesia and Pain Medicine, and the American Society of Anesthesiologists' Committee on Regional Anesthesia, *Executive Committee, and Administrative Council, J Pain* 17(2):131, 2016.

Cleveland Clinic: *Incentive spirometer*, 2022. https://my.clevelandclinic.org/health/articles/4302-incentive-spirometer.

Clore, A., et al:. Early feeding tube placement in burn patients and the impact on nutritional outcomes, Journal of BurnCare & Research, 40(0): S176, 2019.

Colwell J, Goldberg M: *Wound, Ostomy and Continence Nurses Society (WOCN) core curriculum: ostomy management*, 2nd ed., Philadelphia, PA, 2021, Wolters Kluwer.

Conde M, Adams S: Overview of the management of postoperative pulmonary complications, *UpToDate*, 2020. https://www.uptodate.com/contents/overview-of-the-management-of-postoperative-pulmonary-complications. Accessed 3/25/2021.

Connor BT: Best Practices: CAUTI prevention, *American Nurse Today*, 2018. https://www.myamericannurse.com/wp-content/uploads/2018/02/ANT_BestPractices_CautiPrevention.pdf. (Accessed 2 March 2021).

Cooney MF: Postoperative pain management: clinical practice guidelines, *J Perianesth Nurs* 31(5):445, 2016.

Corbett MC, Bizrah M: Chemical Injuries of the Ocular Surface, *Focus-The Royal College of Opthalmologists Quarterly Magazine*, April 2018. https://www.rcophth.ac.uk/wp-content/uploads/2018/04/College-News-April-2018-Focus.pdf. (Accessed 19 February 2021).

Crowley M: Preoperative fasting guidelines, *UpToDate*, 2019. https://www.uptodate.com/contents/preoperative-fasting-guidelines.

D

Daniels JF: Purposeful and timely nursing rounds: a best practice implementation project, *JBI Database System Rev Implement Rep* 14(1):248–267, 2016.

Davis C, et al.: A multisite retrospective study evaluating the implementation of the Pasero Opioid-Induced Sedation Scale (POSS) and its effect on patient safety outcomes, *Pain Manage Nurs* 18(4):193, 2017.

Davis E, et al.: Epidemiology of vancomycin-resistant *Enterococcus faecium* and *Enterococcus faecalis* colonization in nursing facilities. *Open Forum, Infectious Diseases 7*(1), 2020. ofz553.

Daw W, et al.: *Poor inter-observer agreement in the measurement of respiratory rate in children: a prospective observational study BMJ Paediatrics Open* 1, 2017, e0001.

Deibert W: *Virtual Sitters Can Improve Patient Safety and Reduce Unbudgeted Hospital Costs, 2021, Healthcare IT Today.* https://www.healthcareittoday.com/2019/10/01/virtual-sitters-can-improve-patient-safety-and-reduce-unbudgeted-hospital-costs/. Accessed 4/12/2021.

Diabetes Australia: *Insulin,* 2020. https://www.diabetesaustralia.com.au/living-with-diabetes/medicine/insulin/#:~:text=It%20peaks%20approximately%201%20hour%20later%2C%20and%20lasts,hours%20and%20last%20for%206%20to%208%20hours. (Accessed 5 January 2021).

Delawder JM, et al.: Predictive Validity of the Cubbin-Jackson and Braden Skin Risk Tools in Critical Care Patients: A Multisite Project, *Am J Crit Care* 30(2):140–144, 2021.

Delmore BA, Ayello EA: Pressure injuries caused by medical devices and other objects: a clinical update, *Am J Nurs* 117(12):36, 2017.

Demchuk A, Chatburn RL: Performance Characteristics of Positive Expiratory Pressure Devices, *Respir Care* 66(3):482–493, 2021.

Dhalwani N, et al.: Association between polypharmacy and falls in older adults: a longitudinal study from England, *BMJ Open, Geriatric Medicine Research* 7(10), 2017. https://bmjopen.bmj.com/content/7/10/e016358. Accessed February 21, 2021.

Doughty D, Sparks B: Wound-healing physiology, In Bryant RA, Nix DP, editors: *Acute and chronic wounds: current management concepts, ed 5,* St Louis, 2016, Mosby.

Doughty DB, McNichol LL: General concepts related to skin and soft tissue injury caused by mechanical factors. In McNichol LL, et al., editors: *Core curriculum: Wound management,* ed 2, Philadelphia, PA, 2022, Wolters Kluwer.

Drake MG: High-flow nasal cannula oxygen in adults: an evidence-based assessment, *Ann Am Thorac Soc* 15(2):145–155, 2018.

Drislane FW: *Convulsive status epilepticus in adults: Management,* 2022. http://www.uptodate.com/contents/convulsive-status-epilepticus-in-adults-management#H232906673.

Drutz J: *Standard immunizations for children and adolescents: Overview,* 2020, *UpToDate.* https://www.uptodate.com/contents/standard-immunizations-for-children-and-adolescents-overview/print#!. (Accessed 5 January 2021).

Dykes PC, Hurley AC: Patient-centered fall prevention, *Nursing Management* 52(3):51–54, 2021.

E

Earlam AS, Woods L: Moisture-associated skin damage: The basics, *American Nurse Journal* 17(10):6, 2022.

Eglseer D, et al.: Dysphagia in hospitalized older patients: associated factors and nutritional interventions, *J Nutr Health Aging* 22(1):103, 2018.

Eltorai A, et al.: Clinical effectiveness of incentive spirometry for the prevention of postoperative pulmonary complications, *Resp Care* 63(3):347–352, 2018a.

Eltorai A, et al.: Perspectives on incentive spirometry utility and patient protocols, *Resp Care* 63(5):519–531, 2018b.

E Phlebotomy Training: Order of Draw Explained: Clearing Out any Confusion, ND. https://www.ephlebotomytraining.com/phlebotomy-order-draw-explained/ Accessed 3/29/21.

European Pressure Ulcer Advisory Panel (EPUAP) and National Pressure injury Advisory Panel (NPIAP), and Pan Pacific Pressure Injury Alliance: Treatment of pressure ulcers/injuries: Quick Reference Guide, Emily Haesler (ED). EPUAP/NPIAP/PPPIA, 2019a.

European Pressure Ulcer Advisory Panel (EPUAP) and National Pressure injury Advisory Panel (NPIAP), and Pan Pacific Pressure Injury Alliance: Treatment of pressure ulcers/injuries: Clinical Practice Guideline. The International Guideline, Emily Haesler (ED). EPUAP/NPIAP/PPPIA, 2019b.

F

Fan EMP, et al.: Nasogastric tube placement confirmation: where we are and where we should be heading, *Proceedings of Singapore Healthcare* 26(3):189, 2017.

Fasugba O, et al.: Systematic review and meta-analysis of the effectiveness of antiseptic agents for meatal cleaning in the prevention of catheter-associated urinary tract infections, *Journal of Hospital Infection* 95(3):233–242, 2017.

Fehlberg EA, et al.: Impact of the CMS No-Pay Policy on Hospital-Acquired Fall Prevention Related Practice Patterns, *Innovation in Aging* 1(3), November 2017.

Fekete T: Catheter-associated urinary tract infection in adults, *UpToDate*, 2021. https://www.uptodate.com/contents/catheter-associated-urinary-tract-infection-in-adults. Accessed 7/9/22.

Fernandez L, et al.: Use of negative pressure wound therapy with instillation in the management of complex wounds in critically ill patients, *Wounds* 31(1):E1, 2019.

Ferrer M, Torres A: Epidemiology of ICU-acquired pneumonia, *Curr OpinCrit Care* 24(5):325–331, 2018.

Fumarola S, et al.: Overlooked and underestimated: medical adhesive-related skin injuries. Best practice consensus document on prevention, *J Wound Care* 29(Suppl 3c):S1–S24, 2020.

G

Gabriel A, et al.: Wound Irrigation – an overview, *MedScape*, 2021. https://emedicine.medscape.com/article/1895071-overview.

Gokay P, et al.: Is there a difference between the STOP-BANG and the Berlin Obstructive Sleep Apnoea Syndrome questionnaires for determining respiratory complications during the perioperative period? *J Clin Nurs* 25(9-10):1238, 2016.

Goldberg S, et al.: Practical management of a regional anesthesia-driven acute pain service, *Advin Anesth* 35:191, 2017.

Goldberg M, et al.: Management of the adult patient with a fecal or urinary ostomy—An executive summary, *Journal of Wound Ostomy & Continence Nursing* 45(1):50–58, 2018.

Goldstein BG, Goldstein AO: Topical corticosteroids: Use and adverse effects, *UpToDate*, 2022. https://www.uptodate.com/contents/topical-corticosteroids-use-and-adverse-effects.

Gong Y, et al.: The effect of clamping the indwelling urinary catheter before removal in cervical cancer patients after radical hysterectomy, *J Clin Nurs* 26(7-8):1131–1136, 2017. Epub 2017 Mar 7.

Gorman G, et al.: Physical activity, exercise and aging, *Wellbeing* 4(7):1–19, 2014.

Gorski L: *Phillip's manual of IV Therapeutics: Evidence based practice for infusion therapy*, ed 7, Philadelphia, 2018, FA Davis.

Gorski LA, et al.: Infusion therapy standards of practice, *Journal of Infusion Nursing* 44(Suppl. 1):S1–S224, 2021. https://doi.org/10.1097/NAN.0000000000000396.

Gorski LA: *Phillip's manual of IV therapeutics: Evidence based practice for infusion therapy*, (8th ed.)., 2023, FA Davis.

Goudar BV, et al.: Early removal versus conventional removal of nasogastric tube after abdominal surgery: a prospective randomized controlled study, *International Surgery J* 4(1):229, 2017.

Goulart CB, et al.: Effectiveness of topical interventions to prevent or treat intravenous therapy-related phlebitis: A systematic review, *J Clin Nurs* 29(13-14):2138–2149, 2020.

Gould CV et al.: Guideline for prevention of catheter-associated urinary tract infections - 2009, update 2019, Healthcare Infection Control Practices Advisory Committee, Centers for Disease Control and Prevention. https://www.cdc.gov/infectioncontrol/pdf/guidelines/cauti-guidelines-H.pdf 3/2/2021.

Grass G, et al.: Feasibility of early postoperative mobilization after colorectal surgery: A retrospective cohort study, *Int J Surg* 56:161, 2018.

Grigoriadis K, et al.: Comparison of the feasibility and safety of nasotracheal suctioning with curved edge catheter versus conventional suction catheter in critically ill subjects: a prospective randomized crossover trail, *Resp Care* 60(12):1826–1833, 2015.

Grodner M, et al.: *Nutritional Foundations and Clinical Applications: A Nursing Approach*, 8th Edition, 2021, Elsevier.

Growdon ME, et al.: Viewpoint: The Tension Between Promoting Mobility and Preventing Falls in the Hospital, *JAMA Internal Medicine* 177(6):759–760, 2017.

Gudgel DT: Recognizing and Treating eye Injuries, American Acdemy of, *Opthalmology*, 2019. https://www.aao.org/eye-health/tips-prevention/injuries. Accessed February 19, 2021.

Gudgel D: *How to put in eye drops*, 2018, American Academy of Ophthalmology. Accessed February 19, 2021. https://www.aao.org/eye-health/treatments/how-to-put-in-eye-drops.

Gunes UY, Efteli EU: Does errors made during indirect blood pressure measurement affect the results? *Int J Caring Sciences* 9(2):520, 2016.

Gupta K, et al.: Risk factors for opioid-induced respiratory depression and failure to rescue: a review, *Curr Opin Anaesthesiol* 31(1):110–119, 2018.

Gupta P, et al.: Bundle approach used to achieve zero central line-associated bloodstream infections in an adult coronary intensive care unit, *BMJ Open Quality* 10(1), 2021, e001200.

Gwenhure T: Procedure for eye irrigation to treat ocular chemical injury, *Nursing Times [online]* 116(2):46–48, 2020.

H

Haesler E: Evidence summary: pressure injuries: preventing heel pressure injuries with prophylactic dressings, *Wound Practice & Research* 25(94):210, 2017.

Hall KR, Stanley AY: Literature Review: Assessment of Opioid-related Sedation and the Pasero Opioid Sedation Scale, *J Perianesth Nurs* 34(1):132–142, 2019.

Harding M, et al.: *Lewis's medical-surgical nursing: Assessment and management of clinical problems*, 11th ed., St. Louis, MO, 2020, Elsevier.

Harding MM, et al.: *Medical surgical nursing, assessment and management of clinical problems*, ed 11, St. Louis, Mo, 2021, Mosby.

Harman S, et al.: Palliative care: The last hours and days of life, *UpToDate*, 2020. https://www.uptodate.com/contents/palliative-care-the-last-hours-and-days-of-life/print. (Accessed 31 December 2020).

Health Research and Educational Trust (HRET): *Preventing patient falls: A systematic approach from the Joint Commission Center for Transforming Healthcare project*, Chicago, IL, 2016, Health Research & Educational Trust. http://www.hpoe.org/Reports-HPOE/2016/preventing-patient-falls.pdf. (Accessed 22 February 2021).

Heffner A, Androes MP: Overview of central line access, *UpToDate*, 2020. http://www.uptodate.com/contents/overview-of-central-venous-access?-source=search_result&search=central+line&selectedTitle=1%7E150. (Accessed 31 December 2020).

Hernandez AN, Singh P: *Epidural anesthesia*, NIH-National Library of Medicine, 2022, StatPearls. https://www.ncbi.nlm.nih.gov/books/NBK542219/. (Last Update 9 March 2022).

Higgins J, et al.: Comparing the Braden and Jackson/Cubbin Pressure Injury Risk Scales in Trauma-Surgery ICU Patients, *Critical Care Nurse* 40(6):52–61, 2020.

Higginson R, et al.: Airway management in the hospital environment, *British Journal of Nursing* 25(2):94–100, 2016.

Hill A, et al.: The effects of awareness and count duration on adult respiratory rate measurements: An experimental study, *J Clin Nurs* 27:546–554, 2018.

Hitchcock J, Haigh DA, Martin N, Davies S: Preventing medical adhesive-related skin injury (MARSI), *British Journal of Nursing (Mark Allen Publishing)* 30(15):S48–S56, 2021.

Hockenberry MJ, et al.: *Wong's nursing care of infants and children*, ed 11, St Louis, 2019, Mosby.

Hodin R, Bordeianou L: Inpatient placement and management of nasogastric and nasoenteric tubes in adults, *UpToDate*, 2019. https://www.uptodate.com/contents/inpatient-placement-and-management-of-nasogastric-and-nasoenteric-tubes-in-adults.

Hoffman RS, Weinhouse GL: Management of moderate and severe alcohol withdrawal syndromes, *Up-To-Date*, 2021. https://www.uptodate.com/contents/management-of-moderate-and-severe-alcohol-withdrawal-syndromes.

Hotaling P, Black J: Ten top tips: Honing your pressure injury risk assessment, *Wounds International* 12(1):8, 2021.

Huether S, et al.: *Understanding pathophysiology*, ed 7, St Louis, 2020, Elsevier.

Huggins, J., et al: Thoracostomy tubes and catheters: Indications and tube selection in adults and children, 2020 update. https://www.uptodate.com/contents/placement-and-management-of-thoracostomy-tubes-and-catheters-in-adults-and-children. Accessed January 9, 2021.

Hull R, et al.: Heparin and LMW heparin: Dosing and adverse effects, *UpToDate*, 2019. https://www.uptodate.com/contents/heparin-and-lmw-heparin-dosing-and-adverse-effects/print. (Accessed 5 January 2021).

I

Ignatavicius D, et al.: *Medical-Surgical Nursing: Concepts for Interprofessional Collaborative Care*, 10th ed., St. Louis, 2021, Elsevier.

Infusion Nurses Society (INS): *Policy and procedures for infusion therapy*, ed 5, Norwood, MA, 2016, INS.

Infusion Nurses Society (INS): *Infusion Therapy Standards of Practice*, 8th ed., Norwood, MA, 2021a, Infusion Nurses Society.

Infusion Nurses Society (INS).: Infusion therapy standards of practice, *Journal of Intravenous Nursing* 44(15), 2021b.

Institute for Healthcare Improvement (IHI): *The ABCs of reducing harm from falls*, 2017. http://www.ihi.org/resources/Pages/ImprovementStories/ABCsofReducingHarmfromFalls.aspx.

Institute for Healthcare Improvement (IHI): Ventilator-associated pneumonia, 2021. http://www.ihi.org/Topics/VAP/Pages/default.aspx. (Accessed 20 March 2021).

Institute for Safe Medication Practices (ISMP): *Acute care guidelines for timely administration of scheduled medications*, 2011. http://www.ismp.org/Tools/guidelines/acutecare/tasm.pdf. (Accessed 5 March 2021).

Institute for Safe Medication Practices (ISMP). ISMP Targeted Medication Safety Best Practices for Hospitals. ISMP; 2022. https://www.ismp.org/guidelines/best-practices-hospitals.

Institute for Safe Medication Practices (ISMP): *ISMP guidelines for optimizing safe subcutaneous insulin use in adults*, Horsham, PA, 2017, The Institute for Safe Medication Practices.

Institute for Safe Medication Practices (ISMP): *Part II: Survey results suggest action is needed to improve safety with adult IV push medications*, 2018. https://www.ismp.org/resources/part-ii-survey-results-suggest-action-needed-improve-safety-adult-iv-push-medications. (Accessed 1 January 2021).

Institute for Safe Medication Practices (ISMP): *Safety enhancements every hospital must consider in wake of another tragic neuromuscular blocker event*, 2019. https://www.ismp.org/resources/safety-enhancements-every-hospital-must-consider-wake-another-tragic-neuromuscular.

Institute for Safe Medication Practices (ISMP): *2018-2019 targeted medication safety best practices for hospitals*, 2020a. https://www.ismp.org/guidelines/best-practices-hospitals. (Accessed 1 November 2021).

Institute for Safe Medication Practices (ISMP): *2020-2021 targeted medication safety best practices for hospitals*, 2021. https://www.ismp.org/sites/default/files/attachments/2020-02/2020-2021%20TMSBP-%20FINAL_1.pdf. (Accessed 15 March 2021).

Institute for Safe Medication Practices (ISMP): *Oral dosage forms that should not be crushed*, 2020b. https://www.ismp.org/recommendations/do-not-crush. (Accessed 13 March 2021).

Institute for Safe Medication Practices (ISMP): *NRFit: A global "fit" for neuraxial medication safety*, 2020c. https://www.ismp.org/resources/nrfit-global-fit-neuraxial-medication-safety.

International Dysphagia Diet Standardization Initiative (IDDSI): *Complete IDDSI Framework – Detailed Definitions*, 2017. https://iddsi.org/Documents/IDDSIFramework-CompleteFramework.pdf. (Accessed 21 December 2020).

International Organization for Standardization (IOS): *Enteral feeding systems: Design and testing*, 2020. https://www.iso.org/obp/ui/#iso:std:iso:20695:ed-1:v1:en.

Internet Book of Critical Care: *Airway and Respiratory Management of the Suspected COVID Patient*, 2020. https://www.coronavirus.in.gov/files/Airway%20and%20Respiratory%20Management%20of%20the%20Suspected%20COVID%20Patient%20graph.pdf. (Accessed 30 March 2021).

Irving SY, et al., The American Society for Parenteral and Enteral Nutrition: Pediatric nasogastric tube placement and verification: Best practice recommendations from the NOVEL project, *Nutrition in Clinical Practice* 33(6):921–927, 2018.

International Organization for Standardization (ISO): *Small bore connectors for liquids and gases in healthcare applications—part 6: connectors for neuraxial applications, ISO 80369-6*, 2016 https://www.iso.org/standard/50734.html. (Accessed 16 March 2021).

J

Jackson L, Owens M: Does oral care with chlorhexidine reduce ventilator-associated pneumonia in mechanically ventilated adults? *Br J Nurs, 13* 28(11):682–689, 2019.

Jacob J, et al.: Prevention of intravascular catheter-related infections, *UpToDate*, 2019. http://www.uptodate.com/contents/prevention-of-intravascular-catheter-related-infections. (Accessed 31 December 2020).

Jaszarowski KA, Murphree RW: Wound cleansing and dressing selection, In *Wound Ostomy and Continence Nurses Society Core Curriculum: wound management*, Philadelphia, 2016, Wolters Kluwer.

Jaszarowski K, Murphree RW: Wound cleansing and dressing selection, In McNichol LL, et al., editors: *WOCN core curriculum wound management*, 2nd ed., Philadelphia, PA, 2022, Wolters Kluwer.

Jeffcoate WJ, et al.: Current challenges and opportunities in the prevention and management of diabetic foot ulcers, *Diabetes Care* 41:645, 2018.

Johns Hopkins Medicine: *Health Library –Epilepsy and Seizures*, 2021. http://www.hopkinsmedicine.org/healthlibrary/conditions/nervous_system_disorders/epilepsy_and_seizures_85,P00779/. (Accessed 10 April 2021).

Jones KJ, et al.: Evaluation of automated video monitoring to decrease the risk of unattended bed exits in small rural hospitals, *Journal of Patient Safety* 17(8):e716–e726, 2021.

Judd M: Confirming nasogastric tube placement in adults, *Nursing* 50(4):43–46, 2020.

K

Kallionen N, et al.: Sources of inaccuracy in the measurement of adult patients' resting blood pressure in clinical settings: a systematic review, *J Hypertens* 35:421, 2017.

Kampman K, Jarvis M: American Society of Addiction Medicine (ASAM) national practice guideline for the use of medications in the treatment of addiction involving opioid use, *J Addict Med* 5:358, 2015.

Kane-Gill S, et al.: Clinical practice guideline: safe medication use in the ICU, *Crit Care Med* 45(9), 2017, e877.

Karaca T, Korkmaz F: *A Quasi-experimental Study to Explore the Effect of Barrier Cream on the Peristomal Skin of Patients With a Tracheostomy Ostomy Wound Manage* 64(3):32–39, 2018.

Kaya N, et al.: Ventrogluteal site injection: A systematic review, *International Journal of Caring Sciences* 9(3):1168, 2016.

Kiel D, et al.: Falls in older persons: risk factors and patient evaluation, *UpToDate*, 2020. https://www.uptodate.com/contents/falls-in-older-persons-risk-factors-and-patient-evaluation. (Accessed 22 February 2021).

Kirkwood P: Chest tube removal (assist), In Weigand D, editor: *AACN Procedure Manual for High Acuity, Progressive, and Critical Care*, 7th Edition ed 7, 2017. St. Louis.

Kisting MA, et al.: Lose the whoosh: an evidence-based project to improve NG tube placement verification in infants and children in the hospital setting, *J Pediatr Nurs* 46:1–5, 2019.

Koc BB, et al.: Effectiveness of Early Warming With Self-Warming Blankets on Postoperative Hypothermia in Total Hip and Knee Arthroplasty, *Orthop Nurs* 36(5):356–360, 2017.

Kohbodi G, et al.: *Ventilator-associated pneumonia*, 2022. StatPearls (Internet), National Library of Medicine, NIH. https://www.ncbi.nlm.nih.gov/books/NBK507711/.

Kowal K, DuBuske L: Overview of skin testing for allergic disease, *UpToDate*, 2020. https://www.uptodate.com/contents/overview-of-skin-testing-for-allergic-disease/print. (Accessed 3 January 2021).

Koyfman A, et al.: Targeted Temperature Management (Therapeutic Hypothermia), *The Heartorg MedScape*, Jul 26, 2019.

Krasner DL: Wound pain: impact and assessment, In Bryant RA, Nix DP, editors: *Acute and chronic wounds: current management concepts, ed 5*, St Louis, 2016, Mosby.

Kuy S, et al.: Research Letteer: Incidence of Catheter-Associated Urinary Tract Infections With Compliance With Preventive Guidelines, *JAMA Surgery* 155(7):661–662, 2020.

L

Larkin T, et al.: Influence of gender, BMI, and body shape on theoretical injection outcome at the ventrogluteal and dorsogluteal sites, *Journal of Clinical Nursing* 27(1-2):E242, 2018a.

Larkin T, et al.: Comparison of the V and G methods for ventrogluteal site identification: muscle and subcutaneous fat thickness and considerations for successful intramuscular injection, *Int Journal Ment Health Nurs* 27(2):631, 2018b.

Larrow V, Klich-Heartt E: Prevention of ventilator-associated pneumonia in the intensive care unit: beyond the basics, *Journal of Neuroscience Nursing* 48(3):160–165, 2016.

Lawrence K, et al.: The CAUTI prevention tool kit: A professional and collaborative project of the Wound, *Ostomy and Continence nurses, J Wound Ostomy Continence Nurs* 46(2):154, 2019.

Lesser RP, et al.: *Status Epilepticus, BMJ Best Practice*, 2018. https://bestpractice.bmj.com/topics/en-us/464. (Accessed August 2020).

Letchford E, Bench S: Ventilator-associated pneumonia and suction: a review of the literature, *British Journal of Nursing* 27(1):13–18, 2018.

Lewinsohn L, et al.: Official American Thoracic Society/Infectious Diseases Society of America/Centers for Disease Control and Prevention clinical practice guidelines: Diagnosis of tuberculosis in adults and children, *Clinical Infectious Diseases* 64(2):e1–e33, 2017.

Lewis S, et al.: *Medical-surgical nursing: assessment and management of clinical problems*, ed 11, St Louis, 2019, Elsevier.

Lewis, K., & Jeffrey, L. (2023). Wound irrigation. In *StatPearls (Internet)*. Treasure Island, FL: StatPearls Publishing, March 19, 2023.

Lewis K, Pay JL: *Wound Irrigation, StatPearls [Internet]*, Treasure Island (FL), 2021, StatPearls Publishing. Jan. 2020 Aug 16. https://pubmed.ncbi.nlm.nih.gov/30860757/. (Accessed 1 April 2021).

Lilley LL, et al.: *Pharmacology and the nursing process*, ed 8, St Louis, 2020, Mosby.

Liperoti R, et al.: The present and future: herbal medications in cardiovascular medicine, *J Am Coll Cardiol* 69:1188, 2017.

Lip G, Hull R: Overview of the treatment of lower extremity deep vein thrombosis (DVT), *UpToDate*, 2020. https://www.uptodate.com/contents/overview-of-the-treatment-of-lower-extremity-deep-vein-thrombosis-dvt.

Liu M, et al.: Fear of falling is as important as multiple previous falls in terms of limiting daily activities: A longitudinal study, *BMC Geriatrics* 21:350, 2021.

Wen-Liang Lo, et al.: Dysphagia and risk of aspiration pneumonia: A nonrandomized, pair-matched cohort study, *J Dent Sci* 14(3):241–247, 2019.

Lord L: Enteral access devices: Types, function, care, and challenges, *Nutrition in Clinical Practice* 33(1):16–38, 2018.

Lourens GB: Complications associated with epidural catheter analgesia, *Nurse Pract* 41(10):12, 2016.

Lourida I, et al.: Activity interventions to improve the experience of care in hospital for people living with dementia: A systematic review, *BMC Geriatrics* 20:131, 2020.

Lung Health Institute: *Incentive Spirometry Benefits*, Feb 10, 2017. https://lunginstitute.com/blog/incentive-spirometry-benefits/#:~:text=There%20are%20several%20incentive%20spirometry%20benefits.%20Using%20your,lungs%20exchange%20oxygen%20and%20carbon%20dioxide%20more%20effectively. (Accessed 24 February 2021).

M

MacKay S, et al.: Fear of Falling in Older Adults: A Scoping Review of Recent Literature, *Can Geriatr J* 24(4):379–394, 2021.

Manges M, et al.: Hourly rounding and medical-surgical patient falls: A review of the literature, *International Journal of Science and Research Methodology* 17(2):85–95, 2020.

Mann W: *Overview of preoperative evaluation and preparation for gynecologic surgery*, UpToDate, 2020. https://www.uptodate.com/contents/overview-of-preoperative-evaluation-and-preparation-for-gynecologic-surgery. (Accessed 25 March 2021).

Mara A: *Hospital Infection Control: Proper isolation procedures*, 2017. https://www.infectiousdiseaseadvisor.com/home/decision-support-in-medicine/hospital-infection-control/proper-isolation-procedures/. (Accessed 9 March 2021).

Marian T, et al.: Measurement of oxygen desaturation is not useful for the detection of aspiration in dysphagic stroke patients, *Cerebrovasc Dis Extra* 7(1):44, 2017.

Marsden J: How to perform irrigation of the eye, *Nurs Stand* 30(23):36, 2016.

Marsh N, et al.: Observational Study of Peripheral Intravenous Catheter Outcomes in Adult Hospitalized Patients: A Multivariable Analysis of Peripheral Intravenous Catheter Failure, *J Hosp Med* 3(2):83–89, 2018.

Martin E, et al.: French validation of the Revised Algase Wandering Scale for Long-Term Care, *Am J Alzheimers Dis Other Demen* 30(8):762, 2015.

Masato H, et al.: Prophylactic pentazocine reduces the incidence of pruritus after cesarean delivery under spinal anesthesia with opioids: a prospective randomized clinical trial, *Anesthes Analg* 124(6):1930, 2017.

Masood M, et al.: Association of standardized tracheostomy care protocol implementation and reinforcement with the prevention of life-threatening respiratory events, *JAMA Otolaryngeal Head Neck Surg* 144(6):527–532, 2018.

Matiasek J, et al.: Negative pressure wound therapy with instillation: Effects on healing of category 4 pressure ulcers, *Plastic and Aesthetic Research* 5(9):36, 2018.

Mattox E: Complications of peripheral venous access devices: prevention, detection, and recovery strategies, *Crit Care Nurse* 37(2), 2017, e1.

Matz M W., et al: *Patient handling and mobility assessments, ed 2, The Facility Guidelines Institute.* http://www.fgiguidelines.org/wp-content/uploads/2019/10/FGI-Patient-Handling-and-Mobility-Assessments_191008.pdf, 2019. Accessed March 9, 2021.

Mayo Clinic: Healthy Lifestyle: Walker Tips, 2019. https://www.mayoclinic.org/healthy-lifestyle/healthy-aging/multimedia/walker/sls-20076469 Accessed 12/21/20.

McClave S, et al.: ACG clinical guidelines: nutrition therapy in the adult hospitalized patient, *Am J Gastroenterol* 111(3):315, 2016.

McCulloch D, et al.: *General principles of insulin therapy in diabetes mellitus UpToDate*, 2020. http://www.uptodate.com/contents/general-principles-of-insulin-therapy-in-diabetes-mellitus.

McDonald S, et al.: Preoperative education for hip and knee replacement, *Cochrane Review*, May 2014. https://www.cochrane.org/CD003526/MUSKEL_preoperative-education-hip-or-knee-replacement. (Accessed 25 March 2021).

McDonald E: *Clinical practice guidelines for clostridium difficile infection in adults and children: 2017 update by the Infectious Diseases Society of America (IDSA) and Society for Healthcare Epidemiology of America (SHEA)*, 2018. https://www.idsociety.org/practice-guideline/clostridium-difficile/.

McFarland A: A cost utility analysis of the clinical algorithm for nasogastric tube placement confirmation in adult hospital patients, *Journal of Advanced Nursing* 73(1):201, 2017.

McLenon J, Rogers MAM: The fear of needles: A systematic review and meta-analysis, *JAdv Nurs* 75(1):30–42, 2019. Epub 2018 Sep 11.

McNeill Lauren: Back to basics: how evidence-based nursing practice can prevent catheter-associated urinary tract infections, *Urologic Nursing* 37(4):204, 2017.

Medline: *ENFit® enteral feeding connectors:Making safer connections*, 2022, Medline Industries. https://www.medline.com/capabilities/clinical-nutrition/enteral-feeding-connectors/.

Medline.: *ENFit® enteral feeding connectors*, 2023. https://mdlnmfedev.medline.com/capabilities/clinical-nutrition/enteral-feeding-connectors/#:~:text=ENFit%C2%AE%20addresses%20patient-side%20connections%20between%20feeding%20tubes%2C%20administration,Click%20to%20explore%20Making%20the%20transition%20to%20ENFit%C2%AE.

Meghani SH, Vapiwala N: Bridging the critical divide in pain management guidelines from the CDC, NCCN, and ASCO for cancer survivors, *JAMA Network*, 2018. https://jamanetwork.com/journals/jamaoncology/article-abstract/2682591.

Meiner S, Yeager J: *Gerontologic nursing*, ed 6, St Louis, 2019, Mosby.

Meisenberg B, et al.: Implementation of solutions to reduce opioid-induced oversedation and respiratory depression, *Am J Health Syst Pharm* 74(3):162, 2017.

Metheny N: AACN practice alert. Initial and ongoing verification of feeding tube placement in adults, *Critical Care Nurse* 36(2):e8–e13, 2016.

Metheny N, et al.: A review of guidelines to distinguish between gastric and pulmonary placement of nasogastric tubes, *Heart & Lung* 48:226–235, 2019.

Metheny N: Preventing aspiration in older adults with dysphagia, Consult Geri, Issue 20, 2020. https://hign.org/consultgeri/try-this-series/preventing-aspiration-older-adults-dysphagia. Accessed February 20, 2021.

Metheny N: Preventing aspiration in older adults with dysphagia, *Consult Geri*, 2021. Issue 20. https://hign.org/consultgeri/try-this-series/preventing-aspiration-older-adults-dysphagia. (Accessed June 2022).

Miake-Lye IM, et al.: Inpatient fall prevention programs as a patient safety strategy: a systematic review, *Ann Intern Med* 158(5 Pt 2):390–396, 2013.

Mitchell E, et al.: *Principles of ultrasound-guided venous access, UpToDate*, 2020. http://www.uptodate.com/contents/principles-of-ultrasound-guided-venous-access.

Modi S, et al.: Wells criteria for DVT is a reliable clinical tool to assess the risk of deep venous thrombosis in trauma patients, *World J Emerg Surg* 11:24, 2016.

Moyer R, et al.: The Value of Preoperative Exercise and Education for Patients Undergoing Total Hip and Knee Arthroplasty: A Systematic Review and Meta-Analysis, *JBJS Rev* 5(12), 2017 Dec. e2.

Mussa CC, et al.: AARC clinical practice guideline: Management of adult patients with tracheostomy in the acute care setting, *Respiratory Care*, 66(1), 156–169, 2021. https://rc.rcjournal.com/content/66/1/156.

Mwakanyanga ET, et al.: Intensive care nurses' knowledge and practice on endotracheal suctioning of the intubated patient: A quantitative cross-sectional observational study, *PLoS ONE*, 13(8), 2018.

N

Nagappa M, et al.: Opioids, respiratory depression and sleep-disordered breathing, *Best Pract Res Clin Anaesth* 31(4):469, 2017.

Nagy A, et al.: The effectiveness of the head-turn-plus-chin-down maneuver for eliminating vallecular residue, *Codas* 28(2):113, 2016.

National Health Service (NHS): *Sudden confusion: delirium*, 2018. https://www.nhs.uk/conditions/confusion/. (Accessed 19 January 2021).

National Foundation of Swallowing Disorders: *Swallowing disorder basics*, 2020. https://swallowingdisorderfoundation.com/about/swallowing-disorder-basics/. (Accessed 29 June 2019).

National Institute for Health Care Excellence (NICE): *Epilepsies: Diagnosis and management*, 2020. https://www.nice.org.uk/guidance/cg137/chapter/Appendix-E-Pharmacological-treatment. (Accessed 10 April 2021).

National Quality Forum (NQF): *Patient safety 2015, final technical report*, Washington, DC, 2016, Author.

Nazarko L: Choosing the correct wound care dressing: an overview, *J Comm Nurs* 32(5):42, 2018.

Nelson A, Baptiste AS: Evidence-based practices for safe patient handling and movement, *Orthop Nurs* 25(6):355, 2006.

Nelson AL, Algase DL: *Evidence-based protocols for managing wandering behavior*, New York, 2007, Springer Publishing.

Nelson A: *Assessment riteria and care plan for safe patient handling and movement*, Tampa, Fl., updated, 2008. http://www.mtpinnacle.com/pdfs/SafePatientHandlingAssessment_Algorithms_031209.pdf.

Netsch DS, et al.: Negative pressure wound therapy, In Bryant RA, Nix DP, editors: *Acute and chronic wounds: current management concepts*, ed 5, St Louis, 2016, Mosby.

Netsch DS: Refractory wounds, In Wound Ostomy and Continence Nurses Society, editor: *Core curriculum: wound management*, Philadelphia, 2016, Wolters Kluwer.

Neubauer N A, et al.: What do we know about strategies to manage dementia-related wandering? *A scoping review Alzheimers Dement (Amst)* 10:615–628, 2018.

Nijland L, et al.: Subcutaneous or intravenous opioid administration by patient-controlled analgesia in cancer pain: a systematic literature review, *Support Care Cancer* 27(1):33–42, 2019.

Nuckols T, et al.: Clinical effectiveness and cost of a hospital-based fall prevention intervention: The importance of time nurses spend on the front line of implementation, *J Nurs Adm* 47(11):571, 2017.

Nulens E: *Chapter 7: Isolation of communicable diseases. Guide to Infection Control in the Hospital*, 2018, International Society for Infectious Diseases. https://www.isid.org/wp-content/uploads/2018/07/ISID_InfectionGuide_Chapter7.pdf. (Accessed 9 March 2021).

O

O'Malley B, et al.: Project SITUP: An interdisciplinary quality improvement initiative to reduce aspiration pneumonia, *J Nurs Care Qual* 33(2):116–122, 2018.

Occupational Safety and Health Administration (OSHA): Infectious disease: final rule, 29 CFR Part 1910, Fed Reg 75:87, 2011.

Occupational Safety and Health Administration (OSHA): Bloodborne pathogens and needlestick prevention, n.d(a). https://www.osha.gov/SLTC/bloodbornepathogens/index.html. Accessed 1/3/21.

Occupational Safety & Health Administration (OSHA): Worker safety in hospitals, OSHA Publication, n.d.(b). https://www.osha.gov/dsg/hospitals/. Accessed March 11, 2021.

Occupational Safety and Health Administration (OSHA): Safety and health topics: hazardous drugs, n.d(c). https://www.osha.gov/SLTC/hazardous-drugs/controlling_occex_hazardousdrugs.html. Accessed March 15, 2021.

Occupational Safety & Health Association (OSHA): Safe patient handling—preventing musculoskeletal disorders in nursing homes, OSHA Publication 3108, 2014. https://www.osha.gov/Publications/OSHA3708.pdf. Accessed March 11, 2021.

Olson E, et al.: *Surgical risk and the preoperative evaluation and management of adults with obstructive sleep apnea*, 2022. https://www.uptodate.com/contents/surgical-risk-and-the-preoperative-evaluation-and-manage-ment-of-adults-with-obstructive-sleep-apnea.

Oncology Nursing Society (ONS): Toolkit for safe handling of hazardous drugs for nurses in oncology, 2018. https://www.ons.org/clinical-practice-resources/tool-kit-safe-handling-hazardous-drugs-nurses-oncology. Accessed 12/28/2020.

Ousey K, Edward K: Perioperative warming therapy for preventing surgical site infection in adults undergoing surgery, *Cochran Database of systematic Reviews (online)*(6), 2015. https://www.researchgate.net/publication/300563089_Perioperative_warming_therapy_for_preventing_surgical_site_infection_in_adults_undergoing_surgery. (Accessed 27 February 2021).

P

Padula CA, et al.: Prevention of medical device-related pressure injuries associated with respiratory equipment use in a critical care unit, *J Wound Ostomy Continence Nurs* 44(2):138, 2017.

Pagana KD, et al.: *Mosby's diagnostic and laboratory tests reference*, ed 15., Mosby, 2021, St. Louis.

Painchart L, et al.: Particulate contamination associated with the manipulation of drugs in glass ampules: A literature review, *Annales Pharmaceutiques Francaises* 76(1):3, 2018.

Palese A, et al.: "I am administering medication-please do not interrupt me": Red tabards preventing interruptions as perceived by surgical patients, *J Patient Safe* 15(1):30, 2019.

Park JI, et al.: Risk factors associated with the fear of falling in community living elderly people in Korea,: role of psychological factors, *Psychiatry Investig* 14(6):894–899, 2017.

Pasero C: Unconventional use of a PCA pump: nurse-activated dosing, *J perianesthes Nurs* 30(1):68, 2015.

Pastino A, Lakra A: *Patient controlled analgesia*, StatPearls, 2022, NIH-National Library of Medicine. https://www.ncbi.nlm.nih.gov/books/NBK551610/.

Patel KV, et al.: High Prevalence of falls, fear of falling, and impaired balance in older adults with pain in the US: findings from the 2011 National Health and Aging Trends Study, *J Am Geriatr Soc* 62(10):1844–1852, 2014.

Patel DA, et al.: Patient-reported outcome measures in dysphagia: a systematic review of instrument development and validation, *Dis Esophagus* 30(5):1–23, 2017.

Panayi AC, et al.: Evidence based review of negative pressure wound therapy, *World Journal of Dermatology* 6(1):1, 2017.

Perez D, et al.: Physical restraints in intensive care—An integrative review, *Australian Critical Care* 32(2):165–174, 2019.

Petrofsky J, et al.: Use of low level of continuous heat as an adjunct to physical therapy improves knee pain recovery and the compliance for home exercise in patients with chronic knee pain: a randomized controlled trial, *J Strength Cond Res* 30(11):3107, 2016.

Petrofsky J, et al.: The efficacy of sustained heat treatment on delayed-onset muscle soreness, *Clin J Sport Med* 27(4):329, 2017a.

Petrofsky JS, et al.: Use of low level of continuous heat and ibuprofen as an adjunct to physical therapy improves pain relief, range of motion and the compliance for home exercise in patients with nonspecific neck pain: a randomized controlled trial, *J Back Musculoskelet Rehab* 30(4):889, 2017b.

Picard C: Hemorrhage control, a fundamental skill: a review of direct pressure, dressings, wound packing, and bandages for life-saving, *Can J Emerg Nurs* 40(2):26, 2017.

Pickett J: Closed chest-drainage system, In Weigand D, editor: *AACN Procedure Manual for High Acuity, Progressive, and Critical Care*, 7th Edition ed 7, St. Louis, 2017, Elsevier.

Pieper B: Pressure Ulcers: impact, etiology, and classification, In Bryant RA, Nix DP, editors: *Acute and chronic wounds: current management concepts*, ed 5, St. Louis, 2016, Mosby.

Pierson F, Fairchild S: *Principles & techniques of patient care*, ed 6, St Louis, 2017, Saunders.

Powers J, et al.: Development of a competency model for placement and verification of nasogastric and nasoenteric feeding tubes for adult hospitalized patients, *Nutrition in Clinical Practice* 36:517–533, 2021.

Pozuelo-Carrascosa DP, et al.: Subglottic secretion drainage for preventing ventilator-associated pneumonia: an overview of systematic reviews and an updated meta-analysis, *European Respiratory Review* 29(155), 2020.

Pranit C.: *Tube thoracostomy management, 2020 update*. http://emedicine.medscape.com/article/1503275-overview#a5. Accessed January 9, 2021.

Prutkin J: ECG tutorial: Basic principles of ECG analysis, UpToDate, 2019a. https://www.uptodate.com/contents/ecg-tutorial-basic-principles-of-ecg-analysis.

Prutkin J: ECG tutorial: Electrical components of the ECG, UpToDate, 2019b. https://www.uptodate.com/contents/ecg-tutorial-electrical-components-of-the-ecg/print.

Q

Quigley PA, et al.: Outcomes of Patient-Engaged Video Surveillance on Falls and Other Adverse Events, *Clin Geriatr Med* 35:253–263, 2019. https://doi.org/10.1016/j.cger.2019.01.005. Accessed 4/13/2021/.

Quinlan P, et al.: Effects of localized cold therapy on pain in postoperative spinal fusion patients: a randomized control trial, *Orthop Nurs* 36(5):344, 2017.

R

Radecki B, et al.: Inpatient fall prevention from the patient's perspective: A qualitative study, *Applied Nursing research* 43:114–119, 2018. Oct, Epub 2018 Aug 7.

Ramponi DR: Chemical burns of the eye, *Advanced Emergency Nursing* 39(3):193, 2017.

Ramundo JM: Principles and guidelines for wound debridement. Wound debridement, In McNichol LL, et al., editors: *WOCN core curriculum wound management*, (2nd ed.)., Philadelphia, PA, 2022, Wolters Kluwer.

Ratliff CR: Descriptive study of the frequency of medical adhesive–related skin injuries in a vascular clinic, *J Vasc Nurs* 35(2):86, 2017.

Rea K, et al.: A technology intervention for nurses engaged in preventing catheter-associated urinary tract infection, *CIN* 36(6):305, 2018.

Reeder G, Kennedy H: *Overview of the acute management of ST-elevation myocardial infarction, UpToDate*, 2020. https://www.uptodate.com/contents/overview-of-the-acute-management-of-st-elevation-myocardial-infarction. (Accessed 21 February 2021).

Regier NG, Gitlin LN: Towards defining restlessness in individuals with dementia, *Aging Ment Health* 21(5):543–552, 2017.

Respiratory Therapy Zone: How to use an Acapella Flutter Valve (Step-by-Step Guide), 2021. https://www.respiratorytherapyzone.com/acapella-flutter-valve/#:~:text=Here%20are%20the%20indications%20for%20using%20this%20device%3A,aerosolized%20medications%20to%20patients%20receiving%20bronchial%20hygiene%20therapy 122/19/2020.

Restrepo R, et al.: Incentive spirometry: 2011, *Resp Care* 56(10):1600–1604, 2011.

Ritchie M, et al.: Chest Tubes: Indications, sizing, placement, and management, *Clinical Pulmonary Medicine* 24(1):37–53, 2017.

Rittenberger and Callaway: Temperature Management and Modern Post–Cardiac Arrest Care, *New England Journal of Medicine*, 2013. https://umem.org/files/uploads/1311241245_N_Engl_J_Med_2013_Rittenberger.pdf. (Accessed 26 February 2021).

Rolfe S: The importance of respiratory rate monitoring, *Br J Nurs* 228(8):504–508, 2019. https://doi.org/10.12968/bjon.2019.28.8.504.

Rosenquist R: Use of opioids in the management of chronic non-cancer pain, *UpToDate*, 2022. https://www.uptodate.com/contents/use-of-opioids-in-the-management-of-chronic-non-cancer-pain.

Royal College of Anesthetists: Best Practice in the Management of Epidural Analgesia in the Hospital Setting, August 2020. https://fpm.ac/uk/sites/fpm/files/documents/2020-09/Epidural-AUG-2020-FINAL.pdf. Accessed March 16, 2021.

S

Sabado J, and Pittiruti M: Principles of ultrasound-guided venous access, UpToDate, 202019. http://www.uptodate.com/contents/principles-of-ultrasound-guided-venous-access Accessed 12/31/2020.

Sadule-Rios, et al.: Off to a good start: bedside report, *MEDSURG Nursing* 26(5):343, 2017.

Sanchez MG, Perez ER: *NIH-National Library of Medicine*, 2022, StatPearls. https://www.ncbi.nlm.nih.gov/books/NBK554550/.

Santos SC, Woith W, Freitas MI, et al.: Methods to determine the internal length of nasogastric feeding tubes: an integrative review, *Int J Nurs Stud* 61:95–103, 2016.

Sasa R: Evidence-based update on chest tube management: Is your practice current? *American Nurse Today* 14(4):10–14, 2019.

Sawaf A, et al.: Seizure precautions, In *StatPearls*, 2021, StatPearls Publishing. https://www.ncbi.nlm.nih.gov/books/NBK536958/?report=printable.

Schaeffer A, et al.: *Complications of urinary bladder catheters and preventive strategies*, UpToDate, 2021a. https://www.uptodate.com/contents/complications-of-urinary-bladder-catheters-and-preventive-strategies. (Accessed 9 July 2022).

Schaeffer A, et al.: *Placement and management of urinary bladder catheters in adults*, UpToDate, 2021b. https://www.uptodate.com/contents/placement-and-management-of-urinary-bladder-catheters-in-adults.

Schallom M, et al.: Head-of-bed elevation and early outcomes of gastric reflux, aspiration, and pressure ulcers; a feasibility study, *Am J Crit Care* 24(1):57, 2015.

Schmitz D, et al.: Imperative instruction for pressurized metered-dose inhalers: provider perspectives, *Resp Care* 64(3):292, 2019.

Schoene D, et al.: A systematic review on the influence of fear of falling on quality of life in older people: Is there a role for falls? *Clinical Interventions in Aging* 14:701–719, 2019.

Schreiber M: Nursing care considerations: the epidural catheter, *MEDSURG Nursing* 24(4):273, 2015.

Schünemann HJ, et al.: American Society of Hematology 2018 guidelines for management of venous thromboembolism: prophylaxis for hospitalized and nonhospitalized medical patients, *Blood Advances* 2:3198–3225, 2018.

Schwartz SR, et al.: Clinical practice guidelines (update): Earwax (cerumen impaction) executive summary, *Otolaryngol Head Neck Surg* 156(1):14, 2017.

Seifi S, et al.: Accuracy of pulse oximetry in detection of oxygen saturation in patients admitted to the intensive care unit of heart surgery: comparison of finger, toes, forehead and earlobe probes, *BMC Nurs Open* 17(15), 2018.

Seres D: *Nutrition support in critically ill patients: Enteral nutrition, UpToDate*, 2021. https://www.uptodate.com/contents/nutrition-support-in-critically-ill-patients-enteral-nutrition. (Accessed 22 March 2021).

Severo JM, et al: Risk factors for falls in hospitalized adult patients, an integrative review, Rev Esc Enferm USP 48(3):537, 3014.

Shaz B, et al.: *Transfusion Medicine and Hemostasis: Clinical and Laboratory aspects*, ed 3, Science Direct, 2019, Elsevier.

Shealy KM, et al.: Evaluation of the prevalence and effectiveness of education on metered-dose inhaler technique, *Resp Care* 62(7):882, 2017.

Shindul-Rothschild, et al.: Beyond the pain scale: provider communication and staffing predictive of patients' satisfaction with pain control, pain management nursing, *Pain Manage Nurs* 18(6):401, 2017.

Sinha A, et al.: Condom catheter induced penile erosion, *Journal of Surgical Case Reports* 10:275, 2018.

Sivevski AG, et al.: Neuraxial Anesthesia in the Geriatric Patient, *Front Med (Lausanne)* 5:254, 2018.

Smetana G: Preoperative medical evaluation of the healthy adult patient, UpToDate, 2020. https://www.uptodate.com/contents/preoperative-medical-evaluation-of-the-healthy-adult-patient. Accessed 3/25/2021.

Smith A et al: Monitoring sedation in patients receiving opioids for pain management, J Nurs Care Qual 29(4):345-53, 2014. https://pubmed.ncbi.nlm.nih.gov/24686040/.

Smith G, et al.: Epilepsy update: part 2: nursing care and evidence-based treatment, *AJN* 115(6):34, 2015.

Sng B, Sia A: Maintenance of epidural labour analgesia: the old, the new and the future, *Best Pract Res Clin Anaesth* 31:15, 2017.

Soh SL, et al.: Falls efficacy: Extending the understanding of self-efficacy in older adults towards managing falls, *Journal of Frailty, Sarcopenia and Falls* 6(3):131–138, 2021.

Sood M: *Chronic functional constipation and fecal incontinence in infants, children, and adolescents: Treatment*, 2020. Retrieved from https://www.uptodate.com/contents/chronic-functional-constipation-and-fecal-incontinence-in-infants-children-and-adolescents-treatment.

Soudy DA: Therapeutic Hypothermia in improving Neurological outcome after Cardiac Arrest, *Journal of Neurology, Neurological Science and Disorders* 4(1):001–007, 2018.

Soule BM: Evidence-Based Principles and Practices for Preventing Surgical Site Infections, Joint Commission, *International*, 2018. https://www.jointcommissioninternational.org/-/media/jci/jci-documents/offerings/advisory-services/infection-prevention-and-control/jci_ssi_toolkit.pdf?d-b=web&hash=51FCBF18BC050870C6721734A67F79ED. (Accessed 26 February 2021).

Spencer SH, et al.: Enteral tube administration of oral chemotherapy drugs, *J Oncol Pharm Pract* 26(3):703–717, 2020. Apr Epub 2020 Jan 19.

Springer G: When and how to use restraints, *Am Nurs Today* 10(1), 2015. www.americannursetoday.com/use-restraints/. (Accessed January 2021).

Stellar J, et al.: Medical Device–Related Pressure Injuries in Infants and Children, *Wound Ostomy Continence Nurs* 47(5):459–469, 2020.

Stevens S: How to irrigate the eye, *Community Eye Health* 29(95):56, 2016.

Stewart D: *Pearls and pitfalls of patient-controlled analgesia*, 2017, U.S. Pharmacist. https://www.uspharmacist.com/article/pearls-and-pitfalls-of-patientcontrolled-analgesia.

Stotts NA: Wound infection: diagnosis and management, In Bryant RA, Nix DP, editors: *Acute and chronic wounds: current management concepts*, ed 5, St Louis, 2016, Mosby.

Strohfus P, et al.: Evidence calls for practice change in intramuscular injection techniques, *Journal of Nursing Education and Practice* 8(2):83, 2018.

Suliman M, et al.: Knowledge, attitude, and practice of intensive care unit nurses about physical restraint, *Nurs Crit Care* 22(5):264, 2017.

Sullivan R, et al.: Evaluation of a modified version of the Norton Scale for use as a pressure injury risk assessment instrument in critical care, *WOCN* 47(3):224, 2020.

Swanson T, et al.: Ten top tips: identification of wound infection in a chronic wound, *Wounds International* 6(2):22, 2015.

Szekeres M, et al.: The short-term effects of hot packs vs therapeutic whirlpool on active wrist range of motion for patients with distal radius fracture: a randomized controlled trial, *J Hand Ther*, 2017. published online September 8.

T

Takayama A, et al.: A comparison of methods to count breathing frequency, *Resp Care* 64(5):555–563, 2019.

Tamowicz B et al: Mechanical methods of venous thromboembolism prevention – from the guidelines to the clinical practice, Polish Archives of Internal Medicine, Published online 2019, file:///C:/Users/Pat/Downloads/VTEMechanicalprophylaxisPAMW2019.pdf. Accessed 4/14/2021.

Tan ECK, et al.: Medications that cause dry mouth as an adverse effect in older people: a systematic review and metaanalysis, *J Am Geriatr Soc* 88(1):76, 2018.

Taylor SJ, et al.: Feeding tube securement in critical illness implications for safety, *Br J Nurs* 27(18):1036–1041, 2018.

Teruya J: *Red blood cell transfusion in infants and children: administration and complications, Up to Date*, 2020. https://www.uptodate.com/contents/red-blood-cell-transfusion-in-infants-and-children-administration-and-complications/print#. (Accessed 28 December 2020).

Thayer D, et al.: Prevention and management of moisture-associated skin damage (MASD), medical adhesive-related skin injury (MARSI), and skin tears, In McNichol LL, et al., editors: *WOCN core curriculum wound management*, 2nd ed., Philadelphia, PA, 2022, Wolters Kluwer.

The Joint Commission. Managing medical device-related pressure injuries, 2018, issue 43. https://www.jointcommission.org/resources/news-and-multimedia/newsletters/newsletters/quick-safety/quick-safety-43-managing-medical-devicerelated-pressure-injuries/. Accessed 3/27/ 2021.

The Joint Commission (TJC): *2020 Comprehensive accreditation manual for hospitals: the official handbook*, Oakbrook Terrace, IL, 2020a, The Commission.

The Joint Commission (TJC): Provision of Care, Treatment and Services (Hospital and Hospital Clinics/Hospitals) - Restraint and Seclusion - Enclosure Beds, Side Rails and Mitt, 2020b. https://www.jointcommission.org/standards/standard-faqs/hospital-and-hospital-clinics/provision-of-care-treatment-and-services-pc/000001668/. Accessed February 22, 2021.

The Joint Commission (TJC). 2022 Hospital National Patient Safety Goals, 2022, [Oakbrook Terrace, IL. https://www.jointcommission.org/standards/national-patient-safety-goals/hospital-national-patient-safety-goals/?msclkid=eaf4fa35a92a11ecb72283f5782f590e. Accessed March 21, 2022.

The Joint Commission (TJC): *Most commonly reviewed sentinel event types*, 2021a. https://www.jointcommission.org/-/media/tjc/documents/resources/patient-safety-topics/sentinel-event/most-frequently-reviewed-event-types-2020.pdf?db=web&hash=6739433300D8DA4CF9F69DEB79B3A-2BE#:~:text=The%20most%20frequently%20reviewed%20sentinel%20events%20by%20The,Falls%20Unintended%20Retention%20of%20a%20Foreign%20Object%20%28URFO%29.

The Joint Commission (TJC): Pain Management Standards for Accredited Organizations, 2021b. https://www.jointcommission.org/topics/pain_management_standards_hospital.aspx. Accessed April 5, 2021.

The Joint Commission (TJC): *Provision of care, treatment and services (hospital and hospital clinics/hospitals) - Restraint and seclusion - Enclosure beds, side rails and mitts*, 2022. https://www.jointcommission.org/standards/standard-faqs/critical-access-hospital/provision-of-care-treatment-and-services-pc/000001668/.

The Joint Commission (TJC): *2023 National Patient Safety Goals*, Oakbrook Terrace, IL, 2023, The Joint Commission. https://www.jointcommission.org/standards/national-patient-safety-goals/.

Thomas G, Pohl MA: *Blood pressure measurement in the diagnosis and management of hypertension in adults, Up To Date*, 2020. https://www.uptodate.com/contents/3879#. (Accessed 29 December 2020).

Thomas L, et al.: Aspiration prevention: A matter of life and breath, *Nursing* 49(3):64, 2019. 2019.

Touhy T, Jett P: *Toward healthy aging*, ed 10, St Louis, 2020, Elsevier.

Tracheostomy Education: *Subglottic Suctioning: Benefits, Covid-19 and Manual versus Automatic*, 2020. https://www.tracheostomyeducation.com/subglottic-suctioning-covid-19/. (Accessed 30 March 2021).

U

Uhl L: *Pretransfusion testing for red blood cell transfusion*, Up to Date, 2022. https://www.uptodate.com/contents/pretransfusion-testing-for-red-blood-cell-transfusion.

Ukleja A, et al.: Standards for nutrition support: Adult hospitalized patients, *Journal of Parenteral and Enteral Nutrition* 33(6):906, 2018.

Urden L, et al.: *Priorities in critical care nursing*, ed 8, St Louis, 2020, Elsevier.

United States Department of Health and Human Services Centers for Medicare & Medicaid (DHHS): *Updated guidance on medication administration, Hospital Appendix A of State Operations Manual*, Baltimore, 2020, Department of Health and Human Services.

US Department of Health and Human Services (DHHS), Centers for Medicare and Medicaid Services: *Updated guidance on medication administration*, 2020. *Hospital Appendix A of State Operations Manual*.

US Department of Veterans Affairs: *Safe Patient Handling and Mobility (SPHM)*, 2016. https://www.publichealth.va.gov/employeehealth/patient-handling/index.asp.

US Department of Veterans Affairs: *VA National Center for Patient Safety – Falls Toolkit*, 2019. https://www.patientsafety.va.gov/professionals/onthejob/falls.asp.

U S Food and Drug Administration (USFDA): Blood glucose monitoring devices, 2019. http://www.fda.gov/medicaldevices/productsandmedicalprocedures/invitrodiagnostics/glucosetestingdevices/default.htm. Accessed 12/29/2020.

U. S. Food and Drug Administration (FDA): A guide to bed safety bed rails in hospitals, nursing homes and home health care: the facts, 2017. https://www.fda.gov/medical-devices/hospital-beds/guide-bed-safety-bed-rails-hospitals-nursing-homes-and-home-health-care-facts. Accessed February 22, 2021.

Uusi-Rasi K, et al.: Exercise and vitamin D in fall prevention among older women: a randomized clinical trial, *JAMA Intern Med* 175(5):703, 2015.

V

VA Healthcare: Implementation Guide for Fall Injury Reduction, VA National Center for Patient Safety Reducing Preventable Falls and Fall-Related Injuries, 2015. https://www.patientsafety.va.gov/docs/fallstoolkit14/falls_implementation_%20guide%20_02_2015.pdf, Addessed February 22, 2021.

VanBlarcom A, McCoy MA: New nutrition guidelines: Promoting enteral nutrition via a nutrition bundle, *American Association of Critical-Care Nurses* 38(3):46–52, 2018.

Ventocilla M: *Ophthalmologic approach to chemical burns treatment and management*, 2019, Medscape. http://emedicine.medscape.com/article/1215950-treatment. (Accessed 19 February 2020).

Virk H, Wiersinga J: Current place of probiotics for VAP, *Critical Care* 23:46–48, 2019.

W

Walsh B, Smallwood C: Pediatric oxygen therapy: a review and update, *Resp Care* 62(6):645–661, 2017.

Wanderer JP, Rathmell JP: Perioperative Medication Management, *Anesthesiology* 126:A21, 2017.

Wang L, et al.: Is Bladder Training by Clamping Before Removal Necessary for Short-Term Indwelling Urinary Catheter Inpatient? A Systematic Review and Meta-analysis, *Asian Nurs Res (Korean Soc Nurs Sci)* 10(3):173–181, 2016.

Wang R, et al.: The impact of tracheotomy timing in critically ill patients undergoing mechanical ventilation: A meta-analysis of randomized controlled clinical trials with trial sequential analysis, *Heart Lung* 48(1):46–54, 2019.

Wang Z-R, Ni G-X: Is it time to put traditional cold therapy in rehabilitation of soft-tissue injuries out to pasture? *World Journal of Clinical Cases* 9(17):4116–4122, 2021.

Waters J: Chest tube placement (assist), In Weigand D, editor: *AACN Procedure Manual for Critical Care*, ed 7, St. Louis, 2017, Elsevier.

Weinberger J, Cipolle M: Mechanical Prophylaxis for Post-Traumatic VTE: Stockings and Pumps, *Current Trauma Reports* 2(1):35–41, 2016.

Wells PS, et al.: Use of a clinical model for safe management of patients with suspected pulmonary embolism, *Ann Intern Med* 129:997–1005, 1998.

Wheatley I: Respiratory rate 3: how to take an accurate measurement, *Nurs Times* 114(7):11–12, 2019.

Wiegand D: *AACN procedure manual for high acuity, progressive, and critical care*, ed 7, St Louis, 2017, Elsevier.

Wolf P: Epilepsy and the Sensory Systems, *Epilepsy Curr* 16(6):369–372, 2016.

Wolf Z, Hughes R: Best practices to decrease infusion-associated medication errors, *J Infu Nurs* 42(4):183, 2019.

Wound Care Society: Complete Guide For Hydrocolloid Dressings, November 23, 2016, 2016a. http://woundcaresociety.org/complete-guide-hydrocolloid-dressing. Accessed January 27, 2021.

Wound Care Society: Alginate Dressing: a Complete Guide, November 16, 2016, 2016b. http://woundcaresociety.org/alginate-dressing-complete-guide. Accessed January 27, 2021.

Wound Ostomy and Continence Nurses (WOCN) Society: *Guideline for prevention and management of pressure ulcers, WOCN clinical practice guidelines series*, Mount Laurel, NJ, 2016a, The Society.

Wound, Ostomy and Continence Nurses Society (WOCN): *Core Curriculum: Continence Management*, Philadelphia, 2016b, Wolters Kluwer.

Wound, Ostomy, and Continence Nurses Society (WOCN). Clinical Guideline: Management of the adult patient with a fecal or urinary stoma. Mount Laurel, NJ, 2017.

Wound, Ostomy, and Continence Nurses Society (WOCN): Basic Ostomy Skin Care: A Guide for Patients and Health Care Providers, 2018, Mt. Laurel, NJ. https://www.ostomy.org/wp-content/uploads/2018/11/wocn_basic_ostomy_skin_care_2018.pdf. Accessed 3/14/20.

Wu Y, et al.: Characterizing human skin blood flow regulation in response to different local skin temperature perturbations, *Microvasc Res* 111:96, 2017.

Z

Zakaria A, et al.: Impact of a suggested nursing protocol on the occurrence of medical device-related pressure ulcers in critically ill patients, *Journal of Nursing & Midwifery* 9(4):924–931, 2018. https://doi.org/10.15452/CEJNM.2018.09.0025.

Zhu J, Weingart S: Prevention of adverse drug events in hospitals, UpToDate, 2022. https://www.uptodate.com/contents/prevention-of-adverse-drug-events-in-hospitals.

Zupec-Kania B, O'Flaherty T: Medical nutrition therapy for neurologic disorders, In Mahan LK, Raymond JL, editors: *Krause's food nutrition and the nutrition care process, ed 14*, Philadelphia, 2017, Elsevier.

Note: Page numbers followed by *f* indicate figures, *t* indicate tables, and *b* indicate boxes.